The Science and Practice of Middle and Long Distance Running

The popularity of distance running as a sport, and a recreational activity, is at an all-time high. Motivated by the desire to achieve a personal best, remain healthy, or simply complete an event, distance runners of all ages and abilities actively seek out advice from experienced coaches and sport scientists. This is also reflected in the growth of programmes of education for young coaches and aspiring sport scientists in recent years. There are a multitude of different approaches to training distance runners; however, the basic principles and ingredients required for success are applicable to any distance runner. The science that underpins the training and physical preparation of distance runners has developed considerably in recent years. The most experienced and successful coaches in the distance running community rarely have the opportunity to share their tried and tested methods of training. Similarly, the novel work of sport scientists is often only accessible to elite runners, their support teams and academia.

The Science and Practice of Middle and Long Distance Running links together the science and coaching artistry associated with preparing distance runners for events ranging from 800 m up to ultra-marathon distances. It combines the latest scientific evidence, published by world-leading sport scientists, with the sound training principles and strategies adopted by experienced coaches. The book translates cutting-edge scientific research from the fields of physiology, biomechanics, psychology and nutrition into practical suggestions for achieving success. Important topical issues and contemporary practices related to health and performance are also addressed. This book is an essential addition to the library of any distance runner, coach or sport scientist.

Richard C. Blagrove, PhD, SFHEA, ASCC, CSCS is Lecturer in Physiology and Programme Director of the MSc Strength and Conditioning at Loughborough University, UK. Richard is an Accredited Strength and Conditioning Coach and Certified Strength and Conditioning Specialist and was previously Director of the UK Strength and Conditioning Association. He has provided coaching support to middle- and long-distance runners for almost 15 years, including several Olympians and athletes who have won medals at major international championships. He gained a PhD from Northumbria University investigating the utility of strength-based exercise in post-pubertal adolescent distance runners and has delivered over a dozen invited presentations on the physical preparation of runners.

Philip R. Hayes, PhD, CSci is Senior Lecturer at Northumbria University, where he gained his PhD and has worked since 1991. During that time, he has spent 14 years as Programme Leader on the BSc. (Hons) Applied Sport and Exercise Science. His main research interest is the role of muscular strength (acute and chronically) and its role in (i) running performance, (ii) offsetting fatigue-related changes in gait, (iii) overuse injuries. Phil is a UK Athletics Level 4 middle-distance running coach, coaching for a local athletics club. He has coached GB U23, GB Students, GB U20, and GB U18 runners, along with Inter-Counties, British Universities and England Schools medallists. Previously, he has been the UK Athletics Regional Coach (North East England) for Endurance Events. Phil has also provided sport science support to numerous local athletes, some of whom have competed at international championships including the Olympics, World Cross-Country Championships and Commonwealth Games.

THE SCIENCE AND PRACTICE OF MIDDLE AND LONG DISTANCE RUNNING

Edited by Richard C. Blagrove and Philip R. Hayes

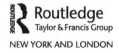
Routledge
Taylor & Francis Group

NEW YORK AND LONDON

First published 2021
by Routledge
52 Vanderbilt Avenue, New York, NY 10017

and by Routledge
2 Park Square, Milton Park, Abingdon, Oxon, OX14 4RN

Routledge is an imprint of the Taylor & Francis Group, an informa business

© 2021 Taylor & Francis

Library of Congress Cataloging-in-Publication Data
A catalog record for this book has been requested

ISBN: 978-0-367-54358-7 (hbk)
ISBN: 978-0-367-42318-6 (pbk)
ISBN: 978-1-003-08891-2 (ebk)

Typeset in Bembo
by Apex CoVantage, LLC

CONTENTS

FIGURES

TABLES

CONTRIBUTORS

Kelly J. Ashford, PhD, SFHEA, is currently Research Associate and Project Manager at the University of British Columbia–Okanagan. She has previously held lectureship roles at Cardiff Metropolitan University and Brunel University London, as well as undertaking a series of senior leadership roles (e.g., Programme Director, Deputy Head of School – Learning and Teaching) at the latter. Kelly attained her PhD from Brunel University London, where she investigated the attentional processes underlying skill disruption in situations of heightened stress. Her current research examines the critical role of attention in skilled individuals across a variety of settings (e.g. sport and education) with the intention of developing and refining novel interventions to enhance performance.

Christopher A. Bramah, PhD, MCSP, is a physiotherapist and researcher at both the Manchester Institute of Health & Performance and the University of Salford. As a Physiotherapist, Chris has worked for British Athletics and Team GB, supporting their endurance athletes throughout numerous championships, including the 2016 Rio Olympic Games, the 2017 London World Championships, IAAF Diamond League events and several international high-altitude training camps. Alongside his work in athletics, Chris operates a private physiotherapy clinic, Extra Mile Health, where he provides physiotherapy support to athletes across multiple different sports. Chris's current research investigates the biomechanical characteristics of high-performance endurance running, with his PhD focusing on the biomechanics of running-related injuries and gait retraining. He has published multiple peer-reviewed articles in academic journals and presented his work at both national and international conferences. Chris also provides consultancy biomechanical assessments across a range of sports, including professional football clubs, British Triathlon and British Athletics.

Meghan A. Brown, PhD, FHEA, SENr, is a lecturer in sport and exercise nutrition at Birmingham City University and contributes to undergraduate and postgraduate courses across the Department of Sport and Exercise as well as research activity in the Centre for Life and Sport Sciences. Meghan has provided nutrition support to a variety of athletes across different levels as a registered sport and exercise nutritionist. She has many research interests, but predominantly in nutrition and exercise metabolism; specifically, nutritional interventions to promote sport and exercise recovery which was the focus of her PhD at Northumbria University. Meghan has worked closely with dancers and has a special interest in energy availability and the specific requirements of female athletes.

Nicola Brown, PhD, is an associate professor in female health at St Mary's University, Twickenham. She is also a member of the Research Group in Breast Health at the University of Portsmouth which is well known within the commercial sector, with research projects funded by many of the major lingerie, sports bra, and sporting apparel manufacturers around the world. Recent projects Nicola has been involved in include investigation of sports bra use, sports bra preferences, breast pain and bra fit issues in exercising females, breast education of adolescent schoolgirls, and the relationship between breast size and body composition. These projects aim to increase scientific knowledge of breast health issues and to inform effective strategies for optimising health and performance of female athletes and exercisers.

Georgie Bruinvels, PhD, is a research scientist at Orreco and a visiting research associate at St Mary's University, Twickenham. Georgie co-created the FitrWoman Female Athlete Programme at Orreco and has worked extensively with elite athletes in both Olympic and professional sports. Georgie's real passion is to break down barriers for women in sport by increasing education and driving research. Her primary aim is to empower women with the tools to know how to support their health and performance. Georgie obtained her PhD from University College London. Specific areas of current research include understanding the physiological impacts of different hormonal profiles in female athletes, including the aetiology of menstrual symptoms and how hormonal contraception and menstrual dysfunction may impact readiness and health.

Stuart Butler, MSc, MCSP, BSc (Hons), is a chartered physiotherapist and the medical lead at England Athletics. He has over 15 years' experience working with track and field athletes of all abilities from local club runners to internationals. He has a MSc from the University of Southampton and undertook his BSc at Middlesex University in sports rehabilitation. He led the athletics medical teams at the Glasgow and Gold Coast Commonwealth Games and has travelled extensively with GB Athletics teams of all ages. He presently works in private practice in Surrey and continues to facilitate the England Athletics Coach and Athlete Development program. He has a keen interest in biomechanics and running efficiency, as well as hamstring muscle injuries and, more specifically, proximal hamstring tendinopathies. He has written blogs for the *British Journal of Sports Medicine* and is active in health promotion (both physical and mental) of running.

Jennie Carter, BSc (Hons), IOC PGDip, SENr, is a lecturer in sport and exercise nutrition at Birmingham City University and a registered Sport and Exercise Nutritionist (SENr). She has 10 years' experience of working in the applied field of sports nutrition with athletes, including a variety of football and cricket clubs. She is currently studying a PhD researching nutrition within professional academy football players at Birmingham City University.

Arturo Casado, PhD, MSc, OLY, RFEAC (Spain Athletics accredited level 3 coach), is a Spanish former professional middle-distance runner specialised at 800 m and 1500 m and (accredited) coach of international-level runners. His PhD study focused on high performance in long-distance runners (deliberate practice and training intensity distribution of the best Kenyan and Spanish long-distance runners). As an athlete, he was European outdoor 1500 m champion in Barcelona 2010 and competed three times at the World Championships (Helsinki 2005, Osaka 2007, Berlin 2009), twice making the final (2005, 2007). He is currently working as a lecturer at International University, Isabel I de Castilla, in the area of training development, and teaches on the MSc High Performance in Sports for the Spanish Olympic Committee. He has published several scientific articles on pacing and training intensity distribution in middle- and long-distance running events, has been invited to deliver numerous presentations on training for distance-runners, and currently leads an international research project funded by World Antidoping Agency.

Tom Clifford, PhD, FHEA, SENR, is a lecturer in physiology and nutrition at Loughborough University. He previously worked at Newcastle University as a teaching fellow and lecturer in sports and exercise nutrition and metabolism. Tom is an accredited sport scientist with the British Association of Sports and Exercise Sciences and a registered sports nutritionist. He has provided nutrition consultancy to a range of sports, including Rugby Union, Triathlon, and Paralympic Swimming. He gained a PhD in health and exercise nutrition from Northumbria University, investigating the role of beetroot in health and exercise. His current research is investigating the health and well-being of professional football players and nutritional interventions to accelerate recovery.

Matthew Cole, PhD, SFHEA, SENr, is Associate Professor in Sport and Exercise Nutrition at Birmingham City University and Course Leader for the BSc (Hons) Sport and Exercise Nutrition degree programme. His main research interests lie in endurance sport, having initially studied his MSc in sport and exercise nutrition at Loughborough University before subsequently completing his PhD at the University of Kent, investigating the influence of different nutrition interventions on cycling efficiency. Matt has provided nutrition support to a variety of elite athletes and teams, as well as being part of the anti-doping team at the London 2012 Olympic Games.

Ceri E. Diss, PhD, FHEA, CSci, is a reader in biomechanics and Programme Convenor of the MSc in Sport and Exercise Sciences: Biomechanics at the University of Roehampton, UK. She was also an elite long-distance runner and has represented Wales and Great Britain in many road races, one of which was the 1991 World 15 km Road Championships. She gained her PhD from Cardiff Metropolitan University, UK, investigating the age-based biomechanics of male running gait. She has analysed the biomechanics that underpins the gait of over one hundred athletes ranging from recreational to elite-level runners with the aim of reducing the incidence of injury. From 2005 to 2018 she worked for the running footwear company Sweatshop in training their staff in gait analysis. Her recent research has focused on joint coordination changes in running gait with age and gait retraining to reduce knee pain.

Karla L. Drew, PhD, MBPsS, is Lecturer in Sport and Exercise Psychology at Staffordshire University. She gained a PhD from Liverpool John Moores University exploring the junior-to-senior transition in sport, particularly looking at interventions to support athletes through the transitional process. Karla is also a trainee sport psychologist, undertaking a Qualification in Sport and Exercise Psychology (QSEP) with the British Psychological Society. She provides psychological support to athletes from a range of sports and levels. Karla also has experience as an elite athlete, representing the Great Britain athletics team in heptathlon.

Andy Galbraith, PhD, SFHEA, is Senior Lecturer in Exercise Physiology at the University of East London. Andy has 15 years' experience providing exercise physiology support to a range of athletes, including Olympic, World Championship and Commonwealth medallists. He gained a PhD from the University of Kent, investigating the use of critical speed in endurance training and performance. His research focuses on the physiology of endurance performance, with current research projects investigating a range of methods to reduce the oxygen cost during endurance running, including the use of altered stride rates and compression garments. Andy is a keen runner; having competed over middle distances as a junior, he is now a regular marathon runner.

Esther Goldsmith, MSc, is a sport and exercise physiologist working for sports and data science company Orreco Ltd, and for Sport and Health Services at St Mary's University. Esther gained her master's degree from St Mary's University, Twickenham, where her research focused on running economy during the menstrual cycle. Since graduating, Esther has worked with professional sports teams and individuals in a wide range of settings; from laboratory-based physiological testing, to online menstrual cycle consultancy, to point-of-care blood biomarker testing. In her work, Esther also delivers presentations and education sessions regarding female physiology, considerations when working with female athletes, and the menstrual cycle in relation to sport and training. Esther is also an active researcher, focusing primarily on the female athlete.

Tom Goom, BSc, MCSP, is a physiotherapist and international speaker with a passion for running injury management. He qualified in 2002 and currently works as the clinical lead for The Physio Rooms in Brighton, where he treats runners of all levels. Tom has gained a worldwide audience with his website running-physio.com and has become known as *The Running Physio* as a result! He's heavily involved in running-related research and enjoys translating and sharing findings to help clinicians and athletes with their injuries. Currently he works as a clinical advisor on a number of running-related research projects to help ensure these studies have a useful impact in practice.

Daniel A. Gordon, PhD, SFHEA, is Principal Lecturer in Exercise Physiology at Anglia Ruskin University, Cambridge, UK, where he is course leader for the BSc Sport and Exercise Science. Dan has published extensively in the field, with his work focusing on the factors which limit maximal oxygen uptake, endurance physiology, and menstrual function and exercise. He has acted as a consultant physiologist across a range of sports including GB Paralympic endurance runners, Trans-Atlantic rowers, ultra-marathon runners and big-city marathon runners. As an athlete, Dan competed in three sports at an international level competing for GB as a swimmer, 400 m track runner and a track cyclist. He competed as a cyclist at the Athens 2004 Paralympic Games and still holds a world cycling record which has stood for 17 years.

Brian Hanley, PhD, SFHEA, FECSS, is Senior Lecturer in Sport and Exercise Biomechanics at Leeds Beckett University. As a former competitive distance runner, his particular research interests are in the area of elite athletics, especially race walking and distance running, as well as the pacing profiles adopted by endurance athletes. He is also interested in musculotendon profiling of athletes to appreciate internal limiting and contributing factors affecting performance, longitudinal studies measuring the technical development of junior athletes as they progress to become senior athletes, sports technology and competition structure. Brian led on the scientific aspects of the Biomechanics Research Projects at the IAAF World Championships, London 2017 and the IAAF World Indoor Championships, Birmingham 2018, as well as being Event Director for distance running events (London) and pole vault (Birmingham). Over the past 15 years, Brian has provided biomechanical support to athletes from around the world in their preparation for global championships.

Mark R. Homer, PhD, is Senior Lecturer in Exercise Physiology at Bucks New University. He is an applied sport scientist with many years' experience within elite British sport. Mark provided physiology support to the Great Britain Rowing Team in preparation for and during the Beijing, London and Rio de Janeiro Olympic Games. After leading the Science and Medicine team during the Tokyo 2020 cycle, he worked as a practitioner with British Swimming while writing articles for several high-profile magazines and websites. Mark's doctorate was titled 'The Physiology of Elite Rowing Performance: Implications for Developing Rowers' and his research interests include the distribution of endurance training.

David R. Hooper, Ph.D., CSCS*D, joined Jacksonville University as an assistant professor in 2017 following 2 years at Armstrong State University in Savannah, Georgia. He received his PhD in kinesiology from Ohio State University in 2015 and has been a certified strength and conditioning specialist since 2007. He has authored or co-authored over 40 peer-reviewed publications and over 50 abstract presentations at regional, national and international conferences. While his interests are diverse, Dr Hooper is particularly interested in exercise endocrinology, including its applications in the form of biomarkers to assess recovery, as well in the context of performance enhancing drug use. In addition, he enjoys providing sport science support to athletes, sport nutrition, and strength and conditioning as a whole.

Glyn Howatson, PhD, FBASES, FACSM, FHEA, ASCC, is Professor of Human and Applied Physiology at Northumbria University, Newcastle, UK. He holds fellowships with the American College of Sports Medicine and British Association of Sport and Exercise Scientists and is an accredited strength and conditioning coach. He has over 200 peer-reviewed publications where much of his work focusses on understanding the stress-recovery-adaptation continuum using training and nutritional interventions to manipulate human physiology. His work as an applied physiologist and a researcher has contributed to the support of athletes that include professional football and rugby, and European, World and Olympic medallists. He continues to work closely with colleagues in the English Institute of Sport and Olympic Sport across a number of areas of research and innovation. Importantly, these interactions are motivated by the desire to provide meaningful impact to athletes and support staff that result in tangible performance improvements.

Louis P. Howe, PhD, ASCC, is Lecturer in Sport Therapy at Edge Hill University. Prior to this role, he held lecturing positions at the University of Cumbria and St Mary's University. Before transitioning into academia, Louis worked as a strength and conditioning coach at Royal Holloway, University of London, providing strength and conditioning services to international athletes as part of the university's Student Talented Athlete Recognition Scheme (STARS). Additionally, his private business specialised in the physical preparation of international track and field athletes. As part of both roles, Louis has helped prepare numerous athletes for the British Athletics Championships, European Athletics Championships, Pan American Games, Commonwealth Games and Olympic Games. He is an accredited strength and conditioning coach with the UK Strength and Conditioning Association (UKSCA) and a graduate sport rehabilitator with the British Association of Sport Rehabilitators and Trainers (BASRaT). Louis has a PhD from Edge Hill University.

Philip E. Kearney, PhD, FHEA, is Lecturer in Motor Skill Acquisition, Coaching and Performance and Course Director for the MSc Applied Sports Coaching at the University of Limerick, Ireland. He received his PhD from the University of Limerick in 2009, investigating how applying skill acquisition principles could accelerate the development of children's fundamental movement skills. He then taught at the University of Chichester from 2009 to 2017, where he was Programme Coordinator for the BSc Sport Science and Coaching. Phil returned to the University of Limerick in 2017. A Fellow of the Higher Education Authority, Phil's research and teaching focus is on skill acquisition and youth sport, particularly in the context of developing track and field athletes. Phil also holds the Athletics Coach qualification from UK Athletics, and his coaching is focused on developing sound fundamentals in young adolescents. Phil is a co-founder of Movement and Skill Acquisition Ireland (@MSAIreland).

Steve Macklin is Head Endurance Coach at Aspire Academy in Qatar, working with the country's top U20 talent. He is also working as the running coach for some of Pentathlon Ireland's Olympic athletes in preparation for the Tokyo Olympics in 2021, having coached two of those athletes to top 8 finishes at the Rio Olympics. He has previously held roles at Athletics Ireland as a Regional Development Officer, National U20 Endurance Coach and National Endurance Coordinator. Steve is an accredited Athletics Ireland Level 3, USATF Level 3 and IAAF Level 5 Endurance Coach. He has provided coaching support to middle- and long-distance runners for 21 years to date, including two Olympians and athletes who have competed at major international championships at U18 and U20 levels. His experience as an endurance coach includes work with athletes from a range of different countries and cultures and runners of all age groups.

Carla Meijen, PhD, CPsychol, FHEA, AFBpsS, Registered Psychologist, is Senior Lecturer in Applied Sport Psychology at St Mary's University, UK. She is a Health and Care Professions Council registered sport and exercise psychologist and a British Psychological Society chartered psychologist. She received her PhD from Staffordshire University, where she focused on challenge and threat states in athletes. She has a keen interest in endurance performance inspired by her work providing brief mental support at running events. Her research focuses on self-regulatory factors of endurance performance and implementing psychological strategies in endurance settings.

Izzy S. Moore, PhD, FHEA, is Reader in Human Movement and Sports Medicine at Cardiff Metropolitan University. Her research has focused on understanding how and why we move the way we do, from both a performance and an injury perspective. She obtained her PhD on economical running from the University of Exeter and has since led several injury epidemiology projects working directly with sporting governing bodies to inform injury prevention and management policies. In addition, she specialises in running-related rehabilitation and has received national and international research awards within the field.

Arran Parmar, MRes, ASCC, is a PhD student at Northumbria University currently researching the aetiology and demands of high-intensity interval training in well-trained middle- to long-distance runners. Alongside his studies, Arran currently works as Head of Strength and Conditioning and Sport Science for Leicester Riders Basketball and is an accredited strength and conditioning coach. He has previously provided sport science, performance analysis, and strength and conditioning support to athletes of various disciplines and backgrounds, including endurance cyclists, boxers, and footballers, among others.

Charles R. Pedlar, PhD, FBASES is a practicing sport scientist and researcher with extensive experience working in high performance systems, motivated to optimise the health and performance of male and female athletes. Charlie has previously held positions at the British Olympic Association and the English Institute of Sport and is currently Chief Science and Research Officer at Orreco, an associate professor at St Mary's University, Twickenham, and an honorary associate professor at the Institute for Sport, Exercise and Health at UCL. Charlie is passionate about distance running and has worked with many Olympians. Charlie is co-organiser of Marathon Medicine, the Virgin London Marathon's conference on the science and medicine of distance running.

Jessica Piasecki, PhD, MSc, BSc (Hons), is a member of the Musculoskeletal Physiology Research group at Nottingham Trent University. She has over 6 years of experience working within physiology research projects. Her interests began in bone health, predominantly in female athletes and how nutrition and menstrual cycles influence bone mass and geometry. Dr Piasecki also has strong research interests in musculoskeletal health during ageing and how exercise may or may not counteract these affects, the main subject area of her PhD. She has been involved in running several large-scale multi-cohort studies investigating changes during ageing and has numerous publications around these topics. Dr Piasecki is also an elite distance runner who has a personal best marathon time of 2:25:28 and has openly shared her own experiences with relative energy deficiency in sport (RED-S) as a younger athlete. Jessica now coaches and mentors a number of athletes with their training and energy balance to ensure they avoid the drastic implications of RED-S.

Paul J. Read, PhD, ASCC, CSCS*D, PGCE, is General Manager of the Institute of Sport, Exercise and Health in London and an associate professor at the University of Gloucestershire. He previously held roles as a clinical lead researcher and Head of the Athlete Assessment Unit at Aspetar Sports Medicine Hospital, Qatar, Senior Lecturer in Strength and Conditioning at St Mary's University, and Program Director of Strength and Conditioning at the University of Gloucestershire. Paul is an accredited strength and conditioning coach with both the UKSCA and NSCA and has consulted with Olympians, professional and international athletes in a range of disciplines. Paul has also authored over 100 research publications in the fields of sports medicine, science and strength and conditioning. His research focuses on assessment strategies of lower limb neuromuscular control in both injured and non-injured athletes and enhancing the efficacy of return to sport assessment strategies following ACL reconstruction.

Andy Renfree, PhD, is Principal Lecturer in Sport and Exercise Science at the University of Worcester where he teaches on subjects related to exercise physiology and interdisciplinary determinants of sport performance. He gained his PhD through using decision-making theory to explain the way in which exercise intensity is regulated during self-paced exercise. His current research interests include affect-based training prescription, determinants of fatigue, and training quantification and monitoring. A former middle-distance runner himself, he has won English Junior and Scottish Senior titles over 3000 m and 1500 m on the track.

Justin D. Roberts, PhD, CSci, SFHEA, is Principal Lecturer in Exercise and Health Nutrition at the Cambridge Centre for Sport and Exercise Sciences, Anglia Ruskin University. He has previously held academic roles at the University of Hertfordshire and Brunel University (Sport and Exercise Nutrition) and Victoria University, Melbourne (Nutritional Therapy). Justin is an accredited sport and exercise physiologist (with the British Association for Sport and Exercise Sciences, BASES), chartered scientist (CSci) and current BASES Laboratory Director. He is also a registered nutritional therapist with the British Association for Nutrition and Lifestyle Medicine (BANT) and the Complementary and Natural Healthcare Council (CNHC). With over 25 years' applied experience across a range of sports and levels (recreational to world-class), Justin utilises an evidence-based, functional approach to nutrition. Having gained a PhD in applied exercise metabolism and nutrition at Brunel University, Justin's research focuses on nutritional strategies to enhance metabolic flexibility and adaptive recovery from exercise, including polyphenol and protein-targeted approaches. Furthermore, having undertaken numerous endurance and multi-stage events, including long-distance triathlons, he is also interested in pre-probiotic and food-based strategies to support exercise-related gastrointestinal function.

Kate L. Spilsbury, PhD, ESSA AES, ASpS2, is a performance scientist at the Queensland Academy of Sport and Practicum Manager for the School of Human Movement and Nutrition Sciences at the University of Queensland. She previously worked at the English Institute of Sport, where she held the role of lead physiologist for British Athletics. There, she supported multiple high-performance athletes and coaches in preparation for both the London 2012 and Rio 2016 Olympic Games and Paralympic Games, in addition to other major international championships. Kate completed her PhD at Loughborough University, in partnership with the English Institute of Sport. Her research investigated tapering strategies for elite endurance running performance. Kate is an accredited exercise scientist and an accredited sport scientist (Level 2) with Exercise and Sport Science Australia. She is currently working with some of Australia's best swimmers and researching strategies to optimise adaptation to training and to enhance performance.

Leif Inge Tjelta, Dr. Philos. Professor Emeritus, is Lecturer in Coaching and Performance Development of the MSc in Sports Science at the University of Stavanger. Leif is a former distance runner at a national level and has more than 40 years of experience as a coach for middle- and long-distance runners at club, national and international levels. He has been Norwegian distance coach in the European Championships, World Championships and

Olympic Games. He gained his Dr. Philos. from the University in Stavanger investigating 'The Training Process in Distance Running at an International Level. Analysis of Training Volume, Training Intensity and Demands to Physical Capacity' (in Norwegian: Treningsprosessen i distanseløp på internasjonalt nivå. En analyse av treningsmengde, treningsintensitet og krav til fysisk kapasitet).

Stacy Winter, DProf, CPsychol, CSci, is Senior Lecturer in Applied Sport Psychology at St Mary's University in Twickenham, London. She is a chartered psychologist with the British Psychological Society, a chartered scientist with the Science Council, and a British Association of Sport and Exercise Sciences accredited practitioner. Stacy has worked extensively with both endurance runners and coaches for over 10 years. She has provided psychology support to middle- to long-distance Olympians, athletes who have represented their countries at all the major championships, and across track, road, and cross-country events. Stacy is also an active researcher, primarily focused on the professional practice of sport psychology. She gained her professional doctorate from the University of Central Lancashire and has since published many research articles. Specific areas of current research interest include the development of practitioner qualities, psychosocial interventions, and the well-being impacts of performance sport.

PREFACE

The popularity of distance running as a sport, and a recreational activity, is at an all-time high. At the elite end of the sport, competition is fierce, with runners striving to improve by small margins in their quest to secure places on their national team and win medals at championships. For example, in the final of the women's 800 m at the Athens Olympic Games in 2004, 0.13 sec separated first from fourth place. Recreational runners have many different reasons for participating in the sport, including to improve their health, gain a sense of achievement and satisfaction and socialise with friends. Irrespective of the level of participation, runners share a mutual passion for the sport and a desire to remain injury-free and achieve their goals. It is common for runners of all ages and abilities to actively seek advice on the best ways to train, optimise their recovery and avoid injury. Social media discussion forums have similar questions posted almost daily by runners who are looking for answers to their performance and injury related questions. For example, 'What is the best way to progress my training?' 'Should I be doing weight training?' 'Will wearing compression garments help my recovery?' 'What is the best thing to eat after my run?' The internet is also awash with online 'gurus' and fellow runners who are quick to offer advice and share their experiences; however, much of this is based on anecdotes and opinions that lack any scientific basis. Additionally, in recent years there has been a large growth in the provision of programmes of education for running coaches and aspiring sport scientists, which need to be supported by high-quality resources. Our primary motivation for writing this book was to address the most common topics and questions of interest to distance runners and coaches by inviting world-leading sport scientists and practitioners to share their knowledge and wisdom.

There are a multitude of different approaches to training distance runners; however, the basic principles and ingredients required for success are applicable to any distance runner. Moreover, our understanding of the science that underpins the training and physical preparation of distance runners has developed considerably over the last decade. The most experienced and successful coaches and practitioners working with distance runners rarely have the opportunity to share their tried and tested methods. Similarly, the novel work of sport scientists is often only accessible to elite runners and those in academia. In this book, we set out to link together the science and coaching artistry associated with preparing runners for middle- and long-distance events/races. It combines the latest scientific evidence, published by world-leading sport scientists, with the sound training principles and strategies adopted by experienced coaches and practitioners. We attempt to translate cutting-edge scientific research from the fields of physiology, biomechanics, psychology and nutrition into practical suggestions for achieving success. Important topical issues and contemporary practices related to health and performance are also addressed.

We have split this book into three parts. Part I addresses the science that underpins success in distance running from a multi-disciplinary perspective, including physiology, biomechanics, nutrition and psychology. Part II covers effective training practices and how runners can best physically prepare themselves to participate/compete in their chosen event(s). Part III focuses on several current and important issues associated with training for distance running and discusses specific considerations for sub-populations of runners. We have attempted to present readers with a summary of the latest research associated with each topic, issue or population of runner, and provide recommendations that runners and coaches can implement in their own training and practice. The scope of the book covers the middle- (800 m–3000 m) and long-distance events (5 km–marathon), with much of the content also applicable to ultra-distance events (>4 hours). We occasionally use the term 'endurance running', which we define as events/races lasting longer than 30 min (Saris et al., 2003).

It was our goal to bring together a group of sport scientists and applied practitioners who each had extensive experience in research and/or directly supporting middle- and long-distance runners. As you will read in the List of Contributors for this book, we certainly believe we have achieved this. Most of the authors who have contributed to this book are widely considered world-leading experts in their specialist areas of work with distance runners, and in many cases their work spans both research and applied practice. We are incredibly grateful that they were willing to share their work and perspectives on preparing distance runners with us. It has been a privilege working with each of them on this project, and we hope you enjoy reading and applying the content as much as we have.

Rich and Phil

PART I

The Scientific Bases of Training and Performance

1

PHYSIOLOGICAL DETERMINANTS OF MIDDLE- AND LONG-DISTANCE RUNNING

Philip R. Hayes and Daniel A. Gordon

Highlights

- Middle- and long-distance running events are determined by a complex mix of factors.
- The highest rate of energy production that can be maintained for the race duration and the ability to convert that into movement determine middle- and long-distance performance.
- The aerobic system is the main energy system used in middle- and long-distance running.
- The anaerobic system is important for middle-distance races and coping with changes of pace within a race.
- Appropriate training can improve all of the factors that determine middle- and long-distance performance.

Introduction

Running is one of the most popular global sporting and leisure-time activities (Hulteen et al., 2017). The popularity of running has grown in recent years with the creation of events such as the parkrun, a weekly, free-to-enter 5-km run, which began with 13 runners back in 2004 and now has 5 million registered runners worldwide. Around the world, runners not only run for the social and health benefits, both physiological and psychological, but also to challenge themselves, run new personal bests and, at the highest level, win global titles and break world records. Whatever stage they are at, the performances of all these runners are achieved through the same physiological processes. This chapter covers these processes. It begins with the link between running performance and energy supply, before presenting a model of factors that determine running performance, each of which are subsequently explained.

Bioenergetic Pathways

First identified nearly 100 years ago (Hill and Lupton, 1923), a hyperbolic relationship exists between race duration and the running speed that can be sustained for a given distance (Figure 1.1a). This is often referred to as the power-duration model, or, in the case of running, the speed-duration model. This relationship reflects the upper limit of human performance, but it is important to remember that it is generated from different runners, each of whom will have their own unique individual profile (Figure 1.1b). Individual profiles are perhaps a more realistic depiction of running capability. The speed-duration model, sometimes referred to as a bioenergetic model, can be explained by the rate at which the different cellular metabolic pathways produce energy. Superficially, this is true, but a complex series of co-ordinated, repeated, muscle actions are required to generate the force needed to attain, and maintain, a given running speed. These muscular contractions, fuelled by cellular metabolic processes, which, in the case of the aerobic system, require integrating with the cardiovascular and pulmonary systems to supply the necessary oxygen.

The faster the running speed, the greater the rate at which the active muscles must produce force, and by extension the metabolic systems produce the required energy. The 'currency' for the generation of force in the muscle is adenosine tri-phosphate (ATP) which when hydrolysed releases the energy used in cross-bridge cycling. The amount of ATP stored in skeletal muscle is very low (~20–25 mM·kg^{-1} muscle); however, a series of regulatory mechanisms, generally referred to as energy systems or metabolic pathways, prevent its catastrophic decline (Joyner, 2016) and complete degradation. These three distinct, yet interconnected metabolic pathways operate concurrently but at different rates. Collectively, they operate to meet the instantaneous energy demands of the muscle (Sahlin et al., 1998; Kang et al., 2014). It is the different rates and durations over which these pathways produce ATP that give rise to the speed-duration relationship.

The first pathway (ATP-PCr) involves the regeneration of ATP through the splitting of the high-energy phosphate, phosphocreatine (PCr). This immediate source of energy has a rapid

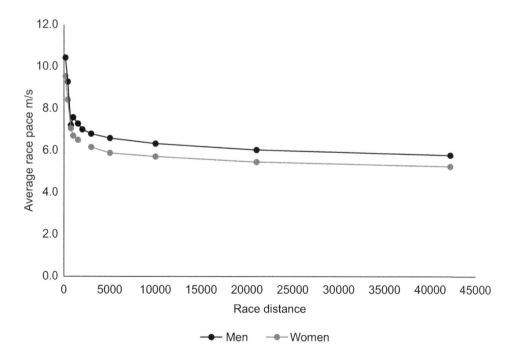

FIGURE 1.1a Men's and women's world record running speeds

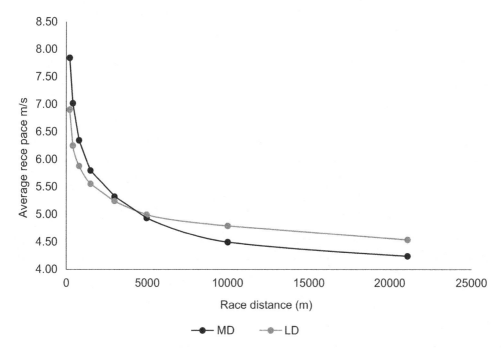

FIGURE 1.1b Comparison of running speeds of a middle-distance (MD) and long-distance (LD) runner

rate of ATP re-synthesis (~9 mM·kg^{-1}·dm^{-1}·s^{-1}) and during maximal exertion is almost completely depleted in approximately 10 sec (Hirvonen et al., 1987). The second pathway (glycolytic) involves the breakdown of stored carbohydrates, mainly in the form of muscle glycogen but also blood glucose, under 'anaerobic' conditions, resulting in ATP re-synthesis and the formation of pyruvate and then lactate. The rate of energy release from glycolysis is, however, slightly slower than that from PCr degradation, with a peak turnover rate of approximately 6–9 mM·kg^{-1}·dm^{-1}·s^{-1}. Compared to the ATP-PCr pathway, glycolysis has a greater capacity for ATP re-synthesis, with glycogen stores of around 250 mM·kg^{-1}. Both the PCr and glycolytic pathways are anaerobic, meaning that oxygen, although present in the muscle, is not used in the chemical reactions resulting in ATP re-synthesis. The final metabolic pathway is aerobic (mitochondrial) respiration, which by contrast does require the use of oxygen to re-synthesise ATP from the breakdown of carbohydrates, fats and, under some extreme circumstances, proteins. There is a greater ATP yield from the aerobic pathway; the breakdown of one molecule of glycogen through glycolysis results in a net gain of 3 ATP, compared to a further 34 ATP produced from mitochondrial respiration. This increased energy yield comes at the price of a considerably reduced rate of ATP production at ~1.32 mM·kg^{-1}·dm^{-1}·s^{-1}. If the rates of ATP release were plotted graphically, a hyperbolic relationship would be observed that largely explains the hyperbolic relationship between average race speed and time.

Until now these energy pathways have been defined separately, but as previously highlighted, they operate concurrently. For example, during a middle-distance track event, the athlete would be using energy derived from all three of the metabolic pathways. As race distance increases, so too does the relative contribution from the aerobic system (see Table 1.1).

TABLE 1.1 Relative energy system contribution by time and race distance

Race distance (m)[a]	% $\dot{V}O_{2max}$	% Aerobic	% Anaerobic	Race duration (s)[b]	% Aerobic	% Anaerobic
800	115–130	60–70	30–40	75	51	49
1500	105–115	80–85	15–20	90	56	44
3000	~100	85–90	10–15	120	63	37
5000	95–100	90–95	5–19	180	73	27
10000	90–95	97	3	240	79	21
Marathon	75–80	99.9	0.1			

Note: This will depend on race duration.

Source: [a] Sandford and Stellingwerf (2019). [b] Gastin (2001).

It is important to note, however, that the duration of the race, not the distance, determines the relative contributions. For example in male and female 1500-m runners of a similar relative standard, the aerobic-to-anaerobic contributions were 75:25% and 83:17% respectively (Hill, 1999). One further point to note is that all of the middle- and long-distance events are predominantly aerobic, even the 800-m race, and can therefore be considered as 'endurance' events.

Models of Performance

Several models have been developed to explain the principal determinants of endurance running (e.g. Joyner, 1991; Bassett and Howley, 2000). These models generally focus on three main components, namely $\dot{V}O_{2max}$, running economy and the fractional utilisation of $\dot{V}O_{2max}$ or a measure of maximum metabolic steady state. These three factors explain approximately 70–80% of middle- (Blagrove et al., 2019) and long-distance running performance (McLaughlin et al., 2010). Models such as this can be considered metabolic models. Paavolainen et al. (1999a) added neuromuscular factors, which included neural control, muscle force and elasticity, and running mechanics, to the traditional metabolic factors. The model proposed in this chapter (see Figure 1.2) is an amalgamation of these models to account for recent literature. In this model, race pace is dependent upon two key factors: the maximum rate of ATP (metabolic energy) production that can be sustained for the duration of the race and the running economy, which can be thought of as the ability to convert the metabolic energy into movement. Both running economy and the maximum sustainable rate of ATP production are multifactorial. The maximum sustainable rate of ATP production depends upon the exercise duration; the shorter the duration, the greater the rate that can be sustained. At intensities above the maximum metabolic steady state, the aerobic system cannot produce ATP fast enough to meet the demands of exercise. In this situation, the shortfall, or deficit, is offset by utilising the anaerobic capacity; however, this is not sustainable because when the anaerobic capacity is depleted, fatigue occurs and the athlete has to slow down (see Burnley and Jones, 2018 for a detailed discussion of fatigue at different exercise intensities). In the middle-distance events, running speeds considerably above maximal metabolic steady state can be sustained for the race duration; therefore, the aerobic system cannot produce ATP fast enough to fuel muscular contractions, and anaerobic ATP production becomes an important factor. As race distance increases, the running speed sustained reduces, becoming closer to

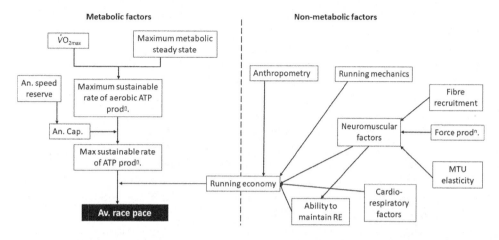

Metabolic factors   **Non-metabolic factors**

FIGURE 1.2 Deterministic model of middle- and long-distance running performance

An. = anaerobic, ATP = adenosine triphosphate, Av. = average, Cap. = capacity, MTU = muscle-tendon unit, prodⁿ. = production, RE = running economy, $\dot{V}O_{2max}$ = maximal oxygen uptake

the speed at maximal metabolic steady state, thereby increasing the importance of maximal metabolic steady state, while the reverse is true of anaerobic ATP production.

Maximal Oxygen Uptake ($\dot{V}O_{2max}$)

$\dot{V}O_{2max}$ is often defined as the maximum rate at which oxygen can be taken in and used by the body (Bassett and Howley, 1997), but it can also be thought of as the maximum rate of ATP production via the aerobic pathway (Medbø et al., 1988). In heterogeneous groups, there is a strong negative relationship between $\dot{V}O_{2max}$ and race performance (Costill et al., 1973), i.e. runners with a bigger $\dot{V}O_{2max}$ have faster times. By contrast, in homogeneous groups of well-trained runners, $\dot{V}O_{2max}$ is a poor predictor of performance (Conley and Krahenbuhl, 1980). This seeming contradiction can be explained by considering that to run a 2 h 15 min marathon, assuming 'average' running economy, a runner would be required to sustain a $\dot{V}O_2$ of approximately 60 mL·kg^{-1}·min^{-1} for the entire race (Bassett and Howley, 2000). This value is higher than the $\dot{V}O_{2max}$ of many recreational runners. A high $\dot{V}O_{2max}$ is therefore a pre-requisite to be an elite runner but not necessarily a determining factor in elite runners.

The extraction of oxygen from that atmosphere through to its use within the mitochondria is a multi-stage process. Oxygen enters the lungs and diffuses into the bloodstream, where it binds with haemoglobin, the quantity of oxygen transported will depend upon the quantity of haemoglobin. The rate at which oxygen is transported around the body depends upon the maximum cardiac output ($\dot{Q}_{max}$), with the final step being the extraction and use of oxygen by the working muscle. Each of these stages could potentially limit $\dot{V}O_{2max}$ and will be considered briefly (see reviews: Levine, 2008; Lundby et al., 2017). The ability of the working muscle to extract and use oxygen is considered to be a 'peripheral' limitation, while all of the others are considered as 'central' limitations.

Except for chronic respiratory diseases, at sea level the lung is not generally considered to be a limiting factor in exercise, even maximal exercise (Dempsey et al., 1984). A minor exception to this is some elite runners, who have exceptionally high cardiac outputs. These athletes have such high rates of pulmonary capillary blood flow that there is insufficient time for haemoglobin to be fully re-saturated, causing arterial desaturation (Dempsey et al., 1984). Altitude reduces the atmospheric partial pressure of oxygen (PO_2), decreasing the diffusion gradient and thereby reducing haemoglobin saturation (Schoene, 2001). The oxygen carrying capacity of blood (CaO_2) is dependent upon the quantity and saturation of haemoglobin. Manipulating the haemoglobin content of blood by venepuncture with or without subsequent reinfusion has been shown to reduce (Gordon et al., 2014) or increase (Buick et al., 1980) $\dot{V}O_{2max}$ respectively. This is the basis of the illegal (under the sporting laws) practices of blood doping or taking erythropoietin (EPO). $\dot{Q}_{max}$ is the product of maximum heart rate (HR_{max}) and maximum stroke volume. A near perfect linear relationship exists between $\dot{Q}_{max}$ and $\dot{V}O_{2max}$. No differences in HR_{max} exist between elite runners, recreational runners and untrained individuals, therefore the difference in $\dot{Q}_{max}$ is due to the larger stroke volumes of runners (Levine, 2008). In whole body exercise, the ability of the heart to supply blood to the working muscle, is thought to be the limiting factor in maximum oxygen consumption (Richardson et al., 1999). Even at $\dot{V}O_{2max}$, the mitochondrial capacity for oxidative phosphorylation exceeds the ability to supply oxygen to the working muscle (Lundby et al., 2017). In middle- and long-distance running, it is maximum cardiac output, specifically maximum stroke volume, that is considered the main limiting factor in $\dot{V}O_{2max}$.

Given that $\dot{V}O_{2max}$ sets the upper limit for endurance performance (Bassett and Howley, 2000), it is unsurprising that a great deal of attention has focused on how to increase it with training. Middle- and long-distance runners use varying quantities of both interval training and continuous running as training methods. In untrained and lesser-trained individuals, low intensity exercise is sufficient to improve $\dot{V}O_{2max}$ (Midgley et al., 2006a), suggesting that both continuous and interval training are effective. By contrast in well-trained individuals, interval training is more effective (Milanović et al., 2015), with intensities between 95% and 100% $\dot{V}O_{2max}$ recommended (Midgley et al., 2006a). In the last decade, short (<30 sec) high-intensity intervals have become a popular method of training to improve $\dot{V}O_{2max}$; however, their effectiveness in well-trained athletes remains equivocal (Weston et al., 2014). Longer interval training repetitions (3–5 min) generate the largest increases in $\dot{V}O_{2max}$ (Bacon et al., 2013), with a recent meta-analysis showing that only relatively large volumes (>15 min) of long interval training repetitions (>2 min) were more effective than continuous training (Wen et al., 2019). It is important to note that most of these findings are from studies on, at best, moderately trained individuals. Very few studies exist on well-trained runners, but they do corroborate the general findings of large volumes of longer repetitions, with the added caveat of the need for greater intensities (Midgley et al., 2007). Increases in $\dot{V}O_{2max}$ arising from interval training are due mainly to an increased $\dot{Q}_{max}$, resulting from a greater stroke volume (Montero et al., 2015).

The general consensus is that $\dot{V}O_{2max}$ can be improved with training but reaches a genetic limit, with longitudinal studies on highly trained runners showing no change in $\dot{V}O_{2max}$, despite improvements in performance (Daniels et al., 1978; Legaz Arrese et al., 2005). Despite this consensus, there is evidence of elite runners improving their $\dot{V}O_{2max}$. For example, a former US record holder for 1500 m and the mile improved his $\dot{V}O_{2max}$ from 74.4 mL·kg^{-1}·min^{-1} at the start of the preparation phase to 80.1 mL·kg^{-1}·min^{-1} during the competition phase (Conley et al., 1984). Equally noteworthy is Michael East, a former Commonwealth Games 1500 m champion with a personal best of 3m38.9. Following a two-year intervention to polarise his training intensity distribution, his $\dot{V}O_{2max}$ increased from 72 mL·kg^{-1}·min^{-1} to 79 mL·kg^{-1}·min^{-1} and his 1500 m time improved to 3m32.4 (Ingham et al., 2011).

Maximum Metabolic Steady State

The maximum metabolic steady state is a critical threshold in endurance physiology. Below this point, a metabolic steady state is achieved; above it, the aerobic system cannot produce ATP fast enough to meet the energetic demands of skeletal muscle, necessitating the anaerobic system to meet the shortfall. Running just above, or just below, the maximum metabolic steady state therefore generates very different metabolic, cardiorespiratory and fatigue responses (for a detailed review, see Jones et al., 2019). At intensities above the maximum metabolic steady state, the finite anaerobic capacity begins to be utilised, with exercise duration limited by its availability. Confusingly, the maximum metabolic steady state has been referred to by a variety of different terms, the most commonly used being onset of blood lactate accumulation (OBLA), lactate threshold, lactate turnpoint, maximum lactate steady state, critical speed, gas exchange threshold or anaerobic threshold. These terms are largely a reflection of the measurement technique employed (Jones et al., 2019). There is however, a broad agreement that the maximum metabolic steady state is dependent upon the ability of the mitochondria to oxidised pyruvate (Holloszy and Coyle, 1984). Mitochondrial density and oxidative enzyme content, or respiratory capacity, therefore become key determinants (Granata et al., 2018).

Regardless of the terminology, or protocol used, a strong relationship exists between purported measures of maximum metabolic steady state and middle- and long-distance running performance (Faude et al., 2009). Many studies looking at the physiological determinants of endurance running performance have found maximum metabolic steady state to be a stronger predictor of performance than $\dot{V}O_{2max}$ (e.g. Farrell et al., 1979). In relation to absolute running speeds, athletes with faster times over the same distance exhibit a faster speed at maximum metabolic steady state. For example, in a group of marathon runners with finishing times between 2h 30m and 3h 00m, between 3h 30m and 4h 00m and over 4h 30 m, the speed at lactate turnpoint was 15.5 ± 0.7 km·h^{-1}, 13.1 ± 1.6 km·h^{-1} and 10.9 ± 1.2 km·h^{-1} respectively (Gordon et al., 2017). Long-distance runners generally have a higher maximum metabolic steady state than middle-distance runners (Svedenhag and Sjödin, 1984), with it being as high as 85% $\dot{V}O_{2max}$ in some long-distance runners (Joyner et al., 2020). A high relative maximum metabolic steady state (i.e. occurring at high % $\dot{V}O_{2max}$) was the best predictor ($r = 0.89$) of how long moderately well-trained runners could run at the speed at $\dot{V}O_{2max}$ (Midgley et al., 2006b, 2006c).

Data collected over a 10-year period on the former marathon world record holder Paula Radcliffe showed that her speed at lactate threshold increased from 14.0 km·h^{-1} to 18.0 km·h^{-1}. During this time, her personal best performances from 3000 m up to the marathon concurrently improved (Jones, 2006). These longitudinal gains in maximum steady state, along with proportionately greater gains in muscle oxidative capacity compared to $\dot{V}O_{2max}$, have led to the view that maximum metabolic steady state is more 'trainable' than $\dot{V}O_{2max}$. Despite this apparent 'trainability' and strong correlation with performance, relatively few studies have focused upon the optimum training approach. In a review of 56 studies, most based on cycling in untrained or moderately active individuals, training volume was more important than training intensity in increasing mitochondrial content (Bishop et al., 2019).

Furthermore, mitochondrial training gains do, however, appear to be rapidly lost when training ceases (Granata et al., 2018). The view that volume is more important than intensity has been contested (MacInnis et al., 2019) but parallels the high volumes and training intensity distributions of elite athletes (see Chapter 8) and training data from recreational marathon runners (Gordon et al., 2017). Anecdotally, a wide range of training approaches have been used by athletes including 'tempo runs' at just below maximum metabolic steady state, and both continuous and interval training at just above maximum metabolic steady state (Tjelta, 2016; Joyner et al., 2020). The inclusion of a weekly 20 min run at the speed eliciting a blood lactate of 4 mmol·L^{-1} (a surrogate measure for maximum metabolic steady state) for 14 weeks in highly trained runners resulted in an increase in this speed (Sjödin et al., 1982).

Anaerobic Capacity

Defined as the maximal amount of ATP re-synthesised from anaerobic metabolism by the whole organism (Green, 1994), anaerobic capacity can play a pivotal role in the performance outcome of middle-distance runners in particular. The proportion of energy supplied by the aerobic system increases with increasing race distance; therefore, the contribution from anaerobic capacity is greater in shorter races (Gastin, 2001). This does not, however, discount its relevance in longer races where sudden changes in energy demand, due to changes in pace or terrain, need to be met instantaneously, principally through the anaerobic system. High peak blood lactate values (18.6 $\pm$ 2.1 ad 21.9 $\pm$ mmol·L^{-1} in females and males respectively) have been found in elite 800 m runners post-race, compared to typical values of approximately 3–5 mmol·L^{-1} at maximum metabolic steady state. Unsurprisingly, the anaerobic capacity of middle-distance runners is approximately 30% larger than that of long-distance runners (Medbø and Burgers, 1990).

Due to the difficulty in measuring anaerobic capacity and lower contribution of anaerobic metabolism to total energy production, this physiological determinant has received little research attention. The findings of this research are somewhat varied; weak relationships ($r \leq$ 0.23) have been found between a variety of anaerobic capacity measures and 800 m performance (Craig and Morgan, 1998; Bosquet et al., 2007a) in club-level runners, while a moderate correlation ($r = -0.61$) was found between maximum accumulated oxygen deficit and 800 m time (Ramsbottom et al., 1994). Over 1500 m, in national standard runners, a strong relationship exists between peak blood lactate after a run to exhaustion and 1500 m speed (Ferri et al., 2012). Both long (2 min) and short (20 sec) intervals performed at intensities above $\dot{V}O_{2max}$ improve anaerobic capacity by around 10% in untrained individuals. Scientific evidence regarding the optimum approach to training anaerobic capacity in well-trained middle- and long-distance runners is currently lacking. Improving performance in high-intensity exercise can also be achieved through non-metabolic means with improved muscle membrane potential regulation (Iaia and Bangsbo, 2010) and strength training (Blagrove et al., 2018a).

Anaerobic Speed Reserve

The anaerobic speed reserve (ASR) is the difference between maximum sprinting speed and the speed at $\dot{V}O_{2max}$ (Sandford et al., 2019c). Being competitive in championship middle-distance races requires more than simply being able to produce a high sustainable rate of

ATP production for the race duration. It requires the ability to produce a fast-absolute speed, particularly over 800 m (Sandford et al., 2018) but also the ability to cope with surges in pace (Sandford et al., 2019b). The ASR is sufficiently sensitive to be able to differentiate sub-populations of elite middle-distance runners, with faster 800 m runners having a larger ASR (Sandford et al., 2019c). Theoretically, ASR can be improved by increasing maximum sprinting speed or decreasing speed at $\dot{V}O_{2max}$. As a higher speed at $\dot{V}O_{2max}$ is also associated with better middle-distance performance (Blagrove et al., 2019), the only logical way to enhance ASR is therefore to improve maximal speed. ASR is an emerging concept and could yet provide further insights into successful middle- and long-distance running (a more detailed view can be found in Sandford et al., 2019c).

Running Economy

Running economy is a simple concept and has traditionally been defined as the steady state oxygen or energetic cost of running at any given sub-maximum speed. This approach has been criticised for a number of reasons: (i) it does not allow a comparison between runners at different speeds, (ii) the substrate used will affect the rate of oxygen consumption and (iii) the speeds are absolute and not relative to the individual's maximum metabolic steady state (Fletcher et al., 2009). A more valid approach is to use energy expenditure per unit of distance covered (Beck et al., 2018; Blagrove et al., 2019) at speeds relative to an individual's maximum metabolic steady state (Fletcher et al., 2009; Shaw et al., 2014). This approach enables a comparison of RE at different running speeds and accounts for variations in substrate usage.

Of the key factors that determine distance running performance in athletes of similar ability, running economy (RE) is perhaps the most variable, with inter-individual differences of as much as 30% reported (Daniels, 1985). Morgan et al. (1995) compared RE in four groups of male runners: (i) those who competed at Olympic trials (5 km, 10 km, marathon), (ii) sub-elite runners (~33 mins for 10 km), (iii) regular runners (~40 mins for 10 km) and (iv) active but untrained. Overall, faster runners had better RE, however there was considerable variation within- (~20%) and between-groups (~10%). It was particularly noteworthy that the RE of the most economic untrained runner was similar to the group mean of the Olympic trialists (182.1 vs. 181.9 mL·kg^{-1}·min^{-1}). Notwithstanding this, in homogeneous groups of highly trained runners, running economy is a better predictor of long-distance race performance than $\dot{V}O_{2max}$ (Conley and Krahenbuhl, 1980; Morgan et al., 1989a). Some studies have shown an inverse relationship between $\dot{V}O_{2max}$ and RE when runners are matched on performance (Jones, 2006). This, however, is inevitable given the study design; a low $\dot{V}O_{2max}$ must be compensated for by better RE in order to achieve a similar performance. Irrespective, a runner with excellent RE will produce less metabolic energy at any given running speed than one with poor economy. Fletcher and MacIntosh (2017) provided an excellent illustration of the importance of running economy by analysing the physiology required to run a marathon in 2h 02m 57s, the world record at the time. A runner with average RE (4.38 kJ·kg^{-1}·km^{-1}) would require a $\dot{V}O_{2max}$ of 85 mL·kg^{-1}·min^{-1}, whereas someone with excellent RE (3.77 kJ·kg^{-1}·km^{-1}) would 'only' need 77.5 mL·kg^{-1}·min^{-1}.

Despite its conceptual simplicity and ease of measurement, RE is multifaceted, incorporating anthropometric, neuromuscular, cardiorespiratory and biomechanical factors (for more detail, see Saunders et al., 2004; Barnes and Kilding, 2015b) plus the ability to maintain RE when fatigued (Figure 1.2). Moreover, RE is often incorrectly referred to as 'efficiency'.

Efficiency is the ratio of work done to energy expended. Work is done when the point of force application moves through a distance (Winter and Fowler, 2009). In running, the point of force application is obviously the foot, but it remains stationary while applying force and therefore the net work done is zero. Economy, by contrast, is the measurement of energy expenditure (Saunders et al., 2004), therefore during running it is possible to measure economy, but not efficiency. In essence, running economy is the ability to convert metabolic energy into movement.

The 'trainability' of RE is unclear (Joyner et al., 2020). Improvements in those previously untrained are unsurprising, although the results are somewhat equivocal in trained runners. Longitudinal profiling has shown mixed results in trained runners (Bragada et al., 2010; Galbraith et al., 2014; Kubo, Miyazaki et al., 2015) with improvements in national (Svedenhag and Sjodin, 1985) and world-class runners (Conley et al., 1984; Jones, 2006), adding to the anecdotal belief that good economy is a product of long-term or high-volume training. Experimental training interventions are more likely to be conducted on untrained or recreational athletes. Better runners are generally less willing to alter their training programmes, leaving a dearth of information regarding effective training interventions in high-calibre runners. Consistent with the view that higher training volumes are important, a recent meta-analysis revealed continuous training to be more effective than interval training in improving RE in recreational runners (Gonzalez-Mohino et al., 2020). Furthermore, the meta-analysis revealed some moderating factors, with improvements in RE more likely in training programmes longer than 8 weeks and weekly volumes of more than 105 minutes of continuous running. There were also benefits from interval training, but only where the repetitions were more than 1 minute long and the cumulative weekly interval time exceeded 23.2 min (Gonzalez-Mohino et al., 2020). Strength training is also an effective strategy for improving RE in middle- and long-distance runners (Blagrove et al., 2018a).

Anthropometry

In adult middle-and long-distance races, competitor's stature and mass can range by as much as 30 cm and/or 25 kg respectively (Barnes and Kilding, 2015b). All other things being equal, the absolute oxygen uptake (L·min^{-1}) and energy expenditure scores (kJ·min^{-1}) increase with increasing body mass. To enable inter-individual comparison, scores are usually corrected by body mass (per kg); however, this assumes a linear relationship between either oxygen uptake (or energy expenditure) and body mass. The validity of this assumption has been long been challenged (Tanner, 1949) with alternative approaches such as allometric (i.e. non-linear) scaling recommended (Lolli et al., 2017). Across a wide range of age, mass and activity levels there is a lack of linearity between oxygen uptake and body mass (Lolli et al., 2017) however, in a large sample (N = 71 women; 101 men) of well-trained runners, correcting scores by absolute mass (kg) was better at removing the influence of mass on RE than non-linear scaling (Shaw et al., 2014).

It is not just a runner's mass that can affect their RE but potentially the distribution (e.g. height, limb lengths, segmental masses and volumes) and composition (e.g. bone, fat and muscle) of their mass. The effect of different distributions has been studied by attaching weights to different parts of the body. A given load attached to the foot will increase RE more than when added to the thigh or trunk (Frederick, 1984; Martin, 1985; Myers and Steudel, 1985). This has popularised the idea that a larger distal leg mass will impair economy due to the additional energy required to swing the leg (Barnes and Kilding, 2015b). Elite East African runners have better RE (Saltin et al., 1995; Lucia et al., 2006; Santos-Concejero et al., 2015) compared to other elite runners, which has been proposed to account for their dominance in distance running (Larsen, 2003; Lucia et al., 2006). Their more slender body shape and lower leg circumference compared to similar Caucasian populations (Saltin et al., 1995; Larsen et al., 2004), would, in principle, reduce the energy required to swing the leg, accounting for their better RE. Conflicting evidence exists in support of this, Lucia et al. (2006) compared elite (<13m 50s for 5 km) Eritrean and Spanish runners, finding RE at 21 km·h^{-1} to be related to calf girth but not body mass or body mass index. By contrast, a comparison of elite Eritrean and European 10 km runners (~28 min) found better RE in the Eritreans but no relationship with either limb lengths or circumferences (Santos-Concejero et al., 2015). In a homogenous group of high-calibre Kenyan runners (993 IAAF points), no single limb length or circumference explained RE; rather, it was a complex interplay of anthropometric factors (Mooses et al., 2015). These studies have generally used small sample sizes, although Black et al. (2020) had similar findings in a large heterogeneous sample of runners (N = 71 women; 101 men) concluding that superior RE was associated with slimmer limbs and a slender physique.

One anthropometric factor that has consistently shown a link to RE is length of the Achilles tendon moment arm, which is the horizontal distance from the centre of the calcaneus to the Achilles tendon when the person is seated with the knee and ankle at 90°. Shorter Achilles tendon moment arms confer superior RE through a greater storage and release of elastic strain energy (Scholz et al., 2008; Barnes et al., 2014; Mooses et al., 2015).

Cardiorespiratory Variables

The effect of cardiorespiratory variables on RE has been examined using both inter- and intra-individual comparisons. Across a large sample of habitual runners (N = 69 women; 119 men), stratified by age (20–60 years old) and training volume (10–50 miles·wk^{-1} for women; 10–70 miles·wk^{-1} for men), when running at 9.6 km·h^{-1}, only $\dot{V}_E$ and HR were significantly correlated with RE (Pate et al., 1992). Pate et al. (1992) estimated that 1–2% of RE was due to differences in myocardial work, while approximately 7–8% was due to ventilation. Given the range of participants used in this study (Pate et al., 1992), the use of an absolute intensity ignores differences in relative intensity, making inter-individual comparisons problematic (Fletcher et al., 2009). Increases in $\dot{V}_E$ from the beginning to end of a treadmill 5 km run were the only physiological variable that correlated with the impaired RE (Thomas et al., 1999). Collectively, these data suggest that cardiorespiratory variables account for a small portion of the energy expended during running, although more evidence is required. Following 6 weeks increased training intensity in habitual recreational runners, RE improved in those undertaking either long interval training (4 min reps; 2 min recovery) or continuous running (20–30 mins @ ~93% HR$_{max}$) but not those using short intervals (15 sec reps; 15 sec recovery) (Franch et al., 1998). The improvement in RE was strongly correlated ($r = 0.77$) with the reduction in $\dot{V}_E$ during a standardised sub-maximal run.

Neuromuscular Determinants of RE

Running requires a repeated sequence of co-ordinated voluntary muscular contractions, the energy for which is provided by intra-cellular metabolic processes. RE measures the oxygen consumed and carbon dioxide produced during aerobic re-synthesis of the ATP used. The number of actin-myosin cross-bridges required to produce the necessary force to attain (and maintain) a given running speed will determine the level of muscle activation and energy production needed (Fletcher and MacIntosh, 2017). This is achieved through the interaction of different neuromuscular factors, including muscle fibre recruitment strategy, the ability of the muscle to produce force and the muscle-tendon unit (MTU) to create, store and use elastic strain energy. These are briefly considered next; for a more detailed explanation, see Barnes and Kilding (2015b) and Fletcher and MacIntosh (2017).

Fibre Recruitment

The muscle fibre recruitment strategy, which is a combination of the number of fibres recruited and frequency of recruitment (rate coding), is dependent upon the force-velocity and length-tension relationships (Fletcher and MacIntosh, 2017). Not only does voluntary activation of muscle increase with increasing running speed (Kyrolainen et al., 2005), but also the timing of activation. EMG (muscle electrical) activity of the leg extensor muscles shows increased activation prior to, and during, the braking portion of the stance phase; this is particularly noticeable in the biarticular muscles (i.e. gastrocnemius, hamstrings, rectus femoris). Concomitant with the increase in fibre recruitment is a reduction in contraction time, thereby requiring a more rapid rate of cross-bridge cycling; together these factors will increase the rate of energy expenditure. This illustrates the importance of measuring RE as an energy expenditure ($kJ \cdot kg^{-1} \cdot km^{-1}$) rather than an oxygen cost ($mL \cdot kg^{-1} \cdot km^{-1}$) as energy expenditure increases with running speed while oxygen cost is linear (Shaw et al., 2014; Blagrove et al., 2019c). Faster running speeds, with their shorter contraction times, require the recruitment of fast twitch fibres which are energetically more costly, further increasing the rate of energy expenditure. Well-trained runners show a reduced stride-to-stride variation in EMG than less trained runners; this reduced variation is considered an indicator of more skilled movement (Osu et al., 2002; Chapman et al., 2008). It is unknown whether this is a cause of consequence of their higher trained status, although motor learning studies show reduced variation as individuals improve their skill (Osu et al., 2002).

Force Production

Increasing strength, usually due to an increase in muscle cross-sectional area, theoretically allows each muscle contraction to occur at a lower percentage of maximum strength. This would require fewer muscle fibres to be recruited to produce the force necessary during ground contact, thereby reducing the energy required (Fletcher and MacIntosh, 2017). The endurance running community has been relatively slow to embrace resistance training due to long-standing beliefs that hypertrophic adaptations will reduce mitochondrial density (Chilibeck et al., 1999) and increase energy expenditure (Beattie et al., 2017). In stark contrast to these beliefs, a recent review found overwhelming evidence that RE improved through resistance training (~2–8%), with no discernible gains in mass (Blagrove et al., 2018a). The ability to generate force also decreases after a run to exhaustion (Nicol et al., 1991b; Dierks et al., 2008; Bazett-Jones et al., 2013) and typical training sessions (Riazati et al., 2020), although this has not been directly linked to changes in RE.

Muscle-Tendon Unit Elasticity

Running has been likened to a repeating series of cyclical bounds, during which the leg acts like a spring, compressing during the braking and mid-stance phases of foot strike and then recoiling during push-off (Farley et al., 1993). Within this analogy, as the leg compresses, it stores elastic energy within the series elastic component of the muscle-tendon units, which is subsequently released during the recoil phase. This release of stored elastic energy reduces the amount of force required from the subsequent concentric contraction to propel the runner compared to a concentric-only contraction, thereby reducing the energy expenditure (Ito et al., 1983). A more compliant tendon would, theoretically, be capable of storing and returning higher levels of energy; however, the most economical runners possess stiffer tendons (Dalleau et al., 1998; Arampatzis et al., 2006; Dumke et al., 2010; Rogers et al., 2017). The stiffness of 'the spring' is therefore an important element in both the storage and return of elastic energy and determining ground contact time. A stiffer spring enables a shorter ground contact time and greater return of the stored elastic energy (McMahon and Cheng, 1990). Unsurprisingly, as running speed increases, so too does MTU stiffness (Kyrolainen et al., 2005) facilitating shorter ground contact times and faster rates of force production. The increase in stiffness occurs due to increased pre-activation of motor units prior to ground contact; this is thought to assist with both absorbing the impending impact force and generating the braking impulse (Kyrolainen et al., 2005). Increased muscle activity prior to ground contact would be expected to increase energy expenditure; however, it serves to maintain more optimal length-tension and force-velocity relationships (Lutz and Rome, 1994). Optimising these relationships enables muscle fibres to produce force under (near) isometric conditions which is more energy efficient than concentric actions (Lutz and Rome, 1994; Fletcher et al., 2013). MTU stiffness increases in response to various types of resistance training (Kubo et al., 2001a, 2001b, 2002; Fletcher et al., 2010) and could therefore enhance RE.

Running Mechanics

When watching any middle- or long-distance race, a range of running styles can be observed. Despite an obvious intuitive link between RE and running mechanics (Anderson, 1996) and extensive research on the topic, very little clear-cut evidence exists in support of it. A review of biomechanical factors contributing to RE concluded that it was not possible to definitively identify any variables (Moore, 2016). The majority of research on this topic has been conducted on small ($N < 25$), often homogeneous samples, recording a limited range of variables. The exception to this is a recent study by Folland et al. (2017), which examined 24 different variables in a heterogeneous sample of 97 runners (47 women; 50 men). They found pelvic vertical oscillation during ground contact normalised to height, minimum knee joint angle during the stance phase and minimum pelvic horizontal velocity accounted for 39% of the variation in RE. Chapter 13 on gait retraining addresses the effect of training on running mechanics.

Ability to Maintain RE

Although not explicitly stated, the three parameters of the 'classical' model of endurance running ($\dot{V}O_{2max}$, fractional utilisation of $\dot{V}O_{2max}$ and RE) while trainable, are assumed to be relatively stable on a day-to-day basis. This, however, is not true for RE, which can deteriorate with fatigue. Increases in RE occur towards the end of a long, continuous run, ranging from 60 min to the marathon (e.g. Brueckner et al., 1991; Hunter and Smith, 2007; Garcia-Pinillos et al., 2020) over the course of a 5-km run (Thomas et al., 1999), after a 4 min bout at the speed associated with $\dot{V}O_{2max}$ (Hayes et al., 2011) and after interval training (James and Doust, 1998).

The multifactorial nature of RE makes it difficult to determine the underlying causal mechanism(s) for the increase in RE. To a layperson watching middle- or long-distance races, the apparent fatigue induced changes in the gait of some runners would seem the obvious cause. Kinematic changes in gait do occur towards the end of both continuous, long-distance running (e.g. Nicol et al., 1991a) see also Chapter 2) and also interval training (e.g. Riazati et al., 2020); however, they do not appear to be related to the changes in RE (e.g. Nicol et al., 1991a). This is likely due to the individual variation in kinematic changes, ranging from large to no change (Nicol et al., 1991a; Hunter and Smith, 2007). The weight of evidence points towards neuromuscular factors causing the impairment in RE with increases in muscle fibre recruitment during braking and push-off phases (Nicol et al., 1991a), a decrease in eccentric:concentric EMG ratio – suggesting a reduction in stored elastic strain energy (Abe et al., 2007), reduction in MTU stiffness (Girard et al., 2013; Garcia-Pinillos et al., 2020) and reductions in muscular force production (Riazati et al., 2020). Furthermore, there is a negative relationship between the increase in RE following a 4-min run at speed at $\dot{V}O_{2max}$ and eccentric muscular endurance of the knee flexors (KF), i.e. better eccentric KF endurance resulted in a smaller increase in RE (Hayes et al., 2011). Collectively, these changes suggest a reduced ability to tolerate repeated impact forces, and a loss of stretch-shortening cycle function is most likely to explain the increase in RE with fatigue (Nicol et al., 1991a). The link between being able to maintain RE and race performance has not been investigated but could be an important determinant of middle- and long-distance performance.

Summary

Running, while a seemingly simple activity, is a complex interaction of different physiological systems. Performance in middle- and long-distance events is determined by the highest rate at which ATP can be re-synthesised for the race duration and the ability to convert this energy into movement. All of the middle- and long-distance running events depend primarily on the aerobic system for ATP re-synthesis, and this dependence increases with increasing distance. Despite this, the anaerobic system plays an important role in race situations, allowing an athlete to cope with changes in pace, particularly in the middle-distance races. Running economy, or ability to convert this energy into movement, is a key factor that differentiates runners and is made up of a complex interaction of, mostly, neuromuscular factors. All of the factors that determine middle- and long-distance performance are, to a greater or lesser extent, trainable, enabling athletes of all levels to improve.

2

THE BIOMECHANICS OF DISTANCE RUNNING

Brian Hanley

Highlights

- Running speed is dictated by an athlete's step length and cadence, although step length is more important in differentiating between faster and slower runners and reduces more with fatigue. Being able to increase cadence, however, is often the deciding factor in sprint finishes.
- Of the different components that make up step length, the distance the body travels during flight is the most important. An athlete's flight distance is determined by upward and forward impulse in late stance, which usually decrease with fatigue because of reduced leg stiffness and tolerance to repeated stretch loads.
- Middle-distance runners are more likely to land on the forefoot or midfoot at first contact, whereas marathon runners tend to land on the heel. There are potential performance benefits to landing near the front of the foot through the stretch-shortening cycle and shorter contact times, although these apply less in longer events.
- There are small gains to be made from following rival runners in terms of air resistance, although having air moving around the body for cooling is important in hot conditions. Running uphill is unsurprisingly more energy costly than running on flat courses, but running downhill can risk injury because of the increased load on the knee, hip, and shin muscles.
- Running on soft surfaces, such as in cross-country running, is more difficult than on roads because the non-compliant nature of the surface reduces the effectiveness of the stretch-shortening cycle and is more energy costly because of an increase in leg stiffness to accommodate a reduction in stability.

Introduction

A knowledge of the biomechanics of running is invaluable when describing an athlete's technique, explaining how they speed up or slow down and understanding the external and internal forces that cause their movements. As the outward expression of movement, an athlete's biomechanics translates their underlying physiological, nutritional and psychological processes into running motion, and those who are biomechanically "better" are often those who can manage this transfer more efficiently and economically while reducing injury risk. This chapter provides a brief review of the important aspects of the running stride and its various components, the effects of different footstrike patterns and fatigue on running technique, and how racing conditions such as wind, hills and underfoot surface affect an athlete's biomechanics.

Step Length and Cadence

Running speed is the product of step length and cadence, the latter of which is often referred to as step rate or step frequency. Step length is the distance between successive foot contacts from a specific gait event on one foot to the equivalent event on the other foot and is measured in metres (m). The term "stride length" is sometimes used interchangeably with "step length" (Enomoto et al., 2008); however, stride length is most often used to refer to the distance between a specific gait event on one foot to the equivalent event on the same foot (e.g., Cavanagh and Kram, 1989). Hence, a stride refers to two successive steps (Levine et al., 2012). Cadence measures how frequently the runner completes a step in a given time, usually per second (measured in hertz, Hz). As speed is step length multiplied by cadence, an athlete with a step length of 1.50 m and a cadence of 3.00 Hz runs at 4.5 metres per second ($m \cdot s^{-1}$). To convert $m \cdot s^{-1}$ to kilometres per hour ($km \cdot h^{-1}$), multiply by 3.6. Thus, our runner's speed of 4.5 $m \cdot s^{-1}$ is equivalent to 16.2 $km \cdot h^{-1}$.

It is clear that both step length and cadence are important to running speed. However, cadence tends to vary less between distance runners, ranging from about 2.75 to 3.25 Hz (165 to 195 steps per minute). In middle-distance running, which includes fast starts and bursts of speed (e.g., to reach the bend before other athletes, or avoid being boxed in), athletes have to accelerate to ensure a good position. Increasing cadence in middle-distance races is therefore a performance-determining factor because of these short phases of great acceleration (Reiss et al., 1993). Over 800 m and 1500 m, individuals usually change from sub-maximal to maximum speed by increasing cadence, as step length is already close to its maximum at competition pace (Hunter et al., 2004). Cadence also increases during sprint finishes; for example, when Kenenisa Bekele won the 2007 World Championship 10,000 m, his step length was relatively constant at approximately 1.95 m throughout the race, and it was by increasing cadence during the last lap (from 3.2 Hz to 3.6 Hz) that he was able to achieve such a fast finish (Enomoto et al., 2008). At running speeds outside of the sprint finish, increases in speed normally arise from increases in step length, with an optimal step length and cadence unconsciously chosen by athletes to minimise energy expenditure (Saunders et al., 2004).

Overall, most distance runners have techniques that optimise performance within their physical and anthropometric builds where, ultimately, step length is limited by the athlete's stature and, more specifically, their leg length. Of course, this does not mean that short athletes cannot succeed in distance running; indeed, many of the world's best-ever athletes are shorter than average, e.g., the hugely successful Ethiopian distance runners, Haile Gebrselassie and Kenenisa Bekele, are about 1.65 m tall (5' 5"). Bushnell and Hunter (2007) found that distance runners' sprinting techniques differed from trained sprinters and suggested that this might be because distance runners practise sprint technique less and are unable to change technique greatly to increase cadence during sprint finishes. Coaches are therefore advised to include sprint technique training into competitive distance runners' schedules.

Components of Step Length

Step length is the sum of four distinct but interrelated components. At first contact, the athlete strikes the ground with the foot, and the distance from the whole-body centre of mass (CM) to the foot centre of mass is the first of these components (here, this is termed "foot ahead"). The body then rolls forwards over the support foot until toe-off, in phases that can be most easily summarised as early stance, midstance and late stance. The distance the foot moves from its horizontal position at first contact until toe-off is the second component contributing to step length ("foot movement"). Although this action is vital for correct running gait, foot movement is a relatively small contributor to overall step length and does not differentiate between faster and slower running. The distance from the CM to the foot centre of mass at toe-off is the third of the four components, which I have termed "foot behind". These three components occur during the contact phase, which has a shorter duration in faster running (because it leads to a higher cadence), and decreasing contact time is indeed one way by which distance runners speed up (Bushnell and Hunter, 2007). After the contact phase, the athlete has an airborne period during which the CM will experience a flight distance (the fourth and final component) before first contact occurs on the other foot and the gait cycle is repeated.

In effect, the three most important components of step length are the distance the foot lands in front of the body, the distance the foot is behind the body at toe-off and the distance the athlete travels during flight. To be successful, the athlete must cover sufficient distances during each of these phases, but running faster is not a simple case of increasing any or all of these components. First, the athlete needs to take care that the foot ahead distance is not too great (sometimes termed "overstriding") as the increased braking forces that occur slow the runner more than necessary (Moore, 2016). However, it should be noted that braking at first contact with the ground is normal and, although it often appears in fast-moving elite athletes that the foot is landing directly under the body, it does not, and to physically undertake such actions would adversely reduce step length. Second, the foot behind distance occurs during late stance when the hip, knee and ankle are extending to push the body forwards. However, as with foot ahead distance, the athlete should take care not to deliberately overextend as the increase in contact time not only decreases cadence but also occurs when the lower limb joints are no longer particularly effective. In general, there is little difference in foot ahead or foot behind distances between elite standard athletes. Although the athlete cannot speed up during flight in the absence of anything to push forwards against, and in fact slightly slows down because of air resistance, flight distance contributes so much to step length that it is the biggest differentiator between athletes. When running slowly, by contrast, flight distance can be very small. Merely instructing an athlete to increase any of these distances is unlikely to be productive; rather, it is through training, particularly at fast speeds and supplemented appropriately with technical and resistance training, that the athlete learns to get the right balance for their stature, strength and ability.

Ground Reaction Forces in Running

The importance of the stance phase during running is obvious given it is during ground contact that the body applies an external force to generate forward momentum. In simple terms, a force causes a change in velocity and, when running, different external forces are experienced. These include ground reaction forces in late stance that accelerate the athlete upwards and forwards, air resistance that causes slowing down, and frictional forces that provide grip. A force is a vector, which means that it has a magnitude (measured in newtons, N) and a direction (Winter et al., 2016). It can be quite difficult to analyse forces as single vectors, so in biomechanics, the ground reaction forces between the body and running surface are very often resolved into three directions: vertical (the only direction affected by gravity), forwards-backwards, and side-to-side. When a person stands still on a weighing scale, the value on the display is their vertical ground reaction force (i.e., their weight), although it is normally displayed in the technically incorrect but more familiar units of kilograms or pounds. Because people's weights vary considerably, it is quite normal in biomechanics to present force magnitudes in bodyweights (BW), whereby the forces measured are divided by the athlete's weight. For example, if a runner who weighs 600 N (approximately 61 kg/135 lb) experiences a landing force of 900 N, we could express this as 1.5 BW.

At first contact with the ground, the runner experiences a large impact force of between 2 and 3 BW (Cavanagh, 1990). Because the impact force occurs very early in the gait cycle, the muscles are often unprepared for it and respond through passive deformation of body tissues (Watkins, 2010). This "muscle latency" period lasts about 70 milliseconds, and the combination of relatively large impact forces and the inability of the body to respond fully mean that there is greater variability within limbs, and asymmetry between them, than during the rest of the gait cycle (Hanley and Tucker, 2018). Vertical forces during running tend to increase during early stance with a peak at midstance, associated with controlling the downwards movement of the CM, and preventing any vertical collapse during this weight acceptance phase (Winter and Bishop, 1992); lower limb joint stiffness is therefore a key factor in maintaining posture during this phase (Serpell et al., 2012). Note here that "stiffness", the relationship between the deformation of a body and a given force (Butler et al., 2003), is used to explain in simple terms how much or how little the lower extremity joints bend during stance, rather than tightness or soreness in the muscles after exercise.

Although vertical forces, and side-to-side forces probably more so, are difficult to link with performance (Cavanagh, 1990), the role of forwards-backwards forces are easier to understand in terms of running speed. Both the braking and propulsive forces that occur in this force direction have peak magnitudes of between 0.3 and 0.5 BW (Cavanagh and Lafortune, 1980; Munro et al., 1987), although what is more important is not the peak force but the total force applied during each phase. The product of force and time is impulse, defined as the change in momentum (Winter et al., 2016). Put simply, the larger the negative impulse during braking in early stance, the more the athlete will decelerate, which requires a similarly large positive impulse during late stance to speed up enough to maintain an overall constant speed (Chang and Kram, 1999). Maintaining a constant pace is therefore easier when the braking impulses are kept low, which theoretically occurs with a shorter foot ahead distance (Moore, 2016) and emphasises the biomechanical advantage of avoiding overstriding.

Movements and Muscles Involved in Running

We have already noted that there are effectively two phases that contribute to step length and cadence during running: a contact phase and a flight phase. These arise because each leg goes through a period where it is in stance (the contact phase) and a period in swing, comprising early swing, midswing and late swing. In normal running, each leg's swing phase is longer than the stance phase, and it is during the short time when both legs are in swing that flight time occurs, whereby one leg is in early swing, just after toe-off, and the other leg is in late swing, just before first contact (Novacheck, 1998). This of course means that during normal running, there is no occasion when both feet are in contact with the ground at the same time. For ease of explanation, the following sections will describe joint and body segment movements during the stance and swing phases, although it should be remembered that these are, in reality, interdependent parts of a continuous movement. In addition, as hundreds of muscles are involved in running, only the activity of large muscle groups will be considered.

Muscle Moments and Powers

Before discussing the movements of the body's joints and segments, it is useful to understand a little about the internal forces produced by muscles. Muscles act on bones to create movements at joints via tendons; for example, the soleus muscle in the calf pulls on the calcaneus (heel bone) via the Achilles tendon to plantarflex the ankle. It is often helpful to consider the muscle and tendon as part of one unit, rather than separate, and refer to it as the muscle-tendon unit (MTU). Most of the movements in running are rotational, such as knee flexion, and joint moments (or torques) indicate the amount and direction of rotational force about a joint. These are useful because they describe the relative contributions of different muscle groups during certain movement phases (Enoka, 2008). Calculations of mechanical power are used to complement the joint moment information by measuring the rate of work done by MTUs across a joint (White and Winter, 1985). MTUs that shorten when activated (often described as "concentric") generate power, whereas those that lengthen ("eccentric") absorb it (Vardaxis and Hoshizaki, 1989). Power that has been absorbed in MTUs stores elastic energy that can be later converted to kinetic energy with resulting power generation (Cavagna et al., 1968) through the stretch-shortening cycle mechanism that increases running efficiency (Cavagna et al., 1964). The stretch-shortening cycle is a complicated phenomenon, but in essence it refers to the rapid lengthening and subsequent shortening of an MTU, whereby the early stretch absorbs energy that enhances performance during the concentric phase of activity (Komi, 2000).

In distance running, some joint stiffness is required for optimal usage of the stretch-shortening cycle, although too much or too little can lead to reduced performances and injury (Butler et al., 2003). Greater running economy has been associated with greater lower limb stiffness (Dutto and Smith, 2002) because of a better use of elastic energy, and Arampatzis et al. (2006) found that runners with better economy had a more compliant quadriceps femoris tendon and higher triceps surae (gastrocnemius and soleus) tendon stiffness. It is also possible that less economical athletes have techniques that lead to unnecessary and wasteful vertical motion (Nummela et al., 2007). Similarly, these authors found that shorter contact times were associated with better running economy at several speeds typical of elite 5000 and 10,000 m runners, and reasoned that this was because shorter contact times tend to feature shorter braking phases.

The Swing Phase

The function of the swing phase is to allow the foot to clear the ground after toe-off and be repositioned in front of the CM ready for first contact (Levine et al., 2012). During early swing, the hip flexes so that the thigh moves from a position slightly behind the body to one in front of the body, with considerable activity by the rectus femoris and iliopsoas muscles. Because of the mass of the thigh and its location as the nearest joint to the trunk, this movement of the hip is important to the whole leg's contribution to overall running speed, with Bushnell and Hunter (2007) reporting that distance runners sped up by flexing the hip 14° more during midswing. The knee moves from a straightened angle of about 160° at toe-off to a very flexed position during midswing (55–60°) by concentric activity of the hamstrings, and then straightens again to about 150° in preparation for landing. The main knee extensors on the front of the thigh, the quadriceps femoris group, are mostly responsible for this movement, although runners should note that the hamstrings are often under considerable stress during late swing because of how they act to control knee extension (Chumanov et al., 2011). As well as helping the foot to clear the ground, the decrease in knee angle during swing acts to reduce the leg's moment of inertia (its resistance to rotation), and enhances the flight phase because the recovery leg's energy requirements are lowered (Kong and de Heer, 2008; Smith and Hanley, 2013). Some of the necessary actions taken to clear the ground are made by the ankle, which is plantarflexed at toe-off and moves to a more dorsiflexed position at landing, caused by activity of the tibialis anterior and other shin muscles. Along with the knee extensors, a key role of the ankle plantarflexors is to create high joint stiffness before and after first contact (Hanon et al., 2005) to enhance the stretch-shortening cycle.

The Stance Phase

The purpose of the stance phase is to generate the impulse the body needs to move forwards. At first contact with the ground, the hip is flexed so that the thigh is ahead of the body and then extends to a position behind the body (usually a small amount of hyperextension). The main muscles involved are the hip extensors, comprising gluteus maximus and the three hamstring muscles, which mostly act concentrically during this motion and provide the "drive" for moving forwards. The knee flexes about 15–20° from its more straightened position at first contact until midstance and is associated with enabling a more level path of the CM (Saunders et al., 1953), although it has been found that elite runners flex their knees less and have shorter durations of knee flexion during stance (Leskinen et al., 2009). These differences in knee motion mean elite runners have greater knee stiffness (Heise et al., 2011) and are thus able to use elasticity better, allowing them to achieve faster times in competition and withstand tiredness for longer (Leskinen et al., 2009). This elasticity occurs because the decrease in knee angle at midstance results in energy absorption through the lengthening of the quadriceps femoris, which subsequently shortens to extend the knee and propel the body forwards and upwards.

The ankle lands in a slightly dorsiflexed position at first contact (Buczek and Cavanagh, 1990) and dorsiflexes more in midstance largely because of knee flexion (as the tibia moves forwards relative to the foot). The plantarflexors, such as gastrocnemius and soleus, are an important energy generator as they act concentrically in late stance to create positive impulse. During the stance phase, there are also important foot movements, such as pronation and supination, which are each effectively a combination of rotational movements. These are often described as ankle motions, but they actually occur at the subtalar joint, which is between the talus bone and heel bone (calcaneus), located under it. In general, the runner lands on the outside of the foot (hence the wearing down of this part of the shoe first), pronate during the early, loading part of stance so that the foot is placed flat on the ground, and then supinate (moves the weight back to the foot's outside) during late stance. The function of the prona-tion and supination movements is to place the foot so that it is in the best position to provide support and guide correct movement, for example as a shock absorber (Novacheck, 1998).

Upper Body Movements

The movements of the upper limbs generally act in opposition to the ipsilateral (same-side) lower limbs to counteract moments of the swinging legs around the vertical axis (Hinrichs, 1987; Pontzer et al., 2009). Furthermore, Hinrichs (1987) stated that the arm swing provides a meaningful contribution to lift and subsequently flight, and although the arms do not provide forward propulsion of the CM, they minimise changes in horizontal velocity during stance. However, it is debated as to whether the shoulder muscles are primarily responsible for the swinging motion of the arms, or whether their movement is mostly a passive response to the legs' movements (Pontzer et al., 2009). Regardless of the exact contribution of the upper limbs, and as elbow angles are generally more variable between runners than lower limb angles (Hanley et al., 2011), the ungainly arm movements often adopted even by elite athletes should be avoided in providing balance and propulsion to the body, and they frequently indicate a problem elsewhere in the body.

The movements of the arms complement those of the torso, where the upper part of the trunk can be seen to act in opposite and counterbalancing motion to the lower part (Nova-check, 1998); indeed, trunk rotation in running has been associated with increased efficiency (Bramble and Lieberman, 2004). Pelvic rotation is the way in which the pelvis twists about a vertical axis, moving each hip joint forwards as that hip flexes and backwards as the hip extends (Levine et al., 2012), meaning that less hip flexion and extension are required because a portion of step length is achieved by the forwards-backwards movements of the pelvis instead (Inman et al., 1981). Another important movement at the lower end of the torso is pelvic obliquity, in which one side of the pelvis drops below the other (Levine et al., 2012). This occurs during midstance, where the gluteus medius muscle on the outside of the hip acts to stabilise the pelvis whilst allowing a small drop to occur on the opposite side so that the overall path of the CM does not fluctuate too greatly (Saunders et al., 1953).

Footstrike Patterns

Distance runners make first contact with the rearfoot (heel-striking), midfoot or forefoot (Stearne et al., 2014). Middle-distance runners are more likely to land with an anterior foot-strike pattern (either midfoot or forefoot) (Hayes and Caplan, 2012), with the percentage of athletes making first contact with the rearfoot increasing as the race distance gets longer (Han-ley et al., 2019; Hasegawa et al., 2007). When grouped across sex and race distance, forefoot and midfoot strikers had shorter ground contact times and faster finishing times in 800 m and 1500 m races (Hayes and Caplan, 2012). Similarly, at the 15 km distance of a half-marathon, rearfoot strikers had longer contact times than forefoot and midfoot strikers (Hasegawa et al., 2007) and the shorter ground contact times in forefoot strikers could be seen as a performance benefit from landing more forwards on the foot, possibly because footstrike pattern is a factor that affects the stretch-shortening cycle (Cavagna et al., 1964; Cavagna and Kaneko, 1977). As faster distance runners are more likely to be mid- or forefoot strikers (Stearne et al., 2014), it has been suggested that running economy is positively influenced by effective exploitation of this elastic energy (Di Michele and Merni, 2014). However, Stearne et al. (2014) found no differences for total lower limb mechanical work or mean power between foot-strike patterns when running at 4.5 m·s^{-1}. This might be because whereas forefoot striking has been associated with greater stiffness at the knee, rearfoot striking has been associated with greater stiffness at the ankle (Butler et al., 2003). Indeed, the lower prevalence of midfoot and forefoot striking over longer distances amongst both recreational and world-class marathon runners (Hanley et al., 2019; Larson et al., 2011) could be because carbohydrate oxidation rates are greater during forefoot striking (Gruber et al., 2013b).

Landing on the front of the foot has been proposed as less likely to lead to injury (Kulmala et al., 2013), as it reduces peak impact forces (Cavanagh and Lafortune, 1980; Lieberman et al., 2010). This is because the wider forefoot allows impact forces to be distributed over a larger area (Rooney and Derrick, 2013), although these forces are also reduced during heel-strike in appropriate footwear (Whittle, 1999). However, it is not conclusive that vertical loading forces are directly responsible for lower limb injury (Nigg, 1997), especially given the multiplanar and complicated movements involved in running. Furthermore, whereas rearfoot striking might be associated with certain injuries (e.g., at the knee), forefoot striking is associated with injury to other areas (e.g., ankle) (Kulmala et al., 2013). Higher loads to the gastrocnemius were found in forefoot striking (Shih et al., 2013), and Stearne et al. (2014) stated that forefoot striking thus might actually increase the risk of Achilles tendinopathy and triceps surae injury. It is therefore inadvisable for habitual rearfoot strikers to switch footstrike pattern as it can increase the injury risk to untrained muscles (Stearne et al., 2014).

Effects of Fatigue

It is well understood that one of the main limits on performance in distance running is fatigue, characterised by a reduction in power output and a decline in performance (Kellis and Liassou, 2009). There are three potential sites of failure: those within the central nervous system; those concerned with neural transmission from the central nervous system to muscle; and those within the individual muscle fibres (Bigland-Ritchie and Woods, 1984). Local muscular fatigue occurs because of intensive activity in that muscle (Mizrahi et al., 2000) and is one of many forms of fatigue that affect distance runners. Even though the competitive distances are shorter, middle-distance runners are more susceptible to fatigue in some ways than long-distance runners, possibly because those who specialise over shorter distances have a greater proportion of fast-twitch muscle fibres (Nummela et al., 2008) and because their pacing profiles in championship competition feature several bursts of great acceleration (Hettinga et al., 2019).

Change in running speed is the most obvious outcome of fatigue, resulting from decreases in either step length, cadence or both (Buckalew et al., 1985; Elliott and Ackland, 1981). However, athletes racing over different distances sometimes suffer decreases in only one of these two factors; for example, in a 5 km road race, Hanley et al. (2011) found that the men had reduced cadence only, whereas in a men's 10,000 m track race, Elliot and Ackland (1981) found decreases in step length (from 1.76 m on the second lap to 1.66 in the second-to-last lap), whereas cadence did not change. In a high-quality women's marathon, Buckalew et al. (1985) found that, as faster finishers had longer step lengths, maintenance of step length over the full distance was the deciding factor in the outcome of the race. This means the marathon differs from shorter-distance races (i.e., changes in cadence are not as important for race success) because the physiological changes that occur in the second half mean that maintaining step length is the key to avoiding great reductions in speed to the finish.

Dutto and Smith (2002) reported that during running to exhaustion, leg stiffness decreased with fatigue, and this might have caused step length to increase (rather than because of a conscious decision by the athletes), with a resulting increase in energy cost. A similar decrease in leg stiffness, found during exhaustive running by Hayes and Caplan (2014), was believed to be more likely due to changes in ankle stiffness, rather than at the knee. A decrease in leg stiffness results in a failure to fully use the stretch-shortening cycle (Chan-Roper et al., 2012), such as during the push-off phase in running. Repeated stretch-shortening cycle exercise itself induces fatigue, leading to increased lower leg stiffness to protect passive biological structures (Debenham et al., 2016), and which affects force production as there is a reduction in the amount of storage of elastic energy (Nicol et al., 1991a). It is possible that this reduction is caused by an increase in transition time from stretch to shortening (e.g., between braking and push-off phases) (Nicol et al., 1991a). Indeed, Hayes and Caplan (2012) found that contact times in high-calibre club athletes increased from the first lap to the last lap of both 800 m and 1500 m races, and given its association with cadence, the ability to maintain or decrease contact time in the later stages might be crucial for success. Nicol et al. (1991b) found that longer contact times occurred after a marathon because of increased maximal knee flexion that suggested a reduction in tolerance to repeated stretch loads, which led to increased muscular work when the knee extended during a longer push-off phase to maintain a constant running speed. As this increased work requirement in itself increases the rate of fatigue, the most common outcome of stretch-shortening cycle fatigue is simply for the athlete to slow. In treadmill tests where runners exercised to exhaustion, those athletes who ran for longer were those who had more stable running styles (Gazeau et al., 1997), and it is possible that detrimental changes in stride mechanics can be avoided to some extent through the development of local muscular endurance of key lower limb muscles, particularly the knee flexors and hip extensors (notably, the hamstrings fulfil both of these roles) (Hayes et al., 2004). The changes that occur from running to exhaustion (or considerable fatigue) could lead to overuse injuries (Riazati et al., 2020), and indeed changes often occur to reduce pain in those already suffering patellofemoral pain syndrome (Bazett-Jones et al., 2013). Many of these gait alterations relate to muscle strength before and after high-intensity exercise; by contrast, with regard to changes in joint angles with fatigue over short race distances, Hanley et al. (2011) found that hip, knee, ankle and shoulder angles at both first contact and toe-off did not alter throughout a 5 km road race, and Elliot and Ackland (1981) reported very small or no changes in lower limb joint angles with fatigue in 10,000 m track running. Thus, even when fatigued, many athletes maintain their usual technique and coaches should note that running form, whether "good" or "bad", is not necessarily a robust guide as to whether an athlete is tiring.

Air Resistance

Air resistance occurs when an athlete runs overground and, as noted earlier for external forces, causes a change in the athlete's speed. An athlete running in still air (wind speed of 0.0 m·s^{-1}) experiences a headwind equal to their running speed (Davies, 1980); compared with no wind conditions, headwinds increase total energy consumption, whereas tailwinds decrease it. Very strong tailwinds can cancel out the effects of running through the air, although they can also have a negative effect on the ability to maintain correct running posture (Davies,

1980). Running closely behind rivals is a very common tactic as it allows less physiologically capable athletes to maintain the pace of faster, front-running athletes (Brisswalter and Hausswirth, 2008), and is one of the principles behind pre-arranged pacemakers. Davies (1980) found that the energy cost of overcoming air resistance on a calm day was approximately 4% for middle-distance running (at 6 m·s^{-1}), and 2% for marathon running (5 m·s^{-1}). He recommended athletes shield behind a front runner until the closing stages of a race, although they need to be in very close proximity. However, many athletes deliberately choose to avoid following others too closely as it can eliminate the cooling effects of moving air, especially in hot conditions (Noakes, 2003). Additionally, Kyle (1979) calculated that middle- and long-distance runners reduced energy consumption by only 2–4% by shielding from the wind, and Trenchard et al. (2016) calculated that distance runners in competitive situations actually gain little from drafting. Ultimately, air resistance is very small at speeds below 4.44 m·s^{-1} (Léger and Mercier, 1984), and might be of great importance for the distance runner only in strong headwinds. In weather conditions where the relative humidity is high (at or close to 100% saturation), rainfall can negatively affect performance, particularly in the marathon (Ito et al., 2013). However, as with wearing loose clothing, some athletes might benefit from light rain because of a cooling effect. Overall, the best conditions for distance running are generally a combination of sea-level elevation, little or no wind, cool but dry conditions and athletes of similar ability acting as pacemakers.

Effects of Gradient

Changes in gradient frequently occur in road racing and are a common feature of cross-country and other off-road running. Even though running downhill is generally faster because of gravitational forces contributing to propulsion (Paradisis and Cooke, 2001), it can also have negative consequences. These effects can be exacerbated because athletes are unfamiliar with running downhill and alter their gait to accommodate the slope, including applying more braking impulse than necessary (Gottschall and Kram, 2005). Although it has a lower metabolic cost than running on a level surface (Minetti et al., 1994), running downhill on shallow slopes still requires some positive mechanical energy generation because elastic energy storage is insufficient to meet all energy demands (Snyder et al., 2012).

Aside from the risk of falling, the mechanics of running downhill can also increase the risk of injury. Although not necessarily direct causes of injury, greater vertical impact peak forces were found during downhill running (Gottschall and Kram, 2005; Telhan et al., 2010), and peak tibial impact accelerations increased on downhill gradients because of higher vertical velocities at impact (Chu and Caldwell, 2004). Because of the greater loading in early stance, running downhill increases the load on the knee extensors, hip extensors and anterior and posterior shin muscles (Eston et al., 1995). Appell et al. (1992) stated that this mechanical stress during downhill running causes disruption of the myofibrils in the affected muscles, and the accrued muscle damage can affect running form and muscle function for up to three days afterwards (Chen et al., 2007). The loss of strength in the quadriceps femoris is caused by morphological damage during exercise (Lieber and Fridén, 1993) and is associated with the relative length of the muscle; for example, the quadriceps femoris does more work at its longer length during downhill running than during uphill running (Eston et al., 1995). Small uphill sections (of 1% gradient or less) often have little effect on the maintenance of running speed (Angus and Waterhouse, 2011). However, anyone who has run uphill knows intuitively that it is more difficult than running on level surfaces because energy cost increases with greater inclines (Minetti et al., 1994), with a more forward lean of the trunk and shorter step lengths. Of course, some athletes deliberately choose hilly courses because of the challenge involved, or because hill running suits their abilities. Training to run downhill before competition can help prevent muscle damage (Eston et al., 2000), and coaches are thus advised to include it in their athletes' training regimens.

Cross-Country and Off-Road Running

Running on natural terrain in the form of cross-country running, trail running, orienteering and fell running are popular with athletes of all abilities. On soft ground, the surface absorbs energy and returns little, which can be particularly detrimental to those distance athletes who rely to a greater extent on lower limb muscle elasticity (Canova, 1998). In general, running on surfaces such as sand, grass and trails requires greater metabolic energy expenditure than running on smooth, flat, hard surfaces (Voloshina and Ferris, 2015). Increases in energy cost of between 26% and 72% have been estimated when running in forests (typical of orienteering and trail running), dependent on the underfoot conditions (Creagh and Reilly, 1997). The energy cost of running through long grass on rough terrain is increased because of decreased step lengths, greater hip flexion during swing and larger vertical displacements of the CM (Creagh and Reilly, 1997). Pinnington and Dawson (2001) found that running on sand had a greater energy cost than running on grass and proposed that this was because of a reduction in elastic energy potentiation, caused partly by an increase in contact time. They also suggested that the increase in energy cost could be because sand's compliant nature requires increased leg stiffness that increases muscle activity to stabilise the lower limb joints (Pinnington and Dawson, 2001). Although running on such surfaces might reduce performance (e.g., time to complete a particular distance compared with athletics tracks or roads), they can provide a beneficial training stimulus and can suit some athletes' running styles better than more stable, harder surfaces.

Summary

Running is a highly complex movement, requiring years of refinement to become automated and efficient, and a good understanding of biomechanics is indispensable in trying to improve performance. Although the running stride has been broken down into its various components, a holistic view of an athlete's biomechanics is essential in good coaching. So, for example, understanding that increasing step length is beneficial to performance should be tempered with the risk of overstriding or decreasing cadence. Training improvements in technique take time and are best viewed as part of a whole-body exercise, where what occurs during swing in one leg is seen as complementing what happens during stance in the other. Distance running is, of course, an endurance activity, and external factors such as the effects of wind, hills, surface and rival athletes' tactics can influence the rate of fatigue. Indeed, the manner in which an athlete accommodates these potential challenges can be affected by tiredness, and coaches are recommended to incorporate technically sound practice in training to prepare the body biomechanically for these race elements.

3

COMMON OVERUSE INJURIES IN RUNNERS AND INJURY RISK FACTORS

Christopher A. Bramah

Highlights

- Running poses a considerable risk of injury, with approximately 50% of runners injured annually.
- Achilles tendinopathy, calf strains, patellofemoral pain, iliotibial band syndrome and bone stress injuries are some of the most commonly seen injuries amongst middle- and long-distance runners.
- Injury is thought to be due to an imbalance between load application and a runner's individual load capacity.
- Load application is influenced by biomechanics, footwear, surfaces, lifestyle, sociocultural pressures and training variables, such as volume, intensity and duration.
- Load capacity represents the ability of an athlete, or a specific tissue structure, to cope with the load demands of training.
- Understanding factors influencing load application and load capacity can facilitate appropriate management strategies to reduce the injury risk of running.

Introduction

Endurance running is becoming one of the UK's most popular methods of physical activity, with the numbers of competitive distance runners continuing to rise annually. However, despite the many health benefits, there is a considerable risk of injury associated with running. The overall incidence of running injury is reported to range between 19% and 79% (van Gent et al., 2007) with approximately 50% of runners injured annually (van Mechelen, 1992) and up to 94% of runners reporting an injury across their lifetime (Kluitenberg et al., 2015). Amongst specific types of runners, injury rates of between 27.3% and 84.9% are reported for new runners with no prior experience, 55% for non-competitive recreational runners, 63.9% for track middle-distance runners, 31.7% to 43.2% of long-distance road runners, 31.3% to 52% of marathon runners and up to 77% of cross-country runners (Kluitenberg et al., 2015).

According to a recent consensus publication, a running-related injury is defined as running-related musculoskeletal pain which causes a restriction to, or stoppage of running volume, duration or speed for a minimum of 7 days or three consecutive scheduled training sessions, or that requires a runner to consult a physician or health care professional (Yamato et al., 2015). Although this provides a useful definition for classifying a runner as injured, it should be noted that the experience of pain and associated psychological and physical distress can vary between individuals. Therefore, what constitutes an injury for one individual is unlikely to be the same for others; consequently, each runner should be managed on an individual basis. The aim of this chapter is to explore common running-related overuse injuries and the main reasons that may contribute to these injuries occurring.

Common Overuse Injuries

Of all running injuries, the majority are overuse in nature, with injuries to the knee, lower limb and foot accounting for up to 50%, 40% and 23% of all injuries respectively (van Gent et al., 2007; Kluitenberg et al., 2015; Edouard et al., 2020). The most frequently observed include Achilles tendinopathy, medial tibial stress syndrome, iliotibial band syndrome, patello-femoral pain, plantar heel pain, calf muscle strain injuries and bone stress injuries (Figure 3.1). Although not as frequently observed, many runners may also encounter hamstring strain injuries or hamstring tendinopathies.

Amongst elite-level long- and middle-distance runners, the majority of injuries tend to occur to the lower leg and foot (Edouard et al., 2020). Amongst recreational runners, the knee seems to be the most frequently injured site (Kluitenberg et al., 2015). This may in part be explained by differences in biomechanics and training behaviours between the two, such as foot strike patterns and a greater frequency of speed-based training sessions amongst elite-level runners.

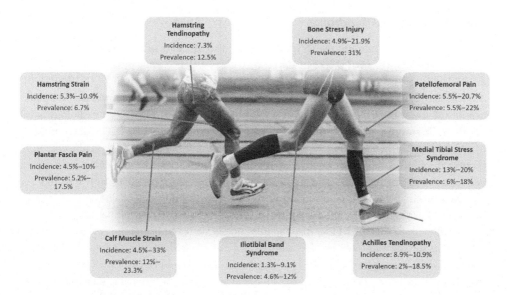

Hamstring Tendinopathy
Incidence: 7.3%
Prevalence: 12.5%

Bone Stress Injury
Incidence: 4.9%–21.9%
Prevalence: 31%

Hamstring Strain
Incidence: 5.3%–10.9%
Prevalence: 6.7%

Patellofemoral Pain
Incidence: 5.5%–20.7%
Prevalence: 5.5%–22%

Plantar Fascia Pain
Incidence: 4.5%–10%
Prevalence: 5.2%–17.5%

Medial Tibial Stress Syndrome
Incidence: 13%–20%
Prevalence: 6%–18%

Calf Muscle Strain
Incidence: 4.5%–33%
Prevalence: 12%–23.3%

Iliotibial Band Syndrome
Incidence: 1.3%–9.1%
Prevalence: 4.6%–12%

Achilles Tendinopathy
Incidence: 8.9%–10.9%
Prevalence: 2%–18.5%

FIGURE 3.1 Incidence and prevalence of common running injuries amongst distance running populations. Incidence refers to the percentage of new cases developed over a given time period, prevalence refers to the percentage of current cases at a given moment in time. Values represent ranges

Within the scientific literature, injury rates are often reported as incidence and/or prevalence rates. Incidence represents the number of new injury cases that occur over a period, while the prevalence represents the number of existing injury cases at a specific moment in time. For example, the number of new injuries sustained by a group of cross-country runners over one or more cross-country seasons would represent the injury incidence, whereas investigating the number of marathon runners who are currently injured represents the injury prevalence.

Achilles Tendinopathy

Achilles tendinopathy is an overuse degenerative condition to the Achilles tendon, occurring most frequently at the mid portion but also affecting the attachment site at the calcaneus (Bula et al., 2008; Cook and Purdam, 2009). The prevalence amongst runners is reported to be up to 18% (Lopes et al., 2012), with some reports suggesting up to 52% of middle- and long-distance runners may experience Achilles tendon pain across their lifetime (Kujala et al., 2005). Injury onset is usually gradual or insidious, thought to occur due to repeated mechanical overload with insufficient recovery. Over time, this may result in disruption of the tendon structure, exacerbating pain and resulting in reduced mechanical function of the tendon (Cook et al., 2016). The average time to symptom recovery is reported to be between 1.5 and 3 months; however, many individuals can experience symptoms for up to 15 months, if not longer (Nielsen et al., 2014b; Mulvad et al., 2018).

Risk factors for Achilles tendinopathy include, but are not limited to, previous tendon injury, increased age, sudden increases to training intensity, volume and frequency and reduced calf muscle strength (O'Neill et al., 2016). All these factors may influence the loads applied to the tendon and the ability of the tendon to withstand and recover from repeated loading.

Medial Tibial Stress Syndrome

Medial tibial stress syndrome (MTSS), also referred to as "shin splints", is an overload syndrome to the lower medial aspect of the shin, with prevalence rates of up to 18% (Pinshaw et al., 1984) and recovery times ranging between 16 days and 18 months (Nielsen et al., 2014b). Pain is usually provoked by activity, easing with rest, and often reproduced on palpation of the lower medial board of the tibia (Winters et al., 2017). The exact pathology is still poorly understood, with some theories suggesting it could represent a fascial traction injury to the periosteum, while others suggest it may be the result of repeated overload to the bone (Franklyn and Oakes, 2015; Winters et al., 2019). Often it can be difficult to distinguish between symptoms of MTSS and those of other injuries, such as tibial stress fractures and chronic exertional compartment syndrome. Therefore, it is important to ensure that an accurate clinical diagnosis is established in order to direct appropriate clinical management.

Specific risk factors for MTSS may include sudden increases in training volumes, changes to running surface and footwear, less running experience, reduced lower limb muscle mass, increased body mass and running biomechanics such as increased impact forces, rearfoot eversion and hip adduction (Moen et al., 2012; Pohl et al., 2008). Additional risk factors reported include increased navicular drop (surrogate measure of foot pronation) and the use of orthotics; however, the latter may be related to underlying biomechanical factors for which orthotics were prescribed, rather than the orthotics themselves (Newman et al., 2013).

Patellofemoral Pain

Patellofemoral pain (PFP), or "runners knee", is an overload condition to the anterior knee, presenting as diffuse pain around or behind the patella aggravated by activities loading the knee, such as squatting, walking up and down stairs and running (Crossley et al., 2016). PFP is perhaps the most common running-related knee injury, with prevalence rates as high as 22.7% (Smith et al., 2018). Recovery times are reported to be on average between 1.5 and 2.5 months. However, in some cases PFP can become a chronic condition, lasting longer than 1 year amongst runners and with up to 50% of people experiencing symptoms for as long as 20 years following initial diagnosis (Nielsen et al., 2014b; Mulvad et al., 2018).

Reported risk factors for PFP include training factors such as sudden increases to training volume, downhill running and greater duration of running, lower limb biomechanics including increased hip adduction and internal rotation, as well as reduced quadriceps strength and hip muscle function, including reduced gluteal muscle strength, delayed and shorter gluteal muscle activity during running and lower rate of force development (Lack et al., 2018; Neal et al., 2016). These risk factors may influence both the magnitude and frequency of joint loading as well as the ability of the lower limbs to attenuate these forces.

Iliotibial Band Syndrome (ITBS)

Iliotibial band syndrome (ITBS) is the second most common running-related knee injury, accounting for up to 14% of all running injuries and presenting as pain localised to the outer knee during running (van der Worp et al., 2012). Historically ITBS has been considered a friction syndrome, whereby repeated knee flexion was thought to cause friction between the outer knee and ITB, resulting in inflammation to an underlying bursa (Jelsing et al., 2013). However, more recently it has been suggested that friction of the ITB is not anatomically plausible, as the ITB is in fact firmly attached to the outer knee. Instead, it has been proposed that ITB syndrome is caused by repeated compression between the structures of the outer knee and the ITB (Fairclough et al., 2007). Regardless of the mechanism, as with many running injuries, ITBS represents a biomechanical overload syndrome to the outer knee.

Known risk factors for this injury remain limited; however, it is predominantly thought to be due to a combination of sudden increases in training volume or duration and lower limb biomechanics increasing the strain placed on the ITB (van der Worp et al., 2012) and resulting in the development of pain. Specific biomechanical patterns associated with ITBS include increased hip adduction and knee internal rotation (caused by inward rotation of the shin, relative to the femur) (Noehren et al., 2007; Mousavi et al., 2019). With the combination of biomechanics and training loads thought to cause an acute overload to the ITB resulting in the development of pain.

Some studies have suggested hip muscle weakness may play a role, reporting symptoms to improve following hip abductor strength training (Fredericson et al,, 2000). However, this has not been supported by further studies, suggesting that hip muscle weakness may occur as a result of injury rather than as a cause (van der Worp et al., 2012).

Plantar Heel Pain/Fasciopathy

Plantar heel pain has a prevalence rate of 17.5% reported to occur in up to 31% of runners (Di Caprio et al., 2010). This injury is considered to be an overuse degenerative condition to the plantar fascia at the insertion to the heel, whereby repeated loading results in a gradual breakdown of the tissue structure. The characteristic presentation is of pain localised to the insertion of the plantar fascia on the heel, often worse on weightbearing after periods of inactivity or following prolonged walking or running (van Leeuwen et al., 2016).

Currently, there are limited high-quality studies reporting risk factors for this injury. Several factors appear to be associated with this condition, including: increased body mass index, the use of spiked running shoes, reduced calf muscle and toe flexor strength, increased dynamic foot pronation, reduced ankle dorsiflexion range of movement as well as both a more pronated foot posture and a high arched foot posture (van Leeuwen et al., 2016). It is possible that these risk factors may increase the biomechanical strain placed upon the plantar fascia during running (van Leeuwen et al., 2016). However, it is important to note these factors are only associations based on examination of individuals who already have the injury; it is therefore difficult to establish cause or effect.

Bone Stress Injury

Bone stress injuries are due to gradual structural failure of the bone tissue, caused by an imbalance between bone loading and the ability of the bone to withstand the applied load (Warden et al., 2014). The severity of bone stress injuries range along a continuum; progressing from stress reactions to stress fracture and, with continued loading, complete fracture. Symptoms usually present as a mild, dull aching sensation during or following activity. As the injury progresses, symptoms can become easily provoked during low-level loading, such as walking, with pain also felt at rest or at night (Warden et al., 2014). Amongst runners, incidence rates are reported of up to 21%, with the most frequently injured areas including the tibia (46% of bone stress injuries), navicular (15%), fibula (12%) and, less frequently, the femur (8%), pelvis (4%) and spine (4%) (Bennell et al., 1996a).

Risk factors for bone stress injury can be broadly categorised into factors which influence bone loading, or the ability of the bone to withstand load (Warden et al., 2014). Factors influencing bone loading include training volume, duration and intensity, running surface, shoes and biomechanics. Each of these can influence the specific bones loaded, the magnitude of the load and how frequently the load is applied, with sudden increases or changes to any of these factors potentially resulting in bone overload structural failure. The ability of the bone to withstand load is largely influenced by the structural integrity of the bone, and therefore factors which reduce the structural properties of the bone leave the bone weaker and more vulnerable to injury. Such factors include low bone density, low body mass index (less than 19), low energy availability, increased training volume, prior bone stress injury, disordered eating or restricted food intake and, for female athletes, late menarche (15 years or older) and menstrual irregularities, such as absent or irregular periods (Tenforde et al., 2013; Kraus et al., 2019). Several studies have shown the greater number of risk factors an athlete has significantly increases their risk of sustaining a future bone stress injury.

Calf Strain Injury (Gastrocnemius and Soleus)

Calf muscle strain injuries can occur to either the soleus or the gastrocnemius muscles, with prevalence rates ranging from 12% to 23.3% and recurrence rates as high as 38% (Rauh et al., 2000). The classic presentation for a gastrocnemius strain is an acute onset of pain localised to the calf muscle belly, with an inability to continue running. Soleus muscle strains often present as a gradual tightening or cramping sensation worsening with activity (Dixon, 2009).

Soleus muscle strains are often underreported or mistaken for simply "a tight calf". However, misdiagnosis of these injuries can lead to significantly longer recovery times and re-injury (Pedret et al., 2015). The soleus muscle is comprised of three distinct intramuscular tendons responsible for the transmission of force during running. If the muscle strain involves damage to the internal tendons, recovery time can be significantly longer, with early return to running risking further tissue damage and re-injury (Pedret et al., 2015).

Currently, only a limited number of studies have investigated risk factors for calf muscle injuries reporting male gender, increased age, higher body mass index and having suffered a previous calf muscle injury as the main risk factors (Green and Pizzari, 2017). It is likely that these risk factors may contribute to biomechanical and neuromuscular maladaptation's reducing the load capacity of the calf complex and increasing the risk of injury (Green and Pizzari, 2017).

Hamstring Tendinopathy

Hamstring tendinopathy presents as deep localised pain in the buttock at the hamstring insertion aggravated by running, lunging and sitting (Goom et al., 2016). Its overall prevalence is reported to be around 12.5% (Lopes et al., 2012). The exact mechanism of injury is poorly understood; however it is thought to be due to excessive loading and compression of the hamstring tendon against the bony insertion at the pelvis (Goom et al., 2016).

Reported risk factors for this injury remain relative sparse, however based on the proposed mechanism of injury, contributing factors are likely to include those that result in a sudden increase in hamstring loads or hamstring lengthening with the hip flexed, such as a sudden increase in faster paced running sessions or hill sessions (Goom et al., 2016).

Hamstring Strain Injury

Hamstring strain injury is less frequently observed amongst distance runners, reported to account for only 6.7% of all distance running injuries (Lopes et al., 2012). Injury onset is usually associated with high speed running, whereby the increased force demands exceed the functional and structural capacity of the muscle resulting in tissue failure (Kenneally-Dabrowski et al., 2019). Injury risk is likely the combined result of exposure to high speed running and reduced capacity of the hamstring muscle to tolerate high forces.

Reported risk factors include structural maladaptation's such as shorter muscle fascicle lengths and increased muscle-tendon unit stiffness, reduced eccentric hamstring muscle strength, older age and a prior history of knee, calf or hamstring strain injury; with a greater risk of re-injury if the athlete has suffered a hamstring strain injury in the last 12 months (Green et al., 2020). These factors may reduce hamstring muscle capacity to tolerate high strains, leaving the athlete vulnerable to injury following sudden increases in high-speed running. Interestingly, recent studies suggest graded exposure to high-speed running results in structural adaptations of the hamstring muscles which may improve the capacity of the hamstrings to tolerate high forces (Mendiguchia et al., 2020). Therefore, in order to reduce the risk of hamstring strain injury, it is recommended to ensure exposure to high-speed running is gradual with the inclusion of eccentric hamstring strength training.

Why Do Runners Get Injured?

Running injuries are thought to be the result of an imbalance between the load applied to an athlete, and the athlete's capacity to withstand the applied load, or load capacity (Figure 3.2). Load application represents the physical, psychological and lifestyle demands that are placed upon the athlete. This may be experienced on a day-to-day basis, within a single running session, or across a training week, month or year. Load capacity represents the ability of the athlete, or a specific tissue structure, to cope with the applied load (Cook and Docking, 2015). This is influenced by a variety of physical, psychological and biological factors such as structural tissue properties, personality traits, mood status, genetics and hormones.

Whether injury occurs depends largely upon the athlete and how the athlete's musculo-skeletal structure responds to the applied loads. Each time an athlete begins a run, they do so with a particular load tolerance capacity. As load is applied to the athlete, this capacity will gradually reduce along a continuum from full capacity, progressing to acute fatigue, microscopic tissue damage, macroscopic tissue damage and ultimately structural tissue failure and injury (Soligard et al., 2016) (Figure 3.2). Simply viewed, if an athlete's capacity to tolerate the applied load is greater than the load applied, or load application ceases before tissue damage occurs, then the athlete will not progress far along this continuum. They will remain

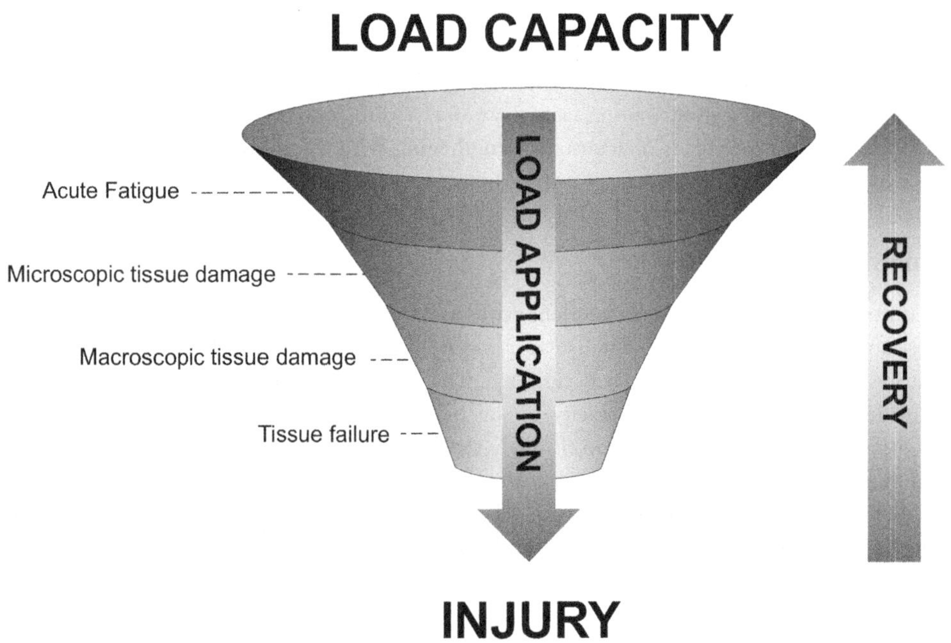

LOAD CAPACITY

Acute Fatigue
Microscopic tissue damage
Macroscopic tissue damage
Tissue failure

LOAD APPLICATION

RECOVERY

INJURY

FIGURE 3.2 Pictorial representation of the interaction between load capacity, load application, recovery and injury development. The gradual narrowing of the funnel represents a gradual reduction in load capacity in response to repeated load application. As tissue capacity reduced, repeated load application results in the gradual progression of tissue damage (Kellis and Liassou, 2009), ultimately leading to injury development. The recovery arrow represents how recovery between load application can lead to a restoration of tissue capacity

uninjured and move onto the next training session. Conversely, if the load applied exceeds the athlete's load capacity, or there is insufficient recovery between loadings, then the load capacity may gradually be reduced, causing the athlete to progress along the injury continuum, increasing the possibility of injury (Figure 3.2).

It is important to note that load is a normal and necessary part of an athlete's training required to develop the physical, psychological and physiological qualities for long-term health and performance. If the load an athlete encounters appropriately challenges these qualities and sufficient recovery is provided between loading bouts, then the athlete is likely to adapt, and their capacity should increase. However, if the load encountered does not sufficiently challenge the athlete or tissue structure, then adaptation is unlikely to occur. In such instances this can have the opposite effect of too much load, resulting in deconditioning and a reduction or weakening of an athlete's load capacity.

This is perhaps one reason why athletes often pick up recurrent injuries or become injured soon after a rest period. During a period of offload, musculoskeletal structures are not subjected to the regular high-impact demands of running, and there is limited stimulus to facilitate the maintenance of load capacity. As a result, tissues start to decondition, becoming weaker and therefore less tolerant to load application. Subsequently, on return to running, load application soon exceeds load capacity, causing the athlete to quickly develop an injury.

The challenge for coaches, athletes and clinicians is to ensure the load encountered is sufficient to develop and maintain the physical qualities and athlete robustness, without causing injury. In order to do so, it is important to understand factors that can influence the load applied to an athlete, as well as factors influencing their load capacity. Identifying such risk factors can allow for appropriate steps to manage the load an athlete encounters and develop their physical capacity to tolerate training and competition demands.

Factors Influencing Load Application

Training Factors

Training variables are perhaps the most important variables influencing the loads encountered by an athlete. During each foot contact of a run, the body is exposed to impact forces upwards of two times body weight with muscular forces considerably greater (Dorn et al., 2012). These forces place the musculoskeletal system under considerable physical stress, with training parameters influencing both the frequency of exposure to loading (such as during high-volume running), as well as the magnitude of the loads encountered (such as during high-speed running). Importantly, how training is structured can have a direct impact upon the development, or detriment, of an athlete's load capacity, through the balance between load application and recovery. Understanding how training parameters influence the stress applied to the body can help athletes, coaches and clinicians to make informed decisions regarding how to safely progress training loads while reducing potential injury-causing effects.

Volume and Duration

Training volume and duration influence the frequency that the body is placed under stress and ultimately the total or cumulative stress encountered. As previously mentioned, during each foot contact of a run the body is exposed to impact forces upwards of two times body weight. Greater duration or volume of running will increase the number of foot contacts experienced and therefore the frequency an individual is exposed to impact forces. Consequently, a greater number of foot contacts means a greater number of loading cycles and greater total applied load.

For example, consider a male runner with a mass of 70 kg and cadence of 180 steps per minute. During a single foot contact, this runner will experience impact forces equivalent to more than 140 kg. For 1 minute of running, impact forces are applied to the body 180 times, meaning a cumulative total force application of 25,200 kg. If the duration of running increases to 30 minutes, the total number of loading cycles rises to 5,400 and the cumulative force encountered across an entire run would exceed 750,000 kg, rising even higher if an athlete was to run a half-marathon or marathon distance. Consequently, the duration or total volume of a run will directly influence the frequency an athlete is exposed to external loading and the cumulative loads they encounter. This can place considerable physical demands on the athlete, resulting in the gradual accumulation of tissue and physical fatigue, progressing along the tissue capacity injury continuum. However, it is important to note that the force encountered per stride (and subsequently the total load encountered during a run) is also influenced by several biomechanical factors. These factors include the type, rate and magnitude of the external forces encountered and kinematic patters, all of which can be influenced by additional factors such as running speed, surface, footwear, anatomy and fatigue, to name a few. To understand fully the total load encountered by an individual, the biomechanical factors need to be considered, alongside the number of foot contacts.

Currently there is no conclusive evidence as to whether there is a threshold of training volume that increases the risk of sustaining a running injury (Nielsen et al., 2012). Some studies suggest that greater miles per week may increase the risk of sustaining an injury (Walter et al., 1989; Macera et al., 1989), while others suggest that athletes who are capable of attaining high training volumes may be less likely to become injured (Bovens et al., 1989). Whether an athlete becomes injured as training volume increases is likely to vary between individuals, dependent upon whether the athlete has the physical capacity to tolerate high training loads or is given sufficient time to adapt to progressively greater training demands. When planning training volumes, it is important to consider whether the athlete has risk factors that may influence their physical capacity to tolerate the planned training loads and allow sufficient time for the athlete to adapt to the demands of training.

Frequency

Frequency of training influences how often load is applied to the body and subsequently how much recovery an athlete has between loading bouts. Some athletes and musculoskeletal structures, such as bone and tendon, can require greater recovery times than others (Warden et al., 2014; Magnusson et al., 2010). Higher frequency of training, such as double day running, may therefore, subject tissues to further load application before they have fully recovered. If tissues have not fully recovered, this can reduce their load capacity entering the next run and subsequently increase the risk of injury development. Exactly how much recovery is required remains unknown and is likely to vary between individuals and within an individual depending on other lifestyle factors, e.g. nutrition.

Intensity

Training intensity represents internal stress experienced by an athlete in response to training demands. The internal stress includes the physical, physiological and psychological stress placed upon the athlete for a given running pace, distance or duration. This can include the muscular force demands, level of oxygen consumption, blood lactate concentrations and perceived physical exertion experienced by the athlete (Bourdon et al., 2017). Training at higher intensities is known to impact upon fatigue accumulation both within a single run and between running bouts.

The accumulation of fatigue may have implications for injury development through its effect upon muscle function, running biomechanics and the load capacity of tissue structures. Several studies have reported fatigue-induced reductions in peak muscle force, rate of force development and muscle fibre conduction velocity (Boccia et al., 2017a; Boccia et al., 2017b; Riazati et al., 2020). Additionally, fatigue-induced biomechanical changes have also been reported, including an extended lower leg at contact, increased ground contact times, increased peak hip adduction and hip adduction range of movement, forward trunk lean and knee abduction angles (Riazati et al., 2020; Winter et al., 2017; Willwacher et al., 2020). These biomechanical patterns are frequently associated with running-related injuries, thought to increase load placed upon specific tissue structures (Bramah et al., 2018; Noehren et al., 2007; Willy et al., 2012a). It is possible that under fatigue, reduced muscle function may contribute to both altered biomechanical patterns and reduced physical capacity to tolerate repeated load application (Riazati et al., 2020). Subsequently the combined reduction in muscle function and alteration to running biomechanics may increase the susceptibility to injury development.

Currently, attempts to monitor training intensity based solely upon running pace have failed to identify any link between pace and injury development (Nielsen et al., 2012). This may largely be explained by the physiological differences between runners, which means the level of intensity for one runner is unlikely to be the same for another (Bourdon et al., 2017). For example, faster or "fitter" runners may be able to sustain a faster pace with a lower physiological intensity compared to a slower, less fit runner. Similarly, for an individual athlete, the physiological intensity of a session can vary from day to day depending upon their cumulative fatigue or health status. This may be influenced by how well they have recovered from the previous session, the addition of external life stressors such as increased work demands, psychological status or whether they are experiencing signs and symptoms of illness.

Although monitoring an athlete's running pace seems an easy way to monitor training intensity, this is likely to lead to inaccurate conclusions about the stress encountered by each individual, as it fails to consider the individual's physiological response to the external training demands as well as to the variable biomechanical loads experienced by each runner. It may instead be better to base measurements of training intensity upon the individual physiological profile of the athlete, such as using heart rate data, rating of perceived exertion or blood lactate concentrations (see Chapter 16). Additionally, through the use of wearable biomechanical technology, it is becoming possible to monitor the biomechanical loads experienced during running (Willy, 2018). If utilised alongside measures of internal training stress (such as rating of perceived exertion and heart rate variability), these methods may provide greater insight to the cumulative stress monitored in real time across a run or training period (Willy, 2018).

Sudden and Rapid Changes

Rather than injury being caused by specific training-related variables, such as volume or speed, injury risk is perhaps greatest when there is a sudden or rapid change in load application. These rises are often termed "acute spikes in training workload", reflecting the change in training for a given week or day compared to the average training that the athlete has completed over several previous weeks and days. In several team sports a sudden increase in total running volume (Murray et al., 2017b; Murray et al., 2017a; Hulin et al., 2016; Jaspers et al., 2018) and volume of high-speed running (Murray et al., 2017a; Murray et al., 2017b) has been shown to significantly increase the likelihood of sustaining an injury. Similarly, within running, several studies have reported injury onset to occur following a sudden or rapid change to weekly running volume and/or training intensity (Winter et al., 2020; Nielsen et al., 2014a; Ferreira et al., 2012). Often, however, the onset of injury in relation to the change in training can be delayed, with injuries occurring up to 4 weeks after the initial change in training (Winter et al., 2020). It is likely that these sudden changes to training load acutely overwhelm the musculoskeletal system, increasing the rate of fatigue and reducing the ability to fully recover prior to subsequent load application. Consequently, there is a gradual progression along the tissue capacity/injury continuum (Figure 3.2), pushing athletes closer to their injury threshold with each subsequent run.

In running, there is a commonly held belief that increasing training loads should follow the "10% rule", whereby training volume is not increased by more than 10% each week. While this may form a useful guide to training progression, there is in fact, no steadfast rule for safely progressing training loads (Damsted et al., 2018; Hulme et al., 2019). Several studies have attempted to identify the relationship between weekly training volume increase and running-related injury (Buist et al., 2008; Nielsen et al., 2014a; Damsted et al., 2019a). Increases of greater than 30% have been reported to increase the risk of injury (Nielsen et al., 2014a; Damsted et al., 2019a); however, no difference in injury rates has been identified when increasing weekly volume by less than 10% or between 10% and 30% (Buist et al., 2008; Nielsen et al., 2014a; Damsted et al., 2018). At present, therefore, current scientific evidence is unable to identify a specific threshold for which a sudden increase in training volume can influence running injury risk (Damsted et al., 2018; Hulme et al., 2019; Damsted et al., 2019a; Nielsen et al., 2014a).

The response to increases in training load will likely vary between individual runners, meaning that some individuals may be more vulnerable to injury than others. This vulnerability is likely to be influenced by multiple factors, including an individual's current level of training as well as their specific load capacity (Hulme et al., 2019). For example, a runner who completes only low weekly training volumes may be able to increase their weekly volume at a greater rate compared to a runner completing high weekly training volumes. This is simply because the runner completing a low weekly training volume may not have reached the limits of their physical capacity and are therefore able to increase training loads at a much greater rate. Conversely, a marathon runner, running 100 miles per week, might be pushing the limits of their physical capacity and as such be more vulnerable to small changes in training load, with even a 10% increase enough to cause injury. Determining the increase in training load a runner can tolerate therefore remains a challenge. Ultimately, a degree of runner, coach and clinician intuition may be necessary to judge the maximal workload potential an athlete can achieve without sustaining an injury (Hulme et al., 2019).

Biomechanics

Running biomechanics influence the loads encountered per stride and the specific tissues loaded during running. When combined with a frequency of load application, such as increasing running mileage, the total load application increases, potentially exceeding the load capacity of specific structures resulting in injury development. For example, the biomechanical pattern of hip adduction has been reported to increase the stress placed upon the patellofemoral joint (Liao et al., 2018). If this stress is repeated over multiple strides, or the load increases due to the biomechanical and neuromuscular response to fatigue, the total load may become greater than the load capacity of the patellofemoral joint, resulting in patellofemoral pain.

Several biomechanical patterns have been reported to increase the stress placed on musculoskeletal structures during running and are associated with running-related injuries. These patterns include increased contralateral pelvic drop, hip adduction, hip internal rotation, elevated breaking and impact forces and an overstride lower limb pattern, characterised by an extended knee and inclined ankle angle at initial contact (Bramah et al., 2018; Napier et al., 2018; Noehren et al., 2007; Davis et al., 2016). Whether injury occurs is likely to be influenced by the frequency biomechanical stresses are applied to the body and whether the specific tissue structures have the capacity to tolerate the elevated loading (Kalkhoven et al., 2020). For those runners who do not have sufficient load capacity, methods should be adopted which aim to improve tissue load capacity and/or reduce tissue loads. Such methods could include a more gradual increase in training load to allow for tissue adaptation and the addition of strength and conditioning focused on improving tissue specific mechanical qualities and physiological function, such as improving muscular endurance, peak force, rate of force development and tendon stiffness (Kalkhoven et al., 2020; Hayes et al., 2004). Alternatively, emerging evidence suggests gait retraining may be an effective method used to influence running mechanics, potentially reducing or redistributing tissue stress away from vulnerable areas (Davis and Futrell, 2016; Bramah et al., 2019; Napier et al., 2019).

Footwear

Running footwear or shoe type influences the biomechanical stress placed on specific musculoskeletal structures (Logan et al., 2010). However, to date, there is no conclusive scientific evidence to suggest a particular shoe type will influence injury risk, or that shoe prescription based on foot posture is effective in reducing injury risk (Knapik et al., 2014; Ryan et al., 2011; Malisoux et al., 2016). Instead, it is possible that injury risk is the result of sudden changes in footwear, resulting in a sudden change or increase in the biomechanical loads applied to specific tissue structures (Ryan et al., 2014; Fuller et al., 2017). Given insufficient time to adapt to the change in stress, or without adequate tissue conditioning prior to a change, tissue structures may be overloaded, leading to tissue damage and failure. For example, a sudden increase in use of track spikes or minimalist shoes will increase the biomechanical demands on the calf and Achilles. If the calf and Achilles are not accustomed to the increased stress, then this may exceed the capacity of these structures, resulting in injury development. This may explain the high frequency of lower limb injuries often observed in early summer, as many athletes suddenly increase the use of running spikes in preparation for the track season, following a prolonged period of trainer and racing flat use throughout the winter months. Therefore, it is recommended that changes in footwear should be gradual and allow time for the body to adapt to the change in biomechanical demands imposed by the specific running shoe.

Surfaces/Environment

Similar to changes in footwear, sudden changes to surfaces or environmental conditions may also pose a risk of injury. A commonly held misconception is that running on softer surfaces will reduce impacts and lower injury rates. This is misleading, however, as different running surfaces will simply impose different biomechanical demands on the body (Dixon et al., 2000; Ferris et al., 1999). For example, although running on softer surfaces has been shown to reduce impact loading rates (Dixon et al., 2000), in order to maintain a given running speed, there is likely to be an increased demand on muscles and tendons (Dixon et al., 2000; Ferris et al., 1999). Subsequently, although changing surfaces may reduce stress on one area of the body, this stress is likely to be redistributed elsewhere and may increase injury risk in other areas. There is, therefore, no one best surface for injury risk reduction. Instead, it may be better to vary running surfaces to allow the development of the physical qualities required for changing surface demands and avoid sudden changes in the volume of training on a given surface.

Training environment is also an important consideration, as this can place varied physical demands on the athlete and also may influence psychological stresses imposed on the athlete. For example, altitude training or warm weather training may increase the physiological stress placed on an athlete. Subsequently, training intensity is likely to be greater, fatigue may occur earlier, and recovery may be compromised. Similarly, changes to social and/or training groups may place an athlete under greater psychological stress through a perceived need to conform to social expectations. This could lead to altered behaviours such as running faster or training harder than normal, development of eating disorders or lack of regard for recovery to impress their peers or conform to a perceived social norm.

Factors Influencing Physical Capacity

Previous Injury

The single greatest risk factor for injury development is having a history of a previous injury (Hulme et al., 2017; van der Worp et al., 2015). It is possible that previous injury may increase the risk of future injury by negatively impacting upon an athlete's physical capacity to tolerate load application. Following an injury, the capacity of the injured tissue is often reduced, due to a combination of structural, biomechanical, physiological and psychological changes in response to the original injury. Such changes may include damage to the tissue structure, loss of muscular strength, changes to neuromuscular coordination patterns, cardiovascular deconditioning, altered gait patterns and fear of re-injury, to name a few.

If the rehabilitation process does not adequately address these maladaptations, then an athlete's physical capacity is likely to be reduced. Following the resolution of pain, the athlete may then return to their previous training routine and stress demands without adequate restoration of their physical capacity. Consequently, load application exceeds physical capacity at much lower levels, causing the athlete to enter a cycle of injury/re-injury (Figure 3.3). This

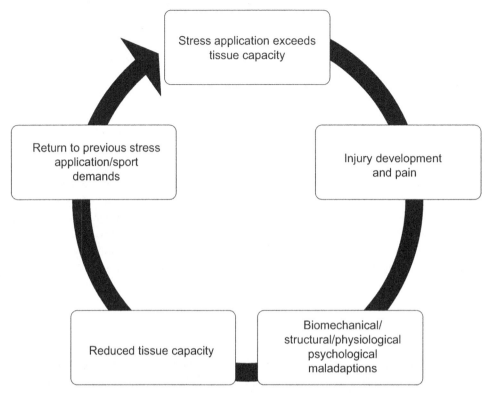

FIGURE 3.3   Cycle of injury/re-injury. In response to an initial injury, failure to adequately address maladaptations following an initial injury results in reduced load capacity on return to sport. Consequently, lower levels of load application are required for injury development

is a common mistake made by many athletes, leading to a cascade of further injuries and the psychological distress of dealing with uncertainty and lack of understanding as to why they can no longer train as they previously have. For this reason, it is essential to ensure an athlete has completed appropriate rehabilitation and has been given sufficient time to gradually build back their training.

Age

Increased age has been reported to be a risk factor for certain types of running-related injuries (van der Worp et al., 2015). In particular, tendon overuse injuries and muscle strain injuries appear to be more frequently observed amongst older runners (McKean et al., 2006). This is perhaps explained by the age-related decline in musculotendon tissue properties reducing the capacity of muscle and tendon tissue to tolerate repeated loading, such as reduced muscle mass and muscle cross-sectional area, reduced muscle power and reduced tendon stiffness (Willy and Paquette, 2019). Appropriate strength and conditioning programmes may therefore be an important component of injury prevention for the older runner in order to maintain muscle tendon tissue properties and prevent injury risk (Willy and Paquette, 2019).

Training Experience

Several studies have reported less experienced runners to be at significantly greater risk of injury than experienced runners (Linton and Valentin, 2018; Kemler et al., 2018; Damsted et al., 2019b). It is thought that with greater training experience, runners are given time to develop their load capacity, meaning their musculoskeletal structures may be better suited to tolerate and recover from repeated load application. Conversely, less experienced runners, or those new to running, may not have developed the physical, physiological and biomechanical qualities necessary to prevent injury. Additionally, through greater training experience, runners may learn to identify the level of load application they can safely withstand, meaning they are better suited to make decisions regarding the need for rest and recovery and when to push their training. Runners with limited experience may not have learnt to identify the limits of load application, leading to poor decision-making and a lack of understanding of the need to recover.

Body Mass Index

Both increased (>25 kg·m^2) and reduced body mass have been associated with an increased risk of running injury development (Hulme et al., 2017). Greater body mass is thought to increase the loads applied to the body during each loading cycle of a run and may also represent a degree of physical deconditioning, as greater body mass index may be the result of a lack of physical activity. Consequently, load application will be greater per running stride and baseline load capacity may be lower and less tolerant to repeated load application.

A low body mass index (<18.5 kg·m^2) is also cited as an injury risk factor and may be a symptom of low energy availability, suggestive of an imbalance between nutrient intake and energy expenditure. Low energy availability will subsequently impair musculoskeletal growth and recovery, contributing to low bone mineral density and resulting in a reduction in structural tissue load capacity (see Chapter 18).

Fatigue

Fatigue is often the result of repeated or prolonged stress application with insufficient recovery in between. The fatigue status of an athlete can dynamically change both within a run and between running sessions, influencing their load capacity at a given moment in time. This may in part explain why some athletes develop injury with seemingly no change in training routine. If a gradual increase in fatigue occurs, then physical capacity may slowly decline, reaching an inevitable "straw that broke the camel's back" moment.

Not only do the physical demands of training influence fatigue, but psychological and lifestyle stressors may also have a large impact upon the fatigue and recovery of an athlete. Factors such as work demands, relationships, pressure from sponsors, prolonged race or competition anxieties, stressful life events, sleep quality, nutrition, lifestyle and mood status may all contribute to stress application and recovery. Therefore, closely monitoring fatigue levels and considering additional sources of fatigue, such as stress, lifestyle changes and sleep patterns, can allow for appropriate adaptation of training routines and intervention to ensure adequate recovery occurs (see Chapter 17).

Relative Energy Deficiency in Sport (RED-S)

Relative energy deficiency in sport (RED-S) is a clinical condition of low energy availability which can affect both male and female athletes. The condition is caused by imbalance between energy intake and energy expenditure, resulting in inadequate energy to support normal physiological functioning (Mountjoy et al., 2018a). This condition is not exclusive to athletes with eating disorders. Due to the high demands of training and competition, it is possible that subtle, unintentional imbalances between energy intake and expenditure may place an athlete at increased risk (Mountjoy et al., 2018a). RED-S can have several health consequences, including impaired metabolic rate, endocrine and menstrual function, reduced bone mineral density, impaired protein synthesis and immune function, as well as negatively impacting upon cardiovascular health (Heikura et al., 2018b; Mountjoy et al., 2018a). This places athletes at considerable risk of long-term health and injury consequences, and in particular is a strong risk factor for bone stress injuries (Thein-Nissenbaum, 2013; Barrack et al., 2017; Heikura et al., 2018b; Mountjoy et al., 2018a). Chapter 18 explores the RED-S syndrome and how to detect and prevent it.

Lower Limb Muscle Strength

Currently there is no conclusive evidence to suggest lower limb muscle strength is a risk factor for running-related injuries. It is important to note, however, that only a limited number of prospective studies have investigated the role of lower limb muscle strength in running injuries (Ramskov et al., 2015; Luedke et al., 2015; Messier et al., 2018; Thijs et al., 2011). Of the limited evidence, studies have reported reduced hip abductor, quadriceps and hamstring muscle strength as risk factors for patellofemoral pain (Ramskov et al., 2015; Luedke et al., 2015), reduced hip abductor strength as a risk factor for medial tibial stress syndrome (Verrelst et al., 2014) and reduced eccentric hamstring muscle strength as a risk factor for hamstring strain injuries. On balance, however, this has not been supported by prospective studies (Christopher et al., 2019; Messier et al., 2018; Thijs et al., 2011; Luedke et al., 2015).

Several studies have reported an association between lower limb muscle strength and running injuries, but due to the nature of these studies, it cannot be concluded whether the observed strength deficits are the cause of the injury or caused by the injury. Studies have identified reduced hip muscle strength amongst runners with Achilles tendinopathy (Habets et al., 2017), patellofemoral pain (Souza and Powers, 2009) and iliotibial band syndrome (Fredericson et al., 2000), as well as reduced calf muscle strength and endurance (both the gastrocnemius and soleus) in runners with Achilles tendinopathy (O'Neill et al., 2019).

Although it is currently uncertain as to whether lower limb muscle strength contributes to running injuries, when considering the physical and physiological demands placed on the body during running, it would seem logical for lower limb muscle strength to have a significant role in injury prevention. During the stance phase of running, the lower limb musculature is required for impact force absorption, control of joint movements and force generation for continued running. Specific muscle forces have been reported to reach up to two times body weight for the gluteus maximus, nine times for the soleus and hamstrings and up to five times body weight for the quadriceps (Dorn et al., 2012), with the soleus muscle contributing to up to 77% of the total force required to accelerate the body into the next stride (Hamner and Delp, 2013). An inability to repeatedly generate and absorb these forces is likely to lead to earlier muscular fatigue, an inability to maintain appropriate biomechanics, reduced force absorption and increased strain placed upon tendons and bones (Milgrom et al., 2007). As such, it seems probable that a minimum strength requirement is necessary in order to protect the musculoskeletal system from injury development (see Chapters 14 and 15 for further discussion and exercise interventions).

Neuromuscular Stability/Core Stability

"Core stability" is perhaps an ambiguous term, often used interchangeably with "core control" or "lumbo-pelvic stability". Originally, the term "core stability" was used to describe the ability of the muscular system to control the position of the trunk and pelvis during dynamic activities (Reed et al., 2012). More recently, however, this concept has been extended to additional body segments such as the feet (McKeon et al., 2015). The term "neuromuscular stability" might therefore be a more accurate reflection of this ambiguous concept, representing the coordinated ability of the nervous and muscular systems to actively stabilise, control and maintain posture of multiple body segments during dynamic activities.

Although there are limited studies investigating runners, reduced neuromuscular control of the trunk and pelvis has been identified as a risk factor for lower limb injuries in several other sports (De Blaiser et al., 2018). It is generally thought that inadequate neuromuscular stability may result in abnormal biomechanical patterns influencing lower limb loading and injury development (De Blaiser et al., 2018; Schmitz et al., 2014). From a running perspective, several studies have reported an association between altered trunk and pelvis running mechanics (Bramah et al., 2018; Noehren et al., 2012; Willy et al., 2012a; Schuermans et al., 2017a, 2017b) as well as foot mechanics (Pohl et al., 2008; Becker et al., 2018) and running-related injuries. However, to what extent these mechanical deficits can be explained by neuromuscular stability, or whether core/neuromuscular training improves these mechanics, remains unknown.

Flexibility

Currently there is no scientific evidence to suggest flexibility influences running injury risk, or that stretching reduces the risk of injury development (Christopher et al., 2019; Hulme et al., 2017). In fact, multiple systematic reviews have suggested there is no injury prevention benefit of stretching (Hulme et al., 2017; Lauersen et al., 2014). Instead, it is possible that athletes who always feel the need to stretch because "muscles are tight" are demonstrating early signs of tissue overload. This may represent an athlete who is not tolerating their current level of load application and should be investigated further.

Lower Limb Structure

Lower limb structure will influence the specific tissues subjected to load during running. Some studies have reported aspects of lower limb structure such as a high arched foot posture, pronated foot posture, increased navicular drop (surrogate measure for foot pronation) and a narrow tibia width to be associated with increased risk of lower limb injuries (Neal et al., 2014; Nunns et al., 2016; Tong and Kong, 2013; Newman et al., 2013). It is thought that structural alignment will influence the biomechanical loads applied to the lower limbs, contributing to injury development. However, there is an argument that provided load application is gradual and there is sufficient recovery between loading bouts, tissues will develop the capacity necessary to tolerate the applied loads. In this instance, injury is more likely the result of an imbalance between load application and recovery, rather than lower limb structure.

Sleep

Sleep is a vital part of the recovery process, with a lack of sleep having negative consequences for physical, psychological and physiological functions influencing injury risk. Physiologically, reduced sleep is reported to negatively impact muscle glycogen stores and hormone production necessary for bone and muscle growth (Finestone and Milgrom, 2008; Fullagar et al., 2015). Consequently, recovery from exercise is likely to be impaired, having detrimental effects upon the capacity of musculoskeletal strictures to tolerate training stress (Finestone and Milgrom, 2008; Fullagar et al., 2015). Several studies have also reported the detrimental effects of reduced sleep on physical and psychological function. Reduced aerobic capacity, muscle strength, muscle power output, increased perceived exercise intensity, fatigue, altered mood status and reduced cognitive function have all been reported to occur following sleep deprivation (Fullagar et al., 2015). As a result, this could lead to a reduction in an athlete's physical capacity to tolerate training loads and impair decision-making and behavioural actions, increasing athlete susceptibility to injury.

For healthy adults, around 7 to 9 hours of sleep per night is considered adequate; however, for athletes with high training and competition demands, as much as 9 to 10 hours may be required (Fullagar et al., 2015). In one recent study, athletes who reported sleeping less than 8 hours per night were found to be 1.7 times more likely to have had an injury when compared to those who slept more than 8 hours (Milewski et al., 2014). Factors such as travel, excessive light, psychological stress as well as pre- and post-competition anxiety or nervousness have all been shown to negatively impact sleep quality (Gupta et al., 2017). Considering the influence reduced sleep quality may have upon injury development, it is recommended that athletes and coaches consider factors that may impact upon an athlete's sleep quality and take appropriate measures to mitigate the associated injury risk.

Psycho-Social Factors

Running injury risk may be influenced by both the psychological status of an athlete as well as sociocultural influences (Messier et al., 2018). Psychological and emotional factors such as low mood status, anxiety, nervousness, depression and increased stress may negatively impact biological processes influencing tissue recovery (Williams and Andersen, 1998). Similarly, personality traits of perfectionism and obsessive behaviours may drive training and lifestyle behaviours leading to greater injury risk, such as obsessing about running mileage and food intake, or ignoring minor injury symptoms (de Jonge et al., 2020; de Jonge et al., 2018). Consequently, athlete psychology can have an impact upon both tissue load capacity and load application (Wiese-Bjornstal, 2010).

It is important to also consider the role of sociocultural influences upon an athlete's psychology status and resulting behaviour. Negative life events, life stressors and social interaction with peers or external sponsors may all lead to increased psychological stress placed on an athlete. These may in turn influence behavioural actions impacting load application and recovery, such as increasing training intensity and frequency, or even reducing recovery time due to external sponsor commitments.

Summary and Recommendations

It may be impossible to truly prevent injury, but steps can be taken to reduce injury risk through ensuring a continued balance between the load demands placed on an athlete and their capacity to tolerate load. It is important to remember that an athlete's response to training loads and their load capacity can vary on a day-to-day basis and will also vary between athletes. Therefore, response to training should be monitored on an individual basis, making adaptations to planned workloads, supplementary conditioning and recovery strategies if necessary. From the perspective of load application, gradual progression of training loads and avoiding sudden and rapid changes to training demands, surfaces, environment, footwear and lifestyle can help develop an athlete's physiological and psychological load capacity while avoiding acute overload which may influence injury risk. Additionally, the inclusion of supplementary resistance training and neuromuscular control exercises and addressing biomechanical contributors to tissue loading may also assist in the development of athlete robustness.

4

NUTRITIONAL REQUIREMENTS FOR DISTANCE RUNNERS

Matthew Cole, Richard C. Blagrove, Meghan A. Brown, Jennie Carter and Justin D. Roberts

Highlights

- Middle- and long-distance running events are largely fuelled by the oxidative metabolism of carbohydrate.
- Carbohydrate intake should be 3–5 g·kg body mass^{-1}·day^{-1} for a runner undertaking low volumes (<1 hour) of moderate-intensity daily training, to 6–10 g·kg body mass^{-1}·day^{-1} for those engaged with high-volume (1–3 hours) running at a moderate-high intensity.
- It is essential that a runner's diet contains an adequate amount of fats (particularly polyunsaturated); however, evidence highlights that high fat–low carbohydrate diets may compromise performance during all but easy running sessions.
- Protein intake should be ~1.0–1.2 g·kg body mass^{-1}·day^{-1} for recreational endurance runners, ~1.2–1.5 g·kg body mass^{-1}·day^{-1} for competitive runners engaging in daily moderate-hard training (~60 min), and ~1.6–2.0 g·kg body mass^{-1}·day^{-1} for elite endurance runners (particularly when undertaking intensive training).
- Runners should aim to consume meals/snacks that contain a balance of nutrients and fluid (~5–7 mL·kg body mass^{-1}) every 3–4 hours throughout the day (5–6 'feeds') to support metabolic regulation and meet caloric requirements.

Introduction

Achieving success in a distance running event is dependent upon the conversion of chemical energy to mechanical energy to sustain a given speed. Middle-distance running events (800 m–3 km) require a high level of energy provision from both aerobic (energy produced in the presence of oxygen) and anaerobic (energy produced without oxygen) sources and rely almost exclusively on carbohydrate to fuel higher-intensity performance. Long-distance running events (5 km–marathon) are heavily reliant on oxygen-dependent replenishment of energy, which requires an adequate delivery of oxygen and availability of carbohydrate and fat as metabolic fuels. Ultra-endurance events (>4 hours) have also increased in popularity over the last decade and present unique physiological challenges in terms of fatigue, hydration and energy demand (Tiller *et al.*, 2019). Fatigue during marathon and ultra-distance running events can often be a consequence of muscle glycogen (carbohydrate) depletion, therefore ensuring that high pre-exercise muscle and liver glycogen concentrations are essential. A runner's diet is of paramount importance for overall health and for provision of essential calories/nutrients to fuel training/racing and to support adaptive processes during recovery from training. Consequently, this chapter aims to provide evidence-based recommendations on appropriate nutrition practices for distance runners.

Energy Metabolism

To understand the nutritional requirements of various distance running events, it is important to first explain how metabolic energy systems resynthesise the high energy compound found in all muscle cells, adenosine triphosphate (ATP). The availability of ATP is critical for all skeletal muscle contractile activity, yet the intramuscular stores of ATP are sufficient to support only a few seconds of exercise (Hargreaves and Spriet, 2018). To maintain ATP levels within working muscles, three metabolic pathways are activated, two anaerobic pathways (substrate-level phosphorylation without oxygen) and an aerobic pathway (oxidative phosphorylation). Metabolism is a dynamic process with relative contribution of each energy pathway during exercise dependent upon the duration and the intensity of activity; however, it is a common misconception that they switch on and off in a sequential or hierarchical order.

During very intense running, such as the first 100 m of a middle-distance race and sprint finishes, most ATP is resynthesised via the anaerobic energy pathways – the phosphocreatine system and anaerobic glycolytic system. The phosphocreatine system has a limited capacity (~10 sec) for ATP resynthesis, whereas anaerobic glycolytic capacity is approximately three-fold higher (Hargreaves and Spriet, 2020). Sustained sprinting (30–60 sec) results in a high reliance on anaerobic glycolysis to maintain ATP levels, which is associated with accumulation of metabolic by-products – lactate and hydrogen ions. Blood lactate concentration reflects the activation of the anaerobic glycolytic system and therefore acts as a useful indicator of exercise intensity. However, there is still a widely held belief that lactic acid causes fatigue, which is incorrect (Brooks, 2001). Rather, it is the metabolites (magnesium ions, adenosine diphosphate, inorganic phosphates and hydrogen ions) and intra-cellular acidosis associated with the breakdown of ATP, phosphocreatine and glycogen during anaerobic metabolism that appear to cause rapid fatigue during high-intensity exercise (Allen et al., 2008). Nutritional strategies (e.g. bicarbonate, beta-alanine) that promote a more alkaline environment and metabolite buffering capacity may therefore provide an avenue for improving performance during middle-distance running events (see Chapter 11).

Distance running events lasting ~2 min and longer derive most of their energy from aerobic processes. Even the men's 800 m event (world record 1:40.91) has a substantial (~60%) aerobic contribution (Duffield et al., 2005). Although oxidative phosphorylation is activated at the onset of exercise, it becomes the major ATP-generating pathway after ~60 sec of exercise. The rate at which oxygen consumption rises at the start of high-intensity exercise to meet the required energy demand via oxidative phosphorylation is known as 'oxygen uptake kinetics', and is an important determinant of endurance performance and highly trainable (Burnley and Jones, 2007). During high-intensity interval training sessions and middle-distance races, intramuscular stores of muscle glycogen and blood glucose (derived from liver glycogenolysis) provide the primary source of energy (Hargreaves and Spriet, 2020).

In the presence of oxygen, pyruvate (converted from glucose) is transported to the mitochondria where it is used to produce acetyl co-enzyme-A, which forms the major entry point for metabolic fuels (fat and carbohydrate) into the Krebs cycle. The Krebs cycle degrades acetyl co-enzyme-A to carbon dioxide and hydrogen, plus resynthesises one molecule of ATP. The hydrogen atoms subsequently enter the electron transport chain that uses oxidative phosphorylation to yield 38 ATP molecules from glucose metabolism, or 129 ATP from a fatty acid. Despite the higher energy yield from a molecule of fat compared to carbohydrate, oxidation of carbohydrate is ~7% more efficient as it generates more ATP per volume of oxygen compared to fat, and the pathways that metabolise carbohydrate are far quicker (Spriet, 2014). This means carbohydrates are the preferred fuel when energy is in high demand. An important adaptation to endurance training, however, is an increased reliance on fat as a fuel for exercise (Achten and Jeukendrup, 2004), which is important for sparing glycogen stores for later in an exercise bout or subsequent sessions.

Oxidative metabolism of carbohydrate and fat provides virtually all the ATP in skeletal muscle for long-distance running performance and continuous moderate-intensity training runs. At higher intensities of exercise (~80–100% maximal oxygen uptake ($\dot{V}O_{2max}$), i.e. 3 km to marathon pace in trained runners) carbohydrate oxidation dominates (Hargreaves and Spriet, 2020). Rates of fat oxidation are highest when the demand for energy is lower at ~60–65% of $\dot{V}O_{2max}$ (i.e. marathon pace in recreational runners, and ultra-distance running intensity). As exercise duration increases, oxidation of intramuscular glycogen and lipid stores decreases, corresponding with an increased reliance on muscle glucose and fatty acid uptake from the blood (van Loon et al., 2001). During prolonged running (> 90 min), liver glucose output can decrease to levels below muscle glucose uptake, resulting in hypoglycaemia ('low blood sugar'). This risk of developing hypoglycaemia can be reduced by ensuring adequate pre-exercise liver glycogen levels and in-event carbohydrate ingestion (Coyle et al., 1983).

Energy Requirements

Consuming enough calories to meet daily energy needs should be a priority for runners. The total daily energy requirement for runners depends upon a variety of factors including age, sex, body mass (BM), body composition, basal metabolic rate, non-exercise physical activity levels and the nature (duration, mode, intensity) of exercise training. 'Energy balance' refers to the ratio between energy intake (from foods, fluids and any supplements) and energy expenditure, calculated as the sum of basal metabolic rate, the thermic effect of food, and the energy expended during non-exercise physical activity and exercise training. A long-term negative energy balance will result in weight loss, and a positive energy balance will cause weight gain. Energy needs can be estimated for active individuals using the Dietary Reference Intake method (Zello, 2006; Box 4.1). The definitions of physical activity in these equations mean that for most recreational and competitive runners, exercise will be classified as 'moderate-vigorous' in nature. This method, and other equations, for estimation of daily energy requirement provide only an approximation of average energy needs, so it should be used as a rough guide.

BOX 4.1 THE DIETARY REFERENCE INTAKE METHOD FOR ESTIMATING ENERGY REQUIREMENT FOR ADULTS (RODRIGUEZ *ET AL.*, 2009). PA = PHYSICAL ACTIVITY

Adult Male

Energy requirement (kcal per day) = 622 − (9.53 × age in years) + {PA × ([15.91 × weight in kg] + [539.6 × height in m])}

Female Adult

Energy requirement (kcal per day) = 354 − (6.91 × age in years) + {PA × ([9.36 × weight in kg] + [726 × height in m])}

PA Level

1.0–1.39	Sedentary, typical daily living activities (e.g. household tasks, walking to bus)
1.4–1.59	Low active, typical daily living activities plus 30–60 min of daily moderate activity (e.g. walking at 5–7 km.h^{-1})
1.6–1.89	Active, typical daily living activities plus 60 min of daily moderate activity
1.9–2.5	Very active, typical daily living activities plus 60 min of daily moderate activity plus an additional 60 min of vigorous activity or 120 min of moderate activity.

Example

21-year-old male well-trained runner performing ~60 min running per day (PA of 1.7) weighing 75 kg and 1.75 m in height:

Energy requirement = 622 − 200 + {1.7 × (1193 + 944)} = 4054 kcal per day*

* This requirement is relevant only to days where the PA level applies, e.g. on rest days (PA of 1.0–1.2) this value is likely to be ~2600–3000 kcal per day.

'Energy availability' is defined as the energy derived from the diet minus exercise and physical activity energy expenditure expressed relative to fat free mass (FFM), providing the amount of energy 'left over' for normal physiological functions (Loucks et al., 2011). Current consensus is that optimal energy availability for healthy physiological function in women is around 45 kcal·kg FFM^{-1}·day^{-1}. For women, 30 kcal·kg FFM^{-1}·day^{-1} appears to represent the lowest threshold of energy availability before physiological systems are substantially perturbated (Mountjoy et al., 2018b). Emerging data also suggests males will also incur deleterious physiological effects during periods of low energy availability, but at a lower threshold of ~20–25 kcal·kg FFM^{-1}·day^{-1} (Koehler et al., 2016; Fagerberg, 2017). High volumes of training often make it problematic for many endurance runners to meet their energy requirements, which can result in periods of low energy availability. Indeed, it has been estimated that 37% of female and 40% of male elite distance runners suffer from a syndrome known as 'relative energy deficiency in sport' (RED-S; Heikura et al., 2017), which is associated with impairments in metabolic rate, menstrual function (for females), bone health, immunity and cardiovascular health (Mountjoy et al., 2014). Readers are referred to Chapter 18, which provides further detail on RED-S and how the syndrome can be avoided.

Macronutrients

Carbohydrate

Carbohydrate is the primary source of energy for moderate and high-intensity exercise and therefore ensuring adequate dietary intake of carbohydrate is essential. Carbohydrate intake should vary according to the nature of the training (and competition) that is being undertaken at any given time. As a general guide, daily carbohydrate requirements for different types of training and event preparation are provided in Table 4.1. Based on these recommendations, an individual weighing 70 kg who runs on most days of the week in the form of continuous runs and interval training sessions (30–60 min in duration) should be consuming approximately 350 g of carbohydrate per day. Chapter 17 provides further detail on the importance, intake and timing of carbohydrate during recovery from training sessions, and Chapter 11 addresses pre-event carbohydrate loading for events lasting > 90 min.

Carbohydrates can be classified as simple (glucose, fructose, sucrose, lactose, maltose, e.g. sugar, honey, jams, energy drinks/gels) and complex (starch, e.g. bread, pasta, wholegrains, potatoes, cereals). As foods from both carbohydrate types can generate similar post-prandial changes in insulin and blood sugar levels, a better classification is the glycaemic index (GI) scale (Donaldson et al., 2010). The GI value of a carbohydrate-rich food is measured on a scale from 0 to 100 that refers to how blood sugar levels rise in the hours post-consumption. Glucose, as a reference, has a score of 100, with values of > 70 considered high GI foods, 55–70 moderate GI foods, and < 55 low GI foods (Atkinson et al., 2008). Examples of high GI foods include potatoes, white bread/baguettes, bananas and cake products. Foods such as green vegetables, beans, wholemeal pasta, nuts, apricots, oranges and apples have a lower GI value. Low GI carbohydrate foods in the hours prior to exercise appears to provide a metabolic advantage over high GI foods due to a higher oxidation of fats in the early stages of exercise and more stable blood glucose levels (Donaldson et al., 2010). Immediately after

TABLE 4.1 Carbohydrate intake guidelines for distance runners during different training and event scenarios

Training/event scenario	Carbohydrate intake
Low volume (<1 hour), moderate intensity	3–5 g·kg BM^{-1}·day^{-1}
Moderate volume (~1 hour), moderate-high intensity	5–7 g·kg BM^{-1}·day^{-1}
High volume (1–3 hours), moderate-high	6–10 g·kg BM^{-1}·day^{-1}
Carbohydrate loading prior to events lasting >90 min	8–12 g·kg BM^{-1}·day^{-1} during 2 days before the event
Recovery following exercise	1.2 g·$hour^{-1}$ in the 4 hours post-exercise

Note: BM = body mass.

Source: Burke et al. (2011); Burke et al. (2017a); Thomas et al. (2016).

exercise, high GI carbohydrate foods appears to be more beneficial to maximise the rate of muscle glycogen resynthesis (Burke et al., 1993).

Fat

Fats are responsible for numerous physiological functions, so they are important for the maintenance of health and optimisation of performance in runners. Fats support important roles in cellular signalling and structural maintenance, nerve function, inflammatory processes, insulation and protection of vital organs, and energy provision. Moreover, it is important that an athlete's diet contains the appropriate amount of essential fatty acids (fats that the body cannot make on its own) and fat-soluble vitamins (A, D, E and K). Although high fat intake and low density lipoprotein (LDL) cholesterol are associated with chronic diseases, fat should certainly not be viewed negatively and low intakes of dietary fat (< 20% of total energy) can negatively impact health and performance (Vitale and Getzin, 2019). Furthermore, cutting out certain food groups that are high in fat, e.g. dairy, can result in micronutrient deficiencies (Close and Morton, 2016). Fats have a higher energy density (9 kcal·g^{-1}) compared to carbohydrate (4 kcal·g^{-1}), therefore care should also be taken not to overconsume foods high in fat over prolonged periods.

Fats are typically classified as saturated and unsaturated; with unsaturated fat further sub-divided into monounsaturated and polyunsaturated fat. Essential fatty acids are considered polyunsaturated fats and are categorised as omega-3 and omega-6 fatty acids. Omega-3-rich foods include oily fish (e.g. salmon, tuna, mackerel), walnuts and flax seeds, and examples of dietary sources of omega-6 fatty acids include vegetable oils, soybeans, eggs, nuts, avocado and meat/poultry/fish. Although the optimal ratio of omega-3/omega-6 fatty acids is 1:1 to 4:1, it is apparent that typical Western diets are heavily deficient in omega-3 fatty acids (Patterson et al., 2012). Therefore, athletes are encouraged to increase weekly omega-3 fatty acid intake, e.g. three portions of oily fish per week (Close and Morton, 2016). Although reducing saturated fats from the diet (particularly processed meats) will likely improve health, they should be replaced with unsaturated fats rather than refined carbohydrate (e.g. bread, pasta, potatoes, Astrup et al., 2011). Finally, hydrogenated fats (or 'trans fat'), are artificially created fats typically used in manufactured food products and the fast food industry. They provide no benefit to health and sports performance, and therefore runners should avoid foods that contain trans fats (Mozaffarian et al., 2006).

Protein

Proteins have many critical roles in the body, including as antibodies, enzymes and messengers, and to provide structure and support for cells. Proteins are composed of amino acids, with nine classified as 'essential' (must be consumed in the diet) and the remainder as 'non-essential' (the body can make its own if required). The current recommended daily allowance of protein for a sedentary non-athlete is 0.8 g·kg BM^{-1}·day^{-1}; however, it appears those engaging in regular endurance exercise require more (Tarnopolsky, 2004). Protein requirements have been estimated at ~1–1.2 g·kg BM^{-1}·day^{-1} for recreational endurance athletes (4–5 × ~30 min runs per week), 1.2–1.5 g·kg BM^{-1}·day^{-1} for competitive endurance athletes engaging in daily moderate-hard training (~60 min), and 1.6–2.0g·kg BM^{-1}·day^{-1} for elite endurance athletes and those performing frequent (≥ 3 times per week) strength training (Tarnopolsky, 2004; Rodriguez et al., 2009; Kato et al., 2016). Regular intake of protein above these amounts does not provide further benefit to endurance athletes (Vitale and Getzin, 2019). Protein requirements for runners can be easily met through a 'food-first' approach. However, supplementary protein may be warranted when logistical challenges are faced, or when liquid meals may be preferred e.g. during acute recovery from training. If athletes choose to use nutritional supplements, they should preferably ensure it has been appropriately batch-tested under a recognised supplement quality assurance program (Maughan, 2013) as verified by an *'Informed Sport'* logo (Smith et al., 2015).

The timing and type of protein that is consumed is equally as important as the absolute daily amount ingested. Athletes should avoid restricting their daily intake of protein foods to mealtimes and instead aim to consume protein 'snacks' throughout the day, particularly before and after exercise (Kerksick et al., 2017). As explained in Chapter 17, protein intakes of 0.25–0.30 g·kg BM^{-1} (~20 g for a 70 kg individual), or 0.4 g·kg BM^{-1} for older adults, is likely to maximise muscle protein synthesis if consumed within the two-hour period after exercise (Moore, 2015). Similarly, dosages of 0.25–0.30 g·kg BM^{-1} (15–30 g for most runners) every 3–4 hours throughout the day (5–6 'feeds') appears to optimise daily protein synthesis rates (Areta et al., 2013; Jäger et al., 2017; Vitale and Getzin, 2019).

In addition to the quantity and timing of intake, the type of protein consumed is also important to consider. Whey protein (the water-soluble part of milk) is a high-quality, easily absorbed protein containing all nine essential amino acids. Crucially, protein sources that contain the essential amino acids known as the branched chain amino acids (leucine, isoleucine and valine) are particularly important, with leucine needed to 'switch on' muscle protein synthesis (Duan et al., 2016). Foods high in milk-based protein result in higher muscle protein synthesis rates post-exercise compared to soya protein (Phillips et al., 2009). Casein (found in milk, yogurt and cheese) is considered a slow-release protein and is therefore beneficial to consume prior to sleep to provide a sustained delivery of amino acids overnight (Res et al., 2012). Animal-based foods (i.e. milk, eggs, cheese, red meat, fish, poultry) provide the most concentrated sources of essential amino acids. Whilst plant-based protein sources (e.g. soy products, tofu, pumpkin seeds, chia seeds, quinoa, lentils, chickpeas, nuts and other grains) contain lower amounts of essential amino acids, for the vegetarian and vegan runner it is possible to consume a diet complete in proteins by making structured and varied food choices (Jäger et al., 2017).

Micronutrients

Vitamins and minerals have many functions that are important for health and running performance, such as energy production, haemoglobin synthesis, maintenance of bone health, repair of damaged tissue, immune function and protection against oxidative damage (Rodriguez et al., 2009). Vitamins and minerals are required only in small amounts; however, except for Vitamin D, they must be consumed through the diet. A list of the major vitamins and minerals important for runners, their physiological functions, recommended daily intake and food sources are shown in Table 4.2. Fat-soluble vitamins (vitamins A, D, E and K) are capable of being stored in the liver and fat cells for later use by other tissues. If dietary intake of these vitamins is low, the body will draw upon its stored reserves, however; if intakes are excessive and stores of these vitamins are saturated, this can cause adverse health issues. Water-soluble vitamins (B vitamins and vitamin C) cannot be stored; therefore, the body cannot draw upon any reserves if intake is low, and excessive consumption is mostly excreted.

Intake of Micronutrients

Inadequate micronutrient intake is known to compromise physical performance and can increase the risk of illness and infection (Lukaski, 2004; Sabetta et al., 2010). Dietary reference values provide the recommended intake of micronutrients for 97.5% of the population; however, regular exercise may increase the turnover and loss of these micronutrients, thus greater intakes of some vitamins and minerals may be required in runners (Woolf and Manore, 2006; Rodriguez et al., 2009). A balanced wholefood diet that contains at least five portions of a variety of fruit and vegetables (see Table 4.2) is usually enough to support the micronutrient requirements of most runners without the need for supplementation. It is also important to remember that increasing the total caloric intake to support the energy demands of training will also increase the intake of micronutrients. Runners are at high risk of developing deficiencies if they: restrict their energy intake, have an unbalanced diet, dislike certain food groups or have allergies and lack sunlight exposure. Runners who fall into one or more of these categories may benefit from additional multivitamin/mineral supplementation (Close and Morton, 2016); however, advice should be sought from a qualified professional concerning the need for supplements. Although a sufficient intake of all vitamins and minerals is important for runners, this section will discuss the micronutrients that runners should pay most attention to.

The B Vitamins

The B vitamins have important roles in regulating energy metabolism, and folic acid and vitamin B_{12} are required to produce new red blood cells. Consequently, a deficiency in the B vitamins can potentially hamper running performance, and low levels of folic acid and vitamin B_{12} can result in anaemia (lack of red blood cells; Lukaski, 2004). Research indicates that exercise may increase the requirements for vitamin B_2 and vitamin B_6; however, it is less clear whether there is an increased requirement for the other B vitamins (Woolf and Manore, 2006). Trained runners who consume a sufficient number of calories to support their exercise and lifestyle requirements tend not to be deficient in the B vitamins (Kaiserauer et al., 1989; Nieman et al., 1989; Habte et al., 2015; Nebl et al., 2019). To obtain adequate amounts of the B vitamins, foods such as wholegrains, fruits, vegetables, and lean meats should be consumed regularly (see Table 4.2).

Vitamin D and Calcium

Vitamin D and calcium are particularly important for growth and repair of bone tissue and regulate nerve impulse transmission and muscle function. A deficiency in one or both of these micronutrients has been associated with low bone mineral density and stress fractures in runners (Nieves et al., 2010; Giffin et al., 2017). Calcium is obtained from the diet (e.g. dairy products, green leafy vegetables and nuts); however, vitamin D is mainly synthesised through sunlight. Runners who live in northern latitudes, spend long periods of time indoors, and train on treadmills or after sunset are therefore at risk of vitamin D deficiency (Close et al., 2013). Consequently, it is recommended that runners actively consume foods high in vitamin D (see Table 4.2) during the winter months, particularly if they are not able to train outdoors during daylight hours. Athletes showing symptoms of insufficiency (e.g. persistent fatigue, mood changes, bone pain, frequent illness), especially during winter months, should have their vitamin D status checked.

Antioxidants

During exercise (particularly of a high intensity), an increase in metabolism accelerates the production of free radicals (or reactive oxygen species). Reactive oxygen species are required for activating cellular signalling pathways that lead to important physiological adaptations; however, they also cause damage to lipids and proteins and contribute towards muscle damage and soreness (Schieber and Chandel, 2014). The main antioxidant micronutrients (vitamins C and E, beta carotene and selenium) and polyphenols mitigate the damaging effects of oxidative stress caused by the release of reactive oxygen species. There has been speculation that athletes require higher amounts of antioxidants in their diet; however, the evidence suggests that this may not the case (Gomez-Cabrera et al., 2008a). In fact, some evidence observed blunted exercise-induced increases in enzymatic antioxidants following supplementation of vitamin C and E, and attenuated training adaptations (Gomez-Cabrera et al., 2008b; Paulsen et al., 2014; Morrison et al., 2015). However, this may apply only to specific nutrients and/or be related to the timing of supplement ingestion (e.g. in close proximity to exercise). Other authors have indicated that fruit-derived polyphenols (>1000 mg·day^{-1} for >3 days) may in fact support antioxidant and anti-inflammatory pathways which may have important implications for endurance or demanding high-intensity events (Bowtell and Kelly, 2019). Further research in this area is warranted, and at present runners should aim to consume a wholefood diet that provides a good variety of fruit and vegetables to meet antioxidant/polyphenol requirements.

Iron

Iron is required to produce oxygen-carrying proteins (haemoglobin and myoglobin) and enzymes involved in energy production. Due to the inflammation caused by running, the hormone hepcidin is upregulated in the hours following exercise, which compromises the absorption of dietary iron (Peeling et al., 2009). Furthermore, the rupture of blood vessels and gastrointestinal bleeding that occurs during running may also affect iron status (Deldicque and Francaux, 2015). For these reasons, iron requirements are ~70% higher for endurance runners compared to non-active individuals (Rodriguez et al., 2009).

Low iron status is common in runners, particularly women (Coates et al., 2017), which can impair muscle function, work capacity and lead to feelings of lethargy (Pasricha et al., 2010). The daily recommended intake of iron for pre-menopausal female runners (18 mg·day^{-1} and 11–12 mg·day^{-1} for hormonal contraceptive users) is higher than for male runners (8 mg·day^{-1}) to account for the regular losses of iron that occur through menstrual bleeding (Deldicque and Francaux, 2015; Pedlar et al., 2018). In adolescents experiencing a period of rapid growth and females who experience heavy menstrual bleeding, daily intake may need to be higher (Bruinvels et al., 2016). Vegetarian runners also struggle to obtain the recommended amount of iron per day due to the lower bioavailability of iron in plant-based foods compared to meat; therefore, iron requirements are 1.8 times higher in vegetarians compared to omnivores (Deldicque and Francaux, 2015). Long-distance runners, especially women, adolescents, vegetarians, and runners training at altitude, should be blood tested regularly to monitor iron status (Sim et al., 2019). Iron supplementation is currently not recommended for runners who have normal iron stores; however, those identified as being iron deficient (including non-anaemics) may benefit from taking an iron supplementation under the recommendation of a medical professional (Rubeor et al., 2018; Sim et al., 2019).

Other Minerals

There are 20 minerals that must be consumed in the diet; however, in addition to those discussed already, zinc and magnesium are most important for runners. Zinc is responsible for growth and repair of tissues, immune function and energy production; therefore, a deficiency affects thyroid hormones, metabolic rate and recovery. Research indicates that athletes, particularly women, have low zinc levels, which suggests they have a higher requirement for zinc compared to those who are physically inactive (Chu et al., 2018). Magnesium plays several crucial roles associated with energy metabolism and regulates neuromuscular function. Endurance training may result in a degree of magnesium deficiency in some athletes (Casoni et al., 1990), highlighting that magnesium requirements for athletes are likely higher than non-active individuals (Bohl and Volpe, 2002; Zhang et al., 2017). Furthermore, high sweat rates without adequate intake of magnesium can cause a deficiency that impairs cardiovascular and neuromuscular function, leading to compromised endurance performance (Nielsen and Lukaski, 2006). However, whilst magnesium supplementation may support hormonal or metabolic demands of training (Golf et al., 1998), there is little evidence that magnesium supplementation directly benefits endurance performance (Terblanche et al., 1992; Zhang et al., 2017). Therefore, athletes who obtain enough magnesium in their diet likely do not require additional supplementation (Wang et al., 2017). If a runner is in energy balance and eats a diet that includes all food groups (see Table 4.2), there is little risk of not meeting the recommended daily intake of minerals. The difference between a safe and a toxic daily intake of minerals is smaller compared to vitamins, and therefore care should be taken when using supplements that minerals are not overconsumed, which can interfere with absorption of other micronutrients (Close and Morton, 2016).

Hydration

During everyday living, euhydration (normal levels of hydration) can be maintained quite easily via behavioural and biological controls (Belval et al., 2019). However, endurance exercise can result in fluid losses that can acutely impair performance (at ~2–3% of body mass) and requires restoration following exercise (Cheuvront et al., 2003). Recommendations for appropriate hydration strategies can be considered before, during and after exercise. In-event/ during exercise considerations are discussed in Chapter 11, and post-exercise guidelines to optimise re-hydration practices are provided in Chapter 17.

Beginning exercise/competition in a euhydrated state is usually easy to achieve if sufficient beverages and meals have been consumed in the hours leading up to the session/event (Sawka et al., 2007). However, if an athlete is in a hot environment they are not fully acclimatised to, they exercise shortly after waking, and/or they have experienced substantial fluid deficits in the previous 8 hours, then an active pre-hydration strategy may need to be used (Sawka et al., 2007). Regularly monitoring hydration status in the hours leading up to a session/event is the best way to determine whether additional fluid is required (Close and Morton, 2016). Within

TABLE 4.2 Main vitamins and minerals, their physiological functions, recommended intake, and food sources

Vitamin/mineral	Physiological function(s)	Recommended daily intake(male/female)	Food sources
Fat-soluble vitamins			
Vitamin A	Antioxidant. Immune function, vision, cell growth and division	0.7 mg/0.6 mg	Cheese, eggs, oily fish, milk, green leafy vegetables, carrots, peppers
Vitamin D	Regulates calcium and phosphate use, bone health, cell differentiation, immunity, muscle function	0.01 mg if confined indoors	Oily fish, red meat, eggs, fortified cereals (*plus sunlight*)
Vitamin E	Antioxidant. Growth and development, maintains skin health and eye function, immunity	4 mg/3 mg	Nuts and seeds, plant oils (corn and olive oil), shrimps
Vitamin K	Blood clotting, formation of some proteins, bone health	~1 μg·kg BM^{-1}	Green leafy vegetables (broccoli, spinach), cauliflower, cereal grain
Water-soluble vitamins			
Vitamin B$_1$ (thiamin)	Carbohydrate and protein metabolism, removal of carbon dioxide, nervous system function	1 mg/0.8 mg	Green peas, fruit, eggs, wholegrain breads, almonds, cereals
Vitamin B$_2$ (riboflavin)	Carbohydrate metabolism, skin and eye health, nervous system function	1.3 mg/1.1 mg	Milk, eggs, mushrooms, broccoli, spinach, bananas, beef, rice
Vitamin B$_3$ (niacin)	Carbohydrate, fat and protein metabolism, skin health, nervous system function	17 mg/13 mg	Meat, fish, eggs, milk, avocados, tomatoes, carrots
Vitamin B$_5$ (pantothenic acid)	Carbohydrate, fat and protein metabolism	~3 mg	Chicken, beef, potatoes, oats, tomatoes, eggs, broccoli, wholegrains
Vitamin B$_6$ (pyridoxine)	Carbohydrate metabolism, forms haemoglobin	1.4 mg/1.2 mg	Bananas, pork, poultry, fish, bread, wholegrains, eggs, vegetables

(*Continued*)

Table 4.2 (Continued)

Vitamin/mineral	Physiological function(s)	Recommended daily intake(male/female)	Food sources
Vitamin B₇ (biotin)	Fat metabolism	< 300 μg	Eggs, kidney, meat
Vitamin B₁₂ (cobalamine)	Carbohydrate metabolism, production of red blood cells, nervous system function	1.5 μg	Meat, fish, milk, cheese, eggs, cereals
Folic acid	Production of red blood cells and some proteins	200 μg	Meat, leafy green vegetables, green peas, cereals, legumes
Vitamin C	Antioxidant. Iron absorption, maintaining skin, blood vessel, bone and cartilage health	40 mg	Oranges and citrus fruit, peppers, strawberries, broccoli, sprouts
Minerals			
Iron	Formation of oxygen transportation proteins and energy-producing enzymes	9 mg/18 mg (11–12 mg for HC users)*	Red meat, beans, nuts, dried fruit, wholegrains, dark-green leafy vegetables, eggs, fortified cereals
Calcium	Regulates muscle function and nerve impulse transmission, bone health, blood clotting	1000 mg	Milk, cheese, yoghurt, green leafy vegetables, soya beans, nuts
Magnesium	Energy metabolism, muscle contraction, nerve transmission	300 mg/270 mg	Meat, dairy foods, fish, green leafy vegetables, nuts, brown rice
Potassium	Fluid balance, cardiac function	3500 mg	Bananas, broccoli, parsnips, sprouts, nuts and seeds, fish, poultry
Zinc	Antioxidant. Immunity, protein digestion, formation of new cell and enzymes	10 mg/7 mg	Meat, seafood, poultry, dairy foods, bread, leafy and root vegetables

Note: BM = body mass; HC = hormonal contraceptive. * Multiply by 1.8 for vegetarians.

a field-based setting, a urine osmolality of <700 mOsmol·kg BM^{-1} and a urine colour that is pale yellow provide an indication of euhydration prior to exercise (Sawka et al., 2007). Validated urine colour charts can be found online; for example, www.usada.org/athletes/substances/nutrition/fluids-and-hydration/. Runners should aim to slowly drink ~5–7 mL·kg BM^{-1} (~400–500 ml for a 70 kg individual) at least 4 hours prior to exercise. If the runner does not urinate or urine is dark, a further 3–5 mL·kg BM^{-1} (~250–300 ml for a 70 kg individual) of fluid should be slowly consumed ~2 hours before the event (Maughan et al., 1996; Shirreffs and Maughan, 1998). Beverages containing a small amount of sodium (460–1150 mg·L^{-1} or 20–50 mEq·L^{-1}) or consumed with a snack containing salt will help fluids to be absorbed (Ray et al., 1998). Attempting to drink more fluid than the aforementioned recommendation does not provide a performance advantage, increases the likelihood of having to urinate during the exercise/event, and in extreme cases risks hyponatraemia (see Chapter 11; Sawka et al., 2007).

The Distance Runners' Diet

The previous sections have provided evidence-based guidelines on appropriate intake of energy, macro- and micronutrients for a runner. Despite consensus in these areas, decisions on what foods to eat, how much and appropriate timings of consumption remain highly individual and depend upon numerous factors including: age, sex, food preferences, food availability, allergies/intolerances, lifestyle, budget, racing and training goals, time of year, training volume and intensity, training modalities, training environment, etc. Intense running sessions can also suppress appetite, and many runners prefer not to exercise within several hours of eating (Kerksick et al., 2018). Therefore, each runner requires a unique and constantly changing nutrition plan that is suited to their own needs (Heikura et al., 2018a). Boxes 4.2 and 4.3 provide two case studies of runners with different nutritional requirements and how their diets might look.

When using a high-carbohydrate availability diet, the percentage of energy contributed from carbohydrate, fat and protein consumed as a proportion of total energy intake in a runner's diet should be roughly 45–55%, 25–35%, 10–15% respectively (Kerksick et al., 2018). Higher percentages of energy derived from carbohydrate (60–70%) have been recommended to support high volumes of training or in the days leading up to a marathon/ultra-distance event (Coyle, 1991). Presenting macronutrient intake targets as percentages can cause confusion due to the differences in the calorie density within macronutrients, which may lead to athletes consuming more or less of each macronutrient than intended (Burke et al., 2011). Furthermore, a runner's diet could comprise an appropriate proportion of carbohydrate (e.g. 50%), but total energy intake may only be 2000 kcal·day^{-1}, which would be insufficient to support energy demands (Rodriguez et al., 2009). It is therefore more appropriate to calculate macronutrient requirements in absolute terms (g·kg BM $^{-1}$·day $^{-1}$), as indicated throughout this chapter.

As carbohydrate is the main fuel used during high intensities of exercise (> 80% of $\dot{V}O_{2max}$), there is a need to ensure adequate muscle glycogen stores prior to hard (i.e. 'tempo', intervals, fartlek) running sessions. It takes approximately 4 hours for carbohydrate to be digested and absorbed into the muscles and liver as glycogen; therefore, wherever possible, pre-session meals should be consumed 4–5 hours prior to runs (Kerksick et al., 2017). Ingesting a light carbohydrate and protein snack ~1 hour prior to intense exercise may also be beneficial (Cade et al., 1991) and provides an option for those who train early in the morning. It is recommended that carbohydrate, protein and fluid intake is spread over the day, evenly spaced (every 3–4 hours) across 5–6 meals or snacks (Kerksick et al., 2018).

Low Carbohydrate–High Fat Diets

High-carbohydrate diets have been researched and recommended for endurance athletes for decades (e.g. Hyman, 1970; Brewer et al., 1988). However, there has been a growing interest in the use of low carbohydrate–high fat (or 'ketogenic') diets over the last 5–10 years (Burke, 2015). A ketogenic diet typically involves consuming < 5% of total energy intake from carbohydrate (<50 g·day^{-1}), 15–20% protein and 75–80% fat (Burke, 2020). High-fat diets (ketogenic and non-ketogenic) have been proposed to improve endurance performance by increasing fatty acid availability and decreasing glycogen utilisation (Volek et al., 2015). Studies have observed similar endurance capacity with high-carbohydrate and high-fat approaches when the exercise intensity remains low (60–70% of $\dot{V}O_{2max}$) (Phinney et al., 1983; Shaw et al., 2019). However, this intensity of exercise is far lower than most runners use during competitive events at all distances up to the marathon. Indeed, at higher intensities of exercise, performance and exercise economy appears to be impaired by following a high-fat diet (Havemann et al., 2006; Burke et al., 2017b) due to an decreased activation of glycogenolysis and the pyruvate dehydrogenase enzyme (Stellingwerff et al., 2006). Although high-intensity training and event performance may be compromised by following a ketogenic diet, there may be beneficial adaptations to fat metabolism by undertaking some training with low glycogen (Hulston et al., 2010). Therefore, an alternative approach is to manipulate dietary fat and carbohydrate within training phases and prior to competitions to take advantage of the potential benefits associated with both types of dietary approach (Burke et al., 2018).

BOX 4.2   CASE STUDY 1

Shelly is a 16-year-old female middle-distance runner who competed for her county last summer. She currently runs four times per week (two interval training sessions at her Athletics Club; one 45 min and one 60 min run both at moderate intensity) plus performs two 30 min strength and conditioning sessions each week. She attends college every day and has a busy social life. She is vegetarian but her parents are unsure whether she is eating a sufficiently healthy diet. Her body mass is relatively stable at 52 kg and her BMI is 20 kg·m^2. She has regular menstrual cycles and has not had any injuries in the last year.

Suggested weekday diet plan:

<u>Breakfast</u> (7:30 am)

Bran flakes (70 g) + semi-skimmed milk (200 ml) + tap water (250 ml)
Energy: 325 kcal, Carbohydrate: 56 g, Protein: 14 g, Fat: 5 g

Mid-Morning Snack (Whilst at College) (10:00 am)

Almonds (20 g) + Greek-style yoghurt (150 g) + tap water (250 ml)
Energy: 318 kcal, Carbohydrate: 8 g, Protein: 13 g, Fat: 26 g

Lunch (13:00 pm)

Red and white quinoa (210 g) + salad tomatoes (85 g) + cucumber (30 g) + 2 Tsp
hummus (~20 g) + baby spinach (80 g) + tap water (300 ml) + dried apricots (50 g)
Energy: 410 kcal, Carbohydrate: 63 g, Protein: 17 g, Fat: 10 g

Pre-Training Snack (16:00 pm)

Medium banana (~100 g) + tap water (300 ml)
Energy: 84 kcal, Carbohydrate: 20 g, Protein: 1 g, Fat: 0 g

17:00–18:00 pm Training

Post-Training Snack (18:30 pm)

Chocolate milk (300 ml) + 4 fig rolls (~84 g)
Energy: 521 kcal, Carbohydrate: 87 g, Protein: 14 g, Fat: 13 g

Dinner (19:30 pm)

Egg noodles (180 g) + tofu (45 g) + broccoli (45 g) + carrots (45 g) + edamame beans
(45 g) + sesame seeds (15 g) all fried in 1 Tsp sesame oil (~4 g) + tap water (500 ml)
Energy: 625 kcal, Carbohydrate: 69 g, Protein: 31 g, Fat: 25 g

Total Daily Breakdown of Key Nutrients

Energy: 2,283 kcal
Carbohydrate: 303 g (5.8 g·kg^{-1}, 53% energy intake), Protein: 90 g (1.7 g·kg^{-1}, 16%
of energy intake), Fat: 79 g (1.5 g·kg^{-1}, 31% of energy intake)
Calcium: 1420 mg, Iron: 30 mg, Zinc: 13 mg, Vitamin B$_{12}$: 4 µg, Vitamin C: 96 mg

BOX 4.3 CASE STUDY 2

Jim is a 54-year-old male recreational long-distance runner who has run six marathons
since he turned 50 years old. He is currently training for a major city marathon in 2
months and aims to break 5 hours. He runs most days and has built his long run back
up to 20 miles on a Sunday morning. Jim and his wife have two teenage children who
play sport most evenings. His full-time job is based in an office, but he often goes out

for the day with his family at weekends. He suffers from mild Achilles tendonitis, which some days prevents him from running. Jim feels he is quite lazy with what he currently eats and often binges on junk food after runs and in the evening. He is 180 cm tall and his current body mass is 75 kg (BMI of 23.1 kg·m²).

Suggested Sunday diet plan:

Breakfast (7:30 am)

> 70 g oats made with 200 ml semi-skimmed milk topped with 160 g strawberries & 2 tsp pumpkin seeds
> 300 ml beetroot juice
> 1 slice wholegrain toast + 1 tsp butter + 300 ml water
> *Energy: 730 kcal, Carbohydrate: 105 g, Protein: 25 g, Fat: 24 g*

9:30–11:30 am – two-hour training run

Post-Training Snack (11:30 am)

> Wholemeal bagel (100 g) + 1 tbsp crunchy peanut butter + 1 banana + 500 ml water
> *Energy: 468 kcal, Carbohydrate: 77 g, Protein: 18 g, Fat: 9 g*

Lunch (13:00 pm)

> Grilled chicken breast mini fillet (50 g cooked in 1 tsp rapeseed oil) + 300 g boiled basmati rice + 80 g boiled broccoli + 90 g boiled carrots + 500 ml water
> *Energy: 516 kcal, Carbohydrate: 87 g, Protein: 27 g, Fat: 7 g*

Mid-Afternoon Snack (16:00 pm)

> Ciabatta (90 g) filled with 1 thick slice of beef (20 g) + 40 g spinach + 1 tsp light mayonnaise + 300 ml water
> *Energy: 291 kcal, Carbohydrate: 44 g, Protein: 15 g, Fat: 6 g*

Dinner (18:30 pm)

> Grilled salmon fillet chunks (80 g cooked in 1 tsp rapeseed oil) + 300 g new potatoes with rosemary + 80 g boiled green beans + 85 g cannellini beans + 500 ml water
> *Energy: 534 kcal, Carbohydrate: 59 g, Protein: 31 g, Fat: 19 g*

Evening Snacks (21:00 pm)

> 90 g natural yoghurt + 140 g frozen mixed berries + 1 tbsp honey + 50 g granola + 30 g raisins
> Smoothie (100 g frozen pineapple, 1 orange, 200 ml semi-skimmed milk, ½ avocado)
> *Energy: 832 kcal, Carbohydrate: 122 g, Protein: 22 g, Fat: 28 g*

Total Daily Breakdown of Key Nutrients

Energy: 3,371 kcal
Carbohydrate: 494 g (6.6 g·kg^{-1}, 59% of energy intake), Protein: 138 g (1.8 g·kg^{-1},
  16% of energy intake), Fat: 93 g (1.2 g·kg^{-1}, 25% of energy intake)
Calcium: 1316 mg, Iron: 20 mg, Zinc: 10 mg, Vitamin B$_{12}$: 7 µg, Vitamin C: 335 mg

Periodised Nutrition

Periodised nutrition refers to "the planned, purposeful, and strategic use of specific nutritional interventions to enhance the adaptations targeted by individual exercise sessions or periodic training plans, or to obtain other effects that will enhance performance in the longer term" (Jeukendrup, 2017). In other words, periodised nutrition is the manipulation of an athlete's diet to best support training prescription and enhance adaptive processes (Stellingwerff et al., 2019). A detailed discussion of the various strategies and approaches to manipulating nutrient availability over the course of a competitive season and training/event week is beyond the scope of this chapter. Readers are referred to several excellent reviews (Jeukendrup, 2017; Burke et al., 2018; Stellingwerff et al., 2019) and case studies (Stellingwerff, 2012; Heikura et al., 2018a) that address this topical area of nutrition. Although all nutrients can be strategically periodised around a runner's training, environment and event/competition schedule, manipulation of the fuels that provide energy for exercise have naturally been the focus of most research in this area. Beyond the recommendations presented in Table 4.1 around high carbohydrate intake before training ('train high'), during competition and post-exercise, several acute interventions that involve reducing carbohydrate availability prior to exercise ('train low') have been investigated (Burke et al., 2018). A brief summary of the main strategies associated with manipulation of carbohydrate availability is provided in Table 4.3.

For long-distance runners preparing for events from the half-marathon to the ultra-marathon, preservation of liver and muscle glycogen stores should be considered part of the training adaptation process. Steady pace training sessions in a fasted or semi-depleted (lowered glycogen) state (the classic 'train low–compete high' approach) during the preparatory and building phases of training may support cellular and enzymatic adaptations associated with increased fat oxidation (Baar and McGee, 2008; Burke et al., 2018). These augmented adaptations may have important benefits for longer duration pace maintenance (as exercise intensity/race pace is typically lower in longer-duration events), particularly following acute glycogen replenishment. However, such practices require careful monitoring to avoid diet-related fatigue and/or immunosuppression.

The approaches described in Table 4.3 can be deliberately used over the course of a training week and mesocycle to ensure high-quality training and boost adaptation. Intuitively, runs above lactate threshold (i.e. 'tempo', intervals and fartlek) performed at a hard-severe intensity are heavily dependent upon carbohydrate, therefore a 'train high' approach would be best, whereas the 'train low' strategy is more suitable for runs where the intensity is below lactate threshold (i.e. medium- to long-duration recovery runs). For example, a high-intensity interval training session would be performed after consuming a carbohydrate-rich meal 4–5 hours prior ('train high'), but a long moderate-intensity run

TABLE 4.3 Common acute strategies associated with manipulation of carbohydrate availability to maximise training/event performance and augment training adaptation

Strategy	Description and method	Purported benefits
'Train high' – adequate carbohydrate availability	• Commence training with adequate muscle and liver glycogen. • Appropriate daily carbohydrate intake (pre- and post-exercise) and option for carbohydrate loading and in-exercise fuelling for long runs (see Table 4.1).	• Ensures intensity targets are met and/or long duration of exercise can be achieved. • Training the gut to avoid gastrointestinal issues.
'Recover high' – rapid carbohydrate refuelling post-exercise	• Intake of carbohydrate following a 'train high' or 'train low' session • 1.2 g·hour^{-1} in the 4 hours post-exercise (~1 g.kg BM^{-1} soon after exercise and repeated hourly) • See Table 4.1 and Chapter 17	• Maximises glycogen storage by taking advantage of increased synthesis following exercise. • Useful to promote glycogen stores for an upcoming session (in <8 hours)
'Train low' – low carbohydrate availability	• Train with low muscle glycogen levels achieved by performing 'double day' training where first run is used to deplete glycogen and second run (at moderate intensity) is performed later in day after minimal carbohydrate (high-fat meals/snacks)	• Activation of cellular signalling associated with mitochondrial adaptation
'Train low' – fasted	• Perform a moderate intensity run following an overnight fast (before breakfast) or >6 hours since last carbohydrate intake. • Consume no carbohydrate in session. • May also be undertaken as part of a 'recover low-train low' strategy or long-term ketogenic diet for added metabolic stress	• Increases metabolic stress during exercise encouraging adaptations associated with glycogen transport (from liver to muscles) and promotion of fat utilisation
'Recover low' – low carbohydrate intake post-exercise/ overnight	• Post-exercise recovery meals/snacks are low in carbohydrate (high-fat and protein) during recovery and/or prior to overnight sleep. • There may be a risk of compromising subsequent high-intensity training, bone health and immune function when carbohydrate is restricted post-run.	• Altered substrate availability post-exercise may enhance upregulation of cell signalling

Source: Jeukendrup (2017); Burke et al. (2018); Impey et al. (2018); Stellingwerff, Morton and Burke (2019).

Note: BM = body mass.

performed the following day could be completed with reduced carbohydrate availability ('train low'). The low glycogen state in the second session could have been achieved via a combination of 'sleep low', 'recover low' and a low daily carbohydrate intake (Stellingwerff et al., 2019).

Summary

Meeting the energy demands of training and event participation should be a major nutritional goal for all distance runners. All but the lowest intensities (60–65% $\dot{V}O_{2max}$) of aerobic exercise rely on carbohydrate as the primary fuel for maintaining ATP levels in skeletal muscle. Therefore, consumption of carbohydrate-rich meals and snacks that total 3–5 g·kg BM^{-1} each day for runners undertaking low volume (< 1 hour per day) training and 6–10 g·kg BM^{-1}·day^{-1} for those logging high volume (1–3 hours per day) of running, should prevent glycogen depletion. Runners should not attempt to remove fat from their diets; however, consumption of foods containing omega-3 fatty acids may need to be increased, and products containing 'trans fats' should be reduced. Low carbohydrate–high fat (ketogenic) diets are inadequate for supporting the fuelling needs of most runners; however, acute periods of low carbohydrate availability during moderate intensity runs ('train low') and recovery periods ('recover low') appears to have short-term utility and can augment training adaptation. Protein intake should be ~1.0–1.2 g·kg BM^{-1}·day^{-1} for recreational endurance runners, 1.2–1.5 g·kg BM^{-1}·day^{-1} for competitive runners engaging in daily moderate-hard training (~60 min), and 1.6–2.0 g·kg BM^{-1}·day^{-1} for elite endurance runners. Runners should aim to consume 5–6 meals/snacks evenly spaced throughout the day (every 3–4 hours) that contain a balance of nutrients and fluid to ensure a state of euhydration (~5–7 mL·kg^{-1}). In the 2 hours after exercise, carbohydrate consumed at a rate of 1.2 g·hour^{-1} and a protein intake of 0.25–0.30 g·kg BM^{-1} should adequately support recovery and adaptation processes. Runners should ensure they consume at least five portions of fruits and vegetables every day to ensure daily recommended intakes of vitamins and minerals are met.

5

PSYCHOLOGY OF DISTANCE RUNNING

Stacy Winter and Carla Meijen

Highlights

- Distance running is unique from a psychological perspective.
- Thoughts, feelings, and behaviours are interlinked and play an important role in distance running performance.
- The role of psychological factors: confidence, motivation, and emotions are discussed in relation to the demands of distance running.
- To facilitate these psychological factors, the evidence surrounding the use of psychological strategies in distance running is outlined.

Introduction

When it comes to middle- and long-distance running events, whether it is the 800 m or a marathon, psychology plays a major role. The psychological effects on performance can be explained through what we think, how we feel, and subsequently the way we behave. This is a cyclical process and a key component to consider is the way our thoughts, feelings, and behaviours are interlinked and influenced by our environment (Bandura, 1997). For example, at the start of a race, a distance runner may become aware of how many other runners there are around them, start to get worried about their positioning, and as a result abandon the conservative pacing strategy they had initially planned. Only minutes into the race, they can get upset and frustrated at themselves. Not having the right approach or mental preparation to deal with the demands of distance running can even lead to drop-out (Antonini et al., 2016). When considering the psychological impacts on endurance running, we therefore need to be aware of how our thoughts influence the decisions we make, as well as how we feel.

There are a wide array of psychological factors that can play a role in distance running. Endurance athletes may recognise the impact of their reasons for running, self-doubts in their ability, feeling nervous before a race, the difficulty in remaining focused when a session does not go as expected, worries about sticking to a race plan, or having thoughts around the urge to slow down or quit. To help manage the psychological factors of motivation, emotions, and self-belief, endurance athletes can draw on psychological strategies such as self-talk, imagery, attentional focus, and goal setting. In this chapter we will explain the role of these psychological factors and outline the evidence around the use of psychological strategies in distance running.

Psychological Factors

Endurance performance is unique from a psychological perspective (Meijen, 2019). A runner requires motivation to put in the training hours, there is a lot of time to think, and it will probably hurt at some stage. Having that much time to think can also provide fuel for self-doubt and other unwanted thoughts, or one might question their pacing strategy or reasons for doing the activity. The next section of this chapter will outline what we currently know about confidence, motivation, and emotions in distance runners.

Self-Belief in Distance Running

Self-belief is one of the important psychological factors that plays a role in distance running. Athletes may question 'Where does my confidence come from?' 'Who influences my self-belief?' and 'Why is it important for my performance?' Self-belief is represented by the psychological concept of self-efficacy (Bandura, 1997). Self-efficacy refers to a judgement about one's own perceived capabilities, or in simple terms, what a distance runner believes they can do. It is important to note that athletes do not possess a single self-efficacy belief; instead, they are dynamic and specific. Firstly, beliefs are dynamic, in that they can and do change based upon the information that is available to a distance runner. For example, beliefs are likely to change based upon how well training sessions have gone, feedback received from coaches, performances in races, and any setbacks experienced, e.g. injuries. Secondly, although typically focused on a task (e.g. running a 5 km), beliefs are specific, in that a distance runner may have a high belief in their ability to execute a race plan or sustain a tough pace, but lower levels of belief in their change of pace or finishing speed.

A distance runner's self-efficacy beliefs develop through the influence of four sources: past accomplishments, vicarious experiences, verbal persuasion, and physiological states (Bandura, 1997). Past accomplishments are the most powerful source and can come from a distance runner's perceptions of the volume and quality of work completed, trusting their training schedule, and success in races. Vicarious experiences are based around modelling from others; for example, observing a runner from the same training group (who the runner perceives to be of similar ability) achieve a personal best. The third source, verbal persuasion, can come either from within (see the section on self-talk later in this chapter) or from feedback and support from those with expertise and credibility to the distance runner (e.g. coaches and training partners). Finally, physiological states refers to perceptions of strength, fitness, pain, and fatigue appraised by the distance runner, in order to successfully meet the task at hand (Anstiss et al., 2018; Samson, 2014).

Efficacy beliefs are important, as they help shape the distance runner's behaviour and thought patterns. For example, athletes high in self-efficacy set themselves more challenging goals, exert greater effort to accomplish tasks, are willing to persevere when faced with difficulties, and experience more positive emotions (Feltz et al., 2008; Moritz et al., 2000). Shaping behaviour and thought patterns is where self-efficacy has been positively associated with sporting performance. However, as Sir Mo Farah highlighted: "It doesn't just come overnight, you've got to train for it and believe in yourself; that's the most important thing" (Abidi, 2012). It is therefore recommended to establish where a distance runner is currently getting their belief from and the subsequent influences on their performance. Novice runners, for example, will have fewer efficacy sources to draw upon compared to the elite distance runner, as these sources are developed and accumulated through a variety of experiences, both positive and negative (Anstiss et al., 2018). A novice runner will need to create an initial sense of belief and develop gradually, compared to the experienced distance runner whose focus could be on reinforcing and strengthening their efficacy beliefs. Psychological strategies can be adopted by both elite and novice distance runners for developing their self-efficacy and will be addressed later in this chapter.

Motivation

Motivation is about wanting (Baumeister, 2016), and what causes us to act in a certain way (Ryan and Deci, 2000). It is, however, not necessarily just about how much (quantity) motivation someone has, but also about the quality of motivation. A question to find out about the quality of a runner's motivation is 'What are the reasons that you take part in running?' or 'Why do you run?' Typically, answers vary from extrinsic factors such as 'I want to beat others', 'I want to win', 'I want to beat a time', 'I want to be faster', to intrinsic factors such as 'I enjoy the feeling and freedom of running' or, as stated by Haile Gebrselassie, "I love running and I will always run" (Quotetab.com, 2020). Self-determined types of motivation (or autonomous motivation), where the runner has more control over their motivation, are associated with more positive outcomes (Deci and Ryan, 2000; Goose and Winter, 2012), including lower perceived susceptibility to injury in marathon runners (Chalabaev et al., 2017). Examples of autonomous motivation are: (i) identified regulation, where a runner can identify with the reasons for doing a task, such as a tough weights lifting session; (ii) integrated regulation, where a runner values a task or a goal because it is meaningful to them; and (iii) intrinsic regulation, where a runner engages in a task for the pure enjoyment. Non-self-determined (or controlled) motivation relates to external regulation, where a runner performs a task because of an external demand, such as completing it for their coach or for an external reward. Finally, introjected regulation is where the athlete engages in a task because they would feel guilty or ashamed otherwise. Neither type of controlled motivation is particularly helpful for enjoyment and long-term engagement with the sport, although external rewards have been found to benefit performance (see McCormick et al., 2015, for a review).

It is also important to consider a distance runner's achievement goals, which represent how they define success from either a task or an ego orientation (Nicholls, 1984). A runner would be task oriented when their main focus is on the development of the self, irrespective of other runners. Whereas a runner would be ego oriented if their main focus was demonstrating superior performances to others. A task orientation has been associated with greater enjoyment, reported satisfaction, engaging in positive achievement, striving through effort, persistence, challenging task choices, and intrinsic motivation (Keegan, 2019). Conversely, an ego goal orientation has been associated with dysfunctional behaviours (e.g. effort withdrawal, low persistence, avoidance of moderately challenging tasks), self-serving attributions for outcomes, greater stress and anxiety, and a tendency towards morally unacceptable behaviours (Keegan, 2019). Furthermore, within training scenarios, high levels of task orientation have been associated with valuing practice and committing to it for development reasons, whereas high levels of ego orientation have been linked to endorsements of avoiding practice and preferring simply to compete (Roberts and Ommundsen, 1996). However, within the context of high-level sport, where a clear emphasis is placed on gaining the normative edge, Hodge and Petlichkoff (2000) found that athletes reported a complementary balance of both the desire to demonstrate superior abilities over others and to develop through personal mastery. It may therefore be suggested that a high ego orientation is not necessarily detrimental to the distance runner, as long as it is combined with a high task orientation.

Emotions

Emotions can also play a big role in distance running. A marathon, for example, can be a rollercoaster of emotions where a runner may experience nerves just before the start, excitement during the first couple of miles, and frustration or despair in the later stages. Emotions are a response to what is happening in the athlete's environment, or a response arising from thoughts in an athlete's mind (Lazarus, 2000). This can include anticipation of an upcoming race, as well as thoughts during and after events. When an athlete faces a demanding situation, like a county cross-country race with qualification for the national championships, they make a judgement of whether there is something at stake ('Is the situation important to me?'), if there is a potential for harm or benefit ('Is there a potential for the situation to help me achieve my goal?'), and what is at stake ('Does it influence my ego ideals, moral values, well-being?'). These judgements are combined with an evaluation of what resources an athlete perceives to have to cope with the demands of the situation, leading to the experience of emotions (Lazarus, 1999, 2000). Typically, when there is a potential for harm and the athlete does not feel that they have the resources to deal with the situation, they are likely to experience a negatively valanced emotion such as anxiety, frustration, despair, or anger. For an athlete, it is helpful to understand what influences their emotions, as these are likely to influence performance (Beedie et al., 2012).

When an athlete experiences an emotion, this can influence their behaviour and decision-making, such as pacing. For example, Paula Radcliffe mentioned: "You see with me, when I'm nervous, I smile and laugh" (Brainyquote, 2020). How athletes perceive and regulate their emotions is a relevant factor to consider. Some runners may perceive a negatively labelled emotion, such as anxiety or anger, to be helpful to performance; for example, feeling anxious before a race could be an athlete's optimal pre-performance state. Whereas other athletes will perceive anxiety to be unhelpful (Beedie et al., 2000; Robazza et al., 2008), resulting in behaviours such as holding back. Being aware of one's emotions and being able to regulate emotional states can influence running performance (Beedie et al., 2012; Rubaltelli et al., 2018). The awareness of which emotional states are helpful to an athlete's performance can be developed through reflective practice. This can help an athlete to engage in emotion regulation to move towards an optimal emotional state, which is beneficial not only to performance, but also to a runner's well-being. To help regulate emotions, runners have reported using goal-setting, recalling of previous accomplishments and how they feel afterwards (Stanley et al., 2012), emotional intelligence (Nicolas et al., 2019), and having a pacer. These have all been shown to benefit positive emotions within distance running (Fullerton et al., 2017).

Summary of Psychological Factors

Thoughts, behaviours, and feelings play a big role in distance running performance. We have specifically considered the psychological impacts of self-belief, motivation, and emotions to highlight the unique demands of endurance events. It is important to develop an awareness of how these psychological factors impact our thoughts, the decisions we make, how we feel, and subsequent behaviours because they can directly impact coach-athlete interactions, training sessions, and performances in races, in addition to athlete enjoyment, satisfaction, and well-being. We can, to an extent, influence these psychological factors through the use of psychological strategies. In the previous section we started to outline ways to facilitate psychological factors and manage the psychological demands of distance running. In the next section we will outline some of the strategies that can help push the psychological limits in running; these include self-talk, imagery, goal-setting, and attentional focus.

Psychological Strategies

Self-Talk

Runners may be familiar with having an internal dialogue, which can be statements you say to yourself out loud or inside your head. This internal dialogue can be automatic or strategic (Hardy, 2006). Automatic self-talk is an internal dialogue that is not planned or prepared, and there is not always an awareness of this dialogue. Whereas strategic self-talk relates to planned statements that serve a purpose to achieve a goal. Using self-talk in a strategic manner has positive outcomes, as it can benefit confidence (Hatzigeorgiadis et al., 2009), emotional states (Lane et al., 2016), pain management, motivation, perceived effort (Blanchfield et al., 2014; Hatzigeorgiadis et al., 2018) and attentional focus (Van Raalte et al., 2015), as well as performance (Barwood et al., 2015). When using strategic self-talk, the distance runner can choose between instructional and motivational types. Instructional self-talk includes statements that focus on technique or form ('Run tall'), tactics (how to pace a race; 'Start steady'), or how to direct attention ('Pay attention where the course gets slippery' in cross-country). Motivational statements can be used to facilitate confidence ('I can do this') and for motivational reasons such as putting in effort ('Try hard!') and psyching yourself up. Ryan Hall provides a great example of the motivational self-talk he uses: "I just tell myself over and over again: You're doing great" (Lobby Havey, 2020). It is helpful to distinguish between these two types of self-talk so runners can be more strategic and specific in their use, and adapt the self-talk according to their needs, rather than rely on one or two general recurring self-talk statements.

Distance runners can develop self-talk plans through the 'IMPACT' approach (McCormick and Hatzigeorgiadis, 2019). This approach works through six steps: (1) identify what you want to achieve, (2) match your self-talk to your needs (considering the type of self-talk, whether instructional or motivational), (3) practice cues with consistency, (4) ascertain which cues work best for you, (5) create specific self-talk plans, and (6) train self-talk plans to perfection. In essence, this approach encourages distance runners to reflect on what they want to achieve and adjust their self-talk accordingly. Throughout this process, it is recommended that different self-talk statements for different parts of a race or training session are identified; for example, in the early stages of a race, a runner might want to focus on their pace and use an instructional self-talk statement ('Focus on my own race'), and for the later stages, a motivational statement such as 'Dig deep' can be helpful. Adapting your self-talk is important, considering that internal dialogues change when the intensity of the exercise increases (Aitchison et al., 2013). When ascertaining which cues/self-talk work best, ensure to notice your self-talk and the effects it has. When practicing different statements, reflect on what is useful and practice in training first. It may take some time to master self-talk plans, which is why there may not be an immediate performance effect. For example, McCormick et al. (2018) did not find an immediate effect of motivational self-talk on ultra-marathon performance, but they found that runners were still using the self-talk strategies after 6 months. The effect of self-talk may also relate to the psychological factors previously covered in this chapter, such as positive emotions, confidence, or improved quality of motivation. Finally, when developing self-talk statements, it is useful to keep them brief and memorable, and to ensure the statements feel right for you and have a motivational or instructional purpose (McCormick and Hatzigeorgiadis, 2019).

Imagery

Imagery is a popular psychological strategy used by athletes across all distance running events. It is defined as: "Using all the senses to re-create or create an experience in the mind" (Vealey and Greenleaf, 2006, p. 248). The most important thing with imagery is using multiple senses, such as what an athlete sees (visual), smells (olfactory), feels (kinaesthetic), and hears (auditory). For example, a distance runner can see where other athletes are around them, smell the fresh air, hear the crowd cheering, and feel their legs striding strongly. From using as many senses as possible, the athlete can imagine an upcoming race or use imagery to reflect back on a previous successful race or training session.

Athletes can choose from two different perspectives when using imagery. Internal (first-person perspective) is when a distance runner would see the image from inside their body, the way their eyes would normally see the situation. Whereas external (third-person perspective) is seeing an image from outside their body, as if viewing themselves on video footage. Athletes have successfully used both imagery perspectives for a number of different reasons, which can be linked to the previously discussed psychological factors in this chapter (Martin et al., 1999). An example is focus of attention, by imagining the correct running technique or execution of a race plan. It can aid drive and commitment by imagining a specific setting that is highly motivating (e.g. standing on a podium receiving a medal). Self-belief can be enhanced through imagining past accomplishments and coping with situations the athlete perceives as challenging, helping them prepare for any race scenario. Finally, images designed to induce relaxation or increase arousal can be used by the athlete to reach their ideal pre-race performance state.

Imagery, just like physical performance, is considered to be a collection of skills that can be improved with practice and experience. The extent to which distance runners can benefit from imagery depends on their ability to create vivid images and control them in a desired way (Vealey and Greenleaf, 2006). For example, some athletes may initially have very blurry images or are able to hold an image in their mind for only a few seconds. The more runners practice their imagery, the more skilful they will become in producing clear, multisensory, and controllable images. To aid the effectiveness of using imagery, the PETTLEP model (Holmes and Collins, 2001) was developed. Each letter of the PETTLEP acronym relates to an element of the real-life situation: Physical, Environmental, Task, Timing, Learning, Emotional, and

Perspective. The authors of PETTLEP conceptualise actual physical performance and imagery on a continuum (Holmes and Collins, 2001). The closer towards the physical end of the continuum, the more effective imagery is likely to be.

Eluid Kipchoge was noted as saying: "Sometimes I dream of running fast and being beaten on the line, then I wake up and realise it was a dream" (Phillips, 2018). Although this quote indicates it was a dream, PETTLEP guidelines can be applied to his real-life scenario of preparing to break the two-hour mark for the marathon distance. For example, Eluid Kipchoge could purposefully imagine his marathon pacing strategy (Task), wearing his racing attire (Physical), using video footage to stimulate vivid details of the Vienna course (Environment), the 4.34 min per mile pace (Timing), incorporating his responses (Emotional), and viewing this internally from what his eyes would see, e.g. the car, projected laser beams, and pacers around him (first-person Perspective). The final recommendation from the PETTLEP model, is that as any Learning takes place, the athlete should update their imagery accordingly to reflect this (Wakefield and Smith, 2012; Williams et al., 2013).

Goal-Setting

Goal-setting has consistently been demonstrated as one of the most effective human behaviour techniques, which both coaches and athletes can employ: "It's so motivating to have goals to aim for and achieve; it gets you out of the door when you might be having second thoughts" (Jo Pavey, timeoutdoors.com, 2020). Specifically, goals can fuel motivation, by encouraging persistence in the pursuit of a runner's aims and helping to direct their attention (Tenenbaum et al., 1999). For example, if a runner has set themselves a goal of decreasing their 1 km repetition time, this may help them focus on what is required, and promote intensity and effort to achieve this outcome. Across all sports, a distinction is made to three types of goals: outcome, performance, and process (Burton et al., 2010). Outcome goals focus on achieving a desired result often at the end of a race, such as finishing in the top three. An athlete is not in total control of reaching their outcome goal, since it depends, at least in part, on the performance of opponents. Performance goals refer to an athlete's individual performance in relation to their own standard of excellence, such as a particular time-based goal or achieving a personal best. An athlete has greater control of achieving a performance goal because other athletes do not directly affect the goal's attainment. Process goals are concerned with how an athlete performs a particular skill, displays a certain technique, or carries out a specific strategy, such as focusing on foot strike, posture, or stride length. These types of goals are directly within the athlete's control. Process goals are especially important, as performance and outcome goals fail to focus on preparing the runner for difficulties that could be encountered. Runners may feel dejected if they are far away from the time-based goal they were looking to achieve, or surprised if it's going much better than expected.

It is recommended that distance runners set all three types of goals for motivational purposes, with an emphasis on performance and process goals to direct attention and positively affect behaviour (Burton et al., 2010). Given the large amount of time athletes spend running, it is important that performance and process goals are set for training scenarios as well as races. Setting goals alone though does not ensure they will impact changes in behaviour and subsequent improvements in performance (Weinberg, 2010). Table 5.1 shows six goal-setting principles that are tailored to a distance runner.

TABLE 5.1 The six principles of effective goal setting for distance runners

Principle	Description
Set specific, measurable goals (Schweickle et al., 2017)	One of the reasons that goals need to be specific is that they also need to be measurable, so that you will know you are making progress towards achieving them. For example, setting the goal of becoming faster or 'Do your best' would not be as helpful as taking 1 minute off your personal best 10 km time within the next 12 weeks.
Make goals challenging, but realistic (Gollwitzer & Oettingen, 2019).	If goals are too easy, you can become complacent because you may feel you can reach the goal without great effort. Conversely, if a goal is too difficult, this can result in failure to attain goals and subsequent feelings of defeat, lack of motivation, and lowered belief in oneself. It is therefore important to assess an athlete's current capabilities, to keep goals realistic, while suitably driving them to reach their respective challenging goals.
Use short- and long-term goals (Kingston & Wilson, 2009).	Long-term goals can provide you with direction and act as dream goals, whereas short-term goals help focus on small improvements. In combination, short-term goals can make a long-term goal seem more achievable by breaking it up into more manageable steps and giving the distance runner a good indication of the progress that they are making.
Write goals down (Weinberg et al., 2019).	To demonstrate commitment to goals, writing them down and displaying them in a prominent place ensures they stay visible and current in your mind.
Develop plans to reach goals (Burton & Weiss, 2008).	Going back to the previous example of taking 1 minute off your personal best 10 km time, this is less likely to happen unless you actively pursue ways of developing new strategies to enhance performance. A key question to ask is: 'What do I need to do to reach my goals?' and identify and incorporate appropriate strategies into training to achieve them.
Evaluate goals (Donovan & Williams, 2003).	Goals are a starting point and should be re-evaluated on a regular basis. For example, you may be exceeding your original goals, and therefore goals should be made more difficult. Conversely, due to, say, injury, it is possible that you may not be near to reaching your goals, so they need to be adjusted. This frequent evaluation will ensure goals remain realistic but challenging and help distance runners keep optimally motivated as they strive to achieve their goals.

Attentional Focus

Finally, how we focus our attention is helpful to consider when distance running. There are different ways of focusing your attention, such as focusing on how the run feels, the weather conditions, pacemakers, or opponents. This is important to consider, as throughout a run a distance runner can adapt their attentional style to optimise performance. Traditionally, a distinction was made between associative (focusing thoughts on bodily sensations) and dissociative (focusing thoughts on external distractions to move attention away from the task) strategies (Morgan and Pollock, 1977), but this has been seen as overly simplistic. More recently, Brick et al. (2014) introduced a five-category model of attentional focus where they identified three categories for associative focus (active self-regulation, internal sensory monitoring, and outward monitoring) and two categories for dissociative focus (active distraction and involuntary distraction). When a runner engages in active self-regulation, their thoughts focus on relaxing their body, their technique, rhythm, or their pacing strategy. Internal sensory monitoring includes focusing on breathing, how the body feels, and muscle tiredness. Whereas a runner who uses outward monitoring focuses on environmental information that is relevant to them, including mile markers, competitors, and split times. A dissociative focus can be involuntary, where a runner distracts themselves by the scenery or irrelevant daydreams. Or it can be active, where the runner's focus is on task-irrelevant thoughts such as talking to others during a run or attending to a task such as planning the interior redecorating of a house in your mind.

Being aware of these five categories is relevant because strategically focusing your attention in a specific way can influence feelings and benefit various aspects of running (Brick et al., 2019). Laura Muir made an interesting distinction between training and racing, regarding her attentional focus: "With training you can get away with it – you know what splits you have to do, so you can just get on with it. But when it comes to racing you need to be really switched on" (Ingle, 2018). Therefore, it is helpful to consider what the context, goal, or aim is when directing your attention. Is it to optimise your pacing, to help reduce anxiety, to develop your running rhythm, or to deal with pain and discomfort? Consider making a plan beforehand, when a particular attentional strategy may be useful. For example, focusing on bodily sensations such as tense shoulders or breathing can help to inform pacing decisions when you are going too fast or too slow. However, focusing too much on bodily sensations throughout a run can increase the perceived effort of a run. A focus on technique can be helpful in situations where a task is difficult or when a runner is fatigued (Samson et al., 2017). Conversely, it is important to note that focusing too much on breathing or technique can interfere with automated running processes and running economy (Schücker et al., 2014; Winter et al., 2014). The act of (periodic) smiling, an active self-regulation strategy, has been found to be useful to help reduce perceived effort and improve running economy (Brick et al., 2018). Voluntary and involuntary distraction can be useful to help distract from painful sensations when the run feels hard, but this can interfere with running fast and can lead to ignoring warning signals of injury. Outward monitoring can be helpful when it comes to pacing, such as being aware of the weather conditions and when one might encounter a head or tailwind, or a twisty section of a cross-country course.

To help integrate these attentional strategies, the first step is to become aware of the various demands of the run, the second step is to identify which attentional strategy would be suitable for these demands, and finally, the athlete can draw upon psychological strategies such as self-talk and imagery to aid switching attentional focus during the distance run.

Summary

Within this chapter we have considered the psychological impacts on distance running and the importance of being aware of how thoughts influence decisions we make, how we feel, and subsequent behaviours. A wide array of psychological factors can play a role in distance running. The role of self-belief, motivation, and emotions were specifically discussed to highlight the unique demands of endurance events and how impactful these psychological factors can be. To facilitate these psychological factors, the evidence around the use of the psychological strategies (self-talk, imagery, goal setting, and attentional focus) in distance running were outlined. To help push the psychological limits in running, these strategies target thoughts, feelings, and behaviours within an endurance setting, influencing the way a distance runner functions or performs. The psychological strategies we have outlined can benefit distance runners from all age groups and experience levels.

You may consider working with a qualified sport psychologist who can assess your specific psychological needs and educate you on the psychological factors and corresponding strategies you could employ. Not only will these strategies be aimed at changing thoughts, feelings, and behaviours impacting distance runner performance, but they may also have a long-term effect on an athlete's perception, which will change how they approach future situations. Finally, we would recommend distance runners practice using the psychological strategies of self-talk, imagery, goal-setting, and attentional focus before and during their runs and training sessions, before adopting a strategy within a competitive scenario. This will allow familiarisation with the psychological strategy, and any modifications required to suit the individual distance runner can be applied before implementing the strategy into a race.

PART II
Training and Event Considerations

6

PHYSIOLOGICAL ASSESSMENT OF MIDDLE- AND LONG-DISTANCE RUNNERS

Andy Galbraith

Highlights

- Assessment options exist for the physiological evaluation of a wide range of laboratory and field-based parameters.
- Laboratory-based physiological assessment should include maximal oxygen uptake ($\dot{V}O_{2max}$), running economy (RE), lactate threshold (LT) and the velocity associated with $\dot{V}O_{2max}$ (v-$\dot{V}O_{2max}$).
- Field-based physiological assessment should include critical speed (CS), the maximum distance that can be achieved at speeds above critical speed (D') and the anaerobic speed reserve (ASR).
- This test battery covers the key determinants which explain differences between athletes in distance running performance.

Introduction

Within medical terminology, a physiological assessment refers to examination into the functioning state of the human body. It follows therefore, that within exercise science terminology, a physiological assessment can be defined as investigation into how the body's various physiological systems respond and adapt to exercise. Following on from Chapter 1, the objectives of this chapter are to describe a battery of valid tests that assess the main physiological determinants of middle- and long-distance running performance, provide reference values for interpretation of test results, and outline how test data can be used to inform training prescription.

Purpose and Benefits

The endeavour for continued performance improvement by athletes highlights the need to recognise mechanisms to optimise athletes' training. Whilst physiological assessments may be conducted for a variety of reasons, a commonly cited rationale for their use includes providing an evaluation of strengths and weakness of the athlete. Such information can then inform training program design, including prescription of individualised optimal training intensities.

Physiological assessment of an athlete may also be useful to monitor and assess the effectiveness of training programmes to understand whether performance is improving, and the associated physiological adaptations are occurring. It has also been suggested an additional benefit of physiological testing for an athlete is that the prospect of regular testing, built into their schedule, may often act as a further motivational influence during a training cycle.

Repeatability of Measures

For data gleaned from physiological testing to be of value to the athlete and coach, it is important that the tests chosen to form part of such assessments are reproducible. This necessitates understanding the extent to which an apparent change in a measure is meaningful and does not lie within the confidence interval for error (Atkinson and Nevill, 1998). Variability in measures of performance can be attributed to technical and biological sources. Technical sources refer to the precision of the instruments utilised, combined with the ability of the tester to operate the equipment efficiently. Biological sources of error within performance tests include cyclic biological variation and motivational changes, which may contribute to small day-to-day variations in test performance of an athlete (Atkinson and Nevill, 1998). A clear understanding of the repeatability of a performance test is important prior to data interpretation. Changes in physiological measures over time may often be small, particularly when working with highly trained athletes; therefore, it is important that a performance test is both sensitive and repeatable, in order to ensure small changes in performance are not masked.

Pre-Test Considerations

In order to minimise the impact of biological sources of error within a performance test, a consistent pre-test routine is important prior to all repeat visits. Where possible, athletes should standardise the time and type of training sessions within the preceding 24 hours of a performance test. Ideally, training within this timeframe should be light recovery-type training. Athletes should avoid fundamental changes to their diet in the days prior to testing and are typically advised to eat no food in the 3 hours before a test. However, it is important that athletes consume adequate fluid in the 12 hours prior to testing. Footwear becomes an important consideration when working with middle- and long-distance runners. Shoes of varying mass may influence the economy of the athlete, therefore influencing the oxygen cost during running (Fuller et al., 2015). Consequently, athletes should be advised to wear the same (or similar) type of shoe for each test session. Environmental conditions should be recorded, with the aim of standardising (as much as possible) conditions across repeat test visits. Finally, an athlete's familiarisation with the test protocols will influence the repeatability of their performance. Therefore, one or more familiarisation sessions should be considered prior to recording test performances.

Laboratory-Based Testing

When conducting a physiological assessment for an athlete, laboratory-based testing provides the opportunity to ensure a greater level of precision. Environmental conditions can be controlled and replicated, whilst calibrated treadmills offer a consistent velocity at each visit. Consequently, the repeatability of laboratory-based physiological assessments has the potential to be high, increasing the sensitivity of such tests to detect small changes in an athlete's performance. However, physiological assessment in a laboratory setting takes place in an environment unfamiliar to most athletes.

Field-Based Testing

For the purpose of this chapter, field testing is defined as tests conducted outside the laboratory environment and do not require specialised equipment for data collection or recording (Maud and Foster, 2006). Physiological assessments should endeavour to closely replicate the athlete's typical exercise conditions. Consequently, field testing is often described as having a higher level of ecological validity than laboratory-based testing (Galbraith et al., 2011). Accordingly, physiological testing conducted in the field may help bridge the gap between the sport scientist, athlete and coach, where field-test protocols better reflect conditions which athletes experience during training and competition (Foster et al., 2006). It has also been suggested that as field testing occurs in the athlete's natural training/competition environment, the sense of 'missing out' on training, by participating in the physiological test, may be reduced. Notwithstanding these advantages, field testing creates distinctive challenges for the sport scientist.

Frequency of Testing

Typically, repeat physiological assessments with middle- and long-distance runners would be scheduled approximately every 3 months, typically around October, January, April and July, to correspond with key transitions in an athlete's seasonal training and competition schedule (Jones, 1998; Galbraith et al., 2014a). However, with the development of field-based test protocols, there is the opportunity for more frequent test points within a training cycle.

Laboratory-Based Physiological Assessment

Assessment options exist for a wide range of laboratory-based physiological parameters which influence middle- and long-distance running performance. This section will focus on three key determinants which have been shown to explain differences between athletes in distance running performance; Maximal oxygen uptake ($\dot{V}O_{2max}$), running economy (RE), and lactate threshold (LT). $\dot{V}O_{2max}$ characterises an individual's maximal rate of aerobic energy expenditure (Jones and Carter, 2000). RE describes the oxygen uptake or energy expenditure required at a given absolute exercise intensity, for example the oxygen uptake required for an athlete to run at 16 km·h^{-1}. The function of $\dot{V}O_{2max}$ and RE generates the velocity associated with $\dot{V}O_{2max}$ (v-$\dot{V}O_{2max}$). LT is a parameter with numerous definitions attached to it, which can present some confusion for the scientific and endurance running communities. In its simplest terms, LT is defined here as the exercise intensity corresponding to the first increase in blood lactate above resting levels (Jones and Carter, 2000).

Assessment Techniques ($\dot{V}O_{2max}$, RE, LT, v-$\dot{V}O_{2max}$)

This chapter adopts the treadmill protocol described by Jones (2006b), which has been used to monitor highly trained middle- and long-distance runners (Jones, 1998, 2006b; Galbraith et al., 2014a). This test has the advantage of enabling the measurement and recording of $\dot{V}O_{2max}$, RE, LT and v-$\dot{V}O_{2max}$ within the same test protocol.

Athletes should be allowed time to complete a self-selected warm-up, which should closely replicate the warm-up routine they use before a typical training session. Prior to the test, the athlete's body mass and stature should be recorded, along with a fingertip capillary blood sample, to determine resting blood lactate concentration.

The treadmill test is administered in two parts:

> *Sub-maximal test*: the first part is a sub-maximal test, using a treadmill gradient of 1% (Jones and Doust, 1996). The initial treadmill belt speed for this phase of the test should be decided individually for each athlete, based on their current fitness level, with the aim of completing 5 to 9 stages during the sub-maximal phase of the test. Typically, the penultimate phase of the test usually equates to a velocity equivalent to that which the athlete can hold during a 60 min hard run. Therefore, the velocity of the penultimate stage may be close to 10-mile or half-marathon race pace, depending on the ability of the athlete. Each stage of the test should be 4 min in duration; however, with highly trained athletes it has been suggested that 3-min stages are appropriate, due to a faster time to achieve a steady state of oxygen consumption within each stage (Jones, 2006a). The treadmill belt speed should be increased by 1.0 km·h^{-1} at the end of each stage; however, for an increased sensitivity of LT determination, 0.5 km·h^{-1} increments may be appropriate (Jones, 2006a). Average heart rate during the final 30 seconds of each stage should be recorded. At the end of each 4-min stage, a capillary blood is collected and, if required, perceived level of exertion using the Borg 6-to-20 scale (Borg, 1998). The sub-maximal test should be terminated when a second breakpoint in blood lactate has been observed (see the interpretation section that follows). Typically, once the participant's blood lactate concentration has normally exceeded 4.0 mmol·L^{-1}, this will have been achieved. Throughout the test, continuous breath-by-breath measurement of the athlete's expired gases should be collected. An active recovery in the region of 10–15 min should follow the termination of the sub-maximal test, prior to the athlete continuing into the second phase of the treadmill test.
>
> *Maximal test*: the second phase of the test is used to determine $\dot{V}O_{2max}$ and the velocity at $\dot{V}O_{2max}$ (v-$\dot{V}O_{2max}$). This test should be started at a 1% gradient and a velocity 2.0 km·h^{-1} below the velocity at which the participant finished the first phase of the test. The treadmill velocity should remain constant throughout this phase of the test, with the treadmill gradient increased by 1% every minute until the participant reaches volitional exhaustion. Throughout the test, continuous breath-by-breath measurement of the athlete's expired gases should be collected, and upon test termination, maximum heart rate recorded.

Maximal Oxygen Uptake ($\dot{V}O_{2max}$)

Interpretation of Test Results and Normative Data

Several methods have been suggested for the calculation of $\dot{V}O_{2max}$. However, when utilising breath-by-breath expired air analysis, a simple method is to report the highest $\dot{V}O_2$ achieved during the test, using a rolling 1-min average (Galbraith et al., 2014a).

Absolute values for $\dot{V}O_{2max}$ are reported in units of L·min^{-1}, however as measures of performance are influenced by the size of the body, a scaled adjustment of the absolute value is common. Traditionally, $\dot{V}O_{2max}$ is scaled to whole body mass in units of $mL\cdot kg^{-1}\cdot min^{-1}$, providing a useful method for comparison of $\dot{V}O_{2max}$ between different athletes. However, a meta-analysis by Lolli et al. (2017) provided evidence against the normalisation of $\dot{V}O_{2max}$ to whole body mass and highlighted the validity of normalising to fat-free mass.

An athlete's $\dot{V}O_{2max}$ score from the treadmill test can be compared to normative data for $\dot{V}O_{2max}$, such as those presented in Table 6.1. This can provide an indication of strengths or weakness within this area, which may then inform future training program design. During repeat assessments, an athlete's $\dot{V}O_{2max}$ score from the treadmill test can be compared to previous scores from the same athlete, providing a useful method to monitor the effectiveness of training programmes and assess whether any adaptation to $\dot{V}O_{2max}$ is occurring.

Application of Test Data

In highly trained runners, it has been suggested that $\dot{V}O_{2max}$ will eventually stabilise, with any further performance improvements, attributed to sustained development of RE and LT. For example, Billat et al. (1999) reported no change in $\dot{V}O_{2max}$, following a 9-week period of endurance training, in a group of highly trained distance runners (mean $\dot{V}O_{2max}$ >

TABLE 6.1 Normative data for $\dot{V}O_{2max}$ ($mL\cdot kg^{-1}\cdot min^{-1}$) for male and female distance runners

	Generalised	Event Specific					
	Middle/Long Distance	800 m	1500 m	5000 m	10,000 m	800–5000 m	10,000 m– Marathon
MALE							
Rabadán et al. (2011)		63.9 ± 3.4 (n = 17)	67.4 ± 4.7 (n = 23)	71.4 ± 3.9 (n = 20)	71.8 ± 6.7 (n = 12)		
Morgan and Daniels (1994)					75.8 ± 3.4 (n = 22)		
Ingham et al. (2008b)		72.4 ± 6.1 (n = 15)	73.3 ± 4.5 (n = 15)				
Smith et al. (2000)						65–80	65–80
Jones (2006a)	65–80						
Galbraith et al. (2014a)	72.5 ± 6.0 (n = 14)						
FEMALE							
Ingham et al. (2008b)		61.6 ± 4.7 (n = 16)	65.2 ± 3.5 (n = 16)				
Smith et al. (2000)						55–65	55–70
Jones (2006a)	55–70						

Note: Values are based on data collected from highly trained runners.

70 mL·kg^{-1}·min^{-1}). Furthermore, Martin et al. (1986) evaluated nine highly trained male distance runners (mean $\dot{V}O_{2max}$ > 70 mL·kg^{-1}·min^{-1}) over a 30-month period, during their preparation for Olympic trials. Across ten repeat treadmill tests, data highlighted no significant change in $\dot{V}O_{2max}$ during this monitoring period, whilst anaerobic threshold increased by 5.6%. In addition, Jones (1998) report no increase in $\dot{V}O_{2max}$ (actually a slight decrease) across a 5-year monitoring period in a world-class female distance runner. However, in contrast Galbraith et al. (2014a) reported a ~5% increase in VO_{2max} following a 1-year period of endurance training in highly trained distance runners (mean $\dot{V}O_{2max}$ > 70 mL·kg^{-1}·min^{-1}). In recreationally trained athletes, $\dot{V}O_{2max}$ improvements of 5–10% have been observed following a 6-week programme (Franch et al., 1998; Carter et al., 1999).

Londeree (1986) used data from elite middle- and long-distance runners to estimate the percentage of $\dot{V}O_{2max}$ that can be maintained for various periods of time. Using these data, it can be estimated that, in highly trained athletes, an 800 m race will require the energetic equivalent of ~120% $\dot{V}O_{2max}$, the 1500 m ~ 110% $\dot{V}O_{2max}$, 5000 m ~96% $\dot{V}O_{2max}$, 10,000 m ~92% $\dot{V}O_{2max}$ and the marathon ~ 85% $\dot{V}O_{2max}$ (Jones, 2006a). Whilst $\dot{V}O_{2max}$ is an important determinant of success for all distance running events, these data highlight that as the competitive distance increases, sub-maximal physiological measures, such as RE and LT, may increase in importance.

Running Economy

Interpretation of Test Results and Normative Data

Reporting the oxygen cost from the treadmill test at a set speed may not provide a fair comparison across athletes of different ages and abilities, therefore it may be useful that RE is calculated over the range of sub-maximal velocities used during the first phase of the treadmill test, by recording the average $\dot{V}O_2$ (mL·kg^{-1}·min^{-1}) for the last minute of each steady-state stage (Galbraith et al., 2014a). Alternatively, reporting the RE at LT speed may provide useful comparisons. Barnes and Kilding (2015a) provide comprehensive normative running economy data for male and female runners of varying ability levels. According to these data:

> Recreationally trained runners at 12 km·h^{-1} report a mean RE of 42.2 mL·kg^{-1}·min^{-1} (range 40.4–45.3) for males and a mean of 43.2 mL·kg^{-1}·min^{-1} (range 38.5–48.1) for females.
>
> Moderately trained runners at 14 km·h^{-1} report a mean RE of 46.8 mL·kg^{-1}·min^{-1} (range 42.0–55.5) for males and a mean of 47.9 mL·kg^{-1}·min^{-1} (range 41.3–53.5) for females.
>
> Highly trained runners at 16 km·h^{-1} report a mean RE of 50.6 mL·kg^{-1}·min^{-1} (range 40.5–66.8) for males and a mean of 54.5 mL·kg^{-1}·min^{-1} (range 46.2–61.9) for females.
> RE can also be reported in units of mL·kg^{-1}·km^{-1}, by inputting the average $\dot{V}O_2$ at the chosen intensity into the following equation (Jones, 2006a):
>
> $$RE\ (mL·kg^{-1}·km^{-1}) = \dot{V}O_2\ mL·kg^{-1}·min^{-1} / (speed\ km·h^{-1} / 60)$$

Normative data for RE in these measurement units have been reported by Jones (2006a) as:

Excellent:	170–180 mL·kg^{-1}·km^{-1}
Very Good:	180–190 mL·kg^{-1}·km^{-1}
Above Average:	190–200 mL·kg^{-1}·km^{-1}
Below Average:	200–210 mL·kg^{-1}·km^{-1}
Poor:	210–220 mL·kg^{-1}·km^{-1}

Finally, RE can be presented as the energy cost of running (rather than the oxygen cost), reported in units of kcal·kg^{-1}·km^{-1} or kJ·kg^{-1}·km^{-1}. Shaw et al. (2014) suggest this provides a more valid index of RE and suggest using the updated nonprotein respiratory quotient equations of Peronnet and Massicotte (1991) to estimate substrate use (g.min^{-1}) during the final minute of each stage. Subsequently, the energy derived from each substrate can be calculated by multiplying fat and carbohydrate usage by 9.75 (40.81) and 4.07 (17.04) kcal (kJ) respectively and presenting RE as the sum of these values, expressed in kcal·kg^{-1}·km^{-1} or kJ·kg^{-1}·km^{-1}.

Normative data for RE reported in kcal·kg^{-1}·km^{-1} are provided by Shaw et al. (2014) who reported data from a sample of 172 highly trained male and female middle/long-distance runners. Data were reported across four speeds ranging from 12.4 to 15.4 km·h^{-1} for females and 13.8 to 16.8 km·h^{-1} for males. RE increased at each speed, with mean values ranging from ~1.14 to 1.18 kcal·kg^{-1}·km^{-1} (4.77 to 4.94 kJ·kg^{-1}·km^{-1}) on average across the four speeds for the subject group. Similar data have been reported by Galbraith et al. (2014a) in a group of highly trained male athletes, with RE values between 1.13 and 1.17 kcal·kg^{-1}·km^{-1} (4.73–4.94 kJ·kg^{-1}·km^{-1}).

Scaling of RE data to an exponent of body mass (BM) is common, with a comprehensive analysis of 172 distance runners by Shaw et al. (2014), reporting that linear scaling of RE to BM^{-1} appeared to be the most appropriate method to remove the influence of body mass on RE in endurance runners.

Application of Test Data

The degree of change in RE following a period of endurance training will depend on the initial fitness level of the individual, with greater scope for a higher magnitude improvement in less highly trained individuals. However high magnitude improvements in RE, following a longitudinal period of endurance training, have still been reported in highly trained individuals, with Jones (1998) reporting a gradual improvement of RE across a 5-year period in a highly trained female distance runner, with values improving from ~200 mL·kg^{-1}·km^{-1} to ~180 mL·kg^{-1}·km^{-1}. The majority of research investigating changes in RE following training has been conducted over relatively short durations (~6–8 weeks). Where already trained runners are concerned, a short period of 'normal' endurance training appears to have little effect on RE (Paavolainen et al., 1999a; Spurrs et al., 2003; Johnston et al., 1997; Turner et al., 2003). However, improvements in running economy can sometimes be observed with short-term training programmes in less-trained individuals. In a recent study, Jones et al. (1999) reported that a 6-week endurance training programme, consisting of continuous and interval running at a speed close to LT, caused a significant improvement in running economy in recreationally active students, with values improving from ~195 mL·kg^{-1}·km^{-1} to ~180 mL·kg^{-1}·km^{-1}. In already-trained runners, it would appear that an additional stimulus above that of typical training is needed in order to generate a short-term improvement in RE. The addition of high-intensity interval running training demonstrated improvements of ~3–7% in RE over the course of a 6- to 8-week training period (Billat et al., 1999; Laffite et al., 2003; Franch et al., 1998; Yoshida et al., 1990). Whilst the addition of explosive strength/plyometric training has been shown to produce ~2–7% improvement in RE across a 6- to 9-week training period (Paavolainen et al., 1999a; Spurrs et al., 2003; Turner et al., 2003).

An improvement in RE will result in the utilisation of a lower percentage of $\dot{V}O_{2max}$ for any given exercise intensity. To put this into context, an athlete with a $\dot{V}O_{2max}$ of 70 $mL \cdot kg^{-1} \cdot min^{-1}$, who displays a RE of 200 $mL \cdot kg^{-1} \cdot km^{-1}$ whilst running at 16 $km \cdot h^{-1}$, would be working at 76% of their $\dot{V}O_{2max}$. A 5% improvement in RE, following a training intervention, would mean the athlete was now only using 72% of their $\dot{V}O_{2max}$ to run at the same speed. Further, as oxygen consumption is directly related to energy expenditure, the athlete would require less energy to run at this speed, preserving energy for later in the race.

Velocity at Maximal Oxygen Uptake (v-$\dot{V}O_{2max}$)

Interpretation of Test Results and Normative Data

v-$\dot{V}O_{2max}$ describes the relationship between $\dot{V}O_2$ at a sub-maximal exercise intensity and $\dot{V}O_{2max}$ and is calculated by solving the regression describing this relationship (Jones, 1998). A simple equation to allow the estimation of v-$\dot{V}O_{2max}$ from the previously described treadmill test was provided by Jones (2006a):

$$\text{v-}\dot{V}O_{2max} \, (km \cdot h^{-1}) = (\dot{V}O_{2max} * 60)/RE$$

Where $\dot{V}O_{2max}$ $(mL \cdot kg^{-1} \cdot min^{-1})$ is calculated as highest $\dot{V}O_2$ achieved during the maximal phase of the treadmill test, using a rolling 1-minute average. Whilst RE $(mL \cdot kg^{-1} \cdot km^{-1})$ is taken as the average $\dot{V}O_2$ achieved during the last minute of each stage of the sub-maximal phase of the treadmill test (taken as an average of this value over the first 4–5 stages). Using the example athlete described in the previous section, who reported with a $\dot{V}O_{2max}$ of 70 $mL \cdot kg^{-1} \cdot min^{-1}$ and a RE of 200 $mL \cdot kg^{-1} \cdot km^{-1}$, the corresponding v-$\dot{V}O_{2max}$ for this athlete can be estimated at 21.0 $km \cdot h^{-1}$.

Normative data for v-VO_{2max} from a cohort of highly trained (mean $\dot{V}O_{2max} > 70$ $mL \cdot kg^{-1} \cdot min^{-1}$) male middle- and long-distance runners were presented by Galbraith et al. (2014a) with values ~19–20 $km \cdot h^{-1}$ across repeat tests over a training year. This is supported by the data from Billat et al. (1999), who report a mean v-$\dot{V}O_{2max}$ of 21.1 ± 0.8 $km \cdot h^{-1}$ in a small group of highly trained ($\dot{V}O_{2max}$ ~72 $mL \cdot kg^{-1} \cdot min^{-1}$) male middle- and long-distance athletes. In female athletes, Jones (1998) reports a peak v-$\dot{V}O_{2max}$ of 20.4 $km \cdot h^{-1}$ during a 5-year case study of a world-class female distance runner. Whilst in recreational athletes, Jones et al. (1999) report values in the region of ~15–17 $km \cdot h^{-1}$ in a group of sports students.

Application of Test Data

v-$\dot{V}O_{2max}$ has been reported as a strong predictor of distance running performance (Morgan et al., 1989a; Jones and Doust, 1998; Jones, 1998), with particular relevance in middle-distance events (Jones and Carter, 2000). Additionally, it has been suggested that the v-$\dot{V}O_{2max}$

provides an optimal speed to train at to stimulate improvements in $\dot{V}O_{2max}$. Training-induced improvements in v-$\dot{V}O_{2max}$ will result in a given percentage of $\dot{V}O_{2max}$ being associated with a faster running speed. Therefore, as a 3000 m race, for example, requires an athlete to run at ~100% of their $\dot{V}O_{2max}$ (Londeree, 1986; Jones, 2006a), the link between an improvement in v-$\dot{V}O_{2max}$ and an increase in race speed becomes apparent. In a purely mathematical example, an increase in v-$\dot{V}O_{2max}$ from 19.0 to 19.2 km·h^{-1} (1% improvement) would lead to a theoretical improvement of ~5 seconds in 3000 m time. The degree of change in v-$\dot{V}O_{2max}$ following a period of endurance training will depend on the initial fitness level of the individual, with greater scope for a higher magnitude improvement in less highly trained individuals. Improvements of ~3–7% have been reported for short- and long-term training programmes respectively, in highly trained athletes (Jones, 1998; Billat et al., 1999). In more recreationally trained athletes, Jones et al. (1999) reported a ~9% increase following a 6-week period of training.

Lactate Threshold

Interpretation of Test Results and Normative Data

LT is a parameter with numerous definitions attached to it, which can present some confusion for the scientific and athletic sporting communities. In a review of research within this area, Faude et al. (2009) identified 25 different LT concepts within published literature. Two thresholds (breakpoints) are commonly used (Figure 6.1), which in theory can be identified from a plot of the blood lactate (y axis) against running speed (x axis) data, obtained during the sub-maximal phase of the treadmill test. However, in practice this can prove problematic, with differences in the LT values identified via these methods, reported across different observers (Yeh et al., 1983).

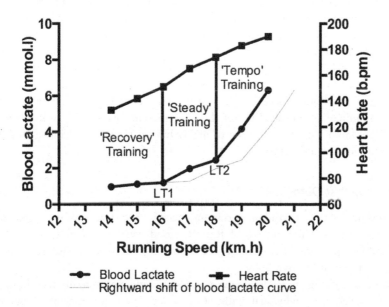

FIGURE 6.1 Example blood lactate and heart rate data from the sub-maximal treadmill test

Lactate threshold: In its simplest terms, the 1st LT (or aerobic threshold) (LT1 on Figure 6.1) is defined as the exercise intensity (running speed) corresponding to the first increase in blood lactate above baseline levels (Jones and Carter, 2000; Jones, 2006a). In an effort to add a level of objectivity to the assessment, LT is often defined as the exercise intensity associated with a fixed blood lactate level, such as 2 mmol·L^{-1}, or identified as the exercise intensity that produces a fixed increase in blood lactate above baseline values, for example a 1 mmol·L^{-1} increase in blood lactate concentration above baseline (Hagberg and Coyle, 1983).

Maximal steady state: The 2nd LT (or anaerobic threshold) (LT2 on Figure 6.1) has been defined as the running speed at which a sudden and sustained increase in blood lactate is observed (Smith and Jones, 2001; Jones, 2006a). This point will sit somewhere between LT1 and $\dot{V}O_{2max}$ and is identified as the second breakpoint seen when plotting the blood lactate vs. running speed relationship (identified as LT2 on Figure 6.1). A fixed blood lactate level of 4 mmol·L^{-1} is also often implemented to identify this threshold. A further frequently used method of identifying this threshold is the D_{max} concept, with Jamnick et al. (2018) reporting a modified D_{max} method as the most valid estimate of maximal steady state.

The exercise intensity at LT is typically reported as a running speed (km·h^{-1}) or a running pace (min:mile or min:km). In addition, it is useful to also report the heart rate in beats per minute (b·min^{-1}) required to exercise at this speed/pace. Due to the numerous different concepts used in the literature to describe LT, presenting normative data is problematic for this parameter. Normative data for LT1 (1 mmol above baseline) from a cohort of highly trained (mean $\dot{V}O_{2max} > 70$ mL·kg^{-1}·min^{-1}) male middle- and long-distance runners were presented by Galbraith et al. (2014a) with values averaging 15.7 ± 1.2 km·h^{-1} (6:09 min:mile) across repeat tests over a training year. In female athletes, Jones (1998) reports LT (a clear threshold increase in blood lactate from a plot of blood lactate against running speed) values ranging from 15.0 (6:26 min:mile) to 18.0 km·h^{-1} (5:22 min:mile) during a 5-year case study of a world-class female distance runner. Whilst in recreational athletes, Jones et al. (1999) report values for LT (a clear threshold increase in blood lactate from a plot of blood lactate against running speed) of 11.2 ± 1.8 km·h^{-1} (8:37 min:mile) in a group of sports students. In a group of trained (mean $\dot{V}O_{2max}$ 65.9 ± 4.2 mL·kg^{-1}·min^{-1}) male junior-distance runners, Tanaka et al. (1984) report values for LT (a marked increase above baseline values) at 14.7 ± 1.4 km·h^{-1} (6:34 min:mile). Finally, Billat et al. (1999) present data for LT2 (velocity at OBLA), at 17.6 ± 1.0 km·h^{-1} in a small group of highly trained ($\dot{V}O_{2max}$ ~72 ml·kg^{-1}·min^{-1}) male middle- and long-distance athletes.

Application of Test Data

A rightward shift of the LT to a higher running speed is characteristic of successful endurance training programmes. This rightward shift of the blood lactate vs. running speed relationship (pale dotted line on Figure 6.1) allows a faster running speed to be sustained at a given blood lactate level (Jones and Carter, 2000).

The degree of change in LT following a period of endurance training will depend on the initial fitness level of the individual, with greater scope for a higher magnitude improvement in less highly trained individuals. However, high magnitude improvements in LT1, following a longitudinal period of endurance training, have still been reported in highly-trained individuals, with Jones (1998) reporting a 20% improvement in LT1 during a 5-year monitoring period in a world-class female distance runner. In contrast, Galbraith et al. (2014a) report little variation (<1%) in LT1 over the course of a training year, in a group of highly trained (mean $\dot{V}O_{2max}$ >70 mL·kg^{-1}·min^{-1}) male middle- and long-distance runners. However, in a group of trained (mean $\dot{V}O_{2max}$ 65.9±4.2 mL·kg^{-1}·min^{-1}) male junior distance runners, Tanaka et al. (1984) report a ~2% increase in LT1 from pre- to post-season. In more recreationally trained athletes, Jones et al. (1999) report a ~6.5% increase in LT, following a 6-week period of continuous and interval running training in a group of sports students ($\dot{V}O_{2max}$ ~50 mL·kg^{-1}·min^{-1}). Training-induced improvements in LT2 (maximum steady state) have also been reported. In a small group of highly trained ($\dot{V}O_{2max}$ ~72 mL·kg^{-1}·min^{-1}) male middle- and long-distance athletes, Billat et al. (1999) report a ~2.5% increase in LT2 (maximum steady state) following a short-term (4-week) training programme, involving interval sessions based around the v-$\dot{V}O_{2max}$.

Jones (2006a) suggest that the speed at LT1 is closely related to the speed that can be sustained over a marathon, whilst the speed at LT2 (maximum steady state) can be maintained for ~60 min in highly trained runners, so it may be closely related to the speed that can be sustained over 10 miles to half-marathon distances (Jones, 2006a).

LT data from the treadmill test also have a useful application in the design of training sessions for athletes. The speed at LT and the heart rate associated with this speed are useful in demarcating transition points between the various exercise intensity zones (Figure 6.1). For example, speeds/heart rates below LT1 may provide useful intensities for easy or 'recovery' training runs. The speeds/heart rates between LT1 and LT2 (maximum steady state) may provide useful intensities for 'steady' running sessions, whilst the speeds/heart rates above LT2 (maximum steady state) may provide useful intensities for training runs set at a more 'tempo' pace (Jones, 2006a).

Training at the LT provides an aerobic training stimulus, whilst enabling blood lactate levels to remain low, allowing high millage runs to be conducted at this intensity. In general, it appears that training at intensities close to or slightly above the LT are important for stimulating improvements in the LT (Carter et al., 1999).

Field-Based Physiological Assessment

Field-based assessment protocols aim to closely replicate the athlete's typical exercise conditions, affording field tests a high level of ecological validity (Galbraith et al., 2011). Field-based assessment, therefore, provides a useful alternative (or enhancement) to laboratory-based testing, when conducting physiological assessment for middle- and long-distance runners. Research describing valid and reliable assessment methods for field-based testing are less prevalent in the scientific literature, but such research has been increasing in popularity in recent years. This section will focus on three key physiological parameters, which can form part of a fitness-testing battery, when working with middle- and long-distance runners: critical speed, D' and the anaerobic speed reserve. A runner's critical speed (CS) has been suggested to reflect the highest sustainable running speed that can be maintained without a continual rise in $\dot{V}O_2$ to $\dot{V}O_{2max}$, whilst D' is notionally the maximum distance that can be achieved at speeds above CS (Jones et al., 2010). The anaerobic speed reserve (ASR) is the speed range from v-$\dot{V}O_{2max}$ to maximal sprint speed (Sandford et al., 2019a).

Assessment Techniques (CS, D')

Galbraith et al. (2011, 2014b) describe a field-based protocol for the assessment of CS and D' which can be conducted in a single visit, an improvement on more traditional multi-visit laboratory-based protocols of CS and D'. Participants should complete three fixed-distance performance trials on a standard outdoor 400 m athletics track. The three performance trials should be conducted over distances of 3600 m, 2400 m and 1200 m (9, 6 and 3 laps respectively), in this order. These distances are selected to result in completion times of approximately 12, 7 and 3 min (Hughson et al., 1984). Participants should aim to complete each trial in the fastest time possible, with the three runs conducted on the same day, with a 30-min recovery period between each run.

An alternate assessment protocol has been described by Kordi et al. (2019), which allows the estimation of CS and D' from just two fixed-distance performance trials (conducted over 3600 m and 1200 m). Kordi et al. (2019) suggest that this 2-point time-trial model can be used to calculate CS and D' as proficiently as a 3-point model, making it a less fatiguing, inexpensive and applicable method for coaches, practitioners and athletes to monitor running performance in a single training session.

Pettitt et al. (2012) describe a third option, suggesting that a single all-out effort over a duration of 3-min can be used to estimate an athlete's CS and D'. This test should again be conducted on an outdoor running track, with the participant wearing a GPS watch. Participants should be instructed to build up to their maximal speed and maintain as fast a running speed as possible throughout the entire test.

Interpretation of Test Results and Normative Data

Participants' CS and D' from the fixed-distance protocols can subsequently be calculated using a range of different mathematical models; see Housh et al. (2001) for a review of different mathematical models available to estimate CS and D'. Arguably the simplest of the available models are the linear models; therefore, this chapter recommends using the linear distance-time model to estimate CS and D' from the fixed-distance, field-based performance trials. This model requires a plot of the three distances (in metres), on the y axis, against the three completion times (seconds), on the x axis. Linear regression can then be used to calculate CS and D' using the following equation, where: d = distance run (m) and t = running time (s):

$$d = (CS \times t) + D'$$

In Figure 6.2 the slope of the regression line describes the athletes CS ($m \cdot s^{-1}$), whilst the y-intercept describes the athletes D' (m).

Participants' CS and D' from the 3-min test are estimated based on the premise that a runner will expend their D' within 2.5 min of the all-out effort; consequently, the mean speed of between 2.5 and 3.0 min will stabilise at CS (Burnley et al., 2006). Therefore, D' from a 3-min running test can be calculated using the following equation (Pettitt et al., 2012), where t = time (sec), $S150$ s = the average speed for the first 150 seconds of the trial ($m \cdot s^{-1}$) and CS is the average speed between 150 sec and 180 sec of the trial ($m \cdot s^{-1}$):

$$D' = t \times (S150 \text{ s} - CS)$$

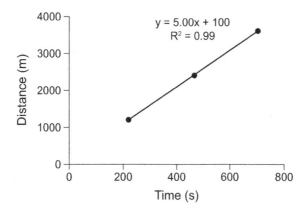

FIGURE 6.2 The linear distance-time model for CS and D', based on data from three fixed-distance performance trials

Note: CS = 5.00 m·s^{-1} and D' = 100 m.

One potential disadvantage of this assessment method, over the fixed-distance trial approach, is the use of a GPS watch. GPS receiver accuracy is dependent on several factors and may vary between testing days, with Pettitt et al. (2012) reporting the accuracy of measurements during their study at ~3 meters.

An athlete's CS describes the highest rate of oxidative metabolism, sustainable without a progressively increasing contribution from phosphocreatine and anaerobic glycolysis (Jones et al., 2010). An athlete's D' is representative of a fixed amount of work (distance) that can be completed once exercise intensity exceeds CS, and is thought to be predominantly a derivative of anaerobic processes (Jones et al., 2010). Although Jones et al. (2010) explain that D' is likely to be related to the 'distance' between an athlete's CS and their VO_{2max}.

Normative data for CS and D' from a cohort of highly trained (mean $\dot{V}O_{2max}$ > 70 mL·kg^{-1}·min^{-1}) male middle- and long-distance runners were presented by Galbraith et al. (2014a). Data were sub-divided to provide normative data from six 800 m runners, mean CS 4.76 ± 0.22 m·s^{-1} and mean D' 162 ± 44 m, and eight marathon runners, mean CS 5.07 ± 0.31 m·s^{-1} and mean D' 94 ± 49 m. Galbraith et al. (2014b) provided data from well-trained (mean $\dot{V}O_{2max}$ > 60 mL·kg^{-1}·min^{-1}) male middle-distance runners, reporting mean CS 4.07 ± 0.28 m·s^{-1} and mean D' 106 m. Triska et al. (2017) reported data for a group of recreationally trained athletes (mean $\dot{V}O_{2max}$ 52.9 ± 3.1 mL·kg^{-1}·min^{-1}), with mean CS of 3.77 ± 0.35 m.s^{-1} and mean D' 225 ± 72 m. Pettitt et al. (2012) provided normative data for a group of well-trained (mean $\dot{V}O_{2max}$ 55 ± 4 mL·kg^{-1}·min^{-1}) female distance runners, reporting mean CS at 4.46 ± 0.41 m.s^{-1} and D' 85.8 ± 40.5 m.

An athlete's CS and D' from the field test can be compared to normative data, such as those presented earlier. This can provide an indication of strengths or weakness, which may then inform future training program design. During repeat assessments, an athlete's CS and D' can be compared to previous scores from the same athlete providing a useful method to monitor the effectiveness of training programmes and assess whether any adaptations to CS and D' are occurring.

Research investigating the degree of change in CS and D' following a period of endurance training are sparse in the scientific literature. Galbraith et al. (2014a) reported small (~2%), but statistically significant, changes in CS during a 1-year training period, in a group of highly-trained (mean $\dot{V}O_{2max} > 70$ mL·kg^{-1}·min^{-1}) male middle- and long-distance runners. CS was lowest during August, reaching a peak in February. The increase in CS appears a small change, although it is important to note that the athletes involved in the study were already highly trained with on average an 8+-year training history prior to the study. In contrast, untrained participants have achieved far larger increases in critical power (10–31%) following a 6- to 8-week period of continuous and/or interval cycle training (Gaesser and Wilson, 1988; Jenkins and Quigley, 1992; Poole et al., 1990). D' showed no statistically significant change throughout a 1-year training period, despite changes of ~24% from August, where D' was at its highest, to November, where D' was at its lowest (Galbraith et al., 2014a). In untrained participants, far greater changes have been reported, with Jenkins and Quigley (1993) demonstrating a significant increase in W' (equivalent to D') of ~49%, following an 8-week cycle training programme.

To improve CS, continuous or interval endurance training appear important (Gaesser and Wilson, 1988; Jenkins and Quigley, 1992; Poole et al., 1990; Vanhatalo et al., 2008), with total distance covered in training and the volume of time spent at intensities greater than LT velocity shown to encourage an increase in CS (Galbraith et al., 2014a). To improve D', a training programme focused on power or sprint training appears important (Jenkins and Quigley, 1993). Due to the ecologically valid testing protocols used in the measurement of CS and D', it has been suggested that the measurement of changes in the distance-time relationship after a training intervention are likely to be of more practical value than the measurements of traditional physiological parameters such as $\dot{V}O_{2max}$ and LT (Jones et al., 2010).

Application of Test Data

Aside from the assessment of physical fitness, the CS and D' values from the test protocols described in this chapter have a variety of potential applications for athletes, coaches and sport scientists. These include prediction of performance, informing racing strategy and the prescription of exercise training.

Prediction of performance: given the previously presented equation, describing the distance-time relationship and it's individual parameters: $d = (CS \times t) + D'$

Jones et al. (2010) explained that the time-to-exhaustion (t) at a specific constant severe-intensity speed (S), that is any speed above CS, may be estimated using: $t = D'/(S - CS)$. Whilst a further re-working of the same equation will allow the estimation of exercise performance capacity (the quickest time an athlete would take to cover a given distance):

$$t = (D - D')/CS$$

For example, the estimation of time to exhaustion for a runner with a CS is 5.0 m.s^{-1} and a D' of 100 m estimates an endurance time at a velocity of 5.1 m.s^{-1} would be 1000 sec, or 16:40 min:sec $(100/(5.1 - 5.0) = 1000)$, and the endurance time at a velocity of 5.3 m.s^{-1} would be 333 sec (5:33 min:sec). This information would be useful for a coach aiming to prescribe a challenging but achievable training session (Jones et al., 2010). For the same runner, the estimated quickest performance time over a 3000 m distance would be 580 sec, 9:40 min:sec

$((3000 - 100)/5.0 = 580)$, whilst over 5000 m would be 980 sec (16:20 min:sec). This information may be useful when considering race pacing strategies. Furthermore, this modelling of performance enables the impact of training-induced changes in CS to be quantified. For example, a 2% improvement in CS for this athlete (a change from 5.0 to 5.1 m.s^{-1}), following a period of training, would correspond to a 19-sec improvement in estimated 5000 m performance time, based on a stable D' of 100 m. Finally, the modelling of estimated performance time from CS and D' may be useful in helping athletes decide where their specialism might lie across the middle and long distances. Jones et al. (2010) explain this concept using two hypothetical female distance runners: athlete A, with a CS of 5.85 m.s^{-1} and a D' of 75 m, and athlete B, with a CS of 5.82 m.s^{-1} and a D' of 95 m. Jones et al. (2010) explain that in a competitive race over 1500 m, it can be calculated (using the exercise performance capacity equation) that athlete B would be fastest of the two athletes. However, at 3000 m, the estimated difference between athletes becomes negligible, and for the 5000 m distance, athlete A would have the advantage (Jones et al., 2010).

Informing racing strategy: data on an athlete's CS and D' may also prove useful when it comes to determining optimal racing strategy (Jones et al., 2010). The distance-time relationship dictates that optimal performance over a given distance (in the severe intensity domain; covering the middle and the shorter long-distance events) can never be achieved if any part of the race is run at a speed below CS (Fukuba and Whipp, 1999) (see the earlier equations on the prediction of performance using CS and D'). Jones et al. (2010) explain that an athlete may use this knowledge to their advantage in a race, by planning race tactics to suit the relative strengths of their CS and D' respectively. For example, a race tactic for an athlete with a high CS and a low D' compared to that of their competitors might be to adopt a front-running strategy, by running at the highest possible speed they can during the race (as dictated by their individual distance-time relationship; see the previous equations for predicting performance). This speed is likely to be above the CS of their competitors, which would require the competitors to run above their CS to maintain pace with the athlete. This would gradually deplete the competitors' D', removing their competitive advantage in a sprint finish. Equally, an athlete with a low CS and a high D' relative to their competitors may be better advised to attempt to slow the race to a pace below their competitors' CS and then use their higher D' towards the later stages of the race in a sprint finish (Jones et al., 2010).

Prescription of exercise training: interval training is a popular mode of conditioning in many sports and involves intermittent periods of work and relative recovery (Morton and Billat, 2004). Interval training has the advantage of enabling a greater amount of high-intensity work to be conducted in a single session than would be possible with continuous training (Margaria et al., 1969). Therefore, designing interval training sessions that are individualised to athletes' specific needs is important. For aerobic training, parameters such as VO_{2max}, v-VO_{2max} and LT have all been used to prescribe individualised training intensities (Berthoin et al., 2006). However, Ferguson et al. (2010) explain that an additional consideration when defining exercise intensity is that CS does not occur at a fixed percentage of $\dot{V}O_{2max}$. Furthermore, between-subject differences in anaerobic capacity result in the D' not representing the same volume of supra-CS exercise in all individuals. The consequence of this is that the exercise intensity experienced during an interval training session will be variable between participants unless CS and D' are accounted for (Ferguson et al., 2010). It has been suggested that an athlete's CS and D' can be used to design interval training; setting interval intensity at a percentage of CS and the number of interval repetitions in accordance with the depletion of D', thereby inducing the desired training load through the interplay between CS, D' and time to exhaustion (TTE). Morton and Billat (2004) describe this principle based on a linear model, explaining that the depletion of D' during work (w) intervals and the restoration of D' during recovery (r) intervals can be estimated as follows: where S = speed and t = time in seconds.

Depletion of D' during work intervals: $(S_w - CS) \times t_w$
Restoration of D' during recovery intervals: $(CS - S_r) \times t_r$

Galbraith et al. (2015) applied this modelling technique to investigate its use in designing track-based interval training sessions for middle- and long-distance runners. Three interval training sessions were designed, with CS and D' subsequently used to model the estimated point (number of repetitions) at which an athlete would fatigue. Although actual and predicted points of exhaustion were not significantly different, a high typical error was observed for all predicted exhaustion times (Galbraith et al., 2015). Whilst its simple design is appealing, the linear model could not closely predict exhaustion during intermittent running and may therefore not be suitable for the accurate prescription of interval training for middle- and long-distance runners.

Assessment Techniques (ASR)

Bundle et al. (2003) first introduced the term 'ASR' into the scientific literature, although in their work the protocol is conducted in a laboratory using a treadmill. The assessment protocol involved the measurement of both anaerobic and aerobic power. The maximum speed supported by anaerobic power was estimated from the highest speed that an athlete was able to maintain for eight steps without a backward drift on the treadmill. This was determined from a series of short high-speed runs at gradually increasing speeds, until the athlete could no longer match the speed of the belt for eight steps (Bundle et al., 2003). The maximum speed supported by aerobic power was determined from a treadmill v-$\dot{V}O_{2max}$ test (see the previously described v-$\dot{V}O_{2max}$ protocol).

A number of field-based assessment techniques have since been proposed for the assessment of ASR, including the recent work of Sandford et al. (2019a, 2019d). In their work, Sandford et al. (2019a) calculated ASR from maximal sprint speed (MSS) and predicted maximal aerobic speed (MAS) performed on an outdoor 400 m athletics track. MSS is assessed via a standing-start 50 m sprint, with athletes performing three maximal efforts with ~3 minutes rest between trials and MSS determined using a sports radar device. On a separate day, a 1500 m time trial was performed for the assessment of MAS (a recent 1500 m race performance time, would be a suitable alternative to a time-trial here).

Interpretation of Test Results and Normative Data

The anaerobic speed reserve can be defined as the speed range an athlete possesses between velocity at v-$\dot{V}O_{2max}$ in the laboratory (or maximal aerobic speed in the field) and maximal sprint speed.

When following the treadmill protocol described by Bundle et al. (2003), ASR is defined as the difference between a runner's maximum anaerobic speed and maximum aerobic speed.

When using the field-based protocol, MAS can be estimated using the following equation (Sandford et al., 2019d):

$$MAS = (1500v - 14.921)/0.4266$$

where 1500v is the athlete's average speed over the 1500 m trial (km·h^{-1}).

The ASR can subsequently be calculated as the difference between MSS and MAS.

An athlete's ASR from the field test can be compared to normative data, such as those presented next. This can provide an indication of strength or weakness, which may then inform future training program design. During repeat assessments, an athlete's ASR can be compared to previous scores from the same athlete, providing a useful method to monitor the effectiveness of training programmes and assess whether any adaptations to ASR (and its components, MSS and MAS) are occurring.

Bundle et al. (2003) report normative data from a small sample of seven trained collegiate athletes (mean $\dot{V}O_{2max}$ 61.7 ± 2.0 mL·kg^{-1}·min^{-1}; range, 53.4–68.0 mL·kg^{-1}·min^{-1}). The mean maximum speed supported by anaerobic power was 31.32 ± 1.44 km·h^{-1} (range, 27.72–37.44 km·h^{-1}). The mean maximum speed supported by aerobic power was 19.08±0.36 km·h^{-1} (range, 17.64–20.52 km·h^{-1}). The mean ASR was 12.24 ± 2.16 km·h^{-1} (range, 8.28–20.16 km·h^{-1}).

Sandford et al. (2019a) report normative data for MSS, MAS and ASR for a group of 19 international standard (800 m PB of ≤ 1:47.50 min:sec, and/or a 1500 m PB of ≤ 3:40 min:sec) male 800 and 1500 m specialists. Mean (± SD) MSS was 33.55 ± 0.64 km·h^{-1}; mean MAS was 22.79 ± 0.39 km·h^{-1} and mean ASR was 12.24 ± 0.79 km·h^{-1}, Sandford et al. (2019a) also partitioned their participants into sub-groups of middle-distance runners, reporting mean data for 'speed types' (400–800 m specialists), '800 m specialists', and 'endurance types' (800–1500 m specialists). The MSS of 400–800 m specialists (35.48 ± 0.30 km·h^{-1}) was faster than the 800 m specialists (33.68 ± 0.63 km·h^{-1}), and 800–1500 m specialists (31.49 ± 0.99 km·h^{-1}). MAS in 400–800 m specialists (22.41 ± 0.62 km·h^{-1}) was slower than both 800 m specialists (22.76 ± 0.50 km·h^{-1}) and 800–1500 m specialists (23.21 ± 0.06 km·h^{-1}). ASR of 400–800 m specialists (14.46 ± 1.00 km·h^{-1}) was larger than 800 m specialists (12.12 ± 0.61 km·h^{-1}) and 800–1500 m specialists (10.13 ± 0.76 km·h^{-1}).

Application of Test Data

The importance of a high ASR to a middle-distance runner can be substantiated by the work of Bundle et al. (2003) and Sandford et al. (2019a, 2019d). Bundle et al. (2003) report that the ASR protocol allows high-speed running performance to be accurately predicted from an athlete's maximum anaerobic and aerobic power. This highlights ASR as an important determinant of performance particularly in middle distance events over 800–1500 m. Sandford et al. (2019a) report that MSS and ASR displayed strong negative ($r = -0.74$) relationships with 800 m performance time. For the international-level athletes tested, a faster MSS (and therefore ASR) is likely to be strongly related to a faster 800 m performance. Interestingly, for the same MSS, a faster MAS or ASR was not strongly related to changes in 800 m time. Sandford et al. (2019a) suggest therefore, that at an elite level, faster 800 m runners will have a larger ASR (as a consequence of a faster MSS), combined with an already established minimum level of MAS. Therefore, once a certain aerobic standard (MAS) is reached, MSS becomes a differentiating factor in elite 800 m runners (Sandford et al., 2019a).

Summary

To measure the important physiological determinants of distance running performance, and thus evaluate a runner's relative strengths and weaknesses, a wide range of laboratory and field-based assessment options exist. Differences in physiological testing profiles between athletes can explain differences in distance running performance. Laboratory-based physiological assessment should include maximal oxygen uptake ($\dot{V}O_{2max}$), running economy (RE), lactate threshold (LT) and the velocity associated with VO_{2max} (v-$\dot{V}O_{2max}$). Field-based physiological assessment should include critical speed (CS), the maximum distance that can be achieved at speeds above critical speed (D') and the anaerobic speed reserve (ASR).

7

MOVEMENT SCREENING AND PHYSICAL CAPACITY ASSESSMENTS

Louis P. Howe and Paul J. Read

Highlights

- Movement screening and physical capacity assessments provide coaches with information that supports the decision-making processes when designing training programmes, by identifying an athlete's strengths and weaknesses.
- Movement screening should be implemented using methods that identify an athlete's level of competence to perform the movement patterns they will be using during strength training.
- When movement faults exist during a screen, an investigatory process should be implemented to identify the cause, which will enable coaches to select corrective strategies that will be successful.
- Physical capacity assessments provide coaches with data to examine athletic performance qualities.
- Strength diagnostic testing assesses an athlete's ability to produce force under varying conditions, while tissue capacity assessments provides data on the ability of the musculotendon unit to tolerate load.

Introduction

A comprehensive assessment of general athletic qualities is a fundamental component in the design of an effective strength and conditioning (S&C) programme. While performance-related tests (e.g. VO_{2max} testing) are associated directly with distance running, movement screening and physical capacity assessments provide valuable information that will also guide training decisions. Although not considered 'sport-specific' in this context, they are 'sport-relevant'. Specifically, movement screening provides coaches with an indication of an athlete's readiness to perform strengthening exercises, while physical capacity assessments support coaches in identifying functional deficits that may (positively or negatively) impact running performance. The aim of this chapter is to provide coaches with the tools to design an effective testing battery that will generate useful data and form the basis of a successful S&C

programme. Additionally, a range of considerations will be discussed to ensure reliable data are collected through the standardisation of testing procedures. Where available, normative data will be provided to support the coach's interpretation of assessment results.

Purpose of Screening and Assessment

Establishing baseline measures for movement skill and physical capacities should be the starting point in the training of relevant general qualities (i.e. strength) that may result in improved running performance and reduced injury risk. The data produced from these tests can inform the training process through the following mechanisms:

1. Identification of functional deficits that may limit performance and increase injury risk. This ensures prioritisation of training for underdeveloped physical qualities, allowing coaches to individualise programme design. For example, decreased strength of the plantar flexor musculature is related to increased risk for developing Achilles tendinopathy (O'Neill et al., 2016). This can be identified during testing of tissue capacity with the calf raise test.
2. Investigate movement quality during fundamental patterns that are relevant to running. For example, poor control of the lumbopelvic region and lower extremity in the frontal and transverse plane during single-leg movements (e.g. single-leg squat) is predictive of displaying the same mechanics during the stance phase of running (Whatman et al., 2011).
3. Determine an athlete's preparedness for loading. This should be the primary objective for screening movement quality. Although competency in bilateral squatting shares few mechanical similarities to running, it does provide insight into whether an athlete possesses acceptable technique prior to loading this movement to improve maximal strength.
4. Establish baseline measures to determine whether a training programme successfully achieves its desired goal. This can be a strong motivational tool for coaches to employ as it allows them to demonstrate to their athletes the "fruit of their labour". As a result, buy-in towards future programmes will be enhanced.
5. Baseline measures recorded during the assessment process can also inform future rehabilitation programmes. Following injury, functional deficits will be present that result in aberrant movement skill (Decker et al., 2002), decreased range of motion (Askling et al., 2006) and diminished levels of strength (Mucha et al., 2017). In addition, coaches may choose to include routine testing as part of pre-injury screening to individualise their return-to-sport criteria.

Accuracy in Testing

Prior to the design of a testing battery, coaches must consider the validity and reliability of each test to determine the accuracy of the results. This information will support the coach's interpretation, allowing for functional deficits to be identified and subsequently targeted during training. Validity, defined in simple terms as the test's ability to measure what it is supposed to measure, should be considered when selecting relevant tests. It is important that coaches select tests that precisely represent the movement skills and the physical capacities they want to measure through screening and assessment, respectively.

Reliability is concerned with a test providing suitable measurement precision and consistency. This is important to ensure a test accurately characterises the athlete's performance within an acceptable level of variability. Understanding the reliability and typical variation in a test allows coaches to determine if observed changes in performance have occurred due to an alteration in the athlete's physical or movement capacity and so represent 'real' change, rather than measurement error. Error in the data recorded may represent biological (variability from the participant while performing a given protocol) or technical error (variability in measuring tools, such as the equipment used) and will vary depending on the test and the manner in which it is performed. The biological and technical error associated with tests can be reduced by standardising protocols. To achieve this, coaches should ensure the same testing equipment is used for each testing session and that the equipment is setup correctly and calibrated as required. Additionally, facilities, athlete clothing and footwear, time of day, the warm-up protocol employed and the instructions provided should be consistent across testing sessions, or large error in test results may be present.

Although access to reliability data is available in published literature, it is important to note that the skill level of the tester, the population sampled and subtle changes in the procedures may influence these values, resulting in the potential for the misinterpretation of findings. Therefore, it is recommended that coaches determine their own measurement error for each test with the population they are working with. A brief example is provided to demonstrate how typical error can be calculated for the calf raise test (described later in this chapter) performed by 11 track and field athletes with 7 days between testing sessions. Table 7.1 presents the scores for each athlete for test days 1 and 2, along with the test-retest difference. Typical error is calculated by dividing the standard deviation of the test-retest difference by $\sqrt{2}$ (Hopkins, 2000). Using the data from Table 7.1, typical error for the calf raise test is 1 repetition, indicating changes in calf raise test scores exceeding a single repetition likely represents a 'real' change in the strength endurance of the ankle plantar flexor musculature.

TABLE 7.1 Single-leg heel raise scores (number of repetitions performed) for 11 athletes from two separate testing days and the between-session absolute difference

	Test Day 1	Test Day 2	Test-Retest difference
Athlete 1	24	23	−1
Athlete 2	12	15	3
Athlete 3	15	16	1
Athlete 4	14	15	1
Athlete 5	16	18	2
Athlete 6	35	33	−2
Athlete 7	17	16	−1
Athlete 8	12	13	1
Athlete 9	22	24	2
Athlete 10	32	35	3
Athlete 11	14	15	1
Mean	19	20	1
Standard deviation	8	8	2

Movement Screening

Movement screening involves analysing an athlete's technical performance across a variety of tasks, with the aim of determining their level of competency. In turn, this provides an indication as to whether an athlete possesses the necessary skill to load the associated movement patterns. For example, an athlete who displays end range of motion spinal flexion during a body-weight squat prior to reaching 90° of knee flexion presents a movement fault relative to the performance criteria associated with the screen (see Table 7.2). If the athlete were to persevere with loading this pattern in an attempt to develop leg strength, injury risk may increase (Siewe et al., 2011) as the spine's tolerance to compressive loading is diminished (Gunning et al., 2001) and shear forces are elevated (Potvin et al., 1991). Instead, the athlete would be better served in addressing the technical issues by removing any functional limitations that exist (e.g. restricted ankle and hip mobility) and devoting time to develop the hip-back disassociation sequencing required to demonstrate a competent squat technique.

Selecting Movements to Screen

Movement screening can be a time-consuming process, taking up to 30 min to complete for each athlete (Bennett et al., 2019). As coaches also often perform a biomechanical analysis (i.e. gait analysis), range of performance tests (i.e. $\dot{V}O_{2max}$ test) and physical capacity assessments, time is a valuable commodity and should be considered when designing a test battery. Movement screens should therefore be filtered to include only movements that qualify an athlete for loading in specific exercises that are likely be prescribed, and can therefore directly inform the training process.

Specificity for exercise selection is an accepted principle for the transfer of training (Brearley and Bishop, 2019). Less commonly appreciated is that movement screens should also be specific to the coaches' intended outcome (i.e. movement quality during exercises that will be loaded) and possess high construct validity. This is particularly relevant when attempting to infer movement quality for one exercise when screening other movement patterns that may appear visually similar. For example, peak knee abduction angle during double-leg squatting is not associated with the same measure during double-leg jump-landing performance (Donohue et al., 2015). It is likely that this occurs due to the task demands being markedly different. In this instance, double-leg squatting presents as a mobility challenge, with considerable sagittal plane motion at the hip, knee and ankle joints required to achieve a deep squat position (Hemmerich et al., 2006), whereas jump-landings require greater eccentric strength to attenuate the larger peak forces (Montgomery et al., 2012). Therefore, if a coach wishes to determine competency for performing squatting and landings, movement screens for each pattern should be included in the testing battery.

When selecting movements to screen, the coach should also consider the way each is performed. Even within the same movement pattern (e.g. squat), slight changes in the constraints related to the task can result in a misleading interpretation of an athlete's skill level relative to a specific exercise. For example, screening the overhead squat with the feet facing directly forward is commonly used during movement screens (e.g. Cook et al., 2014). However, this test offers little insight into an athlete's ability to squat with the arms across the chest and the feet in a self-selected position (McMillian et al., 2016). As the primary aim of movement screening is to determine the runner's readiness for loading within the exercise, the technical features

TABLE 7.2 Guidelines for each example screen, including the performance criteria

Screen	Rationale	Set up	Instructions	Performance criteria
Bilateral drop-landing	Plyometric exercises are commonly recommended for improving distance running performance (Spurrs, Murphy and Watsford, 2003). This screen can be used to determine a runner's readiness to perform double-leg landing exercises (Howe et al., 2020; Lundgren et al., 2016).	Stand upright on the edge of a 0.3 m box with the feet hip-width apart. Arms crossed so each hand touches the contralateral shoulder. Eyes looking directly forward.	"Step off the box and drop directly down ahead of the box, landing simultaneously with both feet. Upon landing, maintain balance, while keeping the arms crossed throughout the landing. Please perform 5 repetitions."	*Anterior view* 1. Feet land between hip and shoulder width apart, facing forward with minimal turn out. 2. Foot contact is symmetrical. 3. Knees remain over the toes throughout. 4. Pelvis remains level and no trunk lean is present. *Side view* 5. Forefoot touches down prior to heel contact. 6. Knee flexes approximately 60–90° following ground contact. 7. The trunk leans forward > 30°. 8. Spine remains in a neutral position. *Additional* 9. Landing sounds relatively quiet.
Single-leg drop-landing	The single-leg drop-landing allows coaches to screen landing skill ahead of prescribing hopping and bounding exercises. The single-leg nature of this screen emphasises the demand on key stabilising muscles around the trunk and hip (Neamatallah et al., 2020), similar to running (Novacheck, 1998).	Stand upright on one leg with the foot on the edge of a 0.3 m box. Arms crossed so each hand touches the contralateral shoulder. Eyes looking directly forward.	"Drop down from the box by leaning forward and landing directly ahead of the box. Upon landing, maintain balance for 2 seconds. Please perform 5 repetitions with the same leg. Once finished, complete 5 repetitions with the alternate leg."	*Anterior view* 1. Foot lands directly under the pelvis, facing forwards. 2. From an anterior view, the knees remain over the toes throughout. 3. Pelvis remains level and no trunk lean is present. *Side view* 4. Forefoot touches down prior to heel contact. 5. Knee flexes approximately 60–90° following ground contact. 6. The trunk leans forward > 30°. 7. Spine remains in a neutral position. 8. No obvious trunk rotation occurs. *Additional* 9. Landing sounds relatively quiet.

(Continued)

TABLE 7.2 (Continued)

Screen	Rationale	Set up	Instructions	Performance criteria
Squat	The squat exercise is regarded as a fundamental movement pattern (Lubans et al., 2010) and is commonly prescribed to develop maximal strength of the leg extensors (Comfort and Kasim, 2007). To perform a full range of motion squat, runners must be able to access hip flexion, abduction and internal rotation range of motion (Swinton et al., 2012) while the knee and ankle concurrently flexes and dorsiflexes, respectively (Hemmerich et al., 2006). Concomitantly, runners must also be able to disassociate hip and spine motion and prevent medial knee displacement under high loads (Myer et al., 2014).	Stand upright with the feet shoulder-width apart and feet turned out approximately 11 and 1 on a clock face. Fingers are interlinked and the hands are placed behind the head with the elbows pointing to the side. Eyes looking directly forward.	"Keeping the feet flat on the ground and the arms parallel to the floor, squat down as low as you can. Hold the bottom position for 1 second, and then return to the start. Please perform 5 continuous repetitions at a controlled pace."	*Anterior view* 1. No change in foot position or alignment. 2. Knees remain over the toes throughout. 3. Pelvis and shoulders remain level throughout. *Side view* 4. Knee flexes to ≥ 90°. 5. Trunk angle is ≤ 10° relative to tibia angle throughout the movement. 6. Spine remains in a neutral position. *Posterior view* 7. Pelvis remains centred over the base of support.
Single-leg squat	Single-leg strength exercises can be used to address between–limb strength differences (Bishop, Turner and Read, 2018) and target key stabilisers of the trunk and lower extremity (Howe et al., 2014). The single-leg squat screen can be used to identify individuals with trunk and hip muscle dysfunction (Crossley et al., 2011; Stickler, Finley and Gulgin, 2015). Additionally, excessive frontal and transverse plane lumbopelvic motion during single-leg squatting is associated with similar movement faults during running (Alenezi et al., 2014; Whatman, Hing and Hume, 2011), which may increase injury risk (Ceyssens et al., 2019, pp. 1–21).	Stand upright on one leg with the foot facing forwards. The non-stance leg is positioned so the knee is flexed to 90° with the hip extended. Shoulders flexed to 90° with the elbows extended. Eyes looking directly forward.	"Keeping the foot flat on the ground, squat down with one leg as low as you can with the arms remaining parallel to the ground. Be sure to keep the non-stance leg slightly flexed throughout. Hold the bottom position for 1 second, and then return to the start. Please perform 5 continuous repetitions at a controlled pace with the same leg. Once finished, complete 5 repetitions with the alternate leg."	*Anterior view* 1. No change in foot position or alignment. 2. Knees remain over the toes throughout. 3. Pelvis and shoulders remain level throughout. *Side view* 4. Knee flexes to ≥ 90°. 5. Trunk angle is ≤ 10° relative to tibia angle throughout the movement. 6. Spine remains in a neutral position. 7. No obvious trunk rotation occurs. *Additional* 8. Balance is maintained throughout.

| Forward lunge | The lunge assesses dynamic flexibility of the hip, knee and ankle joints in the sagittal plane, while controlling the alignment of the trunk, pelvis and lower extremity in the frontal and transverse plane (Crill, Kolba and Chleboun, 2004). Uncontrolled frontal and transverse plane motions during a lunge are strongly related to the same movement faults during the stance phase of running (Whatman, Hing and Hume, 2011). Additionally, some of these movement faults have been associated with elevated injury risk during running (Ceyssens et al., 2019). | Lunge distance is normalised to leg length, calculated as the distance between the anterior superior iliac spine of the pelvis and the medial malleolus of the tibia (measured in supine lying). Tape is placed on the floor to mark the lunge distance (leg length) between the greater toe of the trail leg and the greater toe of the lead leg. Stand upright with the feet hip width apart and facing directly forwards. Hands on hips. Eyes looking directly forward. | "Step forward so the heel lands just ahead of the marker. Upon contact with the ground, drop into a lunge as far as you can before the back knee contacts the ground. Please perform 5 continuous repetitions at a controlled pace with the same leg. Once finished, complete 5 repetitions with the alternate leg." | *Anterior view*
1. Both lead and trail foot face forwards throughout.
2. Knees remain over the toes throughout.
3. Pelvis remains level and no trunk lean is present.

Side view
4. Lead foot remains in full contact with the ground following initial ground contact.
5. Spine remains in a neutral position.
6. Knee flexion for the lead and trail leg is approximately 90°. |
| Romanian deadlift | This screen assesses competency during a hip hinging pattern, whereby athletes must possess dynamic flexibility of the hamstring musculature and sufficient motor control to disassociate movement of the hip and spine. This movement pattern is fundamental for other exercises commonly prescribed to develop leg extensor strength (e.g. Olympic lifts) (Bird and Barrington-Higgs, 2010). | Stand upright with the feet hip width apart and facing approximately forwards. Hold a dowel with an overhand grip and the hands just outside of shoulder width. Eyes looking directly forward. | "Maintaining your spine position, lower the bar down the front of your thighs as far as you can whilst only slightly bending the knees. Hold the bottom position for 1 second, and then return to the start. Please perform 5 continuous repetitions at a controlled pace." | *Anterior view*
1. Bar descends lower than the patella.
2. Bar remains level throughout.

Side view
3. Slight knee flexion occurs during the descent.
4. Tibia remains vertical throughout.
5. Spine remains in a neutral position.

Posterior view
6. Pelvis remains centred over the base of support. |

(Continued)

TABLE 7.2 (Continued)

Screen	Rationale	Set up	Instructions	Performance criteria
Bilateral shoulder elevation	Overhead lifting is commonly prescribed for developing explosive strength (generally through Olympic lifts and variations). This screen provides a measure of a runner's mobility at the thoracic spine and shoulder complex, while establishing their ability to prevent compensatory movements in the lumbar and cervical spine (Howe and Blagrove, 2015).	Stand upright with the feet hip width apart. Arms are by the side with the elbows extended. Eyes looking directly forward.	"Standing tall, lift the arms out to the side until they are directly above your head. Keep the elbows extended throughout the movement and at the top of the movement, the palms should face each other. Please perform 5 continuous repetitions at a controlled pace."	*Anterior view* 1. Upper arm reaches a vertical alignment relative to the ground. 2. Elbows remain extended. *Side view* 3. Arms remain in the frontal plane. 4. Head does not change position. 5. Spine remains in a neutral position. *Posterior view* 6. No obvious signs of shrugging.

of the movement screen should be similar to the associated technical model. It is therefore suggested that coaches carefully consider the constraints imposed on the athlete during the performance of the movement screen.

The coach's approach to training and developing general physical qualities to improve running performance should also assist coaches in selecting relevant movement patterns for screening. In some instances, this may require an assessment of regions of the body that have no direct functional relationship to distance running. For example, coaches that choose to improve a runner's explosive strength through the prescription of weightlifting exercises (e.g. variations of the snatch, clean or jerk) should screen movements that focus on the mechanics of the spine (Howe and Read, 2015) and shoulder complex (Howe and Blagrove, 2015). In this instance, assessing the mobility and coordination of these segments during an overhead movement will inform the coach of the athlete's ability to achieve a successful overhead bar-bell position in preparation for the snatch and jerk exercises and their derivatives. Therefore, a coach's philosophy and their preferential methods to develop strength qualities should also influence the selection of movement screens to inform the training process.

Based upon the physical demands of distance running, and the associated S&C provision that will be required to target 'sport relevant' training adaptations (see Chapter 14), the following movements could be considered for inclusion as part of a comprehensive screening battery. The list presented in the next section should be regarded as a menu for coaches to choose from, with only a small selection of movements being required in most instances. The decision as to what movements to select should be based upon the needs of the athlete, relevant situational context and potential constraints in the training environment, and the programming strategies the coach wishes to employ.

Administering a Movement Screen

A major limitation of movement screening is the requirement to assess numerous components of the performance criteria simultaneously. As such, the level of agreement has been shown to be poor between a tester evaluating movement competency in real time and objective measurements recorded using 3D motion capture (Whiteside et al., 2016). Although real-time movement screening can produce reliable results (Onate et al., 2012), it is recommended that coaches use video analysis when possible to improve accuracy and allow visual test/re-test comparison that may further guide training provision and can act as an effective feedback tool for the athlete. If logistics require coaches to screen in real-time, it is recommended that for each repetition, only one variable from the performance criteria is assessed. This will result in the number of components included in the performance criteria determining the minimum number of repetitions performed for each screen (Gould et al., 2017). If this approach is employed, coaches will avoid the error associated with screening movement with performance criteria's, including several components across only three repetitions in real-time (Whiteside et al., 2016). However, this practice is only appropriate if the athlete has been sufficiently familiarised with the movement pattern and the strategy demonstrated is consistent.

Based upon the need to obtain accurate results from a movement screen, coaches should adhere to the following process:

1. For each screen, a camera should be set up at a distance that captures the entire movement, while accounting for perspective and parallax error (Payton, 2007). It is recommended

that the capture area is marked out for consistency and the distance the camera is positioned from the athlete is measured and recorded to ensure replication for test/re-test purposes. Practically, 3.5 m between the camera and the athlete has been employed for reliably screening movement using 2D video analysis (Howe et al., 2020).

2. For screens that require footage in both the sagittal and frontal plane, coaches can either use two cameras to record footage simultaneously, or, if only a single camera is available, the athlete should perform clusters of repetitions at different angles to the camera to allow for footage to be recorded in various planes.

3. Athletes should wear the same footwear they expect to regularly train in and clothing that allows for anatomical landmarks to be observed (e.g. shorts to mid-thigh length), whilst allowing unrestricted movement.

4. Standardised instructions of how to perform the task should be given using a script that includes only relevant information. A demonstration should also be provided to ensure athletes have a clear understanding for how the task should be performed. See Table 7.2 for a suggested script for each screen.

5. A minimum of three repetitions should initially be performed by the athlete to allow adequate familiarisation. This should be repeated until the athlete reports they are comfortable with the movement and the coach is confident there is sufficient consistency between repetitions to ensure reliable results are recorded. Coaches may need to use this time to reinforce specific test instructions.

Performance Criteria

Movement screens commonly employ a scoring system that allows for a composite score to be calculated through a range of screens (Bennett et al., 2017; Frohm et al., 2012). However, where individual screens may have the potential to identify runners at greater risk of injury (Hotta et al., 2015), the use of composite scores fails to provide the same predictive value (Bring et al., 2018) and also lacks factorial validity (indicating the tests are largely independent of each other and do not screen generic abilities). Furthermore, a composite score fails to help coaches determine competency during each movement pattern. Instead, attention should be focused on the performance of individual screens and the movement faults that may present (Read et al., 2016) and as a result, a pass–fail criterion is suggested for each movement.

Once movements have been selected to screen, coaches must adopt a performance criterion, which athletes can be compared against. The criteria represent the technical features that the athlete should display, providing coaches with a clear guideline for how the movement should be performed. This requires coaches to clarify compulsory features for each screen, so the athlete can be cleared to 'pass' the screen and load the movement. Coaches should therefore filter their performance criteria to include features of the exercise technical model that are fundamental to ensure safe and effective performance of the movement. Table 7.2 presents a performance criterion for each screen presented.

Investigating the Cause of Movement Faults

Following the administration of a movement screen, coaches must determine whether the athlete displays acceptable technique. When an athlete performs a screen that matches all elements of the performance criteria, they have 'passed' the screen. The coach's interpretation should be that the athlete has demonstrated an acceptable level of movement skill and the pattern can be performed with suitable technique so that loading may commence.

When movement faults are present (the athlete fails to perform the movement in a manner that matches all elements of the performance criteria), they have 'failed' the screen and a thorough investigation is required to establish the cause. Due to the complex nature of each movement, using a simplistic approach of equating a movement fault to a functional deficit in the neighbouring anatomical region (e.g. excessive flexion in the spine during the squat equates to weak spinal extensor muscles) in many cases, leads to inaccurate assumptions and unhelpful solutions in an attempt to solve the movement puzzle (Howe and Cushion, 2017). Such an approach in most cases results in the prescription of several corrective exercises that do not address the cause of the movement fault and, therefore, fail to improve movement quality. As time to train is always limited, this strategy not only presents a potential waste of time and resources, but also restricts athletes from completing training that more effectively improves running performance. To avoid this pitfall, a problem-solving process should be implemented to determine the primary cause(s) of the movement fault(s). Figure 7.1 illustrates a four-stage model to systematically investigate the cause of movement faults.

Stage 1 involves having the athlete perform the movement screen with a 'pass' or 'fail' outcome as previously discussed. *Stage 2* requires practitioners to coach the performance of the screen prior to further testing being administered. This allows coaches the opportunity to distinguish between whether a *skill* or *capacity* issue is causing the movement fault. If the athlete can pass the screen following time spent practicing the movement under the coach's guidance, then the athlete is likely to possess the necessary capacities to perform the movement to the standards outlined in the performance criteria. For example, if an athlete performs the squat screen with excessive forward trunk lean, a restriction in ankle dorsiflexion range of motion may be the culprit (Conradsson et al., 2010; Fuglsang et al., 2017). However, if the athlete is made aware of the strategy they are employing and can self-correct without compromising other aspects of technique, enough ankle mobility is present relative to the task demands. In such instances, the skill to coordinate the movement was the underlying cause, with the athlete requiring a more detailed mental template for how the movement should be performed.

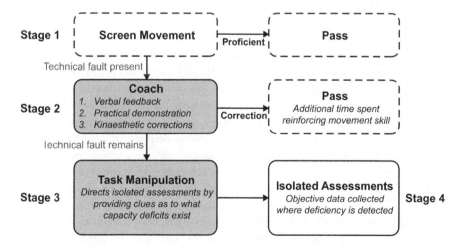

FIGURE 7.1   A four-stage model to systematically investigate movement faults

This process will save a coach's valuable time by decreasing the demand for additional tests and avoid unnecessary prescription of corrective exercise modalities.

In most cases, coaching an athlete how to perform a movement (that may be performed directly after the screen or in a separate session) should last only a few minutes to determine whether a skill issue is present. This suggestion is supported by evidence that drastic changes in technique can occur following basic instruction. Frost et al. (2015) showed performance on a movement screen significantly improved when firefighters were informed of the performance criteria for each movement. However, coaching is more than just explaining technical models. Therefore, packaging information through verbal feedback, demonstrations and the development of kinaesthetic awareness will likely result in greater improvements in movement quality, and in many cases, less time than it takes to explain the performance criteria of a screen. For more information, readers are referred to Cushion et al. (2017).

Stage 3 of this process should guide coaches as to what capacities may be lacking and, as a result, what additional assessments should be employed in *Stage 4*. This is accomplished by manipulating elements of the movement task to gain insight into the underpinning cause. Although an infinite number of options exist, this stage does not need to be extensive or overly complicated. A simple example of how a movement pattern can be manipulated to help identify the primary cause can be to adjust the load or starting position. For example, if an athlete demonstrates a dynamic knee valgus during the single-leg squat screen that does not improve following coaching, weak hip abductor muscles (Crossley et al., 2011) or restricted ankle dorsiflexion range of motion (Dill et al., 2014) may be the cause. In this instance, the coach can manipulate the task in several ways. One option could be to have the athlete perform the movement with both feet together to unload the lower extremity (by using both legs to perform the movement) without changing the mobility demands. If the dynamic knee valgus is no longer apparent, a lack of strength is the likely culprit and the hip abduction strength test should be performed. However, if the dynamic knee valgus remains unchanged, ankle hypomobility may be the cause of the movement fault. This working hypothesis can be further challenged by asking the athlete to perform a single-leg squat with an elevated heel relative to the forefoot (e.g. placing a 2.5 kg weight plate under the heel) to provide the athlete with a greater capacity to translate the knee forward, imitating additional ankle dorsiflexion range of motion. If the athlete can now prevent dynamic knee valgus from occurring during the movement, a restriction in ankle mobility is likely present and the modified weight-bearing lunge test should be performed. Additionally, this information can be used to provide an understanding of how the movement can be regressed. Consequently, Stage 3 develops efficiency in advancing the investigatory process alongside informing programming decisions.

Following manipulations of the task (Stage 3), the investigation process is progressed to Stage 4, where capacities are tested (e.g. mobility, strength, balance) using isolated assessments. For example, during bilateral squatting, the ankle joint dorsiflexes approximately 35° (Hemmerich et al., 2006; Swinton et al., 2012). If an athlete demonstrates restricted ankle dorsiflexion range of motion (i.e. < 35°), squat technique may be compromised (Conradsson et al., 2010; Fuglsang et al., 2017; List et al., 2013). Therefore, objective data obtained during isolated assessments of physical capacities provide information that can be directly compared to the demands of a movement pattern, supporting the interpretation of the findings. Table 7.3 presents isolated assessments used to establish mobility restrictions relevant to the squat screen described in Table 7.2. The interested reader should see Howe and Waldron (2019) for a range of mobility assessments that could be used to identify movement faults in other screens.

TABLE 7.3 Isolated assessments for mobility testing relevant to the squat screen

Test		Start position	Movement	Measurement
Supine active hip flexion test		Laying supine on the ground, with both knees extended and the arms by the athlete's side.	The athlete is cued to maximally bring the knee of the test limb towards the ipsilateral chest, while bending the knee.	Prior to testing, the smartphone is zeroed against a vertical reference (e.g. wall). In the start position, a horizontal line is marked on the athlete's thigh, 5 cm above the base of the patella. At the point of maximal hip flexion, the smartphone is placed proximal to the marked line at the point of maximal hip flexion.
Supine hip abduction test		Athlete lays in a supine position with the legs extended. The test leg is flexed at the hip and knee to 90°.	The athlete maximally abducts at the hip (moves the knee away from the midline of the pelvis) while the coach stabilizes the pelvis, preventing rotation from occurring.	Prior to testing, the smartphone is zeroed against a vertical reference (e.g. wall). At the point of maximal hip abduction, place the phone on the medial surface at approximately mid-thigh.

(*Continued*)

TABLE 7.3 (Continued)

Test	Start position	Movement	Measurement
Active hip internal rotation test	The athlete sits on the edge of a plinth, with the knees flexed at 90° and the lower legs freely hanging off the table. The non-test leg is placed over the lateral edge of the plinth by abducting the hip.	The athlete is instructed to maximally rotate the foot away from (hip internal rotation) the midline of their body, while maintaining a 90° flexed position at the knee.	Prior to testing, the smartphone is zeroed against a vertical reference (e.g. wall) and a horizontal line is made 10 cm above the inferior tip of the lateral malleolus. At the point of maximal hip internal rotation, the smartphone is placed directly proximal to the marked line.
Modified weight-bearing lunge test	The athlete starts in a half-kneeling position, with the pelvis facing forwards and the trunk relatively upright (some forward lean is allowed). The test foot is positioned half a foot length ahead of the knee of the non-test leg, with the knee aligned directly over the foot on the test limb.	The athlete is instructed to reach the knee forward as far as possible, while keeping the knee over the foot, the heel down against the ground and the pelvis facing forward.	Prior to testing, the smartphone is zeroed against a vertical reference (e.g. wall). At the point of maximal ankle dorsiflexion just prior to heel-lift, the smartphone should be placed on the anterior border of the tibia distal to the tibial tuberosity.

Physical Capacity Assessments

Incorporating physical capacity assessments into a testing battery provides coaches with data to examine athletic performance qualities. In turn, this information supports decision-making throughout the training process. The following sections will discuss strength diagnostic and tissue capacity assessments that should be included in the initial athlete assessment and repeated regularly to evaluate progress.

Strength Diagnostics Assessment

Muscular strength plays an important role in the development of the distance runner, significantly contributing to improvements in performance-related measures (Blagrove et al., 2018a) and is associated with reduced injury risk (Lauersen et al., 2014). For the assessment of strength qualities, trunk and lower extremity force production during multi-joint and single-joint tasks provide a global and local indication of neuromuscular capabilities respectively. Table 7.4 illustrates suggested strength assessments, along with equipment requirements and procedures. Table 7.5 provides normative data to support the interpretation of test results (where appropriate).

Maximal Strength

Maximal strength, defined as the maximum force an individual can produce irrespective of time (Tillin and Folland, 2014), is measured directly using specialised equipment (i.e. force platforms and racks). The isometric mid-thigh pull is an example of a test that is commonly used that provides valid and reliable measures of an athlete's peak force development (De Witt et al., 2018). A simple alternative when this equipment is not available is the weight an athlete can lift during an exercise for a specific number of repetitions (Verdijk et al., 2009). Coaches can choose to use either the maximum (concentric) load that can be lifted for a single repetition (e.g. 1 repetition maximum; RM) or a set number of repetitions (e.g. 5 RM testing) to determine maximal strength levels. However, fewer than 10 repetitions should be selected so as to provide an accurate measure of maximal strength (Reynolds et al., 2006).

A key consideration when performing RM testing, irrespective of the number of repetitions performed, is the athlete's skill level on the exercise. To measure leg extensor strength, a variation of the free weight squat exercise is commonly used. However, some athletes do not possess the necessary skill to test maximal strength during the movement pattern (something that would quickly be examined through an appropriate movement screen). As an alternative, coaches may choose to use less complex movements to determine leg extensor strength capabilities. For example, the leg press may be an ideal option for a distance runner as it reduces the demand on the spinal extensor musculature and therefore provides an isolated measure of leg extensor strength. Furthermore, unilateral testing of each leg provides an opportunity to measure limb symmetry. If an athlete presents with no experience of performing resistance training, coaches may choose to delay maximal strength testing until competence in technique under load has been demonstrated.

Explosive Strength

Explosive strength is defined as the maximum force an individual can produce relative to time and is commonly represented as rate of force development (Tillin and Folland, 2014). Explosive strength has been shown to improve distance running performance and maximal sprint speed

TABLE 7.4 Guidelines for example strength diagnostic and tissue capacity assessments

Test	Strength quality	Equipment	Outcome measure	Procedures

Single–leg leg press	Maximal Strength	Leg press machine	1RM
			Between-limb differences
				• The athlete is positioned seated with back fully in contact with the back support and hands holding the allocated handles.
				• Foot position will be determined by the design of the equipment. A general recommendation is at the bottom position, the athlete should have the knee flexed to 90° and the knee directly over the toes and the heel flat against the plate. The foot should face directly forward.
				• The free leg should be held suspended, so it does not interfere with test performance.
				• For each repetition, the athlete starts at the bottom of the movement.
				• The warm up prior to attempting a 1RM should be as follows:
				  • 8 repetitions at 40% estimated 1RM.
				  • 5 repetitions at 60% estimated 1RM.
				  • 3 repetitions at 80% estimated 1RM.
				  • 1 repetition at 90% estimated 1RM.
				    • Three attempts to determine 1RM.
				• Recovery between sets should be 2–5 mins following the 80% 1RM warm-up set.

Countermovement jump	Explosive strength	Smartphone and application	Jump height	• The athlete stands with their hands on their hips and feet hip-width apart. • The athlete explosively descends to a comfortable depth before jumping as high as possible. • Three attempts are permitted with 1 min recovery between jumps.

Test	Quality	Equipment	Measure	Instructions
Drop jump	Reactive strength	0.3 m box Smartphone and application	Jump height Reactive strength index (flight time/contact time)	• The athlete stands with their hands on their hips and feet hip-width apart on top of the 0.3 m box. • The athlete steps off and drops down ahead directly in front of the box. • Both feet should contact the ground simultaneously. • Upon landing, the athlete immediately jumps as high as possible. • Three attempts are permitted with 1 min recovery between jumps.
Hop for distance	Unilateral explosive strength	Tape measure	Horizontal distance Between-limb differences	• The athlete stands on the test leg with the foot behind the start line and the hands on the hips. • The athlete hops forward as far as possible. • The athlete must stick the landing without putting the non-test leg down. • The distance from the start line to the heel should be measured. • The athlete should alternate legs between attempts. Three attempts are permitted for each leg, with 30 sec recovery between hops.
Calf raise	Tissue capacity of calf musculature	0.3 m box	Total repetitions performed Between-limb differences	• Position a box directly in front of a bare wall. • The athlete stands upright on the box with one leg so the heel hangs over the edge of the box and only the ball of the foot is on the box. • Balance is maintained by keeping the finger tips against the wall. • The non-test leg does not contact the test leg, box or wall. • The pelvis should remain level throughout. • Maintaining a neutral knee alignment, the athlete fully plantar flexes the ankle before descending into full ankle dorsiflexion. • The cadence should be 1 sec up and 1 sec down with no bouncing permitted. • The test is stopped when range of motion or cadence is no longer maintained.

(Continued)

TABLE 7.4 (Continued)

Test	Strength quality	Equipment	Outcome measure	Procedures
Single-leg hamstring bridge	Tissue capacity of hip extensor musculature	0.5 m box	Total repetitions performed Between-limb differences	• The athlete lies supine, with the test leg positioned so the heel is on a box, the foot facing directly up, and the knee is flexed to 20°. • Hands are positioned across the chest. • The non-test leg is suspended so the hip and knee are flexed, and the foot is positioned next to the knee. • The athletes are instructed to lift the hips by pushing the heel into the box until the hip extends so that a straight line is formed from the knee to shoulder. • The cadence should be 1 sec up and 1 sec down with no bouncing permitted. • The test is stopped when range of motion or cadence is no longer maintained.
Side bridge	Tissue capacity of lateral trunk musculature	Stopwatch Foam pad	Time Between-side differences	• Athlete is positioned on their side in an extended posture whilst resting on their elbow with the feet on top of each other. • The elbow on the test side should be directly under the shoulder, resting on a foam pad for comfort. • The arm on the non-test side is positioned across the chest so the hand is on the opposite shoulder. • The athlete lifts their pelvis off the ground, bringing the body into a straight line from the feet to the head. • No trunk or pelvic rotation is permitted. • The test is stopped when the athlete can no longer maintain the test position.

| Prone hold | Tissue capacity of posterior trunk musculature | Stopwatch Bench or Plinth | Time | • The athlete lays face down on a bench/plinth so that the belt-line (anterior superior iliac crest of the pelvis) overhangs the bench and only the legs are in contact with the bench.
• With the athlete's hands supporting their upper body, a partner secures the legs by anchoring the lower legs against the bench.
• The athlete then lifts the hands off the floor and crosses the arms over the chest.
• The athlete should be parallel to the ground from head to feet, maintaining a neutral spine position.
• The test is stopped when the athlete can no longer maintain the test position. |
| Double leg hold | Tissue capacity of anterior trunk musculature | Stopwatch Sphygmomanometer (preferably) Fixed pole (e.g. squat rack) | Time | • Athlete lays supine on the ground with the legs extended and hands by their side so that their head is directly in front of the fixed pole.
• The sphygmomanometer cuff is positioned under the centre of the lumbar spine directly under the level of the belly button.
• The cuff is filled to 40 mmHg whilst the athlete is relaxed. This ensures the athlete can maintain a neutral position of the spine throughout the test.
• The athlete is then instructed to bring the arms above head to hold onto the fixed pole. No change in pressure on the cuff should occur.
• With the athlete able to see the sphygmomanometer dial, the athlete lifts both legs off the ground with the knees extended and the heels 2–3 cm off the ground.
• The test is stopped when the athlete can no longer maintain the test position. |

Note: RM = repetition maximum.

TABLE 7.5 Normative data for strength diagnostic and tissue capacity assessment

Test	Poor	Average	Excellent
1RM Single-leg leg press (kg/BM)	<1.0	1.0–1.4	>1.4
Countermovement jump height (m)	<0.30	0.30–0.45	>0.45
Drop jump height (m)	<0.30	0.3–0.45	>0.45
Hop for distance normalised to athlete height (m)	<0.80	0.80–1.00	>1.00
Calf raise (repetitions)	<15	15–30	>30
Single-leg hamstring bridge (repetitions)	<15	15–30	>30
Side bridge (s)	<60	60–120	>120
Prone hold (s)	<90	90–180	>180
Double leg hold (s)	<60	60–120	>120

Note: RM = repetition maximum; BM = body mass.

(Ramírez-Campillo et al., 2014). Measurement in practice commonly includes a variety of jump tests, with peak jump height during a countermovement jump providing an accurate representation of explosive strength (McLellan et al., 2011) and leg power (Nuzzo et al., 2008). However, valid measures of jump height have traditionally required expensive equipment (i.e. force platform or contact mats) that many coaches may not have access to (Buckthorpe et al., 2012). With advances in technology, smartphone applications can now be used to accurately measure jump height (Balsalobre-Fernández et al., 2015). Therefore, jump performance can be assessed across a range of tests using measurement tools accessible for all coaches at a low cost (< £10).

Reactive Strength

Reactive strength is defined as the ability to effectively transition rapidly from an eccentric to concentric muscle contraction utilising a stretch-shortening cycle (Flanagan et al., 2008), and it represents an athlete's plyometric quality. As distance running involves cyclical stretch-shortening muscle actions, it's unsurprising that enhancing reactive strength improves running performance (Ramírez-Campillo et al., 2014; Spurrs et al., 2003). The most common measurement is the reactive strength index (Flanagan et al., 2008), calculated by dividing either jump height or flight time by ground contact time during a plyometric rebound task, e.g. drop jump from a specified height (e.g. 0.3 m) or repeated vertical hopping. As with other vertical jumping tests, specialised equipment has traditionally been a necessity to record measures of reactive strength. However, reactive strength index can also be calculated reliably using smartphone applications (Haynes et al., 2019).

Tissue Capacity

During running, the trunk and lower extremity joint segments are repetitively loaded with each ground contact (Novacheck, 1998). In order to avoid maladaptation occurring and reduce the risk of injury (Cook and Docking, 2015), the muscles surrounding these joints must possess a high load tolerance. Tissue capacity refers to the ability of a musculotendon unit to produce force and tolerate load (Cook and Docking, 2015). Assessments of tissue capacity can provide insight into a specific structure's strength capability through single-joint movements where a prolonged time under tension is the goal of the task. As a result, commonly used assessments require individuals to perform a task for a maximal number of repetitions (Dennis et al., 2008) or hold a certain position for as long as possible (Leetun et al., 2004). Although these tests of strength endurance will provide only a relative indication of maximal strength levels (Reynolds et al., 2006), they require minimal equipment, are simple to administer and provide reliable results (Dennis et al., 2008; Freckleton et al., 2014; Waldhelm and Li, 2012).

Key areas to test for capacity are those associated with injury risk and performance in distance running, such as the trunk (Leetun et al., 2004), hip (Malliaropoulos et al., 2012) and calf regions (Hébert-Losier et al., 2009). For example, the strength of the calf musculature is associated with lower limb injuries (O'Neill et al., 2016) and performance during maximal sprinting (Möck et al., 2018). As maximal sprint speed has been shown to be a determining factor in distance running performance (Sinnett et al., 2001), developing strength qualities in the calf musculature is an important consideration.

Equally, tissue capacity assessments of the hip musculature should also be of interest. Hip abduction strength has been correlated with dynamic knee valgus during running in both injured (Dierks et al., 2008) and healthy individuals (Heinert et al., 2008). Consequently, reduced hip strength has been suggested as an injury risk factor for running-related injuries (Mucha et al., 2017). Furthermore, high levels of hip abduction strength have been shown to increase a novice runner's resiliency to injury when beginning a structured running programme (Ramskov et al., 2015). Unfortunately, testing hip abduction strength requires equipment that a coach may not have access to (i.e. handheld dynamometer). However, poor performance on the single-leg squat screen following coaching, and in the absence of an ankle mobility restriction, likely indicates hip abductor weakness and can be used as a surrogate measure (Crossley et al., 2011). Additionally, the side bridge test relies on lateral trunk and hip abduction strength and consequently is moderately related to hip abduction strength (Leetun et al., 2004). Therefore, coaches can determine whether an athlete presents with weak hip abductors by analysing their performance across several relevant tests. Table 7.4 provides an example of tissue capacity assessments that should be administered, while Table 7.5 displays normative data, and these can be used to support coaches' decision-making processes.

Summary

Movement screening and physical capacity assessments are a fundamental component of the coach's toolkit and should be considered a non-negotiable for use with distance runners. Data collected from these tests provide insight into an athlete's physical profile and should be used to directly influence the training process. Specifically, movement screening allows coaches to determine an athlete's level of preparedness to load relevant movement patterns. This process should be tailored to the athlete's individual needs and the exercises selected to form part of a strength training programme. When movement faults are identified, the four-stage investigatory process presented in this chapter provides a framework for coaches to detect whether a skill or capacity deficit is the primary cause of the suboptimal strategy. Physical capacity assessments should also be administered to determine if the athlete possesses the requisite strength qualities. Examples include measurement of an athlete's maximal, explosive and reactive strength using a variety of strength and jump assessments. Tissue capacity testing also provides useful information regarding a muscle or muscle group's ability to produce and tolerate force and may be helpful in identifying areas that are vulnerable to injury.

8

TRAINING VOLUME AND INTENSITY DISTRIBUTION AMONG ELITE MIDDLE- AND LONG-DISTANCE RUNNERS

Arturo Casado and Leif Inge Tjelta

Highlights

- Training intensity distribution models typically classify runs as (zone 1) below the lactate (or first ventilatory) threshold (moderate-intensity/recovery runs); (zone 2) an intensity between the first ventilatory threshold and maximal steady state (steady and 'tempo' runs, interval training); and (zone 3) intensities above maximal steady state (high-intensity/severe sessions).
- The *pyramidal model* of training is characterised by a decreasing volume of running in zones 1, 2 and 3, respectively: zone 1 contains 80% of the training volume in this model with the remaining 20% performed in zones 2 and 3.
- The *polarised model* of training involves approximately 80% of training volume performed in zone 1, while the remaining 20% is conducted mostly in zone 3 (very little 'steady' pace running).
- Elite distance runners tend to adopt pyramidal or polarised approaches to their training intensity distribution (regardless of the training phase) to build a large aerobic base.
- Examples of the volumes, intensities and frequencies of easy runs, 'tempo' runs and interval training sessions are provided for numerous elite runners, including several who have won medals at major championships.
- One sprint training session per week is recommended for middle-distance runners and a long run each week is a stable component of the training week of runners across events at any time of the season.

Introduction

There are several important variables that can be manipulated in order to create an overload stimulus when designing a training programme; frequency of training, duration or distance of runs, intensity of runs/sessions, and density of training in a given period of time (i.e. recovery time). When planning training in both the long and short term, runners and coaches need to make informed decisions on how far an athlete will run and how fast a run (or repetitions) should be. The training load that a runner is exposed to can impact long-term performance both positively or negatively and can also influence the likelihood of suffering an overuse injury. Determining the optimal training prescription for each individual runner at a given point in time is both a science and an art. However, a great deal of information can be gleaned from analysing the training of highly successful runners and summarising the results of comparative training studies. The aim of this chapter is to describe and analyse the training volume and intensity distribution patterns that emerge from the scientific literature and training of elite middle- and long-distance runners.

Training Volume and Training Intensity Distribution in Distance Running

Concept of Training Intensity Distribution

The combination of training intensity and volume, which is known as training load, can be understood in either absolute or relative terms in relation to the specific capacity tolerated by the athlete. Training load can be considered as either external or internal. External load refers to the actual distance covered, and velocity achieved during a given training session, whereas internal load is deemed as the specific body response to a given training session (i.e., increase of heart rate or blood lactate concentration). While external training load represents an important reference to understand the performance evolution during the training process (Kenneally et al., 2018), it is generally believed that internal load may be the most accurate indicator of the effort made by runners or endurance sport athletes (Seiler and Tønnessen, 2009).

In order to quantify the training load conducted at different intensities relative to the current capacity of each runner, different training zones are created according to either physiological factors – i.e., lactate threshold (maximum steady state), ventilatory thresholds (VT), percentage of the maximum oxygen uptake ($\%\dot{V}O_{2max}$), percentage of the maximum heart rate (%HR) – or perceptual/subjective factors – i.e., rate of perceived exertion (RPE). According to the physiological approach, Skinner and McLellan (1980) developed the triphasic model delimited by both ventilatory thresholds and described the physiological responses throughout the transition from aerobic to anaerobic metabolism generated from an incremental intensity test. Therefore, zone 1 (z1) is represented by intensities below the first ventilatory threshold (VT1), zone 2 (z2) is referred to intensities between the first and second ventilatory threshold (VT2, which is generally associated to maximum steady state) and zone 3 (z3) refers to any intensity conducted above the maximum steady state. According to the perceptual/subjective approach, VT1 and maximum steady state are associated to specific levels of RPE (i.e., level 11 and 14 from the traditional Borg scale (Borg, 1982) represent intensities associated to VT1 and maximum steady state, respectively) (Molinari et al., 2020). Therefore, in order to calculate a particular training intensity distribution (TID) during a given training period, time of training conducted in each training zone is assessed and a specific TID (percentage of the training volume conducted in each zone) is calculated. Both TID and training periodisation, understood as the evolution of training volume and TID during a given season, are essential factors in the design of a training program for endurance runners (Faulkner, 1968).

Training Intensity Distribution (TID) Models

As indicated in Chapter 1, there is a general consensus in the literature regarding the determinant factors of performance in distance running, namely velocity at maximal oxygen uptake (v-$\dot{V}O_{2max}$) (McLaughlin et al., 2010), $\dot{V}O_{2max}$ (Coyle, 1995), maximum steady state (Conley and Krahenbuhl, 1980; Coyle, 1995) and running economy (Conley and Krahenbuhl, 1980). However, there is a lack of consensus regarding the specific training volume and TID required for optimising both performance determinant factors and performance itself in distance runners. In order to achieve it, several TID models have been described within the literature, although five have been considered the most commonly used by runners:

1. The traditional *pyramidal model* is characterised by a decreasing volume of running in zones 1, 2 and 3, respectively. Typically, the z1 contains 80% of the training volume in this model, with the remaining 20% performed at both z2 and z3 (Seiler, 2010).
2. In the *polarised model*, approximately 80% of training volume is performed at z1 while the remaining 20% is mostly conducted at z3 (Seiler, 2010).
3. The *threshold model* is characterised by a higher amount of training volume than in the other models (>20%) conducted at z2 (Seiler, 2010).
4. The *high volume low intensity (HVLI)* model is characterised by high amounts of training conducted in z1 predominantly (Stöggl and Sperlich, 2015).
5. The *Low volume high intensity (LVHI)* model is characterised by high amounts of training conducted in z3 predominantly (Stöggl and Sperlich, 2015).

According to the results of a recent systematic review, both the pyramidal or the polarised model have successfully improved performance in distance runners (Kenneally et al., 2018). Some studies support the use of a pyramidal approach. Esteve-Lanao et al. (2007) found that a pyramidal approach improved performance to a greater extent than a threshold approach in sub-elite distance runners specialised in the 5000 m during a training period of 5 months. Robinson et al. (1991) found that during the preparatory period, 13 nationally ranked male New Zealand distance runners conducted 96% of their training volume below maximum steady state (4 mmol·L^{-1}) and 4% above maximum steady state. In addition, Esteve-Lanao et al. (2005) found that the training of 8 regional- and national-class Spanish runners was following a pyramidal TID, as was the training of nine-time New York Marathon winner Grete Waitz during a 2-year time period (Tjelta et al., 2014). Among other studies supporting the use of a polarised approach, Muñoz et al. (2014) found that although either a polarised or a threshold TID improved performance in 30 recreational runners during an 8-week training period, this improvement was greater in those runners who followed a polarised approach. Furthermore, Stöggl and Sperlich (2014) studied 48 athletes among whom 21 were national-level runners and compared the physiological and performance outcomes of four different TID models during a 9-week training period: HVLI, threshold, LVHI and polarised. Participants who followed the threshold approach displayed greater improvement in performance determinant capacities such as $\dot{V}O_{2max}$, peak velocity and time to exhaustion. Finally, Ingham et al. (2012) reported the improvement in performance from 3:38.9 to 3:32.4 over a 2-year training period of an Olympic 1500 m finalist supposedly due to a shift from a more threshold-oriented to a more polarised-oriented TID.

Quantification of Training Intensity Distribution in Distance Running

Once a decision has been made regarding which TID approach may be optimally used by any middle- or long-distance runner, it is important to know the different ways available to quantify the specific training volume conducted at each training zone, so that it will be possible to control that a given athlete is following the previously selected TID and not a different one. For that purpose, as has been explained previously, either external or internal training loads must be measured according to the training time conducted at each of the different training zones. Regarding the latter, three different methods have been commonly used (Bellinger et al., 2019). Two of these TID quantification methods requires a previous incremental intensity test, which would identify the speed and heart rate associated to both VT through a respiratory gas analysis and heart rate monitoring. This identification is made through the calculation of the gas exchange threshold and the respiratory compensation threshold (Beaver et al., 2016). According to this information, coaches may use any of these two indicators (i.e., either speed or heart rate associated to each VT) to control the intensity conducted by their runners during each training session through the demarcation of the different training zones. Time conducted at each zone will report a specific TID.

Another TID quantification method also used in different studies examining TID in runners (Bellinger et al., 2019; Stellingwerff, 2012) is the session-RPE (s-RPE). This method was created by Foster et al. (2001) and consists in delimiting three training zones according to different levels of the adapted 10-point Borg scale (Borg, 1982); z1= RPE of 1–4; z2 = RPE of 5–6; z3= RPE of 7–10. Runners must complete their RPE training diary 30 min after each training session. According to this indication, the time of each running session is assigned to one of the three zones previously described and a TID quantification can be conducted. Whereas these three methods have been used in different studies, Bellinger et al. (2019) found that TID calculation according to each of these methods during an 8-week training period in well-trained middle-distance runners resulted in different TID models (i.e. running speed-derived TID resulted in a polarised approach, heart rate-demarcated TID resulted in a pyramidal approach and RPE-derived TID resulted in a threshold approach). Therefore, the quantification method used may mislead the interpretation of the training conducted. These authors concluded that each of these methods may be useful for coaches and athletes and can be used during the season according to the type of training sessions conducted (Bellinger et al., 2019). For example, during sessions involving a high amount of changes of pace and short, high-intensity intervals, it is recommended to use the running speed-derived TID as the heart rate-derived approach may not reflect the several changes of pace conducted during these training sessions. However, a heart rate-derived approach may be useful in steady tempo runs or long interval sessions. Additionally, RPE measures may be reported for each part of the session in order to improve its precision as a training load indicator. For example, reporting RPE values for the warm-up, main interval training session and cool down separately may be more valid and precise than just reporting a single value for the whole session.

Given that either speed or heart rate associated to both VT can be obtained only through an incremental intensity test involving either respiratory gas or blood lactate concentration analysis, an alternative field test has been recently validated and may be useful for coaches. The Running Advisor Billat Training has been found to detect both heart rate and speed associated to both ventilatory thresholds through a perceptual-based approach conducted during a three-intensity test consisting on completing 10, 5, 3 and 10 min runs separated by 1 min of passive recovery at values of RPE of 11, 14, 17 and 11, respectively. Paces and heart rate observed at RPE values of 11 and 14 can be associated to VT1 and maximum steady state intensities, respectively (Giovanelli et al., 2019; Molinari et al., 2020). Despite the fact that internal loads are considered the main index to monitor the training process, recent research observed that when monitoring TID according to the pace relative to competition speed in the specific distance being targeted (external training loads), no substantial differences were observed than when the same training content was monitored according to heart rate–derived training zones (Kenneally et al., 2018). Furthermore, these authors suggested that this race pace-based approach may be useful for middle- and long-distance runners' coaches when trying to measure a more specific training load than through a typical triphasic-model approach. For example, many marathon runners conduct high amounts of training at their marathon pace. This pace is just below maximum steady state intensity and relies on the z2, but this zone is wide and the quantifying methods previously shown are not able to account for these specific paces which are considered very relevant on the preparation of distance runners. Similarly, training conducted at z3 can be very different depending on whether it is conducted below, at or above $\dot{V}O_{2max}$ intensities. In the case that training is conducted above $\dot{V}O_{2max}$ intensities, no reference regarding intensity can be provided through heart rate monitoring. In this sense, a race pace-based approach may help to quantify more accurately the training loads conducted at these specific intensities. In conclusion, the combination in the use of the quantifying methods previously described can provide valuable information regarding the training process in middle- and long-distance runners.

Training Periodisation and Intensity Distribution in World-Class Runners

Periodisation refers to the degree of change of training volume and TID over the course of a sport season. Two main different periodisation models have been used in endurance sports, namely, block and traditional periodisation. Traditional or linear periodisation refers to the use of same training contents but with volume decreasing and intensity increasing throughout the season through the implementation of different cycles. Block periodisation involves the split of the training season into shorter periods, or blocks, of highly specific and concentrated workloads (Issurin, 2010). Alternatively, reverse linear periodisation refers to a specific linear periodisation in which volume increases and intensity decreases throughout the season (Boullosa et al., 2020).

Successful elite and world-class middle- and long-distance runners typically follow a traditional linear periodisation in all events with the exception of the marathon in which a reverse linear periodisation was observed (Kenneally et al., 2018). All these programs contain a preparatory, pre-competitive and competitive period. Assuming that the peak of performance is expected to be in the summer, the traditional linear periodisation follows different paths depending on the performance objectives set during the season by coaches. Runners in 800 m, 1500 m, 3000 m steeplechase and 5000 m races can also peak during the winter to compete at indoor competitions. In this case, in the Northern Hemisphere, the preparatory period typically takes from September to December, the pre-competitive period takes from December to January and the competitive period takes from February to March. Then there is another preparatory period from March to May, a pre-competitive period from May to June and a competitive period from June to the end of the season in August or September (Martin and Coe, 1991). Those runners who don't compete at indoor races (including 10,000 m runners) extend the preparatory period until January and try to peak in February and March and excel at some cross-country races. These runners then also usually get into another preparatory period until April or May. Their pre-competitive period takes usually from this time to June. In any case, the presence of frequent competitions throughout the whole season (i.e., cross-country, road, indoor and outdoor races) helps to develop the shape of runners during the training process. The transition period typically takes around 3 weeks of either active or passive recovery (Martin and Coe, 1991). Nonetheless, marathoners usually follow a different path, with a training macrocycle of 4 to 6 months, competing at 2 marathons per year. A typical marathon macrocycle consists of 12 weeks of preparatory period and 10 weeks of pre-competitive and competitive period. Each macrocycle represents the specific preparation of one marathon race. Despite all these descriptions, there is great variability regarding the length of each period depending on the coaching philosophy, competition schedules of each country and other factors (Martin and Coe, 1991).

Despite the caution that should always be taken when giving training advice to distance running coaches based on existing literature (Midgley et al., 2007), the following training descriptions and recommendations are based on articles that have registered the training volume and TID of elite runners over selected training weeks in different periods of the training year (Jones, 2006; Kaggestad, 1987; Leknes, 2013; Rabadán et al., 2011; Stellingwerff, 2012; Tjelta and Enoksen, 2001; Tjelta, 2016), on studies having reported training volume and TID among elite runners based on questionnaires targeted at runners or coaches (Casado et al., 2019a; Casado et al., 2019b; Ferreira and Rolim, 2006; Karp, 2007) and from recommendations made by outstanding distance running coaches either in books (Brook, 1992; Martin and Coe, 1991) or as personal communications specifically conducted for the writing of this chapter.

800 m Event

The 800 m is dependent on great energy contribution from both the anaerobic (34%) and the aerobic (66%) energy system (Spencer and Gastin, 2001), and a male runner at international level must be able to run a 400 m in roughly 45.5 to 47 sec (Martin and Coe, 1991). The event requires in addition a high development of both aerobic and anaerobic capacities as well as speed and muscular strength (Martin and Coe, 1991). It is more difficult to give training recommendations regarding training volume and training distribution in different intensity zones for 800 m runners than for runners competing over longer distances. This is due to TID studies being scarce in the research literature and because outstanding results in the 800 m have been achieved by runners belonging to three sub-groups: (1) 400–800 m runners, (2) 800 m specialist and (3) 800–15,000 m runners (Sandford and Stellingwerff, 2019).

In the first sub-group we find runners like Marcello Fiasconaro, Alberto Juantorena and the world record holder David Rudisha (1:40.19). Rudisha's personal best over 400 m is 45.15. Furthermore, the female world record holder Jarmila Kratochvilova possesses best times of 47.99 and 1:53.25 in 400 m and 800 m, respectively. The weekly average training volume during the preparation period for runners belonging to this sub-group have been reported to be 62.1 ($\pm$17) km.week^{-1} (Sandford and Stellingwerff, 2019). In the second sub-group we find runners like Wilson Kipketer and Vebjørn Rodal. These runners have been reported to run an average of 76.7 ($\pm$18.1) km.week^{-1} (Sandford and Stellingwerff, 2019). In the 800–1500 m sub-group we find runners like Sebastian Coe (1:41.73 in 800 m and 3:29.77 in 1500 m) and Taoufik Makloufi (1:42.61 and 3:28.75). Runners in this category were found to run 118.3 ($\pm$27.5) km.week^{-1} in the preparation period (Sandford and Stellingwerff, 2019). The training volume and TID of the runners in this sub-group are more like the training volume described for 1500 m runners. Training principles across the 800 m sub-groups are lacking in the research literature (Sandford and Stellingwerff, 2019). However, runners in sub-groups 1 and 2 to a greater extent focus on anaerobic training, speed- and strength training compared to excellent 800–1500 m runners.

Vebjørn Rodal, the 1996 Olympic 800 m champion who achieved this title in a time of 1:42.58, can be characterised as an athlete belonging to sub-group 2. In 1996 he ran an average of 72 km.week^{-1} during the preparation period (October to the end of April) (Leknes, 2013). A typical training week for Rodal in the first part of the preparation period (October to the end of January) is listed in Table 8.1.

In the first part of the preparation period, the ratio between anaerobic and aerobic main running sessions were 49% and 51% respectively. In the second part of the preparation period (1 February–30 April), the main running sessions focused on anaerobic training which gave a ratio of 71% anaerobic and 29% aerobic running sessions (Leknes, 2013). The stair/hurdle training in the second part of the preparation period consisted of 50% jumping and running up stairs and 50% different jumping exercises over hurdles and series of different steps. The hurdle/stair training is more intensive than in the first preparation period. Once a week (Friday) the main focus was on speed training over shorter distances with long recovery (Leknes, 2013).

In the pre-competitive period (1 May–30 June) the total running volume was reduced to 60 km/week and the ratio between anaerobic and aerobic running sessions was 77% and 23%, respectively. The anaerobic training sessions were performed over distances from 100 to 600 m. A typical anaerobic training session in the pre-competition period could be: warm-up (4 km progressive running) + stretching + 5 × 100 m strides + 1 × 600 m fast (800 m pace) (8 min recovery) + 4 × 300 m (6 min recovery) (600 m pace) every second very fast + 3 km jog + 3 × 100 m strides. The hurdle/stair training was reduced by 50% compared to the preparation period. The length between the hurdles was longer in this period and the number of jumps fewer. Even though the training in the competition period (1 July to 30 August) was dominated by intensive training sessions and competitions, the total training volume in this period was nearly the same as in the pre-competition period. This was due to long warm-up and jog down before and after competitions. Stair/hurdle training was not performed in every week, and when performed, the volume was lower than in the pre-competitive period.

1500 m and Mile Events

The 1500 m event is characterised by a high aerobic component (84 ± 1%) (Spencer and Gastin, 2001). However, there is a high variability in the weekly training schedules among world-class 1500 m runners. The weekly training volume in the preparation period reported for Spanish middle-distance runners (800 m and 1500 m runners) between 2000 and 2008 (n = 32) were 130–140 km/week (Rabadán et al., 2011). However, the volume reported for 1500 m runners competing at 1500 m and 5000 m has been higher, between 140 and 170 km/week (Tjelta and Enoksen, 2001; Tjelta, 2019, 2016). For this type of runner, it has been recommended to train for 2–4 sessions in z2 and 1–2 sessions in z3 during the preparation period. The z2 sessions can be performed as interval training; for example, the training conducted by three Norwegian brothers (Ingebrigtsen) who achieved a European 1500 m championship title (Tjelta, 2019), or continuous tempo runs (Casado et al., 2019b).

A large amount of training in z2 during the preparation period performed as interval training and/or continuous running is consistent with the findings describing the training conducted by some of the best long-distance runners of the world (Casado et al., 2019b).

TABLE 8.1 Training week in period October–end of January 1996 for Vebjørn Rodal (Leknes, 2013)

Day	Morning session	Evening session
Monday	Progressive running 6 km (z1 and z2) + 20 min with drills	Warm up 4 km progressive (z1 and z2), stretching, some drills + 5 · 80 m strides. 4 · 4 min fartlek (tempo change every 20 s; (1:20 min); then 8 min rec. 4 · 200 m sub 25 s (z1 and z3) (60s). Jog 1 km (z1) + 4 · 100 m strides (z3)
Tuesday	Rest	**Stair/hurdle training** 20 min warm-up (basketball). 10 min stretching. 10–12 different drills. Hurdle training: 8 hurdles 3–4 repetitions · 5 sets. Stair training: 175 stairs, 6 floors. (1) Running up the stairs alternating between 1 step at a time, then 2, then 1. (2) Two-footed jumping up the stairs, 3 steps/jump. (3) Running up one step at a time with high frequency. (4) Single-leg jumping up the stairs 2 steps/jump twice, one with each leg. (5) Two-footed jumping up the stairs, 3 steps/jump. (6) Running up one step at a time with high frequency. Core strength training
Wednesday	6 km progressive running (z1 and z2) + Some strides and stretching	Warm up 4 km progressive (z1 and z2). Stretching. Some drills. 5 · 80 m strides. 12 · 150 m, easy – fast – max, (2 min). (z3) 1 km jog (z1) + stretching
Thursday	Warm up 3 km progressive (z1) Core strength training, Stair/ hurdle and strength training (no weights) 2 · 10 exercises, 20 sec effort, 20 sec rec	5 km progressive running (z1 and z2) 10 · 1 min treadmill running at 24 km/h, (60s) (z3).
Friday	Rest	6 km progressive running (z1 and z2). Stretching + some drills. 6 · 100 m strides. 3 · 200 m maximum effort (22 sec-400 m pace), (4 min). 8 min rec. then 4 · 100 m max (10–11 sec) (4 min) (z3). Jog 1 km (z1) + some strides
Saturday	Rest	6 km progressive running (z1 and z2) **Strength training** (1) Core strength training exercises. 4 · 20 sec (20 sec). (2) Fast knee flexion to 90° 30 kg, 20 repetitions. (3) Step up 30 kg, 2 · 12 repetitions on each foot. (4) Step up 20 kg, 3 · 15 repetitions on each foot. (5) Exercise for hamstrings. 3 · 20 repetitions on each foot. (6) 5 · 30 s split jump. (7) 3 · 30 sec arm oscillation with 2.5 kg in each hand.
Sunday	Easy running 18–20 km (z1)	Rest

Note: z: training zone, recovery time in brackets.

Nonetheless, the number of workouts per week for a 1500 m runner can be very variable regardless of the type of runner. For example, Australian coach Nic Bideau recommends only two sessions per week in z3 (one of them just above the maximum steady state and the other one around VO_{2max} pace) and one at maximum steady state (at the very top end of z2) during the preparatory period which represented 20–25% of the average weekly volume; the remaining training is all in z1 (Nic Bideau, personal communication). This is the training regime of Ryan Gregson, the Australian 1500 m record holder with 3:31:07 who also possesses a best time in 3000 m of 7:42.19. Alternatively, the 2010 European champion over 1500 m, Arturo Casado (co-author of this chapter), guided by the Spanish coach Arturo Martín, conducted three sessions per week at maximum steady state and one in z3, plus one other small session in z3 conducted on hills during the preparatory period of the 2009–2010 season. Casado and Gregson's training weeks during the preparatory period also contained one sprint training session.

The differences in training regimes of middle-distance runners who achieved a similar level of performance are wide, and it is also difficult to determine the relative intensity at which each of these sessions are conducted. Between January and the middle of March 2012, during his preparation period, Henrik Ingebrigtsen, the 2012 European champion in the 1500 m, conducted four of his five high-intensity training sessions per week at maximum steady state intensity (top of z2). The TID during this period, 68.5%, 26% and 6%, of a total volume of 155 km, were conducted in z1, z2 and z3, respectively (Tjelta, 2013). Despite the fact that the absolute intensity for these z2 workouts may be quite fast, the internal load was not too demanding given that he did not surpass the intensity associated to maximum steady state. Apparently, this is the reason why he and his brothers can afford such high frequency of high-intensity training sessions per week. In the case of Bideau's regime, two sessions were conducted at z3 which likely may not allow for a higher number of sessions at z2 during the week. Regardless of the training zone in which each session is performed, according to the training programmes observed in world-class milers, a majority of the 'high intensity' training sessions have to be aerobically oriented during the preparatory period. For example, 8 repetitions of 1000 m with 1 min of active recovery can be either conducted at z2 or z3 depending on the effort made by the athlete. But considering the high total volume of the session and the scarce recovery time between repetitions, it is an aerobically oriented high-intensity training session.

In addition, it is also recommended that one of the weekly high-intensity training sessions conducted during the preparatory period will be near, at, or just above the $\dot{V}O_{2max}$, and there should be another small session dedicated to sprint training in order to develop the maximum speed throughout the season. In the training logs we have observed of world-class milers, examples of these typical training sessions might be something like 5 × 1000 m (3000 m pace) with 3 to 4 min of recovery and 5 repetitions of 100 m (flat-out pace) with 2.5 min of recovery, respectively.

For 1500 m runners it is also cautiously recommended to conduct 2 to 3 sessions per week of strength training during the preparation period (Blagrove et al., 2018a). As the runner progresses into the pre-competition and competition phases, it is recommended to reduce the total training volume, number of sessions and the number of kilometres run in z2 and increase the number of sessions at specific race pace (z3) (Tjelta, 2016). Furthermore, some of the high-intensity sessions conducted in this period should be covered at an 800 m pace. Arturo Casado's training week example conducted during the competitive period is indicated in Table 8.2.

TABLE 8.2 Arturo Casado's training week of 105–110 km conducted during the competitive period in July 2010, three weeks prior to becoming 1500 m European champion

Day	Morning session	Evening session
Monday	6 km (z1) + drills + 3 · 4 · 200 m in ~ 25 sec (60 sec; 3 min rec) + 1 km (z1)	6 km (z1)
Tuesday	6 km at 3:10/km (z2) (4 min) + 6k fartlek (4 · (1 km in 3 min + 500 m in 1:40), 18:40 in total (z2) + 2 km (z1). Most of this workout is conducted at maximum steady state (top of z2).	Rest
Wednesday	6 km (z1) + drills + 4 · 1000 m in 2:30 average (3 min) (z3 just above $\dot{V}O_{2max}$) + 2 km (z1)	6 km (z1)
Thursday	12 km (z1) + gym (resistance training) + drills + 6 · 100 m (running easily, z3)	Rest
Friday	6 km (z1) + drills + 3 · 4 · 300 m (60 sec; 3 min) at 40 sec average (anaerobic capacity, z3) + 1 km (z1)	6 km (z1)
Saturday	15 km (z1) + drills + 6 · 100 m running easily (z3)	Rest
Sunday	6 km (z1) + drills + 8 · 150 m in 16–17 sec (3 min) (with a 4 kg weighted jacket) (anaerobic capacity and power, z3) +1 km (z1)	6 km (z1)

Note: Recovery time in brackets; z = training zone; drills consist of: 2 · 40 m of high knees, butt kicks, straight-leg bounce, forward skip, double leg bounce, forward lung, sprint; gym consists on: 3x (6 · full squat, deadlift, step for each leg, bench press at 50–70% of 1 repetition maximum (RM)), plus other exercises such as hamstring curls, calf raises and core activation exercises.

3000 m Steeplechase, 5000 m and 10,000 m Events

The 3000 m steeplechase, 5000 m and 10,000 m events are predominantly sourced by aerobic contributions. Therefore, these events are similarly trained during the preparatory period, as in those 1500 m runners who also were 5000 m specialists, as was previously described. Ingrid Kristiansen, was the world's best female long-distance runner in the mid-1980s. In 1986 she set world records in the 5000 m (14:37.33) and 10,000 m (30:13.76). During the 49 weeks from November 1985 to October 1986, her average training volume was 155 km.week⁻¹ with a TID of 91%, 4.5% and 4.5% of the total training volume conducted in z1, z2 and z3, respectively (Kaggestad, 1987). The Irish runner Sonia O'Sullivan was world champion in the 5000 m in 1995, and in 1998 she won the long and the shorter distance in the World Cross Country Championships and became European champion over 5000 m and 10,000 m. During the period November 1994 to May 1995, O'Sullivan typically ran an average of 160 km.week⁻¹ conducting many of her runs at a 'steady' pace. During the competition period, she reduced the average weekly training volume to 115–120 km/week (Tjelta and Enoksen, 2001). Spanish distance runner Fernando Carro covered 160–175 km.week⁻¹ during the second preparatory period of the season, between March and June 2019, prior to breaking the Spanish 3000 m steeplechase record in 8:05.69 in July. Typically, each week he conducted a training one session at an intensity above $\dot{V}O_{2max}$ (z3), one session just below $\dot{V}O_{2max}$ (z3), and two more sessions near the maximum steady state (z2). He also conducted a 25 km long run per week on Sunday (Arturo Martín, personal communication). Australian 10,000 m record holder Stewart McSweyn, whose personal best times are 3:31.81, 7:34.79, 13:05.23 and 27.23.80 in 1500 m, 3000 m, 5000 m and 10,000 m, respectively, conducts a very similar training regime during the preparatory period to his partner Ryan Gregson, whose training was previously described. Both athletes are coached by Nic Bideau. The main difference between their training characteristics relies on the greater overall volume (150–160 km.week^{-1} vs. 130–140 km.week^{-1}) completed by Stewart, mainly conducted at z1 (Nic Bideau, personal communication). A training week of his preparatory period is indicated in Table 8.3.

During the last four decades, international distance running has been dominated by runners from East Africa. Billat et al. (2003) studied the training of Kenyan elite runners during a training week in Europe in April 2002. In addition, the runners' training diaries over a period of 8 weeks prior to this week were analysed. The number of runners (n = 20) consisted of 7 women and 13 men. They were all top 30 finishers in the Kenyan Cross-Country Championships in 2002. According to Billat et al. (2003), these runners based their training on either a high-volume pyramidal oriented model (HVPyr-model) or a low-volume polarised oriented model (LVPol-model). Men (n = 6) who used the LVPol-model ran 158 (± 19) km/week and women (n = 6) who used this training model ran 127 (± 8) km/week (88.4% and 11.6% of the total training volume was conducted at z1 and z3, respectively). Men (n = 7) who followed a HVPyr-model ran 174 ± 17 km per week (84.2%, 14.4% and 1.4% of the total training volume were conducted in z1, z2 and z3, respectively). The training volume reported for male HVPyr-model Kenyan runners is in line with the training volume reported for the Norwegian female runner, Susanne Wigene. Wigene finished second in the 10,000 m at the 2006 European Championships. During the training season from November 2005 to the end of August 2006 she ran an average of between 60 and 180 km per week (Enoksen et al., 2011). Between 2000 and 2008, national- and international-level Spanish male long-distance runners (n = 32) reported weekly preparation period training volumes of between 160 and 180 km (Rabadán et al., 2011). Similar to the training characteristics previously described for 1500 m runners, during the pre-competitive and competitive periods the whole training volume is reduced and the intensity is increased. For example, 3000 m steeplechase and 5000 m runners typically conduct one training session per week at 1500 m race pace during these training

TABLE 8.3 A 155–165 km training week conducted by Stewart McSweyn during February 2020 two months after setting an Australian record in the 10,000 m (27:23.80)

Day	Morning session	Evening session
Monday	60 min (z1)	30 min (z1)
Tuesday	20 min warm-up (z1). On grass track, 5 · 1600 m in 4:32 except 4th rep in 4:12 (400 m rec in 1:50–2 min (mainly just above maximum steady state, z3). 20 min cool down (z1).	30 min (z1)
Wednesday	60 min (z1)	30 min (z1)
Thursday	20 min warm-up (z1). maximum steady state run 11.5 km on horse racetrack of thick grass in around 2:58/km (z2). 20 min cool down (z1)	30 min (z1)
Friday	60 min (z1)	Rest
Saturday	20 min warm-up (z1). Hilly 7 km run (3 · 2.3 km loop): the hills are run hard (z3) and in between run at 3:15/km (z2). Three hills per loop – 1 gradual incline that takes ~1:40, one steep incline that takes 45 sec and 1 steep incline that takes 1:10–nine hills in total. 20 min cool down (z2 and z3).	30 min (z1)
Sunday	1 h 45 min easy (z1)	Rest

Note: Recovery time in brackets; z = training zone; easy runs are typically conducted at 4:10/km; (Stewart also conducts 2 easy strength training sessions/week usually 3–4 hours after high-intensity sessions in which he completes resistance training exercises such as half squats and deadlifts, core activation exercises and plyometrics; personal communication of Nic Bideau) phases. Therefore, it is also recommended that runners targeting any of these three events must also compete at lower-distance events during the competitive period and at greater distance events during the preparatory period.

Half-Marathon and Marathon Events

Whereas the half-marathon can be trained using similar principles as those used for the 10,000 m preparation, marathon training differs substantially from the training used for shorter distances. While a linear periodisation is usually conducted by middle- and long-distance runners in shorter events, a reverse linear periodisation is used by marathon runners. This entails conducting the highest volumes (with a high percentage of this volume conducted at marathon pace, just above maximum steady state intensity) during the pre-competitive and competitive periods as the competition is approaching (Boullosa et al., 2020; Kenneally et al., 2018). For example, in order to run under 1 hour at Marugame Half Marathon (Japan) in February 2020, Australian Brett Robinson used similar training during the preparation period to that used by his training partner Stewart McSweyn, previously described, with the only difference consisting in a longer weekly easy run of up to 2 hours and a longer threshold run of up to 16 km (Nic Bideau, personal communication). Nic Bideau recommends that the marathon preparation period should aim to achieve a high performance in shorter events such as 10 km or half-marathon at the end of this 12-week phase. Afterwards, the combined pre-competitive and competitive periods of 10 weeks consist of increasing the training volume conducted in z1 and at specific marathon pace during the following 8 weeks, leaving a two-week tapering prior to the race (Nic Bideau, personal communication).

Regarding overall training characteristics in world-class marathoners, Ingrid Kristiansen's average training volume during the 15 weeks leading up to her world record (2:21:06) achieved in the 1985 London Marathon was 167 km.week^{-1}, with a TID of 90.5%, 5% and 5.5% of the total training volume conducted in z1, z2 and z3, respectively (Tjelta and Kristiansen, 2015). This includes the two last training weeks where the volume was reduced to 131 and 95 km respectively. The 95 km for the last week included the marathon race. According to Billat et al. (2003), the Kenyan female runner Tegla Loroupe used a HVPyr-model (174 ± 17 km.week^{-1}) when she ran 2:20:47 in Rotterdam in 1998 and broke Ingrid Kristiansen's world record. Training volume and TID for Portuguese and French marathon runners (n = 20) over a period of 12 weeks leading up to the Olympic trials in 2000 was registered by Billat et al. (2001). The group consisted of 10 elite (5 male and 5 female) and 10 sub-elite runners (5 male and 5 female). The five elite male athletes ran an average of 206 (± 26) km/week and the sub-elite runners 168 (± 20) km/week. Total weekly running volume was not significantly different for females between performance levels (166 ± 20 km vs. 150 ± 17 for elite and sub-elite, respectively). Overall, these runners conducted 78%, 12% and 10% of the total training volume in z1, z2 and z3, respectively.

A recent study compared the training characteristics of world-class Kenyan (19 male athletes, including some of the best runners in the world) and Spanish long-distance runners (18 male athletes who were some of the best European runners) who were mostly marathon runners. They found that the Kenyan runners accumulated a larger training volume as tempo runs (close to maximum steady state intensity in the top of z2) and short (high-intensity) interval training (z3) than Spanish runners did across their sports careers (Casado et al., 2019a). This research highlighted the relevance of conducting training at, or just below, the maximum steady state intensity in order to optimise performance in long-distance running. Karp (2007) described the training of 2004 U.S. Olympic Marathon trial qualifiers. The number of kilometres per week reported by elite male runners was higher than for national runners (155.6 ± 9.3 vs. 144.2 ± 26.5 km.week^{-1}). For female runners, the training volume was 135.8 (± 31.5) km.week^{-1} for elite runners vs. 111.3 (± 23.3) km.week^{-1} for national runners. A total of 74.8% of the training volume of the best American male marathon runners, and 68.5% for the best female marathon runners, was conducted below average marathon pace. Two Norwegian female runners with personal best times of 2:27:05 and 2:29:12 ran an annual average of 180 and 200 km.week^{-1} (84%, 12% and 4% of the total training volume was conducted in z1, z2 and z3, respectively) during the seasons they ran their best marathon race (2004 and 2008) (Enoksen et al., 2011). Paula Radcliffe, the British female runner, who at the time of writing holds the European record for the marathon with the time of 2:15:25, ran between 192 and 256 km/week (120–160 miles.week^{-1}) when she was in full marathon training (Jones, 2006). Stellingwerff (2012) recorded training and food intake of three elite male marathon runners during the 16 weeks before they ran the marathon in, respectively, 2:11:23, 2:12:39 and 2:16:17. On average, they ran 182 km per week (74%, 11% and 15% in z1, z2 and z3, respectively). The highest training volume reported in a single week was 231 km.

According to Ferreira and Rolim (2006), international-level male marathon runners based their training on either a HVPyr-model or a LVPol-model. Average training volumes in the HVPyr-model were between 200 and 260 km.week^{-1}, with 80–85% of the training volume carried out at a relatively low intensity (60–75% of $\dot{V}O_{2max}$). In the LVPol-model, the weekly training volume was between 150 and 200 km.week^{-1}, with a larger percentage of training conducted at higher intensities (80–87% of $\dot{V}O_{2max}$). Both models have been successfully used by marathon runners who have performed at top international level (Ferreira and Rolim, 2006).

For marathon runners it can be recommended to reduce the training volume by 25% two weeks before the race and by 50% in the competition week, including the marathon competition (Tjelta and Kristiansen, 2015). The training week conducted by Sinead Diver, coached by Nic Bideau, during the pre-competitive period of the marathon training is indicated in Table 8.4. Sinead is an Irish-born Australian long-distance runner who ran 2:24:11 in the 2019 London Marathon despite being 42 years old. Her 10,000 m best time of 31:25.49 at the 2019 Doha World Championships is the over-40s world record. Despite the fact that Diver trains for marathons and McSweyn races 5000 m/10,000 m events, the training programmes share some similarities, for example the hill session conducted on Saturday.

Summary

Distance running coaches are advised to quantify both training volume and TID throughout the training process by means of the implementation of a TID quantification method, for example heart rate, running speed or RPE-derived TID. In addition, it is recommended to use a race pace-based approach to quantify training volume and TID during the pre-competitive and competitive periods in which training at race pace becomes more frequent.

All the aforementioned programmes of world-class middle- and long-distance runners follow either a polarised or pyramidal TID regardless of the event being targeted and the training period being conducted. This fact is in agreement with observations made by two reviews regarding either TID in endurance sports or distance running (Kenneally et al., 2018; Stöggl

TABLE 8.4 A 210–220 km training week conducted by Sinead Diver during February 2020, six weeks prior to a supposed London Marathon which finally was not held due to coronavirus spread

Day	Morning session	Evening session
Monday	60 min (z1)	40 min (z1)
Tuesday	20 min warm-up (z1). On grass track, 8 · 1000 m in 3:10 (200 m jog in 60s) (mainly just above maximum steady state, z3). 20 min cool down (z1).	40 min (z1)
Wednesday	60 min (z1)	40 min (z1)
Thursday	20 min warm-up (z1). 20 km alternating 1 km in 3:10, 1 km in 3:30 (z2 and z3). 20 min cool down (z1)	30 min (z1)
Friday	60 min (z1)	30 min (z1)
Saturday	20 min warm-up (z1). Hilly 7 km run (3 · 2.3 km loop): the hills are run hard (z3) and in between run at 3:15/km (z2) Three hills per loop – 1 gradual incline that takes ~1:40, one steep incline that takes 45 sec and 1 steep incline that takes 1:10–nine hills in total. 20 min cool down (z2 and z3).	30 min (z1)
Sunday	2 h 30 min run with first hour easy and last hour quite hilly and running strongly up the hills (z1 and z2)	Rest

Note: Recovery time in brackets; z = training zones; easy runs are typically conducted at 4:10/km. (Sinead also conducts two easy strength training sessions/week usually 3–4 hours after high-intensity sessions in which she completes resistance training exercises such as half squats and deadlifts, core activation exercises and plyometrics; personal communication of Nic Bideau).

and Sperlich, 2015). In this sense, a huge aerobic base has to be developed in all middle- and long-distance runners (particularly in distances of 1500 m and longer) during the preparatory period through a combination of easy runs, tempo runs and aerobically oriented interval training sessions. For longer-distance events, the training volume has to be greater and the intensity lower. One sprint training session per week is recommended for 800 m and 1500 m runners and in runners targeting track longer events, sprint training should also be present throughout the season. A long run each week, as well as frequent competitions, are observed in all events at any time during the season. Running sessions should be combined with two sessions per week of strength training. During the pre-competitive and competitive periods, runners targeting events other than the marathon have to decrease the training volume and run at race pace and even faster during training. Marathoners should increase their total training volume and conduct greater volumes of race pace training during the pre-competitive and competitive periods.

9

TAPERING AND PEAKING FOR AN EVENT OR MAJOR COMPETITION

Kate L. Spilsbury

Highlights

- This chapter focuses on how to modify training load before an event/competition to optimise performance.
- The expected improvement in endurance running performance from implementing an optimal tapering strategy is ~2–3%.
- The components of training load – volume, frequency and intensity – should be considered separately when designing the taper to achieve the optimal balance between overcoming accumulated fatigue and maximising performance.
- The scientific literature recommends reducing training volume by ~40–60%, whilst maintaining training frequency and perhaps increasing interval training intensity.
- Prior training load and fatigue carried into the taper are important in individualising the strategy and determining the taper duration.
- Optimal tapers should be carefully programmed into the annual training plan to avoid compromising long-term fitness by tapering too often.

Introduction

Most runners train with a long-term goal in mind, such as completing a marathon, setting a personal best time in a specific event, or winning a medal at a major championship. Although a carefully designed and well-executed long-term training programme provides runners with the fitness potential to reach their goal, mistakes in training over the final weeks leading into an event/competition can jeopardise the chance of success. The training that is performed in the period immediately preceding a major event or competition is therefore undoubtedly one of the most important phases of training for runners and coaches to consider. An appropriately designed tapering phase enables a runner to realise the physiological and psychological adaptations that have been accumulated during months of preparatory training. The aims of this chapter are to discuss the science of tapering and peaking, and to articulate the key components of a tapering phase to ensure event/competition day performance is optimised.

Furthermore, the chapter finishes by discussing a number of pragmatic considerations for tapering and peaking, based upon the author's experience of individualising strategies for many successful middle- and long-distance runners over the last decade.

The Science of Tapering

What Is Tapering?

Optimal adaptation to training occurs when the training load is prescribed in an appropriate manner over time. The training programme must provide stimuli large enough to initiate the desired physiological responses, whilst integrating recovery periods sufficient to allow 'super-compensation' to occur and for the adaptations to be realised (Halson and Jeukendrup, 2004; Meeusen et al., 2013; Smith, 2003). During phases of heavy training, the body experiences high levels of physiological stress. This is often coupled with a reduction in between-session recovery time, as endurance athletes typically complete several high-intensity interval sessions per week and sometimes train multiple times in one day. As a result, temporary physiological disturbances can occur, including: muscle glycogen depletion, neuromuscular fatigue, decrements in red blood cell volume and haemoglobin, an imbalance in anabolic and catabolic tissue activities, which ultimately leads to a suppression of performance (Halson and Jeukendrup, 2004; Halson et al., 2002; Hellard et al., 2013; Mujika and Padilla, 2003). Consequently, the challenge for coaches is to programme a change in training load after a heavy period of training that is sufficient to alleviate accumulated fatigue, whilst maintaining or further enhancing physiological adaptation (i.e. supercompensation). This strategy is commonly known as tapering and is used to facilitate the peaking of performance at the appropriate time for an event or major competition. Tapering has been defined as "a progressive, nonlinear reduction of the training load during a variable amount of time, that is intended to reduce physiological and psychological stress of daily training and optimize sport performance" (Mujika and Padilla, 2003).

Physiological Mechanisms

The physiological mechanisms fundamental to the process of tapering have not yet been well defined in endurance runners. This is perhaps due to the complex interaction of the physiological determinants of performance that are associated with endurance running. The available evidence suggests that the tapering period allows for the restoration of enhanced physiological capacities that have been previously suppressed or masked by intensified training, which may then lead to amplified physiological responses to the training completed during the taper (Mujika et al., 2004). Numerous positive physiological changes have been shown to occur during the taper, including metabolic, neuromuscular, hormonal and haematological responses, which may all contribute to enhancing performance (Table 9.1). Positive changes to an athlete's physiological state during the taper are typically accompanied by a number of psychological changes (Table 9.1), which may also be beneficial to improving performance.

Tapering and Performance

Previous research has demonstrated improvements in endurance performance (using competition measures) of between 0.5% and 6.0% in response to tapering in running, swimming,

TABLE 9.1 Physiological and psychological changes during tapering

Physiological Changes	Psychological Changes
Improved running economy	Reduced perception of effort
Increased muscle glycogen	Reduced global mood disturbance
Increased peak blood lactate concentration	Reduced perception of fatigue
Increased muscle strength and power	Increased vigour
Increased oxidative enzyme activity	Improved quality of sleep
Increased blood and red blood cell volume	
Increased circulating testosterone	

Source: Mujika et al. (2004).

cycling and triathlon (Mujika and Padilla, 2003). In endurance runners specifically, improvements in time trial or actual race performance after tapering have been reported in the range of 1.6–3.0% (Houmard et al., 1994; Munoz et al., 2015). The potential performance gain resulting from an optimal tapering strategy could therefore prove extremely valuable for an athlete competing at the elite level. For example, the mean taper-induced improvement in swimming performance was 2.2% at the 2000 Sydney Olympic Games, in events ranging from 50 m freestyle to 400 m medley (Mujika et al., 2002). This was in excess of the differences between the gold medallist and the 4th-placed swimmer (1.6%) and between the 3rd- and 8th-placed swimmers (2.0%) in these events. In athletics, in the men's 1500 m at the Rio 2016 Olympic Games, the difference in finishing times between the winner and 4th position was 0.1% and between 3rd and 8th positions was 0.4%. Therefore, even very small improvements in performance could have a large impact on race outcomes and might be the difference between winning and finishing outside of the medals. It should be noted that tapering is not just reserved for elite athletes, however. Endurance runners of all performance levels can benefit from a taper to achieve their performance goals, whether that be for winning races or to achieve personal best times.

Given the large potential performance improvements from tapering, it is somewhat surprising that there is not an abundance of scientific research studies attempting to predict the optimal taper in endurance runners. This is perhaps due to the complexities of designing and controlling research studies on tapering, and in isolating the effects of the taper on performance. In elite sport, therefore, the design and implementation of tapering strategies has largely come down to the coach and athlete and is predominantly based on their own experiences and intuition (Mujika et al., 2002). However, an increasing number of research studies have investigated various manipulations to training as part of a structured taper, or by way of theoretical mathematical modelling. The findings of these studies will be discussed in more detail to provide general recommendations for optimising tapering strategies.

Components of a Taper

Designing a tapering strategy involves manipulating the training load variables of volume, frequency and intensity over a particular duration in the lead-up to important competition (Houmard, 1991). In endurance runners, the volume of training typically represents the distance covered (km). Training frequency refers to how regularly the training is undertaken and reflects the recovery period between training sessions. Intensity describes the physiological demand of the training and can be expressed in several different ways. Endurance athletes commonly train at relative intensities, running at speeds based on percentages of their own individual maximal aerobic capacity, maximal heart rate or race pace (Jones, 2006). The taper should be a 'natural outgrowth' of regular training, meaning that it should not involve anything drastically different to the athlete's normal program. The only modification made should be to the load. It might be useful to separate training into continuous running (e.g. easy/steady running) and interval training (tempo/high-intensity sessions), when programming for the taper, as the load can be modified in these types of training slightly differently based on the information that follows.

Training Volume and Frequency

Reductions in training volume can be achieved through decreasing training distance (or time), reducing training frequency or a combination of both. Research suggests that dramatic reductions in volume during tapering do not compromise running performance in trained athletes for taper periods of 6 days to 3 weeks (Mujika et al., 2000; Wittig et al., 1989). However, insufficient reductions in training volume undermine the beneficial effects of a taper. A general recommendation involves a reduction in training volume of 41–60% over a 2-week taper to optimise performance (Bosquet et al., 2007b). This represents a fairly large range, so it is important to consider the athlete's training volume in the prior mesocycle. In elite endurance athletes, regardless of event distance, higher weekly training volumes prior to the taper are associated with larger reductions in training volume during the taper (Spilsbury et al., 2015). Athletes undertaking a higher total running volume prior to the taper may require a greater reduction in volume to alleviate accumulated fatigue, compared to those completing lower training volumes prior.

It is not recommended to reduce training volume through reducing training frequency in trained endurance runners. To improve performance, training frequency should not be manipulated during the taper or should be maintained at > 80% of pre-taper levels (Bosquet et al., 2007b). This may help to maintain athletes' daily routines and prevent any 'loss of feel' with regards to running form and technique (Mujika et al., 2000). Elite endurance athletes (800 m to marathon) typically maintain the frequency of high-intensity interval training during the taper (Spilsbury et al., 2015). The frequency of lower intensity continuous (e.g. easy/steady) running is usually maintained at >80% of pre-taper levels, with the exception of elite marathon runners, who reduce training frequency slightly more (~30% reduction) (Spilsbury et al., 2015). This is perhaps due to a larger pre-taper training volume and frequency in marathon runners and therefore a more aggressive taper is required to alleviate fatigue.

Training Intensity

Whilst large reductions in training volume are necessary to alleviate accumulated fatigue from a heavy period of training, the preservation of training intensity during the taper is fundamental to maintaining physiological adaptations and preventing a decline in performance (Bosquet et al., 2007b). High-intensity training in particular must not be compromised during the tapering period and is necessary to achieve an improvement in performance when large reductions in volume and frequency are also implemented (McConell et al., 1993; Mujika, 2010). An increase in the intensity of interval training during the taper may have more profound positive effects on subsequent performance, although a greater overall reduction in training volume may be required to account for the additional physiological stress of this (Shepley et al., 1992; Spilsbury et al., 2019).

Considering the differing manipulations to the component parts of training load (frequency, volume and intensity) discussed earlier, the commonly used description of tapering in terms of a 'reduction in training load' is perhaps too simplistic. This description may lead to the assumption that *all* training load variables are reduced during the taper, when in fact there are intricacies around how each variable should be manipulated (if at all). It is important, therefore, to recognise the different interactions between training intensity, volume and frequency when designing the taper, to achieve a balance that is most favourable to enhancing performance. Adding further complexity to this balance is the pattern of the taper, which describes the manner in which the training load variables are systematically manipulated over time.

Pattern of the Taper

Several different tapering patterns have been researched in an attempt to establish the optimal strategy for performance (Figure 9.1).

Although the term 'tapering' implies that training load is reduced in a progressive manner, it can also be reduced in a non-progressive standardised approach, known as a step taper (Mujika, 1998). However, a sudden and marked decrease in training load is not as favourable as progressive tapering patterns for improving performance (Banister et al., 1999). A linear tapering pattern involves a progressive reduction in training load of equal proportion.

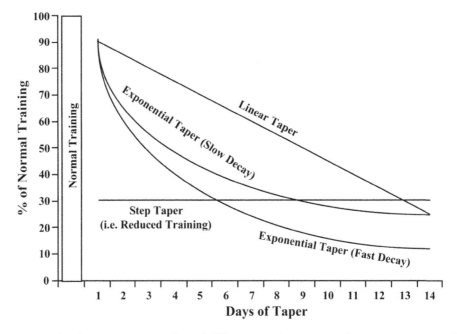

FIGURE 9.1 A schematic representation of different tapering patterns: linear taper, exponential taper with slow or fast time constants of decay of the training, and step taper

Source: Taken from Mujika and Padilla (2003).

However, exponential patterns appear to be the most beneficial of progressive tapers for enhancing performance. In an exponential pattern, training load is reduced dramatically initially before beginning to plateau nearer to competition. Exponential patterns can be implemented with a fast or slow decay of training load reduction. A fast exponential taper is a more effective pattern than a slow decay exponential taper, likely because it results in a lower overall training load than a slow decay over the same taper duration (Banister et al., 1999). A more rapid and aggressive reduction in training volume early in the taper may also help the athlete to overcome the accumulated fatigue from prior training more quickly and allow them to respond more positively to the training completed late in the taper. As an extension to this concept, a more complex 'two-phase' pattern has been investigated using mathematical modelling, whereby an *increase* in training load was implemented during the final 3 days of the tapering period, after an initial reduction over 5 weeks (Figure 9.2; Thomas et al., 2009).

Although the mathematical model predicted that the negative influence of fatigue was completely removed during both tapers, and the positive influence of adaptation to training was enhanced slightly further during a two-phase tapering strategy, performance was improved similarly after both strategies (~4.0%). It was suggested that the two-phase taper might further optimise performance if the second phase contained an increase in work that was specific to the requirements of the upcoming competition, rather than an increase in overall training load *per se*. Given the evidence for large reductions in training volume during tapering (Bosquet et al., 2007b; Houmard et al., 1990; Mujika et al., 2000; Neary et al., 1992; Wittig et al., 1989) and the inclusion of high-intensity training to improve performance (Houmard et al., 1994; Papoti et al., 2007; Shepley et al., 1992), it is possible that the two-phase taper might be more effective if volume remains reduced and only intensity is increased in the final days before competition (Spilsbury et al., 2019). This supports the anecdotal observation that performance often progressively improves from the first round of a major championship to the final, where volume remains low but intensity is high (Thomas et al., 2009).

Taper Duration

Identifying the optimal taper duration poses perhaps one of the greatest challenges for athletes and coaches, and anecdotally, many feel insecure at the prospect of reducing training prior to competition. This anxiety is based on the premise that a prolonged reduction in training

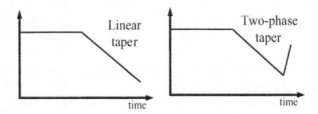

FIGURE 9.2 A schematic representation of linear and two-phase tapering patterns. Both protocols were characterised by a training overload at 120% of normal training for 28 days, followed by a linear taper for approximately 5 weeks. In a two-phase pattern, training load was abruptly increased in the final 3 days of the taper

Source: Taken from Thomas et al. (2009).

load during the taper may start to undo all the hard work that has been put in, resulting in detraining. Detraining can occur during periods of training cessation or from a significant reduction in habitual training load (Mujika and Padilla, 2001a), and is characterised by losses in cardiorespiratory, metabolic and muscular adaptations to endurance training which are detrimental to performance (Mujika and Padilla, 2001a, 2001b). However, a taper period of ~8–14 days appears to be optimal for achieving a balance between reducing fatigue and preventing detraining (Bosquet et al., 2007b). Although some endurance athletes may respond positively to a taper duration from within a much wider range, as little as 6 days up to 4 weeks (Bosquet et al., 2007b). This variability may be due to differences in athletes' physiological responses to reduced training and their individual rate of recovery, in addition to their prior training load (Kubukeli et al., 2002; Smith, 2003) and the amount of fatigue carried into the taper (Bosquet et al., 2007b). However, few experimental studies have attempted to investigate this, perhaps due to the difficulty in quantifying the multifaceted nature of fatigue. Despite this, work by Thomas et al. (2008) using mathematical modelling offers theoretical insight into prior training load and implications for the duration of the tapering strategy. Using computer simulations of training and performance data from elite 100 m and 200 m swimmers over two complete seasons, it was predicted that a 20% increase in training load for 28 days prior to the tapering period would require a longer taper duration (~6 extra days) to improve performance. In contrast, peak performance was achieved within 2 weeks of tapering in triathletes, regardless of whether prior training load was overloaded or whether they were diagnosed as functionally overreached or not prior to the taper (Aubry et al., 2014).

Summary of Recommendations for Programming an 'Optimal' Taper

The first part of the taper should focus on reducing accumulated fatigue, via reducing volume in an exponential fast-decay pattern. This involves dropping the volume quite rapidly initially, before reaching a plateau closer to the race. The general recommendation suggests reducing overall volume by ~40–60% for approximately 2 weeks, but prior training load should be considered, in addition to how an athlete responds to reduced training. Some athletes need to back off more substantially and/or implement a longer taper duration to freshen up, whilst others prefer to back off less and/or complete a shorter taper to prevent feelings of sluggishness. This is likely dependent on the physiology of the individual athlete and may take some trial and error to understand, as currently, there are a lack of physiological tools capable of simply and accurately quantifying athlete fatigue and time course of recovery. Frequency of training should be maintained during the taper where possible. Although slight reductions in the frequency of easy/steady runs of up to 20% may be warranted for athletes undertaking very high training loads in the training phase before the taper. Intensity should not be compromised during the taper and is the key to improving performance. Intensity should be at least maintained in all training runs and sessions, and perhaps even increased slightly towards the end of the taper in high-intensity sessions, when fatigue from prior training has been diminished.

Other Considerations

Whilst the general recommendations from scientific studies have been discussed earlier, a number of additional considerations are important to address when designing a taper. This section will discuss these considerations, which aim to ensure that tapering strategies are appropriately individualised to optimise performance.

Plan Ahead

The competition calendar is often very busy for endurance runners, and racing frequently is common practice for athletes of performance levels. However, chronic adaptation to training and long-term gains in fitness will be limited by implementing 'optimal tapers' too often. Significantly reducing training volume on a regular basis will ultimately compromise the performance level that can be achieved at the most important competition of the year. Therefore, it is important to plan ahead and identify which competitions the athlete will be targeting for the year or the season. Then prioritise them in order of importance, choosing only 1–3 races to implement an optimal taper, with at least 2 months in between them (Le Meur et al., 2012). This will provide enough time for recovery after the first event, whilst still allowing a block of further training and a tapering period before the next major event. For track athletes, the priority races could be an indoor championship early in the year and an outdoor championship in the summer. For marathon runners, it might be a cross-country championship or half-marathon in the winter and a marathon in the spring. Next, consider which of the remaining races may warrant a shorter-duration 'mini taper' (<7 days), where training load is reduced to a lesser extent than an optimal taper. This could be for races where the athlete needs to achieve a qualifying time or selection for a team, or for other important races that they wish to perform well in, but that may not be the major focus. The lowest-priority competitions left on their list are the races which a coach should instruct the athlete to 'train through' and only minimally adjust the training load beforehand, if at all. For these races, it is important to help the athlete manage their expectations and keep the bigger picture of peaking for their major target race in mind, as they may perform sub-optimally without implementing a taper. However, these races are still useful to practice race craft (e.g. pre-race routine and warm-up, tactics, hydration, nutrition, etc.) and can act as a good training stimulus within the overall programme.

Prepare to Be Flexible

The tapering strategy should be individualised and implemented relative to the training that was completed in the previous mesocycle. However, this can often be different to what was originally on the programme. This means practitioners, coaches and athletes might need to be flexible and adjust the modifications to training load that had been planned for the taper. For example, the athlete might have completed a higher load than expected in the previous mesocycle and the taper may need to be longer and/or more aggressive in terms of volume reduction. Alternatively, there may be circumstances where the planned training load could have been interrupted through injury, illness, travel, or other commitments. In this instance, the athlete is unlikely to be suffering from the level of fatigue that was originally anticipated, and performance may be optimised after a shorter and less aggressive taper than planned. The athlete should consistently keep a detailed diary of the actual training load completed (preferably using GPS and heart rate data) and their subjective responses to the training. There are now many online platforms (e.g. TrainingPeaks) to assist with the collection and sharing of this data between athlete and coach/practitioner. This information will help practitioners, coaches and athletes understand the level of fatigue the athlete needs to recover from and will inform the extent to which training load should be manipulated and the taper duration. The data can also be used to evaluate the success of the taper for future races. However, the training load undertaken during a taper should almost always be different leading into each competition. Many athletes tend to want to repeat what they did before their previous competition if it went well. However, it is not advisable to prescribe the same training programme for the upcoming taper as for the previous competition, as it is very likely that the load in the mesocycle prior to that competition was different. A further consideration when planning the taper for young or developing athletes is that their usual load may be restricted in order to protect their rate of development, and they may not yet be training at their full physiological capacity. These athletes are less likely to have the same level of accumulated fatigue to recover from as a more experienced athlete, who is pushing the limits of the training load that they can tolerate. Therefore, developing athletes may not be suffering from the level of fatigue that would cause an acute suppression in performance, and an optimal taper period may not always be warranted.

Since positive performance outcomes can be achieved from a range of taper durations (~1–4 weeks), it's important for athletes and coaches to trial different options whilst taking prior training load and level of fatigue into account. It is worth noting that middle-distance runners typically reduce their training volume in the final phase of training before they begin their taper, as the focus shifts towards higher-quality, more race-specific track work. They may also be implementing a number of mini-tapers for other races in building up to their major competition and therefore may have a lower level of accumulated fatigue to recover from prior to their major event. As a result, this event group would likely respond well to a shorter taper (e.g. 1 week) for optimising performance. In contrast, marathon runners typically complete their highest volume of training in the weeks leading into the taper and therefore a longer taper (e.g. 2–3 weeks) is recommended to dissipate accumulated fatigue.

Specific Programming Considerations

During the taper, it might be useful to programme sessions that the athlete is familiar with. When feeling fresher, they should be able to run more quickly than usual and respond better to the session. Therefore, it might not be necessary to set intensity higher, and faster times should come naturally later in the taper and will give the athlete confidence. However, when the session is going well, the temptation can be to keep going and complete more volume than is necessary. Instructing the athlete to finish the session knowing that they could have done one or two more repetitions of the same quality can help to prevent this. The goal of the final high-intensity sessions in the taper is not to 'empty the tank' but to prime the physiological systems for the race. The athlete needs to be disciplined in adhering to their tapered training programme and be comfortable with completing fewer reps than they are used to for the session. In contrast, programming familiar sessions during the taper could also have the opposite effect on the athlete's confidence and increase anxiety if they are not hitting the times they expect to. Whilst this may help to gauge whether training volume has been reduced enough and allow for adjustments to the taper in real time, it may create added pressure for the athlete. For some athletes, it could help to programme subtle differences in the composition of quality sessions for each taper or have a small selection of different taper sessions to prevent athlete anxiety from making direct comparisons.

Many athletes take a rest day from running every 7–10 days during regular training. It is important to consider where a rest day should be programmed in relation to the competition day. Some athletes prefer to take a rest day 2–3 days before the competition, whilst others prefer to take the day off immediately before the competition. Trial and error will be required to find out which rest-day strategy helps them to feel the most fresh and ready to perform on the day of the race. For most athletes, the final training session before race day involves some easy running with either surges at race pace within the run or a series of 4–6 strides at race pace afterwards. This is to keep the body primed for what to expect in competition, without inducing too much fatigue to recover from. If the race takes place in the evening, you could also consider programming a short walk or an easy 'shakeout' run (10–20 min) in the morning to increase blood flow to the muscles and prevent feelings of sluggishness later in the day. A further consideration when planning the rest day is whether long travel to the event is required. It might not be possible for the athlete to train on the day of travel, and therefore they may be forced to take this as a rest day. It is worth noting that even if the athlete is not training that day, there may still be an element of travel fatigue, and therefore a travel day is not a true rest day. For example, air travel often involves a considerable amount of 'time on feet' in queues and dragging heavy luggage. This is interspersed with long periods of sitting uncomfortably and can involve an earlier wake-up time or later bedtime than the athlete is used to. This should be factored into the taper, with a lighter training day beforehand and a short walk or shakeout run on arrival, if time permits. Travel to a race can be an extra source of stress for the athlete, but this can be minimised by ensuring that travel plans are organised and communicated well in advance.

Another consideration is when the taper should begin if there are multiple rounds of competition over several days. This is particularly relevant for middle-distance runners. If the performance standard of the athlete is high enough that they are able to progress through early rounds with ease, the taper should be planned so they peak for the semi-finals or finals. If not, you should plan to start the taper on countback from the heats/early rounds. If the athlete is successful at qualifying in these rounds, the races themselves will be a large enough stimulus to maintain fitness and sharpness for the duration of the championship, despite the volume being very low.

The discussion in this chapter has focused on tapering the running aspect of training. However, it is common practice among competitive endurance runners to include strength and conditioning activities in their training programme (Blagrove et al., 2020b) and this aspect of training load should be factored into the taper. As with running training, no new strength and conditioning exercises should be introduced during the taper, as unfamiliar exercises can induce muscle soreness and additional fatigue (Connolly et al., 2003). There is limited research on tapering strength and conditioning training for endurance performance, but since training adaptations relating to muscle fibre type distribution, muscle size and strength are typically lost at a slower rate than aerobic adaptations with training cessation (Mujika and Padilla, 2001a, 2001b), athletes should not fear backing off this type of training during the taper. If athletes have been completing two strength and conditioning sessions per week for several months previously, it seems that frequency can be reduced to one session per week during a prolonged competition season without compromising maximal or reactive strength (Beattie et al., 2017). Athletes should avoid completing sets to repetition failure during the taper, as this may delay recovery, and greater improvements in power are apparent when training to non-failure during this period (Izquierdo et al., 2006). If strength and conditioning is not part of the athlete's current training programme, it should not be introduced during the taper.

Nutrition

Most athletes will be aiming to reach their optimal body composition for their major competition. This may require restricting energy intake to create a caloric deficit over a defined period beforehand, as it is not advisable to try to sustain peak body composition all year round (Stellingwerff, 2018). However, it is important to ensure that target body composition is reached *before* the taper begins, as recovery will not be optimal if energy availability is low during this time. On the other hand, careful attention should be paid to energy intake during the taper, as this will need to be adjusted to account for a reduction in energy expenditure due to a lower training volume (especially during longer tapers). Failure to achieve energy balance during the taper may result in undesirable changes in body composition, which can negatively impact performance (see Chapter 18).

It has been widely acknowledged since the 1960s that muscle glycogen is an important metabolic substrate to produce energy for endurance exercise. Increased muscle glycogen has been identified as one of the physiological mechanisms of tapering which may contribute to improved performance (Neary et al., 1992; Shepley et al., 1992). Traditionally, it was thought that a pre-race carbohydrate loading strategy needed to involve a muscle glycogen depleting exercise bout, followed by 2–3 days of low carbohydrate intake (depletion phase), before 2–3 days of high carbohydrate intake (supercompensation phase) (Bergström et al., 1967). However, this strategy is no longer recommended, as the depletion phase may compromise training intensity, which is important to protect during the taper. It could also be a risk to the athletes' health so close to competition, as restricting carbohydrate after exhaustive exercise may result in increased susceptibility to illness (Gleeson et al., 2004). More recently, it has been shown that it is possible to achieve muscle glycogen supercompensation in trained athletes by merely reducing training load and consuming a high-carbohydrate diet (> 50% total energy from carbohydrate) (Walker et al., 2000). The depletion phase is therefore not necessary to increase muscle glycogen during the taper. Chapter 11 explores this strategy in further detail. For further information on matching energy intake to energy expenditure and for advice on nutritional strategies for optimising performance, it may be useful to seek support from a sports nutritionist or dietitian.

Recovery Strategies

Whilst there is some contention in the scientific literature about the regular use of certain recovery strategies during phases of hard training (Kellmann et al., 2018), the taper is the time to maximise physiological and psychological recovery. A wide range of recovery strategies can be utilised, and athletes should use trial and error to determine which combination works best for them. During the taper, athletes should aim to maximise rest and sleep, whilst maintaining good nutrition and hydration. When athletes are completing slightly less training during the taper, it's important to ensure they are not filling their extra time with other fatiguing activities and increasing their 'time on feet'. They may also find it more difficult to sleep when training has been reduced or in anticipation of their competition, so sticking to a good bedtime routine can help. Examples of this include keeping bedtime and waking time regular, avoiding screen time before bedtime, taking a warm shower before going to bed and making sure the sleep environment is dark, cool and comfortable (Kölling et al., 2019). Other recovery strategies that can be considered during the taper include massage, stretching, compression garments and devices, cold water immersion (e.g. ice baths) and whole-body cryotherapy (Kellmann et al., 2018). Chapter 17 discusses the use of these recovery strategies in further detail.

Environmental Influences

Many athletes travel to different countries across the world to compete in their major competition of the year. Some locations can pose environmental challenges, such as high temperatures and humidity or altitude, which may negatively impact on performance if athletes are not appropriately acclimatised (particularly for longer-distance events). For competitions in hot and humid environments, some athletes may to travel to the location in the weeks preceding the event to undergo an acclimatisation process, whilst other athletes might acclimate in artificial environmental conditions before travel (Racinais et al., 2015). The added physiological stress of training in such conditions in the lead-up to competition may require further adjustments to tapering strategies. However, the extent to which training load variables should be modified to ensure optimal recovery is not yet clear (Casadio et al., 2017) and trial and error may be required to determine individual athlete responses.

Altitude training is now commonly incorporated into the training programmes of many endurance athletes, particularly prior to competition. Whilst the body of literature concerning the optimal time to compete after an altitude training block is expanding, little is known about the influence of altitude on the tapering strategy and how further modifications to training might be required to optimise subsequent performance. However, since training sessions at altitude elicit a higher physiological stimulus for the same absolute intensity than at sea level (Friedmann-Bette, 2008), it's likely that athletes may experience greater accumulated fatigue from a training block at altitude. A larger reduction in training volume and/or a longer taper duration may therefore be required after training at altitude to maximise performance on return to sea level (Sharma et al., 2018). Where possible, athletes should experiment with altitude training, tapering and competition prior to utilising altitude before their major competition.

Pacing Strategies

Whilst the taper is crucial to ensure athletes are ready to produce a peak performance, optimal pace selection during the race is critical to the delivery of a peak performance. In non-tactical endurance running races, where athletes aim to complete a fixed distance in the shortest possible time, they must regulate their rate of work output to optimise overall race performance (Tucker and Noakes, 2009). A positive pacing strategy (i.e. faster than even pace start) is typically implemented in events lasting <4 min, whilst pace becomes more evenly distributed in longer events (Tucker and Noakes, 2009). If athletes are unfamiliar with racing in an optimally tapered state, a reduced perception of effort, coupled with high motivation to run fast in a competitive environment, may result in heightened or unrealistic expectations about the level of performance they can achieve. This can lead to poor judgement when it comes to pacing early in the race, and athletes may start too fast and suffer towards the end. It is therefore recommended that athletes take the opportunity to practice pacing strategies in less important competition when mini-tapers are implemented and that athletes should pay attention to split times early in the race, when in an optimally tapered state. However, this may be less relevant for tactical, championship-style races where pace is often very slow initially. Pacing and race strategies are elaborated on in Chapter 12.

Summary

Tapering is a short-term strategy used over approximately the last 2 weeks prior to a major competition. Training volume is usually reduced 40–60%, with frequency and intensity maintained, with a possible increase in interval training intensity. An improvement of approximately 2–3% can be expected in endurance runners following such a taper. When designing a taper training, volume, frequency and intensity should be considered separately to achieve the optimal balance between overcoming accumulated fatigue and maximising performance. Prior training load and fatigue carried into the taper are important in individualising the strategy and determining the taper duration. An optimal taper must be carefully programmed into the annual training plan, as tapering too often can compromise long-term fitness.

10

RUNNING COACHING CASE STUDY AND LESSONS LEARNED

Steve Macklin

Highlights

- Although science heavily informs the principles of training and recovery interventions, individual runners can respond differently to the same training programme for a multitude of reasons.
- A case study approach whereby the unique background, needs and goals of a runner are considered can provide valuable insight into how training can be prescribed on an individual level.
- A longitudinal (3-year) case study is presented for a young male distance runner who won a medal at the European Junior Championships over 5000 m.
- Ten 'lessons learned' for athletes and coaches are described that enable readers to critically develop their own training/practices.

Introduction

Sport science has provided enormous insight over the last few decades into how best to prepare athletes for competition. Although the latest scientific research can provide a platform that guides and informs coaching practices, in the chaos and unpredictability of an athlete's everyday life, the results of well-controlled scientific experiments can have limited applicability. Moreover, it is well recognised that individuals respond differently to the same relative dosage of training; therefore, the results of an intervention (training, recovery, nutritional, psychological) may be different for each athlete. The day-to-day decisions made concerning an athlete's training are therefore the manifestation of sound evidence-based reasoning and the art of coaching the person in front of you. Most of the content contained within this book summarises the latest scientific evidence associated with understanding and developing performance in runners. The primary aim of this chapter is to provide a real-life example of how a runner, at the start of their performance pathway, was carefully developed to reach their personal running goals. This chapter also aims to provide insight into the author's own coaching journey and the 'lesson learned' that have contributed to shaping a coaching philosophy.

Needs Analysis of the Individual Runner

Part I of this book provides a comprehensive analysis of the science that underpins distance running performance, which can inform the physical capabilities that are assessed as part of a testing battery and helps to guide principles of training and recovery. In addition to this understanding, it is also crucial that a thorough analysis of each individual runner is carried out. This is best done in a private meeting with the runner and may also include input from other members of a multi-disciplinary support team (e.g. physiotherapy records, nutritionist reports, etc). The following areas should be considered as part of this initial (or training transition phase) information-gathering process:

- Athlete's background

  - Where they are from and how running fits into their life
  - Sociocultural influences that may be important

- Performance profile (athletes' recent personal best times across a range of distances)
- Athletes' age

  - Chronological age
  - Training age (sport, running and strength training age)
  - Biological age (for under-18s)

- Training history

  - Previous coaches (if relevant)
  - Previous running training volumes, frequencies, intensities, etc.
  - Non-running training (i.e. cross-training, strength training, prehabilitation/conditioning)

- Injury and illness history (doctor and physiotherapy notes ideally referred to, with athlete/parental consent; information provided by other members of the multi-disciplinary support team may help identify likely factors contributing to injury/illness/under-performance)
- Athletes' personal goals/ambitions (short-, medium- and long-term)
- Athletes' expectations of your role as coach
- Lifestyle considerations

  - School/college/employment hours and physical nature of work
  - Family/caring responsibilities
  - Other commitments that may impact recovery, e.g. social life

- Recommendations from other members of the support team (if available)

  - Physiology testing
  - Nutrition report (including body composition if relevant)
  - Strength, capacity and movement assessment
  - Gait analysis

Planning and Goal Setting

In order to plan an effective training programme, it is critical that the long-term goal of the runner is identified first. Identifying the key goals for the year and working backwards from these targets enables planning of mesocycles (1- to 2-month training blocks) and microcycles (5- to 10-day training periods) far easier. These goals should act as a guide but may need to be adapted based upon the athlete's rate of progression and setbacks; therefore, they should not necessarily restrict the day-to-day decision-making process. Goals should be specific, measurable, agreed between athlete and coach, realistic and time-phased (S.M.A.R.T.). The goals for each year should also not lose sight of the longer-term goals for an athlete, particularly in the case of junior runners. Goals are important to help an athlete see a clear direction, aid motivation for training and provide self-belief. Sometimes an athlete will not fully believe that they can achieve a certain goal until a significant other (i.e. coach) shows belief in their ability and capacity to progress. The case study presented later in this chapter provides a sample annual plan (macrocycle) for the athlete, which illustrates the goals that were set and the road map laid out to realise their goal.

Coach-Athlete Relationship

For an athlete to progress and maximise their potential over a long period, the coach-athlete relationship is critical. A good relationship that is open, honest and allows for critical feedback creates 'buy in' from both parties and becomes a key driver of success. For the case study described in this chapter, the coach-athlete relationship was very strong. It was agreed with the athlete that total openness and honesty was important, and good quality feedback to each other was essential to make informed programming decisions. The athlete was extremely honest, reflective and open to sharing how they were feeling. The athlete would ask questions and wished to be educated on the 'why' of the training programme, which enabled a strong coach-athlete relationship to be built.

Physiology Testing

Laboratory physiology testing on a motorised treadmill can provide insight into aerobic determinants of performance to identify areas of physiological deficiency, provide valid monitoring data and gauge potential over various distances. Moreover, physiological testing can provide accurate running speeds and heart rates that coincide with important physiological thresholds for training prescription. Physiological testing data are provided for the athlete in the case study.

Case Study – Junior Distance Runner: Darragh McElhinney

Athlete Background

Darragh lived in a rural location adjacent to undulating and rolling off-road training terrain that was ideal for running. He also had access to a small gym and treadmill at his local school and flat grass fields close by. Darragh was an active child and spend large amounts of time hiking, playing and swimming in his pre-pubertal and pubertal years. At 14 years old he was participating in some running training, but his main sport was Gaelic football (the Irish national sport). The author started coaching Darragh in April 2016 and formulated a plan that would allow him to go through the track season of 2016 playing football and running. He was an extremely self-motivated, ambitious and tough young runner, and it was clear to see that with sensible progression over several years he could perform well on the international stage. He was no different to any other teenager, though, and needed guidance in the areas of preparation, punctuality, behaviour, attitude and self-belief. The long-term goal was to compete for Ireland at an international championship with the goal in his under-20 career of targeting a medal at the European Under-20 Championships in his final year as a junior. The training macrocycle plan for 2017–18 is shown in Figure 10.1. Importantly, Darragh had a very supportive family who backed him fully with his running and helped shape his direction in a positive manner without any pressure.

Injury and Illness History

From April 2016 to July 2019, Darragh suffered the following injuries and illnesses:

- Lower back postural pain during winter 2018 and 2019 which impacted racing more than training
- Missed 6–8 days in total of planned training due to head colds or sore throats
- Missed 12–15 days of total planned training with niggles during this period

Darragh had no other injuries or illnesses throughout his junior ranks, staying remarkably consistent for a long period of time which no doubt contributed largely to his overall success and consistency of improvement.

Physiology Testing

Darragh had a strong mix of endurance, speed and power that allowed him to perform well over distances from 1500 m to 5000 m and had the ability to finish fast in slow tactical races. Table 10.1 and Figure 10.2 show the results of physiology testing for Darragh towards the beginning and end of the 2017–18 season. A sub-maximal incremental discontinuous test was performed (4 min stages at a 1% gradient) to determine blood lactate and heart rate response to increasing running speeds and running economy (expressed as oxygen cost). Table 10.1 shows that Darragh possessed exceptional running economy (< 200 ml.kg^{-1}.km^{-1}) for his age, with improvements at the slower (moderate intensity) speeds following winter training. Figure 10.2 shows that Darragh's lactate threshold occurred at ~17 km.h^{-1}, which informed the highest speed that he should run at during easy/recovery runs (< 17 km.h^{-1}; < 155 beats. min^{-1}). It is important to note that the June 2018 data may have been affected by a busy examination period in the 2 weeks prior to the test, which may explain the deterioration in running economy and blood lactate at the higher speeds.

Long-Term Progression of Training Volume and Intensity

Figure 10.3 displays the volume of running for a sample week in cross-country or track preparation periods, where training emphasis was on developing aerobic qualities. Each sample week represents the highest volume of running for that phase of training each year. Over a period of 3 years in this junior runner (age 16–19 years) weekly running volume more than doubled (164 min.week^{-1} to 359 min.week^{-1}). This increase in running volume has been possible by taking a long-term view of athlete development, which allowed the runner

Athlete name: Darragh McElhinney

Athlete goals:
1) Top 20 finish European Cross-Country (XC) Championships;
2) Qualify for final at World Junior Champs 2008 in 1500 m OR 5000 m;
3) Win All Ireland under-20 (u20) cross-country, All Ireland Schools cross-country, All Ireland Schools track and field (T&F)

Macrocycle 2017-18

Week	Week commencing	Competitions	Importance (1-5)	Event and camp detail	Testing/monitoring	Training phases	Microcycles
1	24.07.17					Recovery	1
2	31.07.17					Recovery	2
3	07.08.17					Conditioning phase	3
4	14.08.17				Physio screen and check	Conditioning phase	4
5	21.08.17			National XC squad	Blood test	Conditioning phase	5
6	28.08.17					Conditioning phase	6
7	04.09.17					Conditioning phase	7
8	11.09.17				Physio screen and check	Conditioning phase	8
9	18.09.17					Conditioning phase	9
10	25.09.17					Conditioning phase	10
11	02.10.17					Conditioning phase	11
12	09.10.17				Physio screen and check	Conditioning phase	12
13	16.10.17	Minor	3	Open International XC	Sub-maximal running test	Conditioning phase	13
14	23.10.17					Conditioning phase	14
15	30.10.17	Minor	3	Belgium XC		Competition 1	15
16	06.11.17				Blood test	Competition 1	16
17	13.11.17				Physio screen and check	Competition 1	17
18	20.11.17	Major	2	National XC		Competition 1	18
19	27.11.17					Competition 1	19
20	04.12.17	Major	1	European XC		Competition 1	20
21	11.12.17					Recovery	21
22	18.12.17					Recovery	22
23	25.12.17					Conditioning phase	23
24	01.01.18				Physio screen and check	Conditioning phase	24
25	08.01.18	Minor	3	Edinburgh XC	Sub-maximal running test	Conditioning phase	25
26	15.01.18					Conditioning phase	26
27	22.01.18					Conditioning phase	27
28	29.01.18	Major	2	AAI Indoor Games		Conditioning phase	28
29	05.02.18					Conditioning phase	29
30	12.01.18					Conditioning phase	30
31	19.01.18	Minor	3	Mun Schools XC		Competition 2	31
32	26.01.18				Physio screen and check	Competition 2	32
33	05.03.18	Major	1	All IRE Schools XC		Competition 2	33
34	12.03.18				Blood test	Recovery	34
35	19.03.18			*Portugal Training Camp*		Conditioning phase	35
36	26.03.18			*Portugal Training Camp*		Conditioning phase	36
37	02.04.18				Physio screen and check	Conditioning phase	37
38	09.04.18					Conditioning phase	38
39	16.04.18					Conditioning phase	39
40	23.04.18				Sub-maximal running test	Conditioning phase	40
41	30.04.18					Conditioning phase	41
42	07.05.18				Physio screen and check	Conditioning phase	42
43	14.05.18	Minor	3	Mun Schools T&F		Competition 3	43
44	21.05.18	Major	2	IFAM Belgium		Competition 3	44
45	28.05.18	Major	2	All IRE Schools T&F		Competition 3	45
46	04.06.18					Conditioning phase	46
47	11.06.18				Physio screen and check	Conditioning phase	47
48	18.06.18					Conditioning phase	48
49	25.06.18	Major	2	National u20 T&F		Competition 4	49
50	02.07.18				Physio screen and check	Competition 4	50
51	09.07.18	Major	1	World u20 T&F		Competition 4	51
52	16.07.18					Recovery	52
53	23.07.18					Recovery	53
54	30.07.18					Recovery	54

Key: Minor competitions (3, 4, or 5); Major competitions (1 or 2); Physio screen and check; Blood test; Sub-maximal running test

FIGURE 10.1 Training macrocycle for the 2017–18 season for Darragh

TABLE 10.1 Summary of rate of perceived exertion and running economy data for two sub-maximal incremental treadmill running tests during the 2017–18 season

Running speed	km.h^{-1}	16	17	18	19	20
	min.km^{-1}	3:45	3:32	3:20	3:09	3:00
Rate of perceived exertion (6–20)	Oct 2017	11	13	14.5	16	17.5
	June 2018	11	14	15	16	18
Running economy (ml.kg^{-1}.km^{-1})	Oct 2017	194	196	197	199	197
	June 2018	183	191	196	206	218

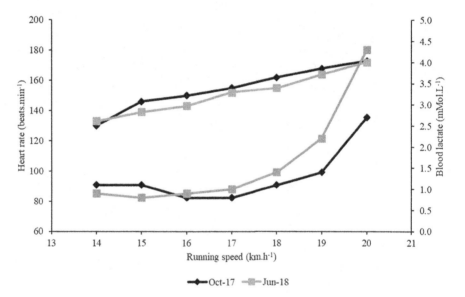

FIGURE 10.2 Heart rate (top lines) and blood lactate (bottom lines) responses during two sub-maximal incremental treadmill running tests during the 2017–18 season

to physically develop and adapt to progressively higher volumes of running. Importantly, Figure 10.3 shows that the increase in running volume has been gradual and avoided rapid jumps in volume from one preparatory phase to the next. This approach requires patience and discipline but, crucially, ensures injury and overtraining is avoided. Moreover, the data reflect a deeper consideration of the individual, including their background, training history, personality and other lifestyle demands.

Table 10.2 provides further technical detail on the nature of the training that took place within the cross-season preparatory phase over three successive years. Subtle increases in the volume and absolute intensity of hard interval and fartlek training sessions are apparent, in addition to the gradual increase in durations of the easy/recovery runs. Furthermore, as aerobic fitness improved over the 3 years, Darragh was able to perform easy/recovery runs at a slightly faster absolute running speed; however, the relative pace remained slow to ensure adequate recovery and freshness for hard running sessions. Mobility, strength and conditioning, and fast strides remained an important and consistent feature of training each year during these off-season preparatory mesocycles.

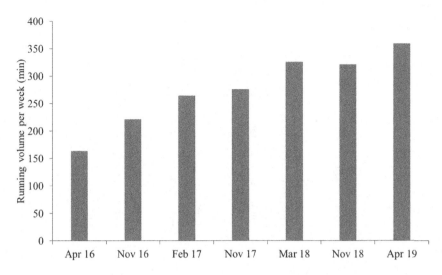

FIGURE 10.3 Long-term changes in running volume taken from a sample week during cross-country or track preparatory periods characterized by high relative volumes of running. Totals exclude warm-ups and warm-downs. Apr = April, Nov = November, Feb = February, Mar = March

As illustrated in Figure 10.4, this increase in total running volume is largely attributed to an increase in moderate-intensity 'easy' running mileage (130 min.week^{-1} to 310 min.week^{-1}). Despite this increase in moderate/recovery running volume, as a relative proportion of total running volume, this type of running has remained approximately the same (Figure 10.4). The distribution of running intensity during these 'off-season' preparatory phases is largely 'pyramidal' in design, with a large base of moderate/recovery running and progressively smaller percentages of running time dedicated to running in heavy/tempo, severe/hard and extreme/speed intensity zones. During preparatory periods of training, this approach develops a strong aerobic base whilst still developing other aerobic qualities (such as maximal oxygen uptake, critical speed and lactate threshold) using tempo, interval and fartlek sessions at around 10 km (or cross-country) race speed. Every training week during these preparatory periods also includes some work (usually part of a longer session) at severe/hard intensities (1500–5000 m speeds), which maintains the aerobic and anaerobic qualities required for dedicated training sessions at these paces later in the training macrocycle. Crucially, the author also believes it is important to include high-intensity (faster than 1500 m pace) and top-end speed work in the training programme year-round (typically 4–8% of training time in preparatory phases). This enables anaerobic and neuromuscular fitness capabilities to be maintained, which are crucial for successful middle-distance track racing, and also provides a strong specific-conditioning stimulus to reduce the risk of musculoskeletal injury during fast running.

Periodisation of Training

Following the general plan of training (see Figure 10.1), Table 10.3 displays the actual volume of running performed at various training intensities across the 2017–18 season. The winter (off-season) training period from October to March places a priority on a consistent phase

TABLE 10.2 Examples of cross-country preparatory training from same time (November) across three successive training years

Day	November 2016	November 2017	November 2018
Monday	30 min easy run on grass and stretching/mobility exercises	Rest	Rest
Tuesday	Rest	Track session: 8 × 1000 m with 90 secs jog recovery in 3.10/ 3.05/3.00/2.55/3.10/ 3.05/ 3.00/2.55 followed by 4 × 200 m in 30 sec with 90 sec jog recovery	60 mins easy run (ave. 14.0 km.h⁻¹), running drills and 8 × 10 sec short hill sprints with 2.5 mins walk recovery
Wednesday	Tempo run on hilly woodland trail: 8 × 1km as 3.40/3.25/3.40/3.25/3.40/3.25/ 3.40/3.20 with 90 sec jog recovery followed by 4 × 30 sec @ 1500 m pace with 90 sec jog recovery	S&C followed by 50 mins easy (ave. 13.9 km.h⁻¹) on grass/trail and 4 × 80 m strides	Tempo intervals (treadmill): 9 × 3 min with 1 min recovery @ 18/19/20/18/19/20/18/19/20 km.h⁻¹, followed by 4 × 1 min hill sprints @ 8% gradient @17–18.5 km.h⁻¹
Thursday	S&C session followed by 40 mins easy run (ave. 13.0 km.h⁻¹) and 4 × 80 m strides	Mobility routine followed by 50 mins easy (ave. 13.9 km.h⁻¹) and 4 × 80 m strides	S&C session followed by 50 mins easy run (ave. 14.5 km.h⁻¹) on grass/trail and 4 × 80 m strides
Friday	40 mins easy run (ave. 13.0 km.h⁻¹), running drills and 8 × 10 sec hill Sprints with 2–2.5 min walk recovery	50 mins easy run (ave. 14.0 km.h⁻¹), running drills and 8 × 10 sec short hill sprints with 2.5 min walk recovery	60 mins easy run (ave. 14.9 km.h⁻¹), running drills and 4 × 80 m strides
Saturday	Fartlek session grass: 2 sets of 30/60/90/2 mins/90/60 30 sec with equal jog recovery between repetitions and 3 min between sets followed by 4 × 80 m fast strides	Fartlek grass session: 2 sets of 30/60/90/2 mins/90/60/30 sec with equal jog recovery and 3 min between sets followed by 4 × 80 m fast strides	Fartlek grass session: 2 sets of 5/4/3/2/1 min with 1 min jog recovery between repetitions and 3 min walk recovery between sets followed by 4 × 80 m fast strides
Sunday	60 mins hilly easy run (ave. 12.8 km.h⁻¹) with last 8 min stride 20 sec/jog easy 40 sec and mobility	80 mins hilly easy run (ave. 14.5 km.h⁻¹) with last 8 min strides 20 sec/jog easy 40 sec and mobility	90 mins hilly easy run (ave. 15.5 km.h⁻¹), with last 8 mins strides 20 sec/jog easy 40 sec and mobility

Note: ave. = average.

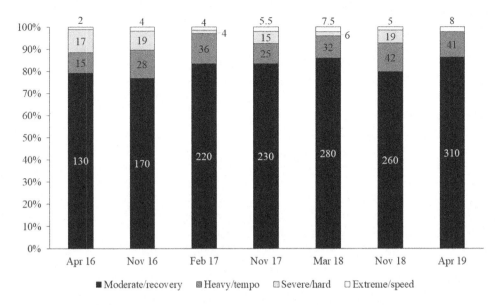

FIGURE 10.4 Training intensity distribution for sample training weeks during cross-country or track preparatory periods. Numbers within bars represent the actual minutes of time spent in each zone. Excludes warm-ups and warm-downs. Moderate/recovery running = below speed at lactate threshold; heavy/tempo = speeds between lactate threshold and ~10 km race pace; severe/hard = speeds between 1500 m and 5 km race pace; extreme/speed = intensities faster than 1500 m pace. Apr = April, Nov = November, Feb = February

TABLE 10.3 Volumes of training at various intensities across a training macrocycle (2017–18)

	Oct 17	Nov 17	Mar 18	May 18	July 18
Moderate/recovery (min)	280	230	280	145	160
Heavy/tempo (min)	15	25	32	13	10
Severe/hard (min)	3	15	6	20	6.5
Extreme/speed (min)	3	5.5	7.5	6	13
Total (min)	**301**	**275.5**	**325.5**	**184**	**189.5**

Note: Excludes warm-ups and warm-downs. Moderate/recovery running = below speed at lactate threshold; heavy/ tempo = speeds between lactate threshold and ~10 km race pace; severe/hard = speeds between 1500 m and 5 km race pace; extreme/speed = intensities faster than 1500 m pace. Oct = October, Nov = November.

of high-volume, moderate-intensity running, with most interval and fartlek training sessions taking place in the 'tempo' or severe (5–10 km pace) intensity domains. As the preparatory off-season period progresses, there is a gradual increase in the volume of interval and fartlek sessions as reflected by the total duration spent in the heavy, severe and extreme intensity zones. During the summer track season (May–August), the volume of running begins to drop (by 40–50% in key race weeks compared to off-season preparatory periods) and the proportion of time spent in higher-intensity training zones (severe and extreme) around target race-pace increases. During July, which included final preparations for the major championships in 2018, the volume of interval running in the extreme zone (faster than 1500 m pace) is approximately double that of the off-season preparatory months (November–March).

Specific Training Phases: General Conditioning

Following an initial meeting with Darragh, a plan was developed that aimed to develop his aerobic base and general level of physical conditioning using a combination of running and football. Because football is an intermittent sport, it provides a strong anaerobic stimulus, therefore the running training prioritised gradually increasing volume rather than intensity. A sample of training week from April 2016 is shown as follows.

Week commencing: 25 April 2016

Monday	Mobility exercises, then 35–40 min easy run on grass, running drills and 4 × 100 m strides
Tuesday	Track session: 3 × 1600 m (lap splits: 90/80/90/80 sec) with 2 min recovery; 2 sets of 10 × 100 m @ 800 m pace (14 sec) with 45 sec jog recovery and 5 min between sets; 4 × 80 m fast strides.
Wednesday	Mobility exercises at home before football match
Thursday	Rest
Friday	Fartlek session in the woods: 15 mins easy warm-up, drills and 4 × 80 m strides; 2 sets of 30/45/60/75/90/75/60/45/30 sec with equal jog recovery and 3 min jog between sets; 4 × 80 m fast strides; 15 min easy warm-down.
Saturday	Mobility exercises at home before football match
Sunday	S&C exercises then 60 min easy run with last 8 min as stride 20 sec/jog 40 sec.

Specific Training Phases: Track Competition 2016

During the early summer months, volume of training was reduced slightly to accommodate increases in training intensity as the priority shifted to key interval training sessions around race pace. The main target race for the summer, during July, was preceded by a lighter-volume training week that included a variety of paces to maintain aerobic qualities and improve anaerobic and race-specific qualities. The tapering and peaking week is shown as follows.

Week commencing: 11 July 2016

Monday	Mobility exercises then 40 min easy run on grass and stretching
Tuesday	Track session: 1600 m tempo (lap splits: 90/80/90/80 sec), 1200 m (3.27), 800 m (2.15), 400 m (62 sec), 200 m (26 sec), all with 4 min recovery.
Wednesday	Mobility exercises, then 40 min easy run on grass and stretching
Thursday	Rest
Friday	20 min easy run on grass, running drills and 6 × 100 m strides
Saturday	Schools International 1500 m (1st in 4.07.15, splits: 73/71/59/43 sec)
Sunday	Mobility exercises, then 30–40 min easy run on grass and stretching

Specific Training Phases: General Conditioning 2016

Following the track season and a short break, the focus returned to building an aerobic base and prioritising structural loading and strength training to enhance resistance to injury. Training here was characterised by a progressive increase in volume with low intensity. Continuous easy running was kept at an intentionally slow relative intensity (i.e. 12–14 $km.h^{-1}$) to facilitate these outcomes and reduce the risk of injury and overtraining later in the season. Running drills and strides were still included regularly to maintain anaerobic qualities and provide a higher-intensity musculoskeletal conditioning stimulus for reducing injury risk during the pre-track season phase. An example of this early preparation phase is shown below.

Week commencing: 12 September 2016 (Week 3 of 2016–17)

Monday	S&C session followed by 35 min easy run (ave.: 13.3 km.h^{-1}) on grass and 6 × 100 m strides
Tuesday	Rest
Wednesday	45 min progression run (mile splits: 7.26, 6.45, 6.34, 6.23, 6.00, 5.49, 5.30) followed by 4 × 80 m strides
Thursday	S&C session followed by 40 min easy run (ave.: 13.3 km.h^{-1})
Friday	35 min easy run (ave.: 13.3 km.h^{-1}) on grass, running drills and 6 × 100 m strides
Saturday	Conditioning circuits (15 min jog before and after)
Sunday	60 min hilly easy run (ave. 12.6 km.h^{-1}) on hills followed by mobility routine

Specific Training Phases: Cross-Country Season Preparation 2016

Table 10.1 provides examples of cross-country preparation training weeks between 2016 and 2019. During this phase, the volume of training was high but now starts to plateau, and the focus shifts to increasing the intensity and quality of aerobic running sessions at around cross-country race intensity (5–10 km track pace) and slightly faster. It was important during this phase that runs between sessions were used as active recovery, and thus the relative intensity was kept strictly low (i.e. 12–14 km.h^{-1}) to ensure adequate recovery and reduce injury risk. Interval and fartlek sessions took place on grass or hilly trail surfaces to closely represent the terrain Darragh would experience in cross-country competition. There was a continued emphasis on strength and conditioning work to maintain musculoskeletal structural integrity.

Hard sessions (interval training, tempo runs and fartlek) usually included repetitions performed at a variety of different running speeds (from maximal sprinting to 10 km 'tempo' pace) throughout the training year. These speeds are all critical to develop in middle- and long-distance runners; therefore, in the author's view, a variety of speeds should be included most weeks in different proportions (depending upon the volume an athlete can handle, the time of year, the primary goal(s) of the session, etc.). By using a variety of paces within a training session, a runner is exposed to several different physiological stimuli that elicit a variety of adaptations. It also prepares them better for races, which tend to involve regular changes in pace and teaches the runner to finish fast whilst under fatigue. For young athletes this session design is also less monotonous and is more challenging than a constant speed session.

Specific Training Phases: Cross-Country Competition (Peaking) 2016

The focus for this phase centred around the main aim for the cross-country season, the European Cross-Country Championships. To facilitate a short-term peak in performance, the volume of training reduced slightly in the 2 weeks prior to the championships and intensity was maintained. The final tapering and peaking week is shown as follows.

Week commencing: 5 December 2016 (Week 15 of 2016–17)

Monday	Rest
Tuesday	Mobility routine followed by 35 min easy run (ave. 13.2 km.h^{-1}) on grass with last 6 min stride 20 sec/jog easy 40 sec
Wednesday	Travel to Dublin. Light session on grass/trail: 2 × 5 min tempo (5.37, 5.33) with 90 sec jog recovery followed by 4 × 1 min with 1 min recovery @ 3 km pace
Thursday	Travel to Rome. 35 mins easy (ave. 12.8 km.h^{-1}) on grass followed by 4 × 80 m strides
Friday	Travel to Sardinia. 10 min easy jog and mobility routine upon arrival
Saturday	Mobility routine and 30 min easy (ave 13.1 km.h^{-1}), running drills and 6 × 100 m strides
Sunday	European Cross-Country Championships under-20 men's race, 39th in 18.04

Specific Training Phases: Track Season Preparation 2017

Following the cross-country season, this training phase was dedicated to further development of aerobic capabilities and maintaining others. Whilst there was a relative reduction in training intensity to accommodate higher volumes of work, the quality of interval training sessions increased slightly, compared to the cross-country preparatory phase.

As a general principle, the author believes in utilising only two key hard sessions in a normal training week (or one hard session plus a race). A truly hard interval or fartlek session usually requires at least 48 hours active recovery (often closer to 72 hours) for most runners, particularly young athletes. Therefore, three days tended to separate the key sessions of the week and at least three days was left between a hard workout and a race. It is important to note that most hard-running workouts contained a relatively high amount of volume most of the year round to develop important aerobic capabilities with smaller dosages of anaerobic work also included. The long run each week, although not a high-intensity running workout, can place quite a high physiological stress on an athlete, particularly at a young age.

Week commencing: 27 February 2017 (Week 27 of 2016–17)

Monday	Rest
Tuesday	Track session: 4 × 1600 m with 90 sec jog recovery in (lap splits: 85/75/85/75 sec reps 1–2; 84/80/76/72 sec reps 3–4) followed by 4 × 200 m in 30/31 sec with 90 sec jog recovery
Wednesday	S&C session followed by 40 min easy run (ave 13.8 km.h^{-1}) on grass and 4 × 80 m strides
Thursday	40 mins easy run (ave. 14.0 km.h^{-1}), running drills and 6 × 10 sec short hill sprints with 2–2.5 min walk
Friday	45 min progression run in the woods followed by 4 × 80 m fast strides.
Saturday	S&C session followed by 40 min easy run (ave 12.6 km.h^{-1}) on grass and 4 × 80 m strides
Sunday	70 min hilly easy run (ave 13.9 km.h^{-1}) with last 8 min stride 20 sec/jog easy 40 sec followed by mobility routine

Specific Training Phases: Track Season 2017

Darragh managed to secure races in several high-quality track meetings during the track season, which provided the opportunity to run fast times. Training volume therefore reduced, and intensity increased to enable peak performance to be reached. Sessions largely involved race-pace intensity efforts; however, some mixed pace work was included to maintain aerobic qualities. The week leading into an important international race over 1500 m is shown as follows.

Week commencing: 22 May 2017 (Week 40 of 2016–17 season)

Monday	40 min easy (ave 12.6 km.h^{-1}), running drills and 3 × 10 sec short hill sprints with 2–2.5 min walk recovery
Tuesday	Track session: 2 × 1600 m (lap splits: 85/75/85/75 sec) with 60 sec jog recovery, 3 × 600 m in 1.39 with 90 sec jog rec, 3 × 400 m in 60 sec with 90 sec jog recovery.
Wednesday	S&C session followed by 40 min easy run (ave 13.3 km.h^{-1}) on grass and 4 × 80 m strides
Thursday	Rest
Friday	Fly to Amsterdam. Mobility routine and 30 min easy (ave 12.6 km.h^{-1}), running drills and 6 × 100 m strides
Saturday	IFAM Meeting, Belgium 1500 m (3.48.05, personal best)
Sunday	Fly to Cork. Mobility routine followed by 30 min easy (ave 12.6 km.h^{-1}) and 4 × 80 m strides

Specific Training Phases: Track Preparation – Portugal Training Camp

A training camp affords an athlete the time to mentally focus on their training, away from the distractions of everyday life, and additional recovery time between training sessions. Moreover, if a training camp is in a warm country, the thermoregulatory adaptations that occur over a period of several weeks may augment performance when the athlete returns to training and racing in a cooler environment. Following an initial period of acclimatisation, Darragh completed a high-volume block of training during this camp. Whilst maintaining the high volume of running, intensity of sessions progressively increased with a larger focus on paces approaching track race speed. Owing to the additional time Darragh had available whilst away on camp, he was also able to separate his running and strength and conditioning training sessions, which he is not usually able to do. Despite the additional time available for training on camp, it is, however, too important not to raise volume and/or intensity of training too much compared to the training that would otherwise be performed at home. It can be tempting on training camps to overload too quickly in the assumption that the recovery process is faster; however, this is not the case. Therefore, the risk of injury, illness and overtraining on a training camp can be high if training load is not managed appropriately.

Week commencing: 26 March 2018 (Week 34 of 2017–18 season)

Monday	AM – 50 min easy run (ave 13.5 km.h^{-1}), hurdle mobility, running drills and 6 × 80 m strides. PM – S&C session.
Tuesday	AM – tempo run on cross-country course: 4 × 8 min with 2 min jog recovery followed by 4 × 100 m strides @ 1500 m pace after. PM – Pilates session.

Wednesday   AM – 50 min easy run (ave 13.2 km.h^{-1}) followed by hurdle mobility and 4 × 80 m strides. PM – gluteal conditioning.

Thursday   AM – 50 min easy run (ave 13.8 km.h^{-1}), running drills and 6 × 10 sec power hill sprints with 2–2.5 min walk recovery.

PM   – S&C routine.

Friday   AM – Hill session: 2 sets of (4 × 90 sec with jog back recovery and 4 × 20 sec with jog back recovery) and 5 min between sets.

PM   – Rest

Saturday   AM – Long run 80 min easy run on trails (ave 14.9 km.h^{-1}), hurdle mobility drills and 6 × 80 m strides

PM   – Mobility/stretching

Sunday   AM – 50 min easy run, running drills and 6 × 10 sec power hill sprints with 2–2.5 min walk recovery.

PM   – S&C session.

Specific Training Phases: Tapering and Peaking

During the tapering and peaking phase (1–2 weeks prior to major competition), training is characterised by a reduction in overall running volume and a maintenance or slight increase in training intensity. The priority each week is given to recovery from hard track sessions, performed at target race pace or faster. The duration of recovery runs drops, and some normal easy/recovery running sessions are removed or significantly reduced due to travel. Some strength and conditioning is included for maintenance of tissue integrity and explosive power.

Week commencing: 2 July 2018 (Week 48 of 2017–18 season)

Monday   Mobility routine followed by 40 min easy run (ave 14.8 km.h^{-1}) and 4 × 80 m strides

Tuesday   Track session: 2 sets of (3 × 800 m @ 5k pace with 45 sec recovery) and 5 min recovery between sets followed by 4 × 200 m @ 1500 m pace with 90 sec jog recovery

Wednesday   Mobility routine followed by 40 min easy run (ave 14.8 km.h^{-1}) and 4 × 80 m strides

Thursday   S&C routine followed by 40 min easy run (ave 14.9 km.h^{-1}) and 4 × 80 m strides

Friday   Track session: 1600 m tempo in 5.10, 3 min recovery, 14 × 200 m in 29/30 secs with 200 m jog recovery, 1600 m tempo in 5.00

Saturday   Travel to Finland. Mobility routine followed by 40 min easy run (ave 14.3 km.h^{-1}) and 4 × 80 m strides

Sunday   Rest (only mobility routine)

Week commencing: 9 July 2018 (Week 49 of 2017–18 season)

Monday   World Junior Championships, Finland
AM   – stadium visit – 20 mins easy run, running drills and 6 × 80 m strides PM – 20 mins easy run and mobility routine

Tuesday	Trail/grass session: 2×3 min @ 10 km intensity with 90 sec jog recovery, 3 min rest, 2×2 min @ 5 km intensity with 2 min rec, 3 min rest, 2×1 min @ 3 km intensity with 60 sec recovery, 3 min rest, 2×30 sec @ 1500 m intensity with 90 sec rec
Wednesday	AM – mobility routine/gluteal conditioning followed by 20 min easy jog
PM	– 20 min easy run, running drills and 4×80 m strides
Thursday	Rest
Friday	AM – 15 mins easy and mobility routine
PM	– 15 mins easy with last 3 min @ 5.30–5.40 per mile pace and last 1 min hard (4.43 per mile pace), 6–7 drills and 4×80 m strides
Saturday	AM – 10 mins easy and mobility routine
PM	– World Junior Championships 5000 m Final, 18th in 14.53.
Sunday	30 min easy recovery run (ave 12.1 km.h^{-1})
Week	commencing: 15 July 2019 (Week 51 of 2017–18 season)
Monday	Rest
Tuesday	50 min easy run followed by running drills 4×80 m strides
Wednesday	AM – 20 min easy run
PM	– 4×800 m in 2.34 with 60 sec jog recovery followed by 4×200 m starting at 30 sec progressing down to 27 sec
Thursday	30 min easy run
Friday	Travel to Sweden. Mobility routine upon arrival.
Saturday	30 min easy run, running drills and 4×80 m strides
Sunday	AM – 20 min easy run
PM	– European Under-20 Championships 5000 m Final, 3rd in 14.06

Performance Progression

Table 10.4 shows Darragh's personal best performances each year between 2014 and 2019. A steady improvement is evident, which reflects the sensible and well-managed progression of training volume over a six-year period. Between 2014 and 2016 Darragh focused on the 1500 m event but gradually increased the number of 3000 m races he participated in with a view to target the 5000 m event in the under-20 age group. By continuing the focus on the 1500 m and 3000 m, the author believes this has enabled Darragh to improve quickly over 5000 m and be competitive in this event at major championships in the future. Importantly, in August 2020, Darragh marked his arrival in senior-level competition by claiming victory over 5000 m in the Irish Senior Championships, defeating an athlete with a best of 13.30 for 5000 m.

TABLE 10.4 Progression of personal best performances for track seasons 2014–19

Year	1500 m	3000 m	5000 m
2014	4:24.34	–	–
2015	4:11.38	9:15.98	–
2016	3:54.50	–	–
2017	3:48.05	8:20.89	–
2018	3:49.45	8:13.80	14:11.80
2019	3:45.12	8:01.48	13:54.10

Lessons Learned From a Coaching Career

This section of the chapter describes ten 'lessons learned' for both runners and coaches that intend to motivate others to reflect upon their own training and practice to better understand how to get the most out of themselves or their athletes. Although these lessons are unique and personal to the author, they aim to help those who are less experienced by sharing wisdom and insight from several decades of coaching runners.

Lessons Applicable to Runners

1. *Attitude*. A runner should be organised, prepared and punctual and should display positive body language, resilience, belief and work ethic. Bring 'your best self' to each day.
2. *Relationships*. Runners should try to connect with their coach, be open and honest, show them a great work ethic and commit to the plan. Surround yourself with people that are positive, of a similar mindset as you and that will help you fulfil your goals in the sport.
3. *Enjoyment*. Enjoy what you do! Running is a sport, and the central tenet to success is enjoying it, being passionate and loving what you do. Doing the work is far easier when you love and enjoy what you do.
4. *Patience and consistency*. Success in endurance sport is reliant on patience, consistency in training/racing and remaining injury/illness free. There are no short cuts; there will be many highs and lows along the journey, but if you are willing to continue on the road to be the best you can be, there are big performances always around the corner with dedication and smart training.
5. *Process*. Have a clear plan on where you want to go and how you are going to get there. This road map is critical in providing direction and also serves as a reminder each day as to why you are doing the work to increase motivation.
6. *Basics*. Athletes must be prepared to complete the basics repetitively, which means performing mundane behaviours for long periods of time. You have only one body, and you must look after it; therefore, perform basic healthy lifestyle behaviours to a high standard (sleep, sound nutrition, hydration, etc).
7. *Accountability*. Athletes must be accountable for their training/race performances and especially for their lifestyle choices.
8. *Adaptability*. Learn to adapt to any situation during training/racing and cultivate this by making training uncomfortable at appropriate times. Having the ability to adapt to unforeseen setbacks and challenges along your journey is also key.
9. *Challenge*. Embrace the challenges thrown at you on your journey and learn from them. Athletes should train hard but not too hard – it is not always about doing more things right but about doing fewer things wrong.
10. *Self-reflection*. This is important for athletes to both foster learning and make improvements. Reflect on your lifestyle choices, your training/racing, your motivation/drive, etc., and make changes where needed. Interact and learn from others but don't continually compare yourself to others.

Lessons Applicable to Coaches

1. *Relationships*. An important part of coaching is building relationships. You are coaching people and not machines; therefore, building a relationship with your athletes should be

the top priority. To bring the best out of an individual, you must therefore focus on the person in front of you.

2. *Resilience*. An athlete's journey involves many up and downs; therefore, coaches must be resilient and prepare themselves to encounter many questions that do not have easy answers. Don't be afraid to fail; this is where we learn. Stick to the process and keep to your plan, and usually it works itself out.

3. *Listen*. Aim to listen twice as much as you speak. Sometimes as coaches we can do all the talking, offer copious amounts of advice, and would be better off listening to our athletes. Allow athletes to be open, honest and offer their reflections and feedback. Listening more can develop trust and buy-in, and enhance motivation.

4. *Excellence*. Normalise excellence by bringing 'your best self' to each day. Also exemplify balance in your lifestyle as a coach. To perform at your best, you must mind yourself as you expect your athletes to.

5. *Change*. If an athlete is not responding to the training you are prescribed, then do not be afraid to change it. Every athlete responds differently to a training stimulus, so experiment to see what works.

6. *Experiment*. No coach can be 100% sure of any training plan, and nobody has the magic formula as it does not exist. Study the sport, learn from athletes and other coaches and find the formula that works. A coach must help an athlete understand the theory behind the training they are doing to increase buy-in and self-belief.

7. *Foundations*. Do not neglect the foundations of athletic development when coaching athletes, i.e. mobility, balance, coordination, agility, speed, strength, etc. This will enable them to handle increases in training volume and intensity.

8. *Coaching style*. Learn from other coaches, but do not try to be like another coach. Be yourself and find your best fit as a coach, whether it be working with grassroots- or elite-level runners.

9. *Learning*. The biggest learning tool for a coach is the athletes themselves. Soak up information from a wide variety of people and resources and then filter what is of most relevance to you and your athletes. Also look outside of the sport for better ways to do things.

10. *Data*. Not everything we can measure is important, and not everything important can be measured. A coach needs to gather relevant data that impacts the training and most importantly aids in improving performance. Coaches should avoid gathering data for the sake of it. Data must be meaningful and contribute to guiding the training/performance process.

Summary

Coaching a runner to achieve their goals and maximise their long-term potential is informed by both a sound understanding of the latest sport science and the art of figuring out what works for an individual athlete. Although science heavily informs the principles of training and recovery interventions, individual runners can respond differently to the same training programme for a multitude of reasons. Prior to designing a training programme, a coach should consider the unique background, needs and goals of a runner via a detailed analysis of their current performance profile, training and injury history, and recommendations from other members of a multi-disciplinary sport science/medicine support team. This chapter provided a summary of the training for a successful junior male runner based upon an analysis of his needs. Ten 'lessons learned' for athletes and coaches are also described that encourage readers to take a holistic and open-minded approach with a runner's development. The recommendations listed encourage behaviours that will enable runners/coaches to learn about 'what works' for themselves/their runners, and the pitfalls to avoid in the journey to becoming the best they can be.

Acknowledgements

The author would like to thank Coach David McCarthy, who guided Darragh for 7 months from January to July 2019 in the run in to his medal at the European Under-20 Championships.

11

SHORT-TERM NUTRITION STRATEGIES TO MAXIMISE EVENT-DAY PERFORMANCE

Justin D. Roberts and Matthew Cole

Highlights

- Carbohydrate loading (8–12 g·kg body mass^{-1}·day^{-1}) in the 48 hours prior to a (ultra-) marathon, in-event carbohydrate intake every 15–20 min (~30–90 g of carbohydrate per hour, <8% concentration) and 'drinking to thirst' (~450–750 mL·hour^{-1}) are all strategies that will likely support performance in events lasting >90 min.
- Nutritional ergogenic aids should not be used by runners as a replacement to sound dietary intake of nutrients, and any supplement deemed appropriate for use by a runner should preferably carry the 'Informed Sport' logo.
- A caffeine intake of 2–6 mg·kg body mass^{-1} consumed approximately 1 hour prior to exercise may enhance endurance performance.
- Sodium bicarbonate supplementation of between 0.2 and 0.4 g·kg body mass^{-1} taken 60–150 min (split into small doses to avoid gastrointestinal disturbances) prior to high-intensity (middle-distance) exercise may improve performance.
- Daily beta alanine consumption of ~65 mg·kg body mass^{-1} over a period of 10–12 weeks has been shown to improve high-intensity running performance.
- Beetroot juice is a natural source of dietary nitrate with acute pre-exercise ingestion (~2–3 hours before exercise) of 5–9 mmol, or 8.4 mmol for prolonged periods (6 to 15 days), required to improve exercise performance.

Introduction

Running is an energetically demanding activity, and several important bioenergetic processes are likely causes of fatigue in middle- (800 m–3 km) and long-distance (5 km upwards) events. As discussed in Chapter 4, middle-distance performances derive their energy from both anaerobic and aerobic metabolism, whereas long-distance events rely almost exclusively on aerobic energy pathways to fuel performance. The anaerobic contribution to energy production is ~30–40% and ~15–30% for the 800 m and 1500 m events respectively (Spencer and Gastin, 2001; Duffield et al., 2005). A high reliance on the anaerobic glycolytic energy pathway in these events is associated with the accumulation of metabolites and a more acidic environment in the muscle that causes rapid fatigue (Allen et al., 2008). Nutritional strategies that promote a more alkaline environment and buffering of metabolites may therefore provide an avenue for improving performance during middle-distance running events.

Almost all the energy production for long-distance running events takes place in the mitochondria of working muscles, which requires an adequate delivery of oxygen and availability of carbohydrate and fat fuels. At fast running speeds (i.e. 10 km race speed and faster), glycogen (carbohydrate broken down) is virtually the sole source of energy; however, at lower intensities of exercise (typical for a recreational marathoner or ultra-distance event), a mixture of carbohydrate and fat is used. Pre- and in-event nutritional strategies that encourage mitochondrial respiration, alter the absorption of fuels into muscles, and that provide a more plentiful supply of energy to sustain running speed therefore have utility in improving endurance performance. Following on from Chapter 4, the aims of this chapter are threefold. Firstly, the chapter will outline how specific pre- and in-event carbohydrate fuelling and hydration approaches can help maximise performance in long-distance running events. Secondly, the chapter examines the potential role of nutritional ergogenic aids in optimising running performance in middle- and long-distance running events with consideration of potential risks and side effects associated with consumption of these supplements. Thirdly, based upon the evidence presented for specific short-term nutritional strategies, recommendations are provided for event/race day preparation.

Pre- and In-Event Nutrition

The nutritional requirements of runners preparing for, and participating in, events of different duration can vary enormously. For example, the nutritional and training demands of a middle-distance runner will be considerably different to a half- or full-marathon distance runner where exercise duration influences caloric and glycogen requirements. The nutritional considerations for a single or multiple-stage ultra-endurance runner may also need to account for metabolic efficiency, immune/inflammatory support, and individual gastrointestinal tolerance. As such, nutritional considerations for distance running events should be undertaken in a personalised and periodised manner as stated previously, in line with the training demands of the runner (Jeukendrup, 2017a).

Consideration to in-event strategies is also warranted, particularly with regards to longer duration sessions or events. Early research demonstrated the correlation between pre-event glycogen stores and exercise duration, which may be particularly relevant when repeated days of training, or event duration, are considered (Costill et al., 1971; Costill and Miller, 1980). Whilst rate of glycogen use is predominantly accelerated with exercise intensity (i.e. as intensity exceeds ~60% $\dot{V}O_{2max}$, glycogen utilization increases exponentially), exercise duration plays a crucial role, considering total glycogen stores are relatively limited. Therefore, in-event nutritional strategies should begin with the pre-training/event period, especially when exercise duration (>60 min) or individual performance is considered. This also has a bearing on pre-event readiness for the runner, including hydration status and offsetting potential gastrointestinal issues in-event.

Carbohydrate Loading and Pre-Event Meals

Classical carbohydrate loading strategies (~7 days prior to event) highlight the importance of high carbohydrate intake coupled with reduced training load (Williams and Lamb, 2008).

For marathon running performance, various mixed carbohydrate loading strategies have been reported, which typically involve an increase in carbohydrate intake 3–6 days prior to an event (Sherman et al., 1981; Hargreaves et al., 2004). Acute carbohydrate loading (in the 2 days prior to event) achieving 8–12 $g \cdot kg^{-1} \cdot day^{-1}$ may be a useful strategy to maximise, or 'supercompensate', glycogen stores prior to events lasting >90 min without the need for longer-term loading approaches (Thomas et al., 2016). For some individuals, particularly in long-duration events, this could positively impact on performance by 2–3% (Hawley et al., 1997; Jeukendrup et al., 2005).

For runners consuming moderately high carbohydrate intakes in their diet prior to an event, a further increase in carbohydrate may not be necessarily beneficial. This is especially the case if a runner is susceptible to in-race gastrointestinal distress, and when pre-event meal planning and in-race fuelling strategies are also considered (Burke et al., 2000; Burke et al., 2011). The key point is to ensure glycogen stores are replenished prior to long-duration running, i.e. half/full marathon distance. Where in-race glycogen depletion is less likely (i.e. 10 km events and shorter), loading strategies are of less importance (assuming adequate initial levels of carbohydrate).

Current guidelines indicate that to maximise long-distance (i.e. marathon) performance, pre-event meal planning should aim for a broad 1–4 $g \cdot kg^{-1}$ carbohydrate to support glycogen lost during overnight fasting (Burke et al., 2011; Vitale and Getzin, 2019). Larger amounts of carbohydrate (up to 4 $g \cdot kg^{-1}$) should be consumed 3–4 hours from the start of an event, with smaller volumes (e.g. 1–2 $g \cdot kg^{-1}$, typically liquid or easily digestible foods) within 2 hours of the event.

Mouth Rinsing

For events < 1 hour, or indeed where runners struggle with long distance in-event gastrointestinal issues, whilst carbohydrate ingestion may not be overly required, the use of carbohydrate mouth rinsing has been suggested as a beneficial strategy (Silva et al., 2013). Mouth rinsing involves swilling a carbohydrate drink around the mouth for 5–10 sec and subsequently spitting it out without swallowing any of the solution. By stimulating taste receptors, it has been proposed that the consequential effect on the central nervous system may positively influence the perception of fatigue, leading to improved performance. Whilst the majority of studies have demonstrated performance benefits in controlled studies with cyclists (Carter et al., 2004), Rollo et al. (2008) have shown that mouth rinsing using a 6% carbohydrate solution compared to placebo favourably influenced self-selected running pace and total distance covered in a 30 min treadmill test. Additionally, Rollo et al. (2011) have also indicated that mouth rinsing (6.4% carbohydrate solution) and ingestion every 15 min can subtly increase distance covered in a 1-hour time trial compared to placebo. A recent review on this area concluded that mouth rinsing could offer a ~2–3% performance effect for short duration bouts (<1 hour) of exercise at moderate to high intensity (>70% $\dot{V}O_{2max}$, Silva et al., 2013).

In-Event Energy Demands and Carbohydrate Requirements

As endurance running events increase in distance, caloric requirements increase, and therefore energy typically needs to be replaced during the event. For events exceeding ~4 hours (i.e. marathon and ultra-distance), a careful balance between intake and gastrointestinal tolerance is needed, particularly in more sensitive individuals. It is apparent that race finishers (particularly faster finishers) tend to ingest higher calories/carbohydrate/fluid/electrolytes compared to slow or non-finishers, particularly in ultra-distance events (Glace et al., 2002; Martinez et al., 2018). Some field studies have reported caloric intakes ~180 kcal·hour^{-1} (Martinez et al., 2018) for marathon distance events (equivalent to ~2 gels per hour), with recommendations for ~150–400 kcal·hour^{-1} for longer-distance events (Tiller et al., 2019) from mixed energy sources.

Whilst mouth rinsing may be effective during shorter-distance events, sustained endurance running (>90 min) will likely require additional carbohydrate ingestion (even when fat metabolism adaptations have been prioritised during training). This is nicely summarised by Burke et al. (2011), indicating that for events lasting 1–2.5 hours, ~30–60 g of carbohydrate per hour (<8% concentration) may optimise energy delivery without undue gastrointestinal 'overload'. Over longer-duration events, a steady provision of easily digestible carbohydrate may help maintain plasma glucose, as well as a sustained use of carbohydrate for energy (and pace maintenance). However, preference is not solely focused on sports drinks, and runners should find a refuelling plan that suits their individual goals including hydration needs and gut comfort based upon various energy sources (Burke et al., 2011). This provides considerable flexibility for the runner, but also indicates the need for regular 'trial and error' during training to establish a personalised approach which may involve a combination of drinks, gels and solid foods (e.g. energy bars, chews, soft fruit). As an example, a typical commercial gel provides ~20–25 g carbohydrate, therefore consuming ~2 gels per hour would generally meet published recommendations, although additional fluid intake is also recommended. Consideration to ingestion timing is also warranted based on individual requirements with the recommendation that regular consumption every 15–20 min may support optimal delivery.

For events lasting >2.5 hours, carbohydrate doses up to 90 g·hour^{-1} are recommended to sustain carbohydrate oxidation rates, although individual tolerance/training experience may influence this upper level; and prior 'nutritional training' is recommended (Jeukendrup, 2014). Numerous studies demonstrate beneficial effects of 'multiple transportable carbohydrates' (MTCs) for optimal carbohydrate delivery, with the indication that ingestion rates of ~1.5 g·min^{-1} or 90 g·hour^{-1} may likely be an upper threshold (Jeukendrup, 2013). By providing mixed sugars (e.g. glucose and fructose, or maltodextrins with added fructose, approximately in a 2:1 ratio) that require different intestinal transporters, the evidence highlights that exogenous carbohydrate oxidation rates are greater compared to single sugar (glucose) use, and may be better tolerated in terms of gastrointestinal symptoms (Jentjens et al., 2004; Jentjens and Jeukendrup, 2005; Jentjens et al., 2006; Rowlands et al., 2012; Roberts et al., 2014). The use of MTCs may also favour water absorption compared to glucose only, with studies supporting their use in overall power output and performance (Currell and Jeukendrup, 2008; Jeukendrup and Moseley, 2010; Rowlands et al., 2012; Roberts et al., 2014), although studies specific to running are limited (Lee et al., 2014). The inclusion of caffeine with sports drinks has also been shown to enhance exogenous glucose oxidation rates (Yeo et al., 2005), increasing carbohydrate availability for exercise (however, research specific to endurance running is warranted). It is important to note that environmental considerations on race day are also relevant. Hydration may become a more important factor during sustained heat exposure, and carbohydrate oxidation rates may be reduced. As such, during hotter conditions, carbohydrate intake should be moderated to reflect this.

In-Event Gastrointestinal Issues

Runners often cite gastrointestinal issues as a common reason for reduced race effort or non-completion (de Oliveira et al., 2014). Prevalence rates vary from a moderate 30–50% of athletes, to over >90% of athletes (particularly in longer-distance, ultra-distance or multi-discipline events), especially when event/environmental demands are more extreme (Jeukendrup et al., 2000; de Oliveira et al., 2014). Individual symptom severity and persistence also appear to vary between runners (suggesting a genetic component), although sustained high-intensity effort or heat exposure may exacerbate gastrointestinal symptoms (Costa et al., 2017). Nausea, bloating, gut cramps and acute diarrhoea are typically the most common symptoms, which can impact on race appetite or desire to maintain hydration practices (de Oliveira et al., 2014). One proposed mechanism is that of reduced blood flow to the gastrointestinal tract during running, which may impact on intestinal transport leading to transient gastrointestinal injury or permeability (Zuhl et al., 2014) and acute endotoxemia. It also appears that fluid restriction can impact on gastrointestinal function (Lambert et al., 2008), which may exacerbate gastrointestinal distress (Costa et al., 2017), highlighting the importance of in-race euhydration. Overconsumption of high-concentration carbohydrate solutions may also be a primary factor in gastrointestinal distress (Costa et al., 2019a, 2019b), along with (potentially unaccustomed) inclusion of in-race foods higher in fibre, fat or protein.

Whilst individualised feeding and hydration strategies should aim to meet recommended hourly delivery targets, self-management of gastrointestinal comfort and/or tolerance during races is clearly needed when gastrointestinal symptoms/severity arise. It is evident that the gut may be 'trained' to progressive and personalised feeding approaches during training (Cox et al., 2010; Jeukendrup, 2014; Jeukendrup, 2017a, 2017b), which may be nutrient specific (e.g. higher carbohydrate loading) and facilitate reduced sensations of fullness, especially if practiced at race-pace. Several practical strategies have been recommended (see Figure 11.1, Jeukendrup, 2017b), along with exclusion, or reduction, of identified foods associated with in-race gastrointestinal distress. Furthermore, strategic inclusion of a low FODMAP (fermentable oligosaccharide, disaccharide, monosaccharide and polyol) foods in the diet may offer targeted support, particularly in runners more susceptible to irritable bowel syndrome-related symptoms (Dis et al., 2018; Wiffin et al., 2019; Gaskell and Costa, 2019). Emerging evidence highlights the potential use of probiotic strategies to reduce gastrointestinal symptom prevalence prior to an event, and in-race (Roberts et al., 2016; Pugh et al., 2019; Leite et al., 2019), which may improve performance during the latter stages of a marathon (Pugh et al., 2019). However, other findings are equivocal (Shing et al., 2014), and (along with other nutrients, e.g. glutamine, colostrum, zinc) indicate the need for further running-specific research.

Hydration and Hyponatraemia

Hydration requirements for endurance runners vary according to individual sweat rate, exercise intensity/duration, environmental heat stress and evaporative cooling processes. Studies have demonstrated that runners can lose ~1.4 L of sweat in a half-marathon, but may consume around 1.1 L of total fluid, resulting in a net loss of 0.3 L (Pereira et al., 2017). Experienced marathon runners have demonstrated body weight reductions of 0.3–1.7% in cool to warm conditions (Cheuvront et al., 2007), despite high fluid intake rates. It is clear that even mild

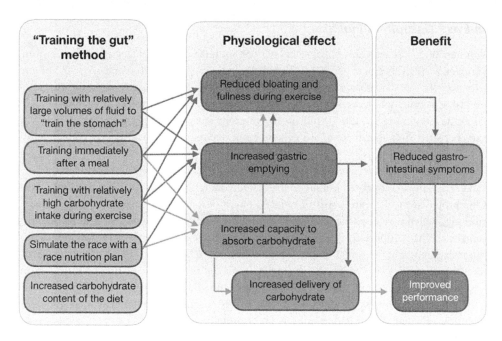

FIGURE 11.1 A summary of methods to 'train the gut', physiological adaptations that may occur and the affect upon performance

Source: Taken from Jeukendrup (2017b).

dehydration (~2% body mass) can impact on exercise performance (particularly in line with reduced race pace in the latter stages of an event), and that minimising or restricting fluid intake can lead to dehydration rates >3.3% (Cheuvront et al., 2007) over marathon-distance events, which can additionally impact on gastrointestinal distress. Post-training, strategic awareness of hyper-hydration practices i.e. ~150–200% exercise-induced body mass losses (particularly with inclusion of moderate-higher dose electrolytes (e.g. sodium) for higher volume intakes) have been shown to sustain positive hydration states in the hours post-exercise (Shirreffs et al., 1996). This may be particularly important during training and leading into events to offset potential pre-race dehydration.

It is evident that in-race dehydration >2% body mass can impact not only on running economy but also cognitive performance, and thermal and physical effort perception (Sawka et al., 2007). During shorter long-distance events, e.g. 10 km to half-marathon, current recommendations are to 'drink to thirst' (Kenefick, 2018). This approach likely minimises the risk of hypo- or hyper-hydration practices, although athletes can refine individual strategies based on basic exercise-induced fluid losses during training runs (particularly under similar conditions where possible to race day). Similar practices have been recommended for longer duration events (Costa et al., 2019b), although environmental conditions (temperature, humidity, physical exposure) and prior acclimation processes should also be considered when aiming to refine hydration strategies. Whilst intakes vary considerably between individuals, recommendations of 450–750 mL·hour^{-1} or 150–250 mL each 20 min may support in-race hydration without undue gastrointestinal overload.

Inclusion of electrolytes (e.g. ~230–690 mg sodium·L^{-1}) as part of hydration formulas may support adequate intestinal water absorption (Jeukendrup, 2011), and offset dehydration during races.

One area of contention, particularly for longer race events (Montain et al., 2001) is that of hyponatraemia (or exercise-associated hyponatraemia; EAH). Over-hydration practices (consuming higher or more frequent volumes of water), high sweat rates, and/or low electrolyte consumption (Sawka et al., 2007) can lead to a relative dilution of blood sodium resulting in hyponatraemia (serum sodium < 135 mmol·L^{-1}; Hew-Butler et al., 2015), which can occur in-race or during post-race recovery. Over-hydration practices may be more applicable to slower, smaller or heavier runners (Sawka et al., 2007; Jeukendrup, 2011). Symptomatic EAH can include nausea, headaches and confusion (also associated with race duration/fatigue), which ultimately can be serious if concomitant with cerebral oedema. Whilst prevalence rates are rare, particularly for sub-marathon distances, runners should aim to consume electrolytes (e.g. 500–700 mg sodium·L^{-1} fluid) as part of their hydration strategy for longer-distance sessions (American College of Sports Medicine et al., 2000). When competing in hot or humid conditions, inclusion of 300–600 mg sodium·$hour^{-1}$ may be warranted (bearing in that most commercial providers fall below these levels per serving) partly to facilitate adequate hydration, and partly to maintain plasma sodium levels. However, it is important to note that whilst plasma sodium levels may be better maintained using electrolyte strategies, this does not guarantee prevention of EAH (Hoffman and Stuempfle, 2015), particularly if over-hydration practices are sustained in-race (Hew-Butler et al., 2015). Therefore, drinking to thirst, and hence avoidance of over-hydration practices, may offer appropriate strategies to minimise the likelihood of EAH (Noakes, 2002; Jeukendrup, 2011; Hoffman et al., 2013).

Nutritional Ergogenic Aids

Should a Runner Use Nutritional Ergogenic Aids?

Whilst ergogenic aids and performance-enhancing supplements can play an important role in both running training and competition, it is important to emphasise that they should be complementary to, rather than in lieu of, both high-quality training and performance diets. Thus, athletes are encouraged to focus their efforts on optimising adequate dietary intake (see Chapter 4) before seeking to consider whether any nutritional ergogenic aid can offer additional improvements in training, recovery or performance. In deciding whether or not to use an ergogenic aid, athletes and coaches should consider implementing a risk-benefit analysis to evaluate the relative weight of scientific evidence and potential performance enhancement vs. the possible risks associated with supplement use (e.g. anti-doping violation, financial costs, risk of excess consumption, etc.).

To mitigate the impact of any potential side effects on the athlete, any supplement use should be ideally trialled in a training environment before committing to use in a competition setting. Where possible, it is advisable to consult with a registered sport and exercise nutritionist (SENr) or sports nutrition professional prior to supplement use and consume products from reputable manufacturers with regular batch-testing (product packaging must carry the 'Informed Sport' logo). Despite widespread use by middle- and long-distance athletes, there remains very few dietary supplements which have been consistently been shown to be ergogenic. An International Olympic Committee consensus statement on supplement use in high-performing athletes (Maughan et al., 2018) suggests that just five supplements – creatine, caffeine, bicarbonate, beta-alanine and nitrates – are considered to have an adequate level of scientific evidence to support their use as performance-enhancing aids. Of these, the former – creatine – has limited value to middle- or long-distance runners, and thus it is beyond the scope of this chapter to discuss its use in sufficient detail.

Caffeine

Caffeine (or caffeine-like substances) has long been used by athletes in the belief that it can improve sports performance. Indeed, until 2004, the International Olympic Committee (IOC) had a tolerance limit of 12 $\mu g \cdot ml^{-1}$ (in urine) imposed on caffeine with serious sanctions for athletes who exceeded this limit (Laurence et al., 2012). Since 2004, the tolerance limit has been lifted (due to its natural occurrence in a wide variety of foods and beverages), resulting in even more widespread use of caffeine as an ergogenic aid (Laurence et al., 2012). Indeed, Desbrow and Leveritt (2007) reported that 73% of Ironman triathletes believed that caffeine enhanced performance.

There is strong evidence that caffeine improves performance in long-distance running events, whilst evidence is lacking for an ergogenic effect during short-term/high-intensity events (Tarnopolsky, 2010). The precise mechanisms responsible for this performance benefit remain unclear, although several theories have been proposed. The long-standing belief of caffeine's ergogenic effect was that caffeine upregulates lipolytic activity, increasing fat metabolism and thus sparing muscle glycogen as a fuel source, which is believed to be a key determinant of endurance performance. This belief stemmed from an observation of a lower respiratory exchange ratio (RER) during endurance exercise, and so the early studies proposed that caffeine increased lipolysis (and thus spared glycolysis through the Randle cycle) via increases in plasma free-fatty acid (FFA) concentrations (Costill et al., 1978; Ivy et al., 1979). However, current evidence suggests that that the ergogenic properties of caffeine are most likely due to a direct effect on the body's central nervous system (CNS) (Tarnopolsky, 2008).

Firstly, it is believed that caffeine can lower an individual's perception of effort through its antagonistic action on the adenosine receptors in the CNS (Solinas et al., 2002). It is proposed that the action of caffeine as a competitive inhibitor to adenosine leads to increases in serotonin and dopamine neurotransmission. According to the central fatigue hypothesis, alterations in CNS serotonin neurotransmission can lead to an increase in the perception of fatigue (Newsholme et al., 1992; Davis, 1995). Thus, if following caffeine ingestion, the serotonin and dopamine levels can be increased during endurance exercise, this has the potential to improve performance. For example, if a runner's perception of fatigue is lower, this could result in running at a faster pace for the same perceived effort.

Furthermore, it has been reported that caffeine improves performance through stimulation of the sympathetic nervous system (Nicholson et al., 1986). This could potentially improve a runner's performance by stimulating the release of sympathetic hormones, e.g. adrenaline, noradrenaline, etc., which may result in a raised heart rate, increased glycolytic activity or attentional focus. More recently, studies have investigated the influence of caffeine and carbohydrate when ingested in combination or within a short period of each other (Cureton et al., 2007; Hulston and Jeukendrup, 2008), as this is common practice amongst many endurance runners. It is suggested that the improvements reported in these studies could be due to caffeine improving the absorption of exogenous carbohydrate into the body (Yeo et al., 2005). As absorption rate appears to be the most significant rate-limiting step for delivery of this carbohydrate source to the active muscle, suggested to be due to saturation of the sodium-dependent glucose transporter (SGLT-1; Jeukendrup, 2004), this evidence provides an alternative mechanism for the potential performance enhancing effects of caffeine. However, whilst some studies have indicated improvements in performance following the co-ingestion of caffeine and carbohydrate (Cureton et al., 2007; Hulston and Jeukendrup, 2008), others have indicated no enhancements (Jacobsen et al., 2001) or differences in carbohydrate metabolism (Ivy et al., 1979; Graham et al., 2008) compared to a placebo.

Regardless, the ergogenic potential of caffeine for distance runners is unequivocal even if the exact mechanism is still disputed. In terms of an adequate dosage for ergogenesis, a review of scientific studies involving caffeine indicates that consumption of 2–6 mg·kg^{-1} body mass of caffeine approximately 1 hour prior to exercise will enhance endurance performance (Tarnopolsky, 2010). This dosage would appear optimal as additional caffeine ingestion provides no further ergogenic potential and increases the likelihood of side effects, e.g. gastrointestinal distress, muscle tremor, insomnia, etc. (Burke, 2008). Additionally, for those athletes participating in more prolonged endurance events, the consumption of a moderate dose of caffeine (<3 mg·kg^{-1} body mass; ~200 mg) in the latter stages of an event has been shown to combat perceptions of fatigue and aid with maintenance of pace (Talanian and Spriet, 2016). It is also worth noting that typical performance improvements are likely to be small (~1–3% for short duration events; ~3–7% for endurance-based races) and that there is large individual variability in responses to caffeine ingestion. Thus, higher/lower caffeine doses, variations in the timing of intake before and/or during exercise and the need for (or lack thereof) a caffeine withdrawal period should be trialled in training prior to competition use (Maughan et al., 2018).

Sodium Bicarbonate

One of the primary causes of fatigue, especially during high-intensity exercise (e.g. middle-distance events), is a decrease in the intra-cellular pH caused by an accumulation of hydration ions, a by-product of anaerobic glycolysis. As a consequence of this increased acidosis, there is a subsequent decrease in glycolytic enzyme activity, calcium sensitivity, and muscle force production which reduces the capacity to sustain (near-)maximal effort (McNaughton et al., 2016). The ingestion of sodium bicarbonate (NaHCO$_3$) creates a more alkalotic environment within the blood, raising blood pH and thus increasing the hydrogen ion gradient between the blood and the muscle. This increased gradient results in greater removal of hydrogen ions from the muscle into the bloodstream, therefore mitigating the effects of hydration ion accumulation within the muscle and reducing muscle fatigue (Carr et al., 2011).

A typical a dosage of 0.3 g·kg body mass^{-1} has been shown to provide the most ergogenic potential (McNaughton, 1992), although there is some individual variance in the most optimal dose for each athlete. Thus, a range between 0.2 and 0.4 g·kg body mass^{-1} is often recommended, with consumption advised anywhere between 60 and 150 min prior to exercise (Carr et al., 2011). Gastro-intestinal discomfort is the most-commonly reported side effect following sodium bicarbonate ingestion, with typical symptoms including feelings of bloatedness, burping and bowel urgency/diarrhoea. These symptoms can be minimised by splitting the dose into several smaller doses over a longer period or co-ingestion with a small, high-carbohydrate meal

(~1.5 g·kg body mass^{-1} carbohydrates; Carr et al., 2011). Given the high prevalence of symptoms among athletes, thorough investigation into the best individualised strategy is recommended prior to use in a competition setting (Maughan et al., 2018). Performance enhancements of ~2% have regularly been reported in short-term, high-intensity efforts of ~60 seconds in duration, with reduced effects as the effort duration exceeds 10 min (Carr et al., 2011).

Beta Alanine

Carnosine is a naturally occurring protein in the muscle known to support high-intensity exercise performance by regulating intracellular pH, increasing calcium ion sensitivity, and acting as an antioxidant (Trexler et al., 2015). Within the muscle, beta-alanine and L-histidine are the precursors for carnosine production. However, substantially less beta-alanine availability makes it a rate-limiting factor for carnosine production (Lancha Junior et al., 2015). Therefore, supplementing beta-alanine has the potential to increase intramuscular carnosine levels and thus enhance muscle buffering capacity, thereby allowing higher-intensity exercise to be sustained for a prolonged period (Maughan et al., 2018).

Rather than acute intake on the day of training or completion, beta-alanine requires a more chronic consumption strategy in order to adequately increase muscle carnosine levels enough for ergogenesis. Daily consumption of ~65 mg·kg body mass^{-1} over a period of 10–12 weeks has been shown to be optimal (Saunders et al., 2017). Paraesthesia, a non-harmful tingling sensation usually reported in the face and hands, is a commonly reported side effect of beta-alanine supplementation (Quesnele et al., 2014; Lancha Junior et al., 2015) although runners are advised to undertake a split dose regimen (i.e. ~0.8–1.6 g every 3–4 hours) in order to minimise the risk of these side effects. As with other ergogenic aids, performance improvements are likely small (~0.2–3%) but potentially meaningful during both continuous and intermittent exercise of 30 seconds up to 10 min.

Dietary Nitrates

Nitric oxide (NO) is free-radical gas with an involvement in many metabolic signalling and regulatory pathways associated with endurance performance. There are two known pathways by which NO is synthesised:

1. Endogenously, the nitric oxide synthase (NOS) dependent pathway requires oxygen and L-arginine to synthesise NO and L-citrulline, with the co-produced L-citrulline recycled back to L-arginine to continue production (Bredt, 1999; Besco et al., 2012).
2. The exogenous intake of inorganic dietary nitrates (NO_3^-) can be reduced to nitrite (NO_2^-) independently of oxygen by anaerobic bacteria in the oral cavity, before being further reduced to NO during acidic and hypoxic conditions such as high-intensity exercise (Modin et al., 2001; Lundberg and Weitzberg, 2009).

Therefore, a nitrate-rich diet high in leafy green and root vegetables (e.g., beetroot, spinach, rocket, etc.) is expected to enhance the NOS independent pathway, thus giving rise to the popularity of concentrated vegetable extract ingestion. It is expected that enhanced NO availability can improve mitochondrial respiration, decreasing both the oxygen and energy cost of submaximal exercise and thus improving endurance performance (Jones et al., 2018). Beetroot juice is the most common source of dietary nitrate supplementation, having been used in most exercise studies (Peeling et al., 2018) owing to its ease of consumption and high concentration of dietary nitrate. Despite a growing body of evidence in recent years supporting its use as an ergogenic aid, our exact understanding of the optimal dosing strategy remains unclear.

There appears to be a dose-response relationship with moderate amounts of dietary nitrate (8.4 mmol; 140 ml) being more effective than low amounts (4.2 mmol; 70 ml); however, this appears to plateau with no increased benefit seen following consumption of larger (16.8 mmol; 280 ml) amounts (Wylie et al., 2013; Hoon et al., 2014). Additionally, Vanhatalo et al. (2010) reported similar improvements in exercise efficiency when participants consumed dietary nitrate both acutely (1 day) or chronically (over 15 days), thus suggesting that regular consumption is not required in order to elicit ergogenic effects. In general, the main body of evidence indicates that acute pre-exercise ingestion (~2–3 hours before exercise) of 5–9 mmol may be necessary to increase exercise economy; however, a larger dose of 8.4 mmol for prolonged periods (6 to 15 days) may be necessary to increase exercise tolerance, particularly in higher-level athletes where performance improvements via nitrate supplementation appear to be harder to obtain (Jones, 2014). In terms of ergogenic potential, performance improvements of 3–5% are typically observed in events lasting 12–40 min, with limited evidence supporting the use of nitrates for shorter-duration efforts.

There appear to be few known adverse effects resulting from dietary nitrate supplementation, although, as with many ergogenic aids, some athletes are more susceptible to gastro-intestinal discomfort than others. Given the paucity of research in the area, athletes are advised to investigate their own optimal dosing strategy in training prior to implementation in competition.

Application to Event/Race Day Performance

The precise pre- and in-event nutritional strategy will be dependent upon both the duration and intensity of an event and, whilst the consumption of certain ergogenic aids may be common across many events, the precise intake strategy will often differ. In addition, it is important to acknowledge that whilst a dose-response relationship exists with most ergogenic aids, 'more' is not necessarily 'better' and, on the contrary, may increase the prevalence and severity of side effects. Moreover, as previously stated, ergogenic aids should be complementary to an appropriately designed competition nutrition strategy – not an 'easy fix' or 'quick win' in the absence of optimal dietary intake. Finally, it should be emphasised that all nutritional strategies should be trialled first in training before implementation in competition. Based upon the discussion presented in this chapter and Chapter 4, Figure 11.2 shows a hypothetical example of the pre- and in-event nutritional strategies that may benefit a marathon runner. Similarly, Figure 11.3 provides a visual representation of how nutritional ergogenic aids could be used by a middle-distance track athlete prior to an event.

Summary

Short-term strategies to maximise in-event performance should be tailored to the individual and practised during training to refine personalised strategies. Evidence highlights the importance of short-term carbohydrate loading in the pre-event period (e.g. 8–12 g·kg body mass^{-1}·day^{-1} in the 48 hours prior) to maximise glycogen stores particularly for longer-duration

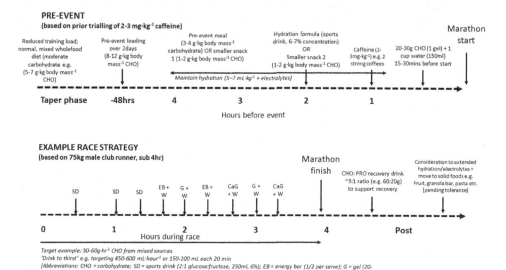

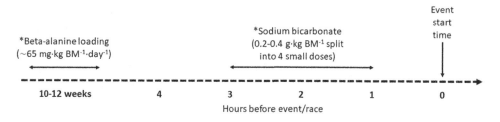

FIGURE 11.2 Pre-event (top schematic) and in-event (bottom schematic) nutritional strategies for a male 75 kg marathon runner

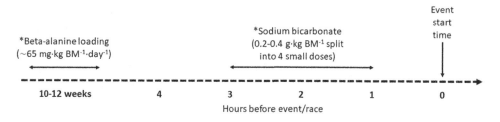

*Note – There is limited evidence supporting the use of both Beta-alanine and Sodium bicarbonate as a co-supplementation strategy. Thus, runners are advised to adopt their preferred selection after trialling in training prior to competition.

FIGURE 11.3 Pre-event nutritional ergogenic aids that could be used by a middle-distance track runner. BM = body mass

events. In-event carbohydrate intake ranging from 30 to 90 g·hour^{-1} pending event distance (>90 mins) and individual tolerance consumed at regular intervals is recommended as part of managing individual pacing. For sustained events, e.g. marathon distance, use of 'multiple transportable carbohydrates' from mixed sources are recommended as part of the fuelling strategy. Likewise, to minimise risk of dehydration, a 'drink to thirst' approach is recommended throughout endurance events with a view of targeting 450–750 mL·hour^{-1}.

Of the plethora of nutritional ergogenic strategies that could be employed for endurance events, it is important that runners recognise that such 'aids' must not replace a personalised *food-first* approach. Only a few approaches likely offer a small-modest performance benefit and should be trialled during training to assess individual effects. Of these, caffeine (2–6 mg·kg body mass^{-1}, taken ~1 hour pre-event, or during the latter stages of an event) and dietary nitrates (e.g. beetroot juice, 8.4 mmol for 6–15 days pre event) may support sustained endurance. In addition, sodium bicarbonate (0.2–0.4 g·kg body mass^{-1} taken 60–150 min in split doses pre-event) and beta-alanine (~65 mg·kg body mass^{-1} over a period of 10–12 weeks pre-event) may support high-intensity (middle-distance) events.

12

STRATEGIC AND TACTICAL DECISION-MAKING IN MIDDLE- AND LONG-DISTANCE RUNNING RACES

Andy Renfree and Brian Hanley

Highlights

- Regulation of pace is a decision-making process that is influenced by knowledge of how far an athlete has left to run combined with an awareness of the internal physiological environment that governs the athlete's state of fatigue.
- The most frequently used pacing strategy to achieve a fast time in the 800 m event involves a positive split approach, characterised by a fast initial 200 m followed by a progressive deceleration over the remainder of the race.
- In track middle-distance events (800 m and 1500 m), remaining close to the leader and avoiding running wide on bends is important for gaining qualification for subsequent rounds or winning a medal.
- In events longer than 800 m, an even pace throughout is recommended to achieve the fastest possible time and finish in a high position.
- Marathon runners are advised to start conservatively (based on their present fitness and target time) to avoid slowing in the second half of the race.
- Running behind a pacemaker or in a pack of runners provides a large advantage by reducing the energetic cost of running and the cognitive burden associated with pace-related decision-making.

Introduction

Middle- and long-distance runners spend many hours preparing for competitive events in an attempt to improve their race outcomes, whether they are faster finishing times or higher finishing positions in races. However, although this training might improve performance potential, there is no guarantee that it will result in enhanced performance itself. To realise performance potential, it is imperative that athletes deploy their physiological resources appropriately over the duration of a race. If they are unable to do this, then they risk premature fatigue and underperformance. The way effort is distributed over the course of a bout of exercise is termed 'pacing'. This chapter reviews the theory that explains how pacing is achieved, describes observations of pacing behaviour that have been published, and ends with some practical recommendations for coaches and runners aiming to improve their pacing ability.

Regulation of Pace

Although various models have been proposed to explain the regulation of pace during exercise, a common theme is that the process requires central regulation by the brain and nervous system (Renfree et al., 2014b). A key component of this regulatory process also appears to be knowledge of the endpoint of exercise (Ulmer, 1996). Indeed, this is intuitively obvious; if you were challenged to a race, the first question you would ask would almost certainly be 'How far?' Knowledge of how much of the race remains is combined with knowledge regarding the condition of the internal physiological environment, gained via feedback from various receptors throughout the body, to decide how quickly to run at any given time (St Clair Gibson et al., 2006). In effect, pace regulation is a decision-making process. Before even starting exercise, the athlete is required to identify an overall strategic approach that will be taken, whereas during exercise the athlete might be required to continually adjust exercise intensity. The athlete must decide whether the current pace is sustainable until the end of exercise without risking catastrophic physiological failure, or whether they are able to run faster. If the change in pace is considered necessary, they must also decide how large this change must be, and they are able to select from all possible paces between zero (i.e., they stop running) and the maximum speed they are able to generate at that point.

There is some controversy as to exactly how the athlete regulates pace during exercise and to what extent this is an unconscious or conscious process. However, regardless of the precise mechanisms, observations of athletes' strategies are remarkably consistent. In situations where the goal is to complete a given distance in the fastest possible time, an even-paced, or negative pace strategy (where the second half of the event is completed more quickly than the first) is generally associated with superior performances (Abbiss and Laursen, 2008). In an analysis of 32 previous world records over the mile run, Noakes et al. (2009) found that the first and last laps were significantly quicker than the second and third laps, which were generally completed at similar speeds. Likewise, in a similar analysis of world record runs over 5000 m and 10,000 m, a consistent pattern was identified whereby the first and final kilometres were run at higher speeds than the middle sections of the races. Furthermore, in a historical analysis of world records over the marathon, it was found that the overall trend was for the performances to become more evenly paced as they became faster in recent years (Díaz et al., 2018). It is noteworthy that in the recent successful sub-two-hour performance by Eliud Kipchoge in Vienna, it was decided to adopt an even-paced strategy with the speed being controlled by a pace car. Indeed, it could even be argued that the use of the car in this way made Kipchoge's task somewhat easier because it reduced the need for self-regulation through decision-making, thereby reducing the cognitive load on the athlete.

The remainder of this chapter aims to discuss methods that both elite and recreational runners can use to improve the quality of their strategic and tactical decision-making relating to pacing, and the ability to maintain these strategies during competition itself. We differentiate between events where the goals are either 'best possible time' or 'highest possible finishing position' and address these aims in three broad sections: middle-distance (800 m–1500 m) events, long-distance (5000 m–10,000 m) events, and road and cross-country races.

Middle-Distance Events

Although the middle-distance running events include the 800 m, 1500 m and 1 mile distances, the optimal pacing strategy for achieving the fastest possible time appear to differ between events. Analysis of pacing displayed by elite male and female 800 m runners during their season's best performances indicates that, in contrast to longer events, these are achieved with a 'positive' strategy characterised by a first-half of the race that is faster than the second (Filipas et al., 2018a). However, differences have been found between men and women. In both sexes, the first 200 m was the fastest of the race, but whereas men demonstrated a further slowing with each subsequent 200 m split, women displayed an almost constant pace for the remainder of the race. Similar findings were reported in an analysis of 26 world record performances over 800 m (Tucker et al., 2006) whereby the average speed in the second lap was significantly lower than in the first in only two individual performances. This finding supports the suggestion that performance in faster events is optimised through a strategy characterised by a fast start, and that the ability to increase speed in the second lap is limited. The precise reasons for this are unclear, although one possible explanation is related to the faster start accelerating oxygen uptake kinetics at the onset of exercise, thereby increasing the aerobic contribution to energy expenditure and sparing anaerobic capacity (Jones et al., 2008).

With regards to the 1500 m and mile events, a study of 32 previous male world records over the mile was described earlier in the chapter (Noakes et al., 2009). In these 32 performances, on only two occasions was the final lap of the race the slowest, an observation that was proposed to provide evidence that pacing strategies are regulated in anticipation of exercise duration, rather than simply reflecting the onset of peripheral muscular fatigue. Regardless of these observations regarding the optimal pacing strategies associated with achieving the fastest possible time, it is evident that athletes do not always prioritise running as quickly as possible as highly as they do achieving the highest possible finishing position, especially in major international championship events. The range of winning times in recent men's 1500 m races at global championships, from 3:27.6 by Hicham El Guerrouj in the 1999 IAAF World Championships to 3:50.0 by Matt Centrowitz in the 2016 Olympic Games, illustrates the range of ways in which races can unfold. To best understand how athletes can adopt strategies that maximise their chances of achieving a high overall finishing position in events where time achieved is of secondary importance, it is necessary to study the relationship between tactical behaviours throughout the race and eventual race outcome.

An analysis of the men's 800 m event at the 2000 Sydney Olympics provides a striking example of the importance of tactical decision-making, especially in races where all competitors are likely to be closely matched in terms of ability. The gold medal was won by Nils Schumann of Germany in a time of 1:45.08, ahead of world record holder Wilson Kipketer of Denmark who gained the silver medal in a time of 1:45.14. However, video analysis of the race revealed that Schumann ran closer to the inside lane throughout most of the race and covered a total distance of 802 m compares to 813 m by Kipketer (Jones and Whipp, 2002). Through calculation of the average speeds maintained over distances covered, it becomes evident that Schumann ran 800 m in 1:44.82 compared with Kipketer's 1:43.46.

The example just described may seem obvious in that, clearly, athletes who run further than necessary put themselves at a significant disadvantage. However, in reality, the situation is likely to be more complex. By simply attempting to run the shortest distance possible, athletes risk putting themselves in a 'box' whereby they may be prevented from following changes of pace initiated by other runners. Furthermore, falling behind other competitors means an athlete needs to run faster over the remainder of the race just to draw level with them. This may be possible if the leading athletes are slowing, but in many championship races (especially 1500 m), the last lap is the fastest of the race, meaning athletes who are in trailing positions need to run faster than competitors who are themselves already running very fast. With these issues in mind, several studies have analysed the relationship between intermediate positioning and race outcome in middle-distance running events at international championships (Casado and Renfree, 2018; Mytton et al., 2015; Renfree et al., 2014a).

An analysis of the heats and semi-finals of the 800 m and 1500 m events at the 2012 Olympic Games calculated the probability of automatic qualification to the next round of competition for athletes in each available position at various intermediate stages of races (Renfree et al., 2014a). Unsurprisingly, athletes with superior seasonal best performances over the distance were more likely to qualify than slower athletes. However, in the 800 m races, there was a striking relationship between intermediate position and likelihood of qualification. By the midway point of the race, athletes already in one of the leading three positions had a 61% probability of qualification. By the 600 m point, this had increased to 84%. In the 1500 m there were more changes in position as races progressed. However, athletes outside one of the automatic qualifying positions by the 1000 m point had less than 50% chance of qualification to the next round. Similar results were found in a subsequent analysis of the middle-distance events at the 2017 IAAF World Championships (Casado and Renfree, 2018). This study also rank-ordered the athletes in terms of absolute speeds over each intermediate race section and found that an even bigger predictor of eventual race outcome was the ability to produce a fast final lap. Therefore, even though intermediate positioning is extremely important throughout races, there could be some opportunity to 'salvage' a bad situation if the athlete develops the ability to finish quickly. This observation is in agreement with earlier work by Mytton et al. (2015), which found medallists in middle-distance swimming and running events at major championships displayed greater variation in pace compared with non-medallists, and that this variation was the result of a greater acceleration in the final stages.

Improving Strategic and Tactical Decision-Making in Middle-Distance Events

Based on the research described so far, it is possible to make some practical recommendations to athletes that may maximise their chances of achieving their physiological potential in middle-distance races. The most obvious strategy is to train appropriately to maximise physiological capacities. Doing so will increase the range of behavioural options available to an athlete at any point in a race due to maintenance of a greater physiological reserve capacity. It is not as though an athlete can simply consciously 'decide' to run faster than they are able to keep up with an opponent! Additionally, athletes need to ensure they make appropriate strategic and tactical decisions.

Strategic decision-making sets the overall approach to the race and is performed in advance of the starting gun being fired. If the goal is simply to achieve the fastest time possible, then analysis of elite performers suggests running the first 200 m of an 800 m race slightly faster than the goal time followed by an even pace or slight deceleration for the remainder is the optimal strategy. In 1500 m races, faster times are associated with a more even pace, or even an acceleration in the final lap. Although seemingly relatively simple to implement, these strategies require accurate assessment of current abilities to set appropriate performance goals. Inappropriately ambitious goals will almost certainly result in premature fatigue and underperformance.

One further issue which has not been discussed thus far relates to the use of other athletes who act as 'pacemakers' by setting the pace in the initial stages of races and are a common sight on the Grand Prix circuit. It is thought that pacemakers serve to benefit athletes by reducing the air resistance encountered, and thereby the energetic cost of running at a given speed. Pugh (1971) demonstrated that overcoming air resistance accounted for 7.5% of energy expenditure when running at 'middle-distance' speed, but that running one metre behind another athlete reduced this by 6.5%. Theoretically, following another athlete during the early and middle stages of a race may conserve physiological reserve capacity until further into the race.

An additional potential benefit of following a pacemaker is that it may reduce the level of cognitive fatigue induced through the requirement for continual pace-related decision-making (Renfree et al., 2015). Rather than need to interpret various environmental and perceptual cues in order to assess and adjust running speed throughout a race, it is likely to be less cognitively demanding to simply do what everyone else does. This so-called 'herd behaviour' (Banerjee, 1992) has been observed in a wide range of human environments and may be a 'hardwired' characteristic that confers some form of advantage. However, it must be emphasised that the consequences can also be negative if an athlete attempts to follow others with superior physiological abilities, and the result is likely to be underperformance.

5000 m and 10,000 m Events

The 5000 and 10,000 m races are the longest track races at major championships, although competitions over these distances are also held on roads. To the casual observer, races over these longer track distances are run with a fairly constant pace, with athletes who cannot keep up gradually fading, and the winner usually being the athlete who possesses best sprint finish. It is certainly true that the endspurt can be crucial in deciding the medal places; for example, Dieter Baumann overtook three rivals to win the men's Olympic 5000 m final in 1992 with a last 100 m in 11.39 s (8.78 m.s^{-1}) (Reiss et al., 1993). However, to get into a position where winning is a possibility, the pacing tactics used beforehand can make a difference in structuring the race to provide an athlete with an advantage over their rivals (Martin and Coe, 1997).

With regard to recent major championship racing, Hettinga et al. (2019) found that 5000 m finalists in major championships ran with negative splits (including medallists and those finishing at the back of the field), although variations in pace were quite considerable (coefficients of variation of 8.5% and 6.9% in men and women, respectively). Thus, pacing profiles in 5000 m racing show an overall even pace for the first 4000 m (Filipas et al., 2018b) but with microvariations in running speed injected into the race that are often adopted by the leading athletes to try to shake off rivals (Thompson, 2007). Using data from the 2008 Olympic Games, Thiel et al. (2012) found that both men and women in the 5000 m finals had variable pacing profiles (running speed dropped very quickly from 7 m.s^{-1} at 100 m to 5 m.s^{-1} at 400 m in the men's race), and thus the authors recommended variable pace training for athletes who aim to perform well in championship races. Aragón et al. (2016) found that these changes in 5000 m race pace mainly took place on the bends, in contrast to the 1500 m where they occurred on the straights, even though this tactic in the 5000 m would seem to be counterproductive given the extra distance that must be run away from the inside kerb.

Although physiologically similar (Duffield and Dawson, 2003), performances over 10,000 m are of course run at a slightly slower pace compared with the 5000 m, but also have fewer variations in pace (Filipas et al., 2018b). For example, Thiel et al. (2012) showed that 10,000 m finalists at the 2008 Olympics had relatively variable pacing profiles (mean pace per lap varied by 3.6% for men and 3.4% for women) and, like in the 5000 m, this was more variable than contemporary world record performances. Hettinga et al. (2019) found that the winners' paces increased noticeably over the last 1000 m (to a maximum of approximately 7.5 m.s^{-1} in the men's race, and 6.25 m.s^{-1} in the women's), having been relatively even paced over the first 9000 m. For example, when Kenenisa Bekele won the 2007 IAAF World Championship 10,000 m, it was the increase in speed during the final 400 m that separated him from the silver and bronze medallists (the gap between 1st and 3rd was only 0.42 s at the bell, but 5.52 s at the finish); he completed the last lap in 55.51 s, equivalent to a mean speed of 7.21 m.s^{-1} (Enomoto et al., 2008). Thus, although even pacing is often considered the best approach for maximising endurance performance, the small physiological differences between world-class athletes mean that strategic pacing is crucial when competing in championship races.

In both the 5000 m and 10,000 m, world record performances are more evenly paced than in championship racing. For example, Thiel et al. (2012) showed that 5000 m world record pacing profiles had very small variations in pace for both men (1.7%) and women (2.5%) and require a different training approach from that needed for the more tactical racing used in major championship finals. Although championship athletes might vary pace because of tactical reasons, it is of course more usual for those outside the world's best to have varied pacing profiles because of how much they slow in the later stages of fast-run races (Filipas et al., 2018b). The tactic of running an even pace throughout a long-distance race is thus recommended for competitive club runners who, like world record holders, aim to achieve their fastest possible time, and in most road races is also the most effective tactic for finishing in a high position.

Marathon and Half-Marathon Events

The marathon differs from shorter-distance races because the unique physiological challenges posed by the duration of the event mean that maintaining speed is a considerable challenge. These changes arise because of glycogen depletion and a subsequent reliance on lipids as a key energy source (O'Brien et al., 1993). In addition, hyperthermia can occur in warm weather (as is frequently the case during Olympic and World Championship marathons) often resulting in a reduction in pace, or drop-out (March et al., 2011). By contrast, cooler weather conditions (5–10°C), which are more common in big city marathons in spring and autumn, are associated with smaller reductions in running speed, particularly in faster runners (Ely et al., 2008). Because of these factors, pacing the marathon well, usually by achieving an even pace or a negative split, is associated with better performances to a greater extent than shorter-distance events (Hettinga et al., 2019). However, even world record performances could have been improved with a greater appreciation of the effects of weather and gradient (Angus, 2014). World records in the marathon are generally obtained on relatively flat courses with favourable weather conditions (Díaz et al., 2019), but the effect of pacemakers must also be taken into account. As noted previously, although using pacemakers is often considered advantageous because they potentially provide a drafting benefit, their value might lie more in the way in which they reduce the psychological load on the lead runners who otherwise would have to focus intently on the pace throughout the race. As a result, recent marathon world records (those since 1988) have been run at very even speeds dictated by pacemakers, and many include a last 5 km that was the fastest part of the race; by contrast, older world records (those set between 1967 and 1988) were achieved through a very fast start but with large drops in speed in the latter part of the race (Díaz et al., 2018). Of course, running an even pace is achievable for physically fit and well-prepared club runners, particularly in big city marathons where the volume of runners can provide unintentional pacemaking opportunities.

Although even pacing is usually the most appropriate approach to take, the reality in World and Olympic marathons is that 95% of men and 87% of women have been found to run slower in the second half of the race (Hanley, 2016); women are generally better at achieving even pacing than men, a finding that has been observed across running abilities (Deaner et al., 2015). However, Santos-Lozano et al. (2014) reported that athlete ability was a better predictor of significant slowing in the second half of the marathon than any sex-based difference. Indeed, World and Olympic marathon medallists of both sexes are more likely to maintain their pace from 10 km onwards (men ~5.4 m.s^{-1}; women ~4.8 m.s^{-1}) and achieve negative splits. Renfree and St Clair Gibson (2013) analysed the pacing profiles of women marathon runners competing in the 2009 World Championships and found that those who started faster than personal best pace had greater decreases in speed than those who started slower than their previous best pace. Marathon runners are therefore advised to start conservatively (based on present fitness and realistic goals) to avoid considerable slowing in the later stages of the race, and coaches who know their athletes are likely to take risks in terms of starting too fast are encouraged to develop a conservative approach to pacing in training (Deaner et al., 2019).

In contrast with the marathon, very little research has been conducted on the half-marathon, despite its considerable popularity with recreational runners. This might be because it is not a standard championship distance, although it is held as a biennial World Championship event. An analysis of six of these World Championship half-marathons showed that athletes generally started quickly over the first 5 km with a gradual slowing until 20 km, after which they increased speed substantially until the finish (Hanley, 2015). What was more interesting from this analysis of pacing was the way in which the athletes formed packs – these varied between those who ran the whole race together, which included teammates and sets of twins, to those who moved between groups ('nomadic pacing'), and those who ran the entire race alone. The results showed that those who ran together for the whole race had the most even paces, with nomadic pacing also working well in this regard. However, those who ran the race alone or quickly dropped off a group were more likely to suffer decreases in running speed between the opening 5 km and the rest of the race. Another interesting aspect of racing that arose from this analysis was the way in which packs of runners tended to slow to the exact same extent between 15 and 20 km, and showed that slowing down is not necessarily an outcome arising from fatigue but can also be a tactic employed to use other athletes as external references for pacing (Renfree et al., 2014b). The fast final 1.1 km confirmed clearly that these athletes were not slowing because of extreme fatigue but because they believed it placed them into a strong position to beat their nearest rivals (Hanley, 2015). An analysis of packing in major championship marathon running showed that whereas the tactic of running in a pack with athletes of similar ability and ambition throughout was beneficial for runners of both sexes (Hanley, 2016), nomadic pacing was less successful compared to world-class half-marathon racing. This is likely due to the greater fatigue that occurs in the second half of the marathon.

Cross-Country Running and 3000 m Steeplechase

Cross-country running has unique pacing characteristics because variations in terrain can affect the running style used, not only making it different from track and road running but often from one course to another, or even within the same course (Canova, 1998). Achieving anything close to a constant speed is difficult in cross-country because the World Athletics rules state that natural obstacles such as hills or logs should be incorporated to create a challenging course. Furthermore, steady pacing is a challenge even for accomplished runners given that no accurate distance markers are used. Laps can also alter in length (often including 'small' and 'large' laps) and time elapsed is not an indication of being close to the finish; for example, the winning time in the men's 12 km race in 2004 was 35:52, compared with 32:45 in 2013 (Hanley, 2014). The lack of a reliable source of pacing information means that the most popular tactic in the senior men's World Cross Country Championships from 2002 to 2013 (over 12 km) was for all athletes to start quickly and try to keep up for as long as possible with the leaders. This approach is perhaps understandable given the slightly unstructured nature of the event and the team competition that makes every finishing position important. However, this pacing approach inevitably means that the high number of athletes who start too quickly end up dropping behind the lead pack after only a few laps and continue to slow throughout the race (Esteve-Lanao et al., 2014).

The current equalised men's and women's race distances of 10 km at the World Cross Country Championships were adopted for the first time in Kampala in 2017, and pacing analyses of those championships showed that men ran with a more even pace than over the previously contested 12 km distance (Hanley, 2018). Instead, they had either an even pace or an increase in speed during the last 2 km, although it should be noted that their pace had still slowed from the initial lap, regardless of finishing position. Hanley (2018) was also the first to analyse women's pacing at World Cross Country Championships, and the increase in race distance led to pacing profiles that were very similar to men. Runners of both sexes should therefore remember that the distance of cross-country races and the terrain involved mean that fast starts are not always necessary, and that the same self-discipline of pacing required in track or road running also applies to off-road racing.

Although it is held on the track, the 3000 m steeplechase resembles cross-country running in that maintaining a constant running speed is hindered by the negotiation of 28 barriers and seven water jumps. Unsurprisingly, the quickest section found in Olympic steeplechase finals was the first half-lap that features no barriers, although better athletes were also quicker over the last lap than any of the preceding ones, leading to an overall U-shaped pacing profile (Hanley and Williams, 2020). In terms of differences within laps, the water jump section tends to be more disruptive of pace in women's racing, which is also characterised by a relatively quicker opening than the men's races (Hanley and Williams, 2020). This might be related to the fact that even world-class women steeplechasers have greater difficulty in negotiating the water jump because they land nearer the barrier on exit, and therefore into deeper water (Hanley et al., 2020).

Summary and Practical Recommendations

This chapter has addressed the mechanisms underpinning the regulation of pacing strategy, as well as some of the commonly observed behaviours during athletic races. Although we have examined a wide range of differing events, there are some obvious similarities. The most obvious is that, in all events longer than 800 m, when the goal is to run as fast a time as possible, an even-paced strategy is most likely to result in realisation of physiological potential. In the 800 m, fast times are typically associated with a positive pacing strategy characterised by a quick initial 200 m followed by a progressive deceleration over the remainder of the race. Therefore, for most events, the recommended strategy may be to determine the goal time and required intermediate splits, and to stay as close as possible to this schedule throughout the race. Although this may seem simple, such a strategy is only likely to be effective if appropriate performance goals are used to inform strategic planning of races. When attempting to run quickly, it is also likely to be beneficial to use pacemakers, if possible. These can have the effect of reducing the energetic cost of running because of the reduction in air resistance encountered and can also reduce the cognitive demands of racing by decreasing the need for pace related decision-making. Even if there are no designated pacemakers for a runner's desired speed, it is still likely to be beneficial to run in packs with other competitors of similar ability.

Athletes ambitious enough to realistically challenge for medals at major championships need to develop an additional skillset, as the ability to run fast times alone is insufficient. Rather, athletes must develop the ability to run at a variable pace and accelerate over the final stages. Given the small time gaps covering athletes at the end of championship races, tactical positioning throughout is of paramount importance. Particularly in the middle-distance events, it is important to be close to the leading positions as the race enters its final stages, and to minimise distance covered by avoiding running wide on the bends. However, there is a risk associated with this approach in that maintaining a position close to the inside line could leave an athlete 'boxed in' if they get trapped behind slower athletes during a break made by other competitors. In this sense, tactical training is an important aspect of distance running to complement the physical preparation required to do well in competition.

13

GAIT RETRAINING FOR PERFORMANCE AND INJURY RISK

Izzy S. Moore, Tom Goom and Kelly J. Ashford

Highlights

- There is no such thing as the 'correct way to run' or 'perfect running form'; a universal style of running does not appear to exist, particularly regarding economical running.
- Gait retraining may need to be undertaken only by some runners, and prescription should be based upon an individual assessment that includes other clinical considerations.
- Male and female runners should be considered separately due to important discrepancies in running biomechanics between the sexes, and the potential influence of breast motion on running economy in females.
- Gait retraining has been used successfully to lower the risk of developing certain injuries and to reduce the pain associated with specific overuse injuries; however, modification of running style redistributes loads, which may increase injury risk in other parts of the body.
- Internal focus of attention verbal cues seems more effective at producing desired technique changes, potentially by invoking constructive conscious control of one's gait to mediate improvements of a habitual movement pattern.
- The overall injury rate is similar between barefoot runners and those who wear trainers; however, small amounts of barefoot running may be useful as a gait retraining, conditioning and rehabilitation approach in some runners.

Introduction

The biomechanics of running has been well researched, with early work dating back to the 1930s. Running, like other movements, is a skill. Yet, our innate ability to run without instruction from an early age means many individuals never receive training specifically relating to this skill. Fundamentally, this means that how most individuals run is a consequence of the body self-organising. Many constraints are placed upon the body as it self-organises, including anthropometrics (height, leg length), injury history, experience and exposure, and although rather a simplistic view, metabolic cost has often been cited as the primary driver of gait selection. Other factors that appear to contribute to movement selection include minimising muscle excitation, effort requirements and reducing the 'jerkiness' of motion (Hreljac, 2000). Theoretically, pain may also contribute to gait selection due to avoidance behaviours. The gait an individual uses is therefore a complex interplay of contributing constraints and drivers.

Two juxtaposing views can be presented by practitioners and researchers that either running gait should be left untouched, or that it must be changed to prevent injury and improve performance. To this end, this chapter will discuss how and when to modify gait and seek answers to the following questions: Is there an economically optimal running technique? Can and should we modify uninjured gait patterns to prevent injury? How can gait retraining be used during lower limb injury rehabilitation? And, is there a role for footwear and barefoot running in modifying gait?

Gait Retraining and Performance

The pursuit of the 'perfect running form' is likely to be a fruitless task, particularly when often sex-aggregated data are used to assess associations between running economy and gait. Females produce greater relative stride lengths (stride length divided by leg length), use higher stride frequencies at the same velocity, opt to use a lower duty factor by spending less time in contact with the ground (Nelson et al., 1977) and have greater pelvic anterior tilt than their male counterparts (Schache et al., 2003). They are, therefore, not using a gait that is a scaled-down version of what males use due to typically being shorter and weighing less.

Adopting a one-size-fits-all approach to running gait has led to different forms of running being advocated and specific values being recommended for certain gait characteristics. For example, there appears to be a gravitation towards wanting runners to produce a cadence of 180 steps per minute, but there is currently no evidence to support this approach. Whilst there is no basis for this, several modifiable intrinsic and extrinsic running biomechanical factors and their effect on running economy have been identified (see Table 13.1), with the propulsive phase being highlighted as having the strongest direct relationships with running economy (Moore, 2016). It is important to note that unless otherwise stated in this section, the term 'runners' is used to represent 'male' runners due to paucity of female-specific studies.

Economical Spatiotemporal Characteristics

From an economical perspective, large changes in stride length and frequency are to be avoided in trained runners. Numerous studies have shown that increasing or decreasing stride lengths and frequencies by >6% increases the volume of oxygen consumed, meaning economy is worsened. In fact, trained runners exhibit incredibly economical stride lengths and frequencies, which tend to be within 3% of their optimal stride length/frequency (Cavanagh and Williams, 1982; de Ruiter et al., 2013). The mathematically optimal stride length/frequency is quantified as the stride length/frequency that would produce the lowest metabolic cost of running. In addition, small changes (<3%) to stride length do not appear to affect running economy (Moore, 2016; Craighead et al., 2014). Therefore, stride length appears to be able to operate within an optimum window, which is 97–100% of the self-selected stride length (Moore, 2016).

In untrained runners, there is likely to be greater opportunity to modify stride length/frequency to reap economical benefits. De Ruiter and colleagues (2013) reported untrained

TABLE 13.1 Modifiable intrinsic and extrinsic running biomechanics and their effect on running economy (RE)

Evidenced effect on RE	Intrinsic			Extrinsic
	Spatiotemporal	Kinetics	Kinematics	
Beneficial	Self-selected stride length (minus 3%)	Greater leg stiffness	Less leg extension at toe-off	Firm, compliant shoe–surface interaction
	Lower vertical oscillation	Alignment of GRF and leg axis during propulsion	Large stride angle	Barefoot or lightweight shoes (<440g)
		Low lower limb moment of inertia	Maintain arm swing	
Conflicting	Ground contact time	Impact force	Foot strike pattern	Orthotics
	Swing time	Anterior-posterior forces	Trunk lean	
Limited or unknown	Horizontal distance between the foot and CoM at initial contact	Impulses	Swing phase	
	Braking/ deceleration time			
	Speed lost during ground contact		Breast kinematics	

Note: GRF = ground reaction force. CoM = centre of mass.

Source: Adapted from Moore (2016).

runners to be 8% away from their optimal stride frequency, suggesting such runners may benefit from a gait retraining intervention to increase their stride frequency towards one that minimises metabolic cost. It is interesting to note that in both untrained and trained runners, the preference is to overstride, i.e. produce strides that are longer than optimal, and therefore produce stride frequencies that are lower than optimal. Anthropometrics such as leg length and height may place constraints on which combination of stride length and frequency can be achieved by an individual; however they are not the primary determinants (Cavanagh and Kram, 1989). It is likely to be a complex interaction between the physiological constraints, energy demand and metabolic cost that lead to an individual self-selecting a given stride length.

Ground contact time is the metabolically expensive phase of the gait cycle (Arellano and Kram, 2014), meaning swing time is the less metabolically expensive phase. Intuitively, this could be interpreted to mean shorter ground contact times and longer swing times are desirable. Associations between the time spent on the ground and running economy have, however, been conflicting (Moore, 2016). Reasons for such conflicting evidence could be the underlying muscle-tendon properties of each runner. Short ground contact times require high magnitudes of force to be produced rapidly. Therefore, this strategy may be suited to individuals with a higher proportion of fast twitch fibres and favour the use of elastic energy storage and return (Lussiana et al., 2019). Conversely, long ground contact times mean force is produced slowly, suggesting a greater reliance on slow twitch muscle fibres, but enables greater forward translation of the centre of mass (Lussiana et al., 2019). Ground contact time has since been shown to be an optimised gait characteristic in male and female runners (although only one female was part of the cohort) (Moore et al., 2019a). This means, like stride length and frequency, male and female runners choose ground contact times that minimise the metabolic cost of running (enhance running economy).

Interestingly, 60% of the male and female runners in a study by Moore and colleagues (2019a) had ground contact times that were slightly shorter than their predicted optimal ground contact time, whilst 40% had slighter longer than optimal times (Figure 13.1). The collective understanding about ground contact time highlights two different strategies: (1) short ground contact times leading to low duty factors; and (2) long ground contact times leading to high duty factors. Duty factor is the proportion of the gait cycle one foot spends in contact with the ground. Trained runners, through a combination of self-optimisation and training, are likely to possess the strategy that works best for their musculoskeletal system but may need slight modifications to fine-tune their gait. An individual assessment of economical running would help inform training requirements for both trained and untrained runners to identify if small or large refinements to technique are warranted.

The amount a runner's centre of mass rises and falls during each gait cycle in the vertical direction is known as vertical oscillation. Increasing vertical oscillation leads to a worsening of running economy (Tseh et al., 2008), possibly because the work performed against gravity is increased (Moore, 2016). However, no study has tried to minimise vertical oscillation and measure the effect on running economy. Minimising vertical oscillation will, however, have repercussions for other gait characteristics given the interaction with spatiotemporal characteristics. In particular, it will reduce stride length (Adams et al., 2018), increase stride frequency (Adams et al., 2018) and lengthen ground contact time (Adams et al., 2018). Further, if stride length, stride frequency and ground contact time have been shown to be optimised gait characteristics in runners, vertical oscillation could also be considered optimised. In support of this, Lussiana and colleagues (2019) identified different magnitudes of vertical oscillation depending upon the duty factor of a runner. Runners with a low duty factor had shorter ground contact times relative to stride time, larger vertical oscillations and lower horizontal centre of mass displacements than runners with a high duty factor. Yet, there was no difference in running economy between high and low duty factor runners. Interestingly, there was an equal proportion of females (40%) in the low and high duty factor groups, showing that both types of strategies can be adopted by females and males. Practitioners should be aware of the potential change in vertical oscillation that accompanies changes in other spatiotemporal characteristics but may not need to target it specifically as an uneconomical gait characteristic.

Economical Kinetics

Early work demonstrated that the vertical force required to support an individual's body mass under gravity, known as body weight, is one of the primary determinants of running economy, along with the time spent applying force (ground contact time) (Kram and Taylor, 1990). However, whilst running at a constant velocity, the average vertical force applied to each stride will always be equal to the body weight of a runner and, thus, cannot be modified during a run to the same extent that ground contact time can be (see the 'Economical spatiotemporal characteristics' section).

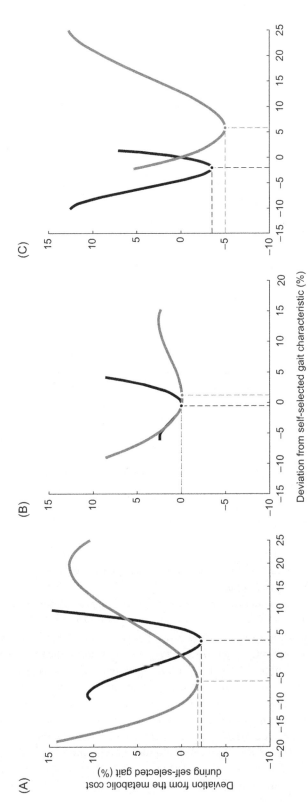

FIGURE 13.1 Relationship between the deviations from self-selected running gait characteristics (%) and from the metabolic cost during self-selected gait (%). (A) Example of self-selected ground contact time longer than optimal. (B) Example of self-selected ground contact time within 1% of optimal. (C) Example of self-selected ground contact time shorter than optimal. Solid grey lines represent leg stiffness. Solid black lines represent ground contact time. Optimal gait characteristics that minimise metabolic cost are identified by circles (black (●) = ground contact time; grey (●) = leg stiffness). Dashed lines highlight the corresponding X and Y values for optimal gait characteristics

Source: Adapted from Moore et al. (2019b).

Running at a constant velocity requires alternating periods of deceleration and acceleration. Reducing the amount of velocity lost during the braking (deceleration) phase of stance would reduce the amount of propulsion (acceleration) required to generate momentum. This would beneficially impact economy, as the propulsive impulse along with the vertical force to support a runner's body weight incur the greatest metabolic cost (Arellano and Kram, 2014).

Understanding the interaction between braking and propulsion has been relatively unexplored in runners, but the seminal work by Chang and Kram (1999), which applied external horizontal forces to the body, identified that braking incurs a lower metabolic cost than propulsion in males and females. Yet, to achieve a constant velocity, braking and propulsive impulses must be equal. It therefore follows that reducing the change in centre of mass velocity during braking would be a beneficial economical strategy to adopt. This strategy appears to be the case only when sex-aggregated data are used (Folland et al., 2017). When females are considered separately, greater velocity changes are associated with better running economy (Williams et al., 1987). Further, through two studies on female beginner runners, Moore and colleagues (2012b, 2016) observed reduced knee extensor moments during braking, greater alignment of their legs with the ground reaction force (GRF) during propulsion, greater propulsive forces and stiffer calf musculo-tendon units as the runners became more economical. However, only the change in GRF alignment was associated with the change in economy, meaning females appear to be able to reduce muscular force requirements during braking and enable a more economical push-off to be produced, potentially through a more efficient stretch-shortening cycle in the calf musculo-tendon unit. The direct relationships observed between propulsive kinetics and economy may in fact be mediated by braking kinetics. It is not known why female and male runners appear to exhibit different braking and propulsion strategies. Studies need to be designed to capture the potential female-specific factors that contribute to this (e.g. breast biomechanics) rather than the continued focus on only the lower limb to understand economical running gait.

Arguably, leg stiffness receives a lot of attention in relation to economical movement. As a quantity derived from a theoretical model of running gait (the spring-mass model), the application is perhaps muddied by a lack of awareness around the assumptions of the model and eagerness to consider this quantity as an actual, tangible gait characteristic. Nevertheless, the storage and reutilisation of elastic energy is seen as a fundamental component of running gait. Therefore, being able to store and/or reutilise more elastic energy by having a stiffer musculoskeletal system intuitively should minimise the volume of oxygen required to produce the level of energy needed to run a given distance.

It was previously thought that greater leg stiffness would lead to superior running economy (Moore, 2016), but this has been shown only in correlational studies (Dalleau et al., 1998) or inferred from knee and ankle flexion angles during stance (Folland et al., 2017; Moore et al., 2014b). Notably, adopting a compliant, crouched running gait ('Groucho running') with exaggerated knee flexion worsens running economy. Yet, like spatiotemporal gait characteristics (e.g. stride frequency, stride length and ground contact time), leg stiffness appears to be a relatively optimised gait characteristic in males and females (Moore et al., 2019a). Furthermore, trained runners appear to have a homogenous leg stiffness modulation strategy involving force production, which is not evident in untrained runners (Bitchell et al., 2019). Both male and female runners predominately favour stiffer limbs than is optimal for running economy, which allows them to produce short ground contact times (Moore et al., 2019a). If this strategy is combined with longer strides than optimal as reported by Cavanagh and Williams (1982), it potentially exposes runners to large braking forces and vertical loading rates. As a result, we recommend individually assessing runners. It is possible that optimising stride length, frequency, ground contact time and leg stiffness using an individual running assessment to improve running economy may also be beneficial for injury risk, if braking forces and impact loading rates are reduced (Hreljac et al., 2000; Napier et al., 2018).

Economical Kinematics

A large number of lower limb kinematics have been associated with running economy in males and females (Moore, 2016), with the act of swinging the leg contributing to 7% of the metabolic cost of running (Arellano and Kram, 2014). Many of the lower limb kinematics have been identified only within one study and often conflicting relationships are presented for the same kinematic variable. For example, high magnitudes of peak knee flexion during stance may be good for economy but could also be bad for economy (Williams and Cavanagh, 1987; Folland et al., 2017). Greater peak knee flexion may indicate faster knee flexion velocities, which are associated with smaller changes in centre of mass velocity during braking and propulsion (Williams et al., 1987), whilst lower peak knee flexion may indicate a stiffer lower limb during stance (see the 'Economical kinetics' section for further detail). Nevertheless, one consistent finding, reported for both male and female runners, is that a better running economy is associated with less leg extension at toe-off (Moore et al., 2012b; Williams and Cavanagh, 1987; Moore et al., 2014b; Cavanagh et al., 1977). This can be achieved through less knee extension, less ankle plantarflexion or a combination of both. It is hypothesised that having a degree of flexion at this point of the gait cycle may allow the muscles to operate at favourable lengths to produce force or that this places the leg in a favourable position going into swing, reducing the degree of movement required and reducing the moment of inertia of the leg.

When considering the initial ground contact from an economical perspective, an individual's habitual foot strike does not appear to be detrimental to their running economy at any speed, so targeting this gait characteristic for endurance runners to aid performance improvements is therefore not supported by evidence. Indeed, for male and female rearfoot strikers, imposing a forefoot strike on them appears to worsen running economy at slow and medium speeds (Gruber et al., 2013b).

Much attention has been directed towards understanding the lower limb contributions to running and running economy, with less known about the torso, head and upper extremities. Hinrichs (1987) was the first to quantify a rotational coupling in angular momentum between the upper and lower extremities. Therefore, swinging the arms enables runners to counter the vertical momentum of the lower limbs, as well as facilitating vertical oscillation of the centre of mass and minimising head, shoulder and torso rotation. As a result, restricting arm movement, by holding them behind your back or on top of your head, increases the metabolic cost of running and thus, worsens running economy (Arellano and Kram, 2011). Collectively, owing to the upper and lower limb coupling, it is recommended that runners are encouraged to maintain their natural arm swing.

As discussed earlier, female runners should be considered separately to male runners. In addition to differences in common gait characteristics, females must consider the interaction of these factors with their breast biomechanics. Unfortunately, this is an under-researched field, but some meaningful advancements have been made in recent years (e.g., Milligan et al., 2015; Milligan, 2013). Breasts move in a three-dimensional figure of eight during each gait cycle. A breast impact shock occurs following each foot strike and can lead to many females suffering breast pain whilst running. Given the rotational coupling of the upper and lower extremities, greater breast motion may lead to greater counteracting motion of the lower limbs. There is growing evidence to support this theory, with breast kinematics being shown to affect knee angle (Milligan, 2013), step length (Milligan, 2013), trunk lean (Milligan et al., 2015) and medio-lateral forces (White et al., 2009). Ensuring female runners have appropriate breast support to minimise breast motion serves two potential functions: (1) eliminating or reducing pain associated with running; and (2) reducing unwanted rotational motion at the lower limb and medial-lateral forces that may contribute to increased metabolic cost (worsening of economy).

Individual Assessment for Economical Running

Optimising running form for economy improvements based on current evidence traditionally requires laboratory-based testing (e.g. motion capture and gas analysis systems). For many this may not be available. However, surrogate measures, such as heart rate and video/app analysis, can be used in combination with freely available software (Moore, 2019) or an automated spreadsheet (Moore, 2020) that can predict the gait with the lowest heart rate response. This software and spreadsheet have been developed to support practitioners for performing high-level testing of individuals with minimal equipment.

Using a combination of a metronome and verbal instructions, such as "run to the beat", practitioners can either manipulate step frequency or ground contact time. To manipulate step frequency, one must first determine the individual's self-selected cadence using a video app or visual inspection. Then set the metronome to a beat that represents their self-selected cadence ±5% and self-selected cadence ±10%. Example formulas to help calculate these are shown in Table 13.2. To manipulate ground contact time, repeat the first step to determine self-selected cadence. Then set the metronome to the self-selected cadence and instruct individuals using the verbal cues provided in Table 13.3. In our laboratory, we have found that providing appropriate time to familiarise individuals to the protocol is crucial before testing. Manipulating ground contact in this way will enable leg stiffness optimisation to also be determined.

In summary, there is a need to consider female and male runners separately due to the conflicting findings and potential effects of breast motion on economical gait characteristics. We argue that there is no such thing as a *perfect running form*, particularly regarding economical running, and whilst associations previously identified are informative, they should not be used as a blueprint of how everyone should run. Instead, we strongly recommend undertaking an individual economical running gait assessment by systematically examining the effects of modifying a specific gait characteristic for each runner. This can be done for cadence, stride

TABLE 13.2 Example cadence manipulation equations

Desired cadence	Calculation	Equation	Cadence to use
90% of self-selected	Self-selected × 0.90	160 × 0.90	144 steps per min
95% self-selected	Self-selected × 0.95	160 × 0.95	152 steps per min
105% self-selected	Self-selected × 1.05	160 × 1.05	168 steps per min
110% self-selected	Self-selected × 1.10	160 × 1.10	176 steps per min

TABLE 13.3 Gait retraining methods for targeted biomechanical variables

Biomechanical variable	Intervention	Verbal instructions			Biofeedback	Performance (P), injury prevention (IP) or injury rehabilitation (IR)	Injury
		Internal	External	Analogy			
Cadence	Verbal cues and metronome or *music*	Match your footsteps to the beat of the metronome (Bramah et al., 2019) Increase the number of times your foot hits the ground by 10% (Adams et al., 2018)	*Run to the rhythm of the metronome* *Run to the beat*		Video self-modelling (Breen et al., 2015; Diss et al., 2018) Wearable foot pod and watch (Willy et al., 2016)	P, IR	Patellofemoral pain syndrome (Bramah et al., 2019) Chronic exertional compartment syndrome (Breen et al., 2015; Diebal et al., 2012) Tibial stress fracture (Willy et al., 2016) Plantar fasciitis (Pohl et al., 2009)
Ground contact time and leg stiffness	Verbal cues and metronome	Make contact with the ground in time with the beat and increase/decrease contact time as much as possible (Moore et al., 2019a)		*Imagine you're running on hot coals* *Imagine you're running in sticky mud*		P	
Increase step width	Verbal cues and biofeedback	Run with a narrower/wider step width (Meardon and Derrick, 2014) *Make sure your knees don't touch* Keep your feet either side of the line (tape on treadmill)		*Imagine you are holding a balloon between your knees*	Mirror	IR	

(*Continued*)

TABLE 13.3 (Continued)

Biomechanical variable	Intervention	Verbal instructions		Analogy	Biofeedback	Performance (P), injury prevention (IP) or injury rehabilitation (IR)	Injury
		Internal	External				
Reduce vertical impact peak force and loading rate	Verbal cues and biofeedback	See forefoot/toe strike cues	Run softer (Chan et al., 2018; Crowell et al., 2010; Crowell and Davis, 2011)	See forefoot/toe strike cues	Vertical force-time curve (Chan et al., 2018) Tibia acceleration-time curve (Crowell et al., 2010; Crowell and Davis, 2011)	IP, IR	General lower limb running-related injury (Chan et al., 2018) Patellofemoral pain syndrome (Cheung and Davis, 2011)
Reduce peak horizontal braking force	Biofeedback and metronome	Match your footsteps to the beat of the metronome (increase cadence)	Run to the rhythm of the metronome		Anterior-posterior force-time curve (Napier et al., 2019)	IR	General lower limb running-related injury (Napier et al., 2018)
Flatter foot angle (midfoot strike) or forefoot/toe strike	Verbal cues	Run with a flat foot (Moore et al., 2019b) Run on your toes (Roper et al., 2016) Run on the balls of your feet (Roper et al., 2016)	Run quietly (Diebal et al., 2012)	Imagine an orange under your arch and squash it on every landing (Franklyn-Miller, 2016) Run like you're trying to squash oranges (Phillips et al., 2017)	Video self-modelling (Breen et al., 2015) Camera feedback	IR	Patellofemoral pain syndrome (Roper et al., 2016) Chronic exertional compartment syndrome (Breen et al., 2015; Diebal et al., 2012)
More vertically aligned tibia at initial contact	Verbal cues	Try to contact that ground with your foot near your body rather than out in front of you		Imagine your leg is a piston (Franklyn-Miller, 2016)	Video self-modelling (Breen et al., 2015) Camera feedback	IR	Chronic exertional compartment syndrome (Breen et al., 2015)

Target	Feedback	Verbal cue		Biofeedback		Condition
Reduce peak tibial acceleration	Verbal cues and biofeedback	Make your footfalls quieter (Creaby and Franettovich Smith, 2016)	Run softer (Creaby and Franettovich Smith, 2016) *Run quietly*	IR	Tibia acceleration-time curve (Crowell and Davis, 2011) Haptic feedback of resultant acceleration (Sheerin et al., 2020)	Tibial stress fracture (Crowell and Davis, 2011)
Reduce knee abduction	Verbal cues and biofeedback	Point your knees towards the wall	*Keep the markers apart (place markers on the outside of the knee)*	IR	Mirror *Video self-modelling*	Iliotibial band syndrome
Reduce hip adduction	Verbal cues and biofeedback	Run with your knees apart pointing straight ahead (Willy et al., 2012b; Noehren et al., 2011) Squeeze your buttocks (Willy et al., 2012b) *Don't let your knees touch*		IR	Mirror (Willy et al., 2012b) *Video self-modelling*	Patellofemoral pain syndrome (Willy et al., 2012b)
Contralateral pelvic drop	Verbal cues and biofeedback	Run with your knees apart pointing straight ahead (Willy et al., 2012b; Noehren et al., 2011) Squeeze your buttocks (Willy et al., 2012b)		IR	Mirror (Willy et al., 2012b) *Video self-modelling Camera feedback*	Patellofemoral pain syndrome (Willy et al., 2012b)

(Continued)

TABLE 13.3 (Continued)

Biomechanical variable	Intervention	Verbal instructions			Biofeedback	Performance (P), injury prevention (IP) or injury rehabilitation (IR)	Injury
		Internal	*External*	*Analogy*			
Increase pelvic external rotation	Verbal cues and biofeedback	Keep your knee pointing forward (Hunter et al., 2014) Keep your foot point forward (Hunter et al., 2014) Reduce your arm swing (Hunter et al., 2014)			External rotation of pelvis angle-time curve (Hunter et al., 2014)	IR	Iliotibial band syndrome (Hunter et al., 2014)
Reducing vertical oscillation	Verbal cues	Keep the body as low to the ground as possible (Adams et al., 2018) Run lower (Eriksson et al., 2011)	*Reduce how much you bounce when you run*		Vertical centre-of-mass displacement with identifiable target value (Eriksson et al., 2011)	IR	Plantar fasciitis (Pohl et al., 2009) (via reductions in instantaneous loading rate)
Upright torso and neutral pelvis	Verbal cues	Rest your chin on a shelf (Franklyn-Miller, 2016) Stand tall (Franklyn-Miller, 2016)			*Camera feedback*	IR	Chronic exertional compartment syndrome (Franklyn-Miller, 2016)
Greater knee and/ or ankle flexion at toe-off	Verbal cues	*Keep your knee slightly flexed at push-off Keep your ankle slightly flexed at push-off*	*Drive forwards Push the treadmill backwards*		*Video self-modelling*	P	

Note: Italics denotes author suggestions. Other information is taken from literature.

Camera feedback can be provided by connecting a camera to a screen in front of the individual running. The camera can be placed at the side or behind the individual to provide them with sagittal and frontal (back) views.

length, ground contact time and leg stiffness using video analysis, heart rate and open-access software to predict the mathematically optimal value that minimises heart rate (a surrogate measure for economy).

Gait Retraining and Injury

The most common running-related injuries that occur are in the lower limb and are chronic in nature, in part due to the repetitive loading that accompanies the act of running. Gait retraining has been proposed as both an injury prevention and injury rehabilitation strategy for lower limb running-related injuries. Whilst gait retraining for performance focuses on improving running economy, when used for injury purposes it focuses on redistributing the load a runner experiences. The external forces that act upon the lower limb cannot be eliminated altogether, but in some instances, they can be attenuated by modifying technique and being transferred to other joints and/or structures. Table 13.3 outlines gait characteristics that can be modified through gait retraining and the specific injuries they are designed to address. Female and male runners have been included in gait retraining studies, with no sex-specific differences in outcomes noted to date, meaning in this section 'runner' refers to both males and females. This section will cover the most common gait characteristics that have been the focus of research.

Is Injury Prevention Possible by Changing Running Gait?

It is widely accepted that injury is multifactorial. Using gait retraining as a preventative strategy assumes a mechanical basis to the development of the injury, where symptoms result from the changes to a tissue, which are associated with overload to that tissue. Based on this assumption, it follows that if we can change the way the musculoskeletal system is loaded (e.g. frequency, direction, magnitude, rate, variability, point of application), the load experienced by the tissue would not exceed its capacity and symptoms would not occur. In support of this approach, Chan and colleagues (2018) demonstrated that a two-week gait retraining intervention to reduce vertical loading rates in untrained runners, prior to a 12-month period of running, led to a 62% lower rate of injury than if no gait retraining was undertaken. The gait retraining approach applied in this intervention encouraged individuals to eliminate the vertical impact peak force, suggesting a forefoot strike pattern was adopted. Lower loading rates mean vertical stiffness of the body is reduced during impact. If a rate-dependent relationship between loading and bone injury is present in humans, like it is for other animals (Burr et al., 1985), then lower loading rates could be associated with lower risk of bony injuries. It is notable that the study by Chan and colleagues (2018) decreased the occurrence of patellofemoral pain and plantar fasciitis but increased the occurrence of Achilles tendinopathy and calf strain possibly due to the higher ankle plantarflexor moments (Nunns et al., 2013) required during forefoot striking. Therefore, individuals with a previous history of calf or Achilles injuries are advised to avoid this type of gait retraining approach. Conversely, individuals with a history of knee injuries may benefit from this gait retraining strategy.

Not all running-related injuries share a clear relationship with load and many injuries may not present with any structural changes to the tissue. The association between tissue changes, such as pathology, and pain is also unclear, with pathology frequently present in asymptomatic individuals (Horga et al., 2019). This calls into question a purely mechanical approach to injury occurrence. Consequently, injury prevention based on the underlying assumption that injury is simply a mechanical issue cannot be universally applied.

In addition, using a gait retraining approach to prevent injuries will likely mean idealising and pursuing a certain running gait. Like performance, and as can be seen in the study by Chan and colleagues (2018), one running gait is unlikely to suit everyone. Whilst these critiques are also true for injury rehabilitation, there is far more supporting evidence that gait retraining reduces pain in symptomatic runners; it may also provide a greater opportunity for a more individually tailored running form to be encouraged.

Rehabilitating Lower Limb Injuries Using Gait Retraining

Pain reduction is undoubtedly one of the most important outcomes for an individual undergoing injury rehabilitation. Gait retraining can be an effective rehabilitation strategy but can be performed only on individuals who are able to run whilst injured. Modifying running gait has successfully reduced pain associated with patellofemoral pain syndrome (anterior knee pain) (Bramah et al., 2019; Esculier et al., 2017; Noehren et al., 2011; Roper et al., 2016; Willy et al., 2012b), iliotibial band syndrome (Hunter et al., 2014) and chronic exertional compartment syndrome (Breen et al., 2015; Diebal et al., 2012). Understanding which gait characteristics to target requires knowledge of anatomy and how it functions, as well as knowledge of the movement that causes pain. There is also the need to consider the anatomy and how it functions with structures proximal and distal to the site of pain. For example, the hip and/ or foot should be considered when assessing patellofemoral pain. Table 13.3 provides an overview of the different gait characteristics that have been targeted, and we will focus on the three most common ones: cadence, tibial acceleration and hip kinematics.

One of the simplest technique changes that has been employed is an increase in cadence, which is usually undertaken with an individual running on a treadmill contacting the treadmill belt in time to the beat of a metronome. Example calculations to manipulate cadence are provided in the 'Individual Assessment for Economical Running' section (p. 192). Typically, between 7.5% and 10% increases in cadence have been used (Bramah et al., 2019; Willy et al., 2016) and are associated with a number of kinetic and kinematic changes (Heiderscheit et al., 2011). For example, the foot is horizontally placed closer to the centre of mass at initial contact, peak horizontal braking and vertical impact forces are reduced, estimated knee reaction forces and work at the knee are lowered, work at the ankle increases and the tibia is more vertically aligned (Heiderscheit et al., 2011; Lieberman et al., 2015). Faded feedback approaches and one-off visits can be used to change cadence. However, it is important to note that large changes to cadence will worsen running economy (Moore, 2016). Encouragingly, even just a 3% increase in cadence can reduce knee pain and, vertical and braking forces during running (Diss et al., 2018), whilst also not being detrimental to running economy (Bruton et al., 2017). Making incremental changes to cadence until perceived pain has reduced would allow a practitioner to potentially mitigate the magnitude of change in running economy by settling on the minimum cadence increase required to reduce pain.

Peak tibial acceleration, sometimes referred to as tibial shock, appears to be higher in female runners who have a history of stress fractures (Milner et al., 2006). It has since become a focus of gait retraining research. Previous work has shown that reducing tibial acceleration also enables male and female runners to reduce instantaneous and average loading rates (Crowell et al., 2010; Crowell and Davis, 2011), which may be beneficial for reducing patellofemoral pain or general lower limb injury risk. Lowering peak tibial acceleration can be achieved with some simple verbal instructions as well as using real-time biofeedback (see Table 13.3). If tibial acceleration can be relayed in real-time, researchers have used a 50% reduction in peak tibial acceleration as a target value (Crowell et al., 2010; Crowell and Davis, 2011). This can be achieved by some runners, but inter-individual variation exists regarding the level that can be achieved. Such variation is also present when changing cadence and foot angles at initial contact. If tibial acceleration cannot be relayed in real time, the verbal instructions used by others means runners are likely to be exhibiting a flatter foot (midfoot) or forefoot strike pattern to produce lower tibial accelerations (Clansey et al., 2014). Therefore, instructing runners to alter their foot strike pattern will likely achieve the same outcome. Shortening stride lengths has also been shown as an effective way to reduce tibial acceleration in male runners (Mercer et al., 2002).

During the stance phase, the lower limb must attenuate the external force it is exposed to. Several kinematic strategies exist to achieve this. Whilst the largest motion of the lower limb is observed in the sagittal plane, a greater number of frontal plane movements have reported associations with injury (retrospectively and prospectively), particularly at the pelvis, hip and knee. The collapsing of the lower limb during ground contact time can be visually seen and quantified as hip and thigh adduction, knee abduction and contralateral pelvic drop. Some of these kinematics are exhibited in runners who have a history of, or develop, iliotibial band syndrome (van der Worp et al., 2012) and who have patellofemoral pain syndrome (Neal et al., 2016). Changing such a movement pattern can be achieved using gait retraining within a relatively short space of time (2 weeks) (Willy et al., 2012b), and may in fact be superior to trying to do so through a strength-based intervention which typically takes 6 weeks (Willy and Davis, 2011). Along with the time requirements, there are two other reasons to favour adopting a gait retraining approach. Firstly, lower limb muscle strength consistently displays very poor-to-no relationship with running kinematics, meaning higher strength is not associated with less or more movement (Baggaley et al., 2015; Schmitz et al., 2014; Fukuchi et al., 2014). Secondly, increasing lower limb muscle strength does not lead to changes in running kinematics (Ferber et al., 2011; Willy and Davis, 2011). If a practitioner feels there is a need to change frontal plane pelvis, hip and knee kinematics, then verbal instructions and biofeedback, rather than strength interventions, will enable a runner to do so.

In summary, gait retraining has been successfully used to reduce the incidence of certain injuries, yet increase the incidence of others, in addition to reducing the pain associated with several overuse lower limb injuries. Modifying a runner's cadence and/or tibial acceleration produces several kinematic and kinetic changes that may contribute to redistributing the load applied to the painful body region. Specific frontal plane lower limb kinematics can also be targeted and altered within a relatively short time.

How to Perform Gait Retraining

Gait retraining means providing instructions and/or feedback to an individual to modify specific gait characteristics. It can be undertaken with either a performance or injury-related goal in mind. Depending upon the goal in mind, different gait characteristics may be targeted. Firstly, we must consider how to perform gait retraining, which applies to both performance and injury goals. Gait retraining starts with a systematic assessment of running gait alongside a clinical examination to determine a runner's goals and needs. A runner's spatiotemporal characteristics, kinematics and kinetics will be examined alongside their symptoms during gait, which may include pain and when it occurs in the gait cycle, as well as how it changes with gait retraining or changing constraints, such as speed and gradient.

Once an assessment is complete, then goals of gait retraining can be created, and outcome measures can be used to determine effectiveness. In the treatment of injury this may involve reducing symptoms during running, or alteration of provocative movement patterns while measures of economy or performance can be utilised if they are the main goal. An integral part to the effectiveness of any proposed gait retraining intervention is the application of appropriate motor learning principles. While it is beyond the scope of this chapter to cover in-depth coverage of these principles, we will present some key considerations for practitioners.

Developing Verbal Instructions

Developing verbal instructions to facilitate bringing about a modified running gait is a challenge. But, it is important to note, all studies employ a verbal instruction during gait retraining, sometimes as the only way to modify gait and other times in combination with biofeedback and/or self-modelling (see Table 13.3). First, a practitioner must decide on which gait characteristic they wish to modify in an individual. It is preferable to select one characteristic at a time, rather than providing an individual with multiple characteristics to focus on. Then the language used to instruct an individual must be considered. Three main types of instructions are typically used: (1) analogy; (2) external focus of attention and (3) internal focus of attention. There are both clinical (Franklyn-Miller, 2016) and coaching (Pedley et al., 2017) examples where analogies are used during gait retraining. However, analogies suffer from a similar issue as external focus of attention instructions, in that they may be ambiguous. They may also lead to unwanted gait changes (Phillips et al., 2017) and produce inconsistent gait responses between individuals (Kleynen et al., 2019). The most common types of verbal instructions used are external and internal focus of attention and the underlying theory is discussed next.

Focus of Attention and Constructive Conscious Control

Wulf and Lewthwaite's (2016) *Optimising Performance Through Intrinsic Motivation And Learning* (OPTIMAL) theory provides an excellent overview of performance-related motor learning. The authors advocate for the use of an external focus of attention, where one's attention is directed towards the movement effect (task outcome) during training to promote skill learning and development, rather than the use of an internal focus of attention where attention is directed towards one's body and its movement (task execution). There is a substantial body of evidence to support this approach e.g., greater throwing accuracy (Lohse et al., 2010), jumping higher (Wulf and Dufek, 2009) or further (Wu et al., 2012).

To date, gait retraining studies have reported employing an external focus of attention verbal cue to manipulate gait (e.g. Chow et al., 2014). However, inspection of the methods (the inclusion of visual feedback alongside the cue) and verbal cues (which include an internally focused section preceding the externally focused section: "we're aiming to change foot strike, so run quietly" (Moore et al., 2019b) or "run with your knees pointing towards the wall") suggests the terminology used has muddied the waters between an external and internal focus of attention. This hybrid model of verbal cueing is often used by clinicians, so whilst the internal aspect may be beneficial, the external portion of the cues have the potential to induce unwanted changes to running technique that consequently may increase loading of the painful body region. Indeed, Moore and colleagues (2019b) have shown that by using this type of cue, a hybrid technique response is produced. Meaning individuals produced technique responses somewhere in between the responses of individuals exposed to either an internal (most effective at producing the desired change) or external cue (least effective at producing the desired change).

This hybrid approach supports a body of work that advocates the importance of utilising an internal focus as a mediator for continuous improvement (Toner and Moran, 2015). Specifically, rather than trusting movements will change based on unconscious trial and error, it has been suggested that increasing somatic reflection (bodily awareness) promotes the refinement of, and/or changes in, habitual movement patterns. Therefore, it appears that the theoretical concept of 'constructive conscious control' is relevant in this context. For example, take a runner who is experiencing a low-level knee pain. Providing a verbal instruction to run without the knee pain, without providing clear, internally focused instructions about what kinematic strategies to adopt (based on clinical assessments) to facilitate this is likely to be unhelpful. Thus, for runners who want to modify gait because of injury, or to improve performance, a clear, unambiguous kinaesthetic reference point (an internal focus) allowing them to refine their running gait in a systematic way may be advantageous. It is important for practitioners to be mindful of the current debate and consider the potential importance and effectiveness of utilising internal focus of attention cues for their clients during gait retraining.

Considerations for the Provision of Gait Training

Literature often uses the same verbal instruction for each runner to allow a hypothesis to be tested. However, within a coaching and clinical setting, individually tailored verbal instructions are encouraged. It is possible that this may mitigate the ambiguity issue associated with externally focused instructions or analogies. Additionally, asking for the individual's interpretation of the verbal instruction is recommended. This may mean using an iterative approach, where trial and error is used before settling on a given instruction. Providing these instructions every 20–30 seconds during the initial stages of gait retraining balances the need to remind individuals, without becoming too annoying for both runner and practitioner (Moore et al., 2019b).

If possible, a period of learning the modified gait should occur over several sessions. A typical approach is to adopt a faded-feedback paradigm, whereby instructions and/or feedback are gradually withdrawn until none are provided and the individual must run with the modified gait unaided. Faded-feedback over eight sessions has been used to good effect to treat running-related patellofemoral pain (Noehren et al., 2011, Willy et al., 2012b). Single-session gait retraining can achieve desired kinematic changes (Moore et al., 2019b; Bramah et al., 2019), but retention of the modified running gait may be more difficult to acquire.

Biofeedback and Self-Modelling

Gait retraining can be performed using a variety of biofeedback methods, whereby gait characteristics are relayed back to an individual as they run. Table 13.3 provides an overview of the different variables that have been simultaneously calculated and visually displayed to individuals whilst running on a treadmill. Many of the biofeedback techniques employed in research require sophisticated, expensive research equipment, such as three-dimensional motion analysis or instrumented treadmills. Encouragingly, there are some simpler, cheaper alternatives. Frontal plane gait characteristics (e.g. hip adduction, step width) can be viewed using a mirror, whilst sagittal and frontal plane (back view) gait characteristics can be viewed by syncing a video camera with a display screen positioned in front of the runner. A practitioner can then move the video camera to the side or back of the individual to highlight target gait characteristics. Another option is the use of wearable technology. Willy and colleagues (2016) were able to use a global positioning system (GPS) watch and foot pod to determine cadence whilst individuals ran outside. The GPS watch was then programmed to display cadence using a faded-feedback paradigm. Wearable technology can also be used to help quantify workload variables and monitor running rather than relying on self-report measures (Stiles et al., 2018). But, the accuracy and reliability of the technology used must also be considered, given the scarcity of validated wearables on the market (Peake et al., 2018).

Self-modelling refers to the observation of yourself successfully performing the desired movement. In the context of gait retraining, this can be achieved by videoing the individual producing the specified technique change and asking them to review this video before they go running. This is a form of 'self-modelling' known as positive self-review (Dowrick, 1999). It has been used to reduce anterior knee pain during a cadence-focused gait retraining intervention and increase confidence in ability to perform the modified gait (Diss et al., 2018). However, the authors recommend the need to use criteria-based progression rather than time-based progression, meaning each individual may need a different number of gait retraining sessions to achieve the desired technique changes.

To potentially facilitate the transference of a newly acquired running technique to other constraints such as different surfaces, footwear or gradient, feedforward self-modelling may be useful. This would require an individual to be filmed performing successfully under these different constraints and providing an individual with such videos. This has been shown to be effective in learning more complex, higher-level moves during trampolining (Ste-Marie et al., 2011), but has yet to be undertaken during running gait retraining. Encouraging results from Zhang and colleagues (2019) have shown that gait retraining on a level treadmill with the aim of reducing tibial acceleration did transfer to overground running and uphill running, but not to downhill running. Runners may need to be reminded to pay specific attention to producing the modified gait during the initial stages of gait retraining to help facilitate future retention.

Gait Retraining in Practice

Gait retraining can be conducted both on a treadmill and overground, yet most of the evidence is derived from treadmill running. Using a treadmill has several advantages: (1) runners can modify gait without worrying about maintaining a specific speed; (2) runners can practice the modified gait at a variety of speeds and/or inclines; (3) biofeedback can be displayed in front of a runner and (4) practitioners can easily view and video multiple steps, providing an opportunity to see gait strategies each runner is employing. Facilitating the transference of the modified gait to overground could be undertaken through the use of feedforward self-modelling. Verbal instructions can also serve as useful reminders that a runner can use when practicing the modified gait during overground running.

Gait Retraining for Performance

Using a biomechanically derived training intervention to enable a runner to change gait char-acteristics, e.g. ground contact time and cadence, seems to be achievable. Indeed, we advo-cate this approach above an exercise/conditioning training intervention in the first instance, as there is very limited evidence showing that exercise- or conditioning-based interventions change desired gait characteristics of a runner (Giovanelli et al., 2017; Gomez-Molina et al., 2018). Conversely, short biomechanical interventions (<15 days) have shown some promising results; for instance, male and female runners may benefit from 15 to 30 minutes of running at higher cadences for 10 to 15 days (Quinn et al., 2019; Morgan et al., 1994). Morgan and col-leagues (1994) reported that runners were able to successfully modify cadence towards their optimal cadence using this type of training approach and improve their running economy. Whilst, these biomechanical changes take about half the training time to produce as physi-ological adaptations do, we recommend caution with using consistent gait modifications for such long periods of time as it may impart a high cardiovascular and musculoskeletal demand, which may not be suitable for all runners.

Producing greater knee and/or ankle flexion at toe-off could be targeted for potential improvements in running economy. A verbal instruction such as 'keep your knee slightly flexed at push-off' (internal cue) or 'drive forwards' (external cue) may lead a runner to modify their toe-off leg orientation. This will need to be monitored visually by recording the runner in the sagittal plane and ensuring the desired technique change is being produced.

Gait Retraining for Injury Rehabilitation

Here we will outline two scenarios for using gait retraining in practice for lower limb injury rehabilitation. Scenario A is a runner coming into the clinic for a one-off visit. Scenario B is a runner engaged in a treatment programme that includes multiple visits to the clinic over a 1-month period.

Scenario A: A male runner presents with patellofemoral pain during running, and assess-ment reveals several gait characteristics which may be increasing load on this body region: the runner has minimal knee flexion at initial contact and their foot lands a large distance in front of their hip, they exhibit high peak knee flexion at mid-stance and a kinetic assessment reveals a high peak braking force. His self-selected cadence running at 12 km·h^{-1} was 158 steps per minute.

Increasing step rate by 10% has been found to reduce overstriding and peak knee flexion (Heiderscheit et al., 2011; Lenhart et al., 2014) as well as being associated with decreased peak braking force (Napier et al., 2019). Recent research has found that just one session of implementing this strategy can be effective in runners with patellofemoral pain (Bramah et al., 2019). In this runner's case we may experiment with 3%, 5%, 7.5% and 10% increases in cadence within the session to determine a strategy that achieves our goals without increasing effort excessively (see Table 13.2 for example calculations). A metronome could be used to create this change, and a GPS watch could provide additional feedback to determine whether the increase was achieved.

Videos would be taken, and kinetic data collected while running with these cues to exam-ine changes in kinematics and peak braking force. Further feedback is then provided to opti-mise the changes. If kinetic data are not available, videos would suffice for this intervention.

In the case of a single session of this nature, providing a runner with ongoing instruction and feedback is important. The runner could continue to use the metronome while running and monitor his cadence using a GPS watch.

Scenario B: A female runner presents with lateral hip pain, and gait analysis reveals two kinematic findings which may increase load on sensitive tissue: increased peak hip adduction and contralateral pelvic drop during the stance phase on the symptomatic leg.

These findings may be associated with a narrow stride width (Brindle et al., 2014); however increasing stride width can be problematic as a narrow stride is thought to minimise energetic cost (Arellano and Kram, 2011). In a clinical setting, this means that we should avoid increasing stride width excessively, and a runner may need more feedback and multiple sessions to optimise this new running technique.

If the knees brush together as a result of increased hip adduction, then cueing, 'don't let the knees touch' can be a simple and effective strategy to reduce hip adduction. Instructing the runner to 'run wider' or to run on either side of a line on a track can also be effective. In addition, increasing step rate has also been found to reduce peak hip adduction, so that can be considered too (Bramah et al., 2019). In our experience, verbal feedback when applying these cues, alongside visual feedback from a mirror or video, is especially important when making these changes, and several sessions may be required with gradually reducing feedback.

In summary, we argue that there is a need to develop constructive conscious control during gait retraining to enable an individual to acquire the desired technique changes to modify their gait. Using an internal focus of attention may facilitate this to a larger extent than an external focus of attention or analogy will. Devising individually tailored verbal instructions is recommended, along with criteria-based progression, whereby individuals are only progressed to another instruction and/or phase of gait retraining if they have achieved the desired technique change. Biofeedback has shown promising results, particularly when included as part of a faded-feedback paradigm, but traditionally biofeedback has required sophisticated computer algorithms and equipment to create. Wearable technology is allowing biofeedback to be undertaken 'in the field', yet currently only selected characteristics can be quantified precisely (e.g. cadence). Self-modelling is encouraged to enable individuals to review successful gait retraining performances to facilitate learning.

Gait Retraining Using Barefoot or Minimalist Footwear

Adding mass to the foot during running will worsen running economy. For every 100 g added to each foot, running economy will worsen by 1% as the metabolic cost of running increases (Frederick, 1984; Fuller et al., 2014). When mass is added to the lower limb, it increases its moment of inertia (resistance to move). The further away from the hip (point of rotation) that the mass is added, the greater the effect on moment of inertia, and thus a more pronounced effect on running economy is observed (Myers and Steudel, 1985; Martin, 1985). However, a review by Fuller and colleagues (2014) reported that running in a shoe weighing less than 220 g (or 440 g per pair) would not lead to a significant worsening of running economy compared to running barefoot. This makes the choice of footwear an important consideration for a runner from an economical perspective, with lighter shoes or no shoes at all (barefoot) being superior.

It is important to note that barefoot running is seen as a specific running form, and minimalist footwear is often recommended as a way of achieving this running form whilst providing protection to the sole of the foot. This means the possible benefits that may be associated with running barefoot or in minimalist footwear are argued by some to not just be a function of removed mass but are due to the 'barefoot running form' being adopted. This is typically described as: reducing your stride length and thus, increasing stride frequency, producing greater knee flexion upon initial contact with the ground, and striking the ground with the ball of your foot (forefoot striking or most likely toe-striking). The reduction in stride length appears to come from the foot being brought closer to the centre of mass at initial contact as the knee flexes more and the tibia rotates forwards, placing the tibia in a near vertical position. Additionally, a forefoot or toe-striking pattern occurs, and the ankle is plantarflexed at initial contact. The combination of the kinematic changes means the effective mass being accelerated upon ground contact is reduced, and there is a distinct lack of vertical impact force in the force-time curve (Lieberman et al., 2010).

Unfortunately, when barefoot running is often discussed, the notion of it being about a *running form* is overlooked or misunderstood. Simply taking your shoes off will not mean a runner will adopt the running form outlined here; there are of course many factors at play. Factors that influence responses to being barefoot are: level of somatosensory feedback (Moore et al., 2014b), pain tolerance, surface stiffness (Allison et al., 2013), and the speed and time a runner is exposed to being barefoot (Moore and Dixon, 2014). The first two factors, somatosensory feedback and pain tolerance, are why exposing individuals to barefoot running may be a useful therapeutic tool during gait retraining and injury rehabilitation. This is because individuals may subconsciously adapt their running kinematics to reduce pain and attenuate forces being applied to the musculoskeletal system. Holistically, this could be a mechanism to explore how an individual 'self-protects' and tries to redistribute lower limb load.

It would appear intuitive that increasing the variability of how individuals modulate load distribution through technique alterations may increase the tissue capacity of the musculoskeletal system, in so much as parts of the musculoskeletal system are now being exposed to higher levels of load than perhaps they would during a runner's normal gait. Exposure to variable loading patterns may explain why runners who use two or more pairs of different trainers during their running programme have a lower rate of injury than those who use just one pair of trainers (Malisoux et al., 2015). Variability can be induced in several other ways (e.g., changing terrain and gradient); however, if practitioners are turning to barefoot running to prevent injury or improve running economy, verbal instructions may be needed to facilitate learning the barefoot running technique.

Regarding injury risk, barefoot runners have similar injury rates to runners who wear trainers (shod runners). However, the most commonly injured body regions differ. Barefoot runners tend to injure the plantar surface of the foot, the calf musculotendon unit and the ankle, whilst shod runners tend to injure their hip, knee and plantar fascia (Altman and Davis, 2016). Load distribution during barefoot and shod running supports these different trends. Barefoot running produces greater ankle plantarflexion moments and ankle joint work compared to shod running, which produces greater knee flexion moments and knee joint work. If runners are interested in transitioning footwear i.e. from shod to minimalist or barefoot, a phased transition should be undertaken over several weeks. This should include gradual exposure to the footwear or removal of it, in addition to exercises to condition the musculotendon units that will be exposed to greater loads. However, it remains debatable whether such a change is likely to lead to improvements in running economy or performance and if these outweigh the notable risk of injury during transition.

Summary

- We recommend undertaking an individual economical running gait assessment rather than drawing upon cross-sectional, correlational studies that appear to present an 'economical running technique'. Pursuing such a running form assumes there is a perfect running form that should be targeted for all individuals, which is not the case.
- Strengthening exercises and the retraining of other movements (e.g. single leg squats) do not translate to gait modifications. Therefore, if a practitioner wishes to target a specific running gait characteristic, gait retraining is recommended. Gait retraining can improve running economy and reduce pain within 15 days, whilst physiological adaptations are shown to take much longer.
- Common gait modifications for injury rehabilitation that can be targeted outside of a research laboratory are: an increase in cadence, a reduction in tibial acceleration, increasing hip adduction and reducing contralateral pelvic drop
- Internal focus of attention verbal cues are more effective at producing desired technique changes, potentially by invoking constructive conscious control of one's gait to mediate improvements of a habitual movement pattern.
- Lightweight footwear (<220 g per shoe) or barefoot running will incur a lower metabolic cost than running in footwear >220 g per shoe. The overall rate or injury is similar between barefoot and shod running, but specific injuries may become more or less common. Practitioners should also be mindful that not all individuals will adopt a 'barefoot running form' by simply taking their shoes off, and therefore the desired gait modifications may not be achieved.

14

STRENGTH TRAINING FOR ENHANCING PERFORMANCE AND REDUCING INJURY RISK

Richard C. Blagrove and David R. Hooper

Highlights

- Strength training activities (resistance training and plyometrics) can enhance middle- and long-distance running performance, maximal sprint speed, and running economy.
- Overuse injuries are common in distance runners. High-intensity strength training performed frequently in short bouts may help reduce the risk of certain types of overuse injury.
- Endurance athletes can be prone to low bone mineral density, and strength training may be a potent stimulus to combat this issue.
- For runners new to strength training, developing movement competency across a wide range of exercises should be prioritised initially.
- Resistance training exercises (e.g. back squat, deadlift, step-ups) should be performed twice per week in the preparation for competition phases or targeted events.
- Plyometric exercises (e.g. skipping, hopping, jumping and bounding) develops neuromuscular qualities relating to the stretch-shortening cycle and offers a high level of transfer to running.

Introduction

> In the winter and spring of 1957 I must have run 2500 miles in training and lifted thousands of pounds in weights.
>
> —*Herb Elliott, Olympic 1500 m Champion, 1960; World Record Holder 1500 m and 1 mile, 1958; quoted in Trengrove (2018)*

The use of weight rooms and gymnasium-based exercises as an adjunct to a distance runner's training programme is not novel. In the 1950s, Percy Cerutty (coach to Herb Elliott), controversially advocated the regular use of heavy weight training for his group of highly successful Australasian distance runners. Peter Snell, the triple-Olympic gold medallist from the 1960s, is also known to have incorporated explosive bounding into his running sessions, and Sebastian Coe was a strong exponent of strength work and circuit training as part of his physical preparation in the late 1970s and 1980s. Although strength and conditioning exercises have been successfully used for decades by distance runners, it is only over the last 20 years that sport scientists have begun to understand the role of the neuromuscular system in endurance running events, and how strength training can be used to enhance performance. The aim of this chapter is to provide a scientific rationale for the inclusion of strength training in the programme of a distance runner and to outline practical recommendations for the implementation of appropriate strength training activities.

The Physiological Basis for Strength Training in Runners

Middle- (800 m–3 km events) and long-distance (5 km–marathon events) running performance is principally limited by the body's ability to deliver oxygen to the working muscles and clear the metabolites that inhibit muscular contraction (Joyner, 1991; Brandon, 1995). From a specificity perspective, the use of extensive and intensive running sessions is logically the best stimulus to drive adaptations to the cardiovascular and metabolic systems to enhance these processes. It may therefore seem counter-intuitive for a distance runner to perform resistance training exercises, which sit at the opposite end of a specificity continuum and largely target neuromuscular-related qualities.

In addition to cardiovascular and metabolic factors, which are crucial to develop in distance runners, the amount of energy that runners use to sustain a given running speed is also known to be an important determinant of performance (Ingham et al., 2008a; Blagrove et al., 2019). The less energy that is required to maintain a given sub-maximal pace, the more 'economical' a runner is said to be, and considerable variability exists between runners (Daniels, 1985). In highly trained runners, economy distinguishes performance more accurately than other physiological determinants of performance such as maximal oxygen uptake ($\dot{V}O_{2max}$) or running speed at a given blood lactate value (Conley and Krahenbuhl, 1980; Allen et al., 1985; McLaughlin et al., 2010). Moreover, running economy appears to become a more important factor in determining performance as race distance increases (DiMenna and Jones, 2016), therefore understanding how this quality can be enhanced is crucial.

Running economy is influenced by a multitude of intrinsic (physiological, morphological, neuromuscular and biomechanical) and extrinsic (technological and environmental) factors (Pate et al., 1992; Barnes and Kilding, 2015a; Moore, 2016). Many of these factors are modifiable using appropriate training interventions, including progressive increases in the volume of running (Mayhew et al., 1979; Morgan et al., 1995; Jones, 2006), and potentially gait re-training strategies (see Chapter 13). Importantly, several neuromuscular (eccentric strength and rate of force development) and structural (tendon stiffness) qualities contribute towards running economy (Barnes et al., 2014; Li et al., 2019). Therefore, training exercises, which specifically target development of these capacities, potentially offer one means of enhancing economy.

The amount of energy required by the muscles of the lower limb to sustain a given running speed is largely dependent upon the magnitude and rate of muscle fibre length change (Fletcher and MacIntosh, 2017). A muscle that remains static (isometric contraction) during the ground contact phase of the running stride will activate less muscle mass (Chow and Darling, 1999) and use less energy compared to a muscle that lengthens (eccentric contraction) upon initial ground contact and subsequently shortens (concentric contraction) during 'push-off' (Fletcher and MacIntosh, 2017). If a muscle were able to remain in an isometric state during the propulsive phase of a stride, the change in muscle-tendon unit length and joint angles (flexion at ankle, knee and hip) could theoretically be achieved using only the tendon. This is far more energy efficient as tendons are highly elastic structures that have a large capacity for storage and return of elastic strain energy.

Strength training typically results in an increase in recruitment of motor units (the muscle fibres that are innervated by a nerve), the rate at which motor units are activated, and tendon stiffness (Folland and Williams, 2007). Therefore, by improving these qualities, the lower limb is able to cope better with the magnitude and rate of force expression required during ground contact to enable muscle fibres to lengthen and shorten to a lesser extent; and for the tendons to accommodate any change in muscle-tendon unit length required (Fletcher and MacIntosh, 2017). Furthermore, possessing a capability to express higher levels of absolute force means that relative force production for tasks requiring sub-maximal sustained levels of force production (such as endurance running) is also lower, which may also contribute to improving running economy. The energy savings that result from improved running economy are therefore likely to enable a faster speed to be achieved over the duration of an event (Beneke and Hütler, 2005; Saunders et al., 2010; Hoogkamer et al., 2016), or a faster finish in the closing stages of a race (Damasceno et al., 2015).

Of the muscles in the lower limb, the ankle plantar flexors (gastrocnemius and soleus) contribute most to generating vertical support force during sub-maximal running and increases in stride length (Dorn et al., 2012). The energetic cost of running is also strongly related to force-length-velocity potential of the soleus complex (Bohm et al., 2019). However, at faster speeds (> 5 m.s^{-1}; $< 3:20$ min.km^{-1}), muscle fascicle shortening rates increase, which reduces the force the ankle plantar flexors can produce due to their force-velocity relationship (Lai et al., 2015). Beyond 7 m.s^{-1} ($< 2:23$ min.km^{-1}), peak ankle plantar flexor force begins to decrease, and running speed is generated to a greater extent by the forces produced by the gluteus maximus, hip flexors and hamstrings (Dorn et al., 2012). This shift in muscle recruitment strategy can help inform choice and prescription of strengthening exercises for the middle- and long-distance runner.

Distance running performances are strongly influenced by aerobic factors. However, the middle-distance events, and competitive races involving surges in pace and sprint finishes, also rely heavily on the capacity of anaerobic energy processes (Thompson, 2017). For an 800 m runner, near-maximal velocities of running are reached during the first 200 m of the race (Reardon, 2013), which necessitates a high capacity of the neuromuscular and anaerobic system. Moreover, possessing greater maximal speed also increases a runner's anaerobic speed reserve, which has been shown to be an important component of success in elite male 800 m running (Sandford et al., 2019a). Whereas strength training adaptations positively influence running economy by reducing the rate of energy turnover within active muscles, high-speed running is predominantly limited by the production of high vertical ground reaction force relative to body weight in a short ground contact time (Weyand et al., 2000). The ability to apply higher levels of force to the ground may also partly explain the improvements that have been observed in middle-distance running performance (1.5–3 km) following a period of strength training (Ramirez-Campillo et al., 2014; Skovgaard et al., 2014; Pellegrino et al., 2016).

Does Strength Training Improve Performance?

Several studies have noted strong relationships between proxy measures of anaerobic power or neuromuscular factors and distance running performance (Houmard et al., 1991;

Paavolainen et al., 1999b; Nummela et al., 2006; Hudgins et al., 2013; Bachero-Mena et al., 2017). This suggests that higher levels of strength are indicative of faster running performances. Correlation findings are useful in helping to explain how much variability in distance running performance can be explained by an anaerobic or neuromuscular factor, but this does not imply that greater strength capabilities can cause an improvement in distance running performance.

At least 25 training intervention studies have investigated whether strength training (heavy resistance training, explosive resistance training, plyometric training, or mixed modality training) can improve performance and/or the physiological factors that are important for distance running, compared to running training only (see the review by Blagrove, Howatson et al., 2018a). Strength training activities performed 2–3 times per week for a period of 6–14 weeks improve measures of strength and explosive power in middle- and long-distance runners (Trowell et al., 2020), and these improvements likely underpin the positive changes typically observed in running economy and performance compared to a programme that involves just running (Beattie et al., 2014; Berryman et al., 2017; Denadai et al., 2017; Blagrove, Howatson et al., 2018a). Importantly, most studies have not observed noticeable changes in body composition (i.e. muscle mass) following a period of strength training (Blagrove, Howatson et al., 2018a).

Neither age nor training status appear to be moderating factors in the degree to which running economy and performance can improve following a period of strength training (Denadai et al., 2017; Blagrove, Howatson et al., 2018a). Indeed, 'possibly beneficial' (−3.5%) changes in running economy were observed in post-pubertal adolescents following 10 weeks of multi-modal strength training compared to a running-only group (Blagrove et al., 2018a). Moreover, masters age (>40 years) runners significantly improved (−6.2%) their running economy at marathon pace after 6 weeks of concurrent strength and endurance training compared to a control group (Piacentini et al., 2013). Similarly, several studies that have used recreational-level distance runners have reported benefits to running economy following a period of strength training (Johnston et al., 1997; Turner et al., 2003; Albracht and Arampatzis, 2013; Festa et al., 2019). These improvements are of a similar magnitude to those observed in highly trained and elite distance runners who were exposed to comparable volumes of strength training (Paavolainen et al., 1999a; Millet et al., 2002; Saunders et al., 2006).

Several reviews have also been conducted summarising the literature that has investigated the effect of strength training interventions on acceleration and maximal speed, concluding that plyometrics (de Villarreal et al., 2012) and resistance-based training (Seitz et al., 2014; Bolger et al., 2015) have a positive effect on sprint performance. The same conclusion was also provided in a recent paper summarising the effects of strength training on maximal sprint speed, specifically in distance runners (Blagrove, Howatson et al., 2018a).

Does Strength Training Reduce Injury Risk?

Overuse type injuries are common amongst runners, with between 18% and 92% of runners per year suffering an injury, and prevalence rates of 7 to 59 injuries per 1,000 hours of running (Hreljac, 2005; Saragiotto et al., 2014). Common overuse injuries include bone-stress injuries, iliotibial band syndrome, shin splints, patellofemoral pain, plantar fasciitis and Achilles tendinopathy (Hreljac, 2005; Francis et al., 2019). Overuse injuries generally require a long time for recovery and are often the reason for stalled progress or runners quitting the sport.

Although a reasonable body of research exists showing strength training provides boosts to running economy and performance, the evidence indicating that long-term strength training lowers the risk of developing an overuse injury is far less convincing. It is therefore surprising that the most popular reason for runners to engage with strength and conditioning activities is the belief that it lowers their risk of getting injured (Blagrove, Brown et al., 2020b).

The underlying reasons that a runner develops an overuse injury are multifaceted and complex. Other than previous injury, very few other risk factors have been consistently identified (Saragiotto et al., 2014). Runners should therefore prioritise strengthening tissues that have previously been injured and address specific movement limitations that may have contributed towards the injury. The risk factors for each type of running injury differ slightly; however, errors in training prescription (i.e. rapid changes in running distance, weekly volume and/or running intensity) increase the likelihood of overuse injury (Hreljac, 2005). It is therefore advisable that runners monitor their training closely and aim to progress training gradually. This also applies to the introduction and progression of strength and conditioning training.

Research investigating risk factors associated with a runner's anthropometry and biomechanics have shown inconsistent results (Ceyssens et al., 2019; Vannatta et al., 2020). Previous work has shown that female runners who sustained overuse injury exhibit larger hip adduction angles during the stance phase of running (Ferber et al., 2010; Milner et al., 2010; Noehren et al., 2012) and greater contralateral hip drop is also associated with common injuries (Bramah et al., 2018). It is therefore advisable that runners (especially women) utilise and practice the practical screening tests highlighted in Chapter 7 to evaluate movement abnormalities and improve neuromuscular control.

Weakness in specific muscle groups has also been linked to certain overuse injuries in runners. Compared to non-injured runners, weaker gluteal muscles have been shown in runners suffering from patellofemoral pain (Cichanowski et al., 2007; Ferber et al., 2011; Finnoff et al., 2011; Luedke et al., 2015), iliotibial band syndrome (Fredericson et al., 2000), shin splints (Becker et al., 2018) and Achilles tendinopathy (Niemuth et al., 2005; Franettovich et al., 2014). Similarly, lower strength in the calf muscle group is associated with a higher likelihood of Achilles tendinopathy (Mahieu et al., 2006; O'Neill et al., 2019). Although this body of work indicates that low levels of strength may predispose runners to overuse injury, several of these studies were not prospective, and therefore reduced strength may be a consequence of an injury, rather than the cause.

An overuse injury occurs when the repetitive and frequent loading placed on a tissue exceeds the capacity of that tissue, which causes pain. Therefore, one logical way of lowering injury risk is to increase tissue capacity, so it can withstand higher volumes of loading. Gradual increases in running volume will progressively expose tissues to more load, and therefore cause the tissue to adapt; however, strength training exercises may provide a more potent stimulus to build structural resilience. Indeed, frequent and brief exposures to high magnitudes of loading appear to be best for driving positive changes in bone mineral density (BMD; Turner, 1998), tendon structure (Malliaras et al., 2013) and ligamentous tissue (Baar, 2017). Moreover, experts have suggested that muscle weakness is an important modifiable risk factor for athletic tendinopathies (O'Neill et al., 2016). Therefore, strength training, which exposes vulnerable tissues to higher magnitude and/or rates of loading compared to running, potentially offers a time-efficient and effective way of increasing strength and lowering the likelihood of an injury.

Bone Stress Injuries

Endurance athletes often exhibit low BMD due to factors related to the female athlete triad in women (see Chapter 18), and similar factors in men. The American College of Sports Medicine suggests that a criteria for low BMD is a Z-score of less than −1, meaning that the BMD is one standard deviation below the average for that person's age, sex and race (De Souza et al., 2014). Prior research has demonstrated that 21.5% of women athletes exhibited a Z-score between −1 and −2, and a further 5.9% less than −2 (Gibbs et al., 2013). A more recent study broke down women collegiate athletes by sport, and noted that 19% of cross-country runners had a BMD of less than −1 (Tenforde et al., 2018). While there is considerably less research in this area in men, a similar percentage was noted in adolescent male runners, of 23.5% of runners with a Z-score of less than −1 (Barrack et al., 2017). These low BMDs are a concern as they have been shown to lead to a heightened risk of stress reactions and/or fractures in women (De Souza et al., 2014) and an analogous process appears to occur in men (Tenforde et al., 2016).

The typical recommendation to stimulate adaptations to BMD is weight-bearing exercise with high impact (Turner, 1998). Thus, it appears paradoxical that individuals participating in high volumes of running; a weight bearing, impact exercise, could exhibit low BMD. This can be explained, at least in part, by low sex hormone concentrations associated with the female athlete triad (De Souza et al., 2014), exercise hypogonadal male condition (Hackney, 2008) or relative energy deficiency in sport (Mountjoy et al., 2014). In these cases, clearly, despite the weight bearing and impact nature of running, the stimulus is insufficient to develop, or even maintain, BMD.

Although low BMD alone is not used to diagnose the presence of osteoporosis – it must be accompanied by a history of stress fractures (De Souza et al., 2014) – the osteoporosis literature is able to provide guidance on how to enhance BMD. While aerobic activity is suggested to be capable of limiting the reduction of BMD, it is stated that progressive strength training is superior to aerobic activity for developing BMD (Benedetti et al., 2018). It is recommended that resistance training should involve the use of heavy loads (>85% of one repetition maximum), as this appears optimal to enhance BMD (Turner, 1998; Watson et al., 2018). Other recommendations related to strength training include loading the hip and spine, as these areas are particularly prone to low BMD and bone development is highly site specific (Benedetti et al., 2018). Thus, exercises such as the barbell back or front squat, lunges or deadlifts would be particularly beneficial.

Training to Reduce Overuse Injury Risk

It has previously been shown that increasing the volume and intensity of strength training is associated with a reduced risk of sports overuse injury (Lauersen et al., 2018), even compared to other types of conditioning such as stretching, proprioception training or a mixed exercise approach (Lauersen et al., 2014). However, these conclusions were largely based upon research in soccer players and documented overuse injuries not typically observed in distance runners. Studies specifically using distance runners have reported no differences in overall injury rates between a group exposed to a strength-related training intervention compared to a placebo-intervention or running only control group (Bredeweg et al., 2012; Baltich et al., 2017; Toresdahl et al., 2020). These investigations used large cohorts of recreational runners over relatively short periods (3–6 months) and unsupervised low-intensity strength or neu-romuscular training interventions ≤4 times per week. It may be the case that higher-intensity loading regimens over longer durations are required for the benefits of strength training to manifest as reductions in overuse injury occurrence. One study noted that eight strengthen-ing and stretching exercises incorporated into the daily warm-up routine of military recruits during 14 weeks of intensive training resulted in a 75% reduction in overuse knee injuries (Coppack et al., 2011). Similarly, a three-week daily hip abductor-strengthening protocol was shown to be effective in decreasing pain and stride variability in runners with patellofemoral pain (Ferber et al., 2011). Strengthening exercises for the gluteal muscles (Earl and Hoch, 2011) and knee extensors (Eapen et al., 2011; Chiu et al., 2012) have also been shown to reduce pain and improve function in physically active non-runners with patellofemoral pain syndrome. The most common site of injury in runners is the knee; therefore, these findings are useful.

Based upon the preceding discussion, the frequency and intensity with which muscle-strengthening exercises are performed seems to be important for reducing the likelihood of overuse injury. Studies have also shown that short-frequent bouts (10–15 min) of neuromus-cular training have the largest preventative effect for lower extremity injury in youth game sport athletes (Steib et al., 2017). It is therefore recommended that short bouts (<20 min) of intense strength training exercise are performed on most days of the week to minimise the risk of overuse injury. Changes to BMD also take several months, therefore regular and con-sistent long-term exposure to strength training is required to observe a reduced risk of bone stress-related injury.

Understanding 'Strength' and How Can It Be Developed

Strength can be defined as the ability to voluntarily apply force under a specified set of move-ment constraints to achieve a specific task outcome (Goodwin and Cleather, 2016). In the context of distance running, task-specific strength describes the way in which force is applied to the ground during each stride. For a runner to become more economical at a given run-ning speed, lower peak forces produce less muscle activation and therefore a lower energy turnover (Fletcher and MacIntosh, 2017). To improve economy, runners therefore need to develop the ability to manage force appropriately at ground contact whilst still producing enough force to overcome gravity and maintain running speed. As the foot remains in con-tact with the ground for 0.15–0.25 sec during running, the rate at which force needs to be developed is high. To develop higher competitive running speeds and maximal sprint speed, greater ground reaction forces need to be produced within shorter periods of time (Weyand et al., 2000). Therefore, selecting exercises that activate larger amounts of muscle mass in the lower limb (to increase motor unit recruitment) and switch muscles on quickly (to improve firing frequency) will help control and produce high forces, and decrease the relative propor-tion of muscle mass required to produce force.

Resistance training exercises are ideal for achieving these outcomes, with moderate-heavy loads and low repetition ranges (3–8 repetitions) required to enhance motor unit recruitment. Light load ballistic exercises using low repetition ranges (3–6 repetitions) are most appropriate for enhancing firing frequency. Plyometric training exercises also expose the body to higher forces than the running stride due to the increase in vertical drop height or the horizontal distance covered with each step. Maintaining a short (~0.2 s) ground contact time during plyometric exercises therefore enhances similar neuromuscular qualities to resistance training with the added benefit of developing stretch-shortening cycle capabilities that include storage and return of elastic energy from tendons.

There has been speculation that performing solely resistance training exercises provides little benefit to performance in runners (Dankel et al., 2017). Three studies, two in recreational-level runners (Damasceno et al., 2015; Karsten et al., 2016) and one in well-trained duathletes (Vikmoen et al., 2016), have, however, observed improvements in time trial performance following a period of resistance training, and several others have shown benefits to running economy (Johnston et al., 1997; Storen et al., 2008; Albracht and Arampatzis, 2013; Piacentini et al., 2013). Given the lack of biomechanical specificity between the force expression during running and traditional resistance training exercises, it is perhaps unsurprising that plyometric training or a multi-activity approach to strength training provides greater benefits to performance, at least in the short to medium term. Possessing greater maximal strength may, however, provide a greater magnitude of improvement in explosive strength capabilities (Cormie et al., 2010; James et al., 2018), which has important implications for the long-term periodisation of training.

Training Specificity

Training sessions and exercises can be represented on 'specificity pyramid' as shown in Figure 14.1. Based upon the principle of specificity, the most effective training to prepare the body for a given race would be to simulate the actual event as closely as possible. Given the lengthy recovery time and tedium associated with this approach, a better training strategy would be to take a longer-term view and use training sessions to develop specific physiological capabilities that underpin performance in the target event. This is also a less exhausting approach than simply mimicking a maximal race effort on a frequent basis; therefore, a greater

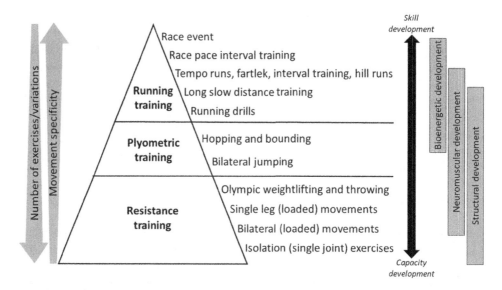

FIGURE 14.1   The training activity specificity pyramid

volume of work can be performed over a given period, which is likely to lead to greater long-term improvements. Running training (interval training, tempo runs, fartlek, long-slow distance running) obviously represent the most specific and important sessions in a runner's programme and generates cardiovascular and metabolic adaptations that enhance the bioenergetic pathways relevant to performance.

Strength training activities (plyometric and resistance training) sit below running training in the specificity pyramid. Unilateral plyometrics (hopping and bounding) have a high level of movement similarity to running; however, the force demands are far greater. Bilateral jumping exercises provide less of a stability challenge compared to unilateral plyometrics; however, the eccentric control requirements and vertical forces are typically higher. Therefore, jumping offers a strong stimulus for neuromuscular development and enhancement of stretch-shortening cycle qualities that are important during running.

Although resistance training exercises should bear some movement resemblance to the running action, it is important to remember that the purpose of these exercises is to overload the neuromuscular system: to increase maximal force production and rate of force development. Therefore, it is important to select the exercises and appropriate stimulus to achieve these outcomes. Similarly, specific strengthening for joints or structures that are vulnerable to injury (e.g. Achilles tendon) requires exercises that isolate and load the area directly. Often these exercises may have no real likeness to the running action but are necessary to build greater resilience and integrity in the tissue. In this regard, it is crucial that exercise selection and programming towards the bottom of the specificity pyramid is adaptation-led, as the priority is development of strength and structural capacity, rather than enhancing bioenergetic processes or the skill of running.

Programming Considerations

Long-Term Planning

It is important that runners address programming of strength training with the same attention to detail as their running training. The manipulation of training variables in a cyclical, non-linear manner over a long period of time (6–12 months) is a well-recognised approach to enhancing strength qualities, compared to a non-periodised approach (Williams et al., 2017). Although a relationship appears to exist between the duration of a strength training intervention and the magnitude of change in running economy (Denadai et al., 2017), there is currently a lack of research that has investigated whether further improvements are possible over periods of longer than a few months. Providing evidence-based guidelines around how strength training should be varied across a long-term period of preparation for an event is therefore problematic.

Figure 14.2 shows a generalised annual plan for a runner who is targeting the Northern Hemisphere track season or an early-autumn road event. Following the completion of an initial battery of movement and strength assessments, it is advisable that runners initially prioritise improving their weaknesses (see Chapter 7). For a runner new to strength training, this will usually be developing movement competency on basic exercises (e.g. squat, hip hinge, step-up, lunge, hop and stick) with their body weight or a light load (≤20 kg) (Blagrove, 2015). Alongside this, runners should focus on specific (isolation/single-joint) exercises or movement patterns than strengthen tissues that have previously been injured and/or areas identified as lacking capacity. Although high volumes of plyometric exercises should be

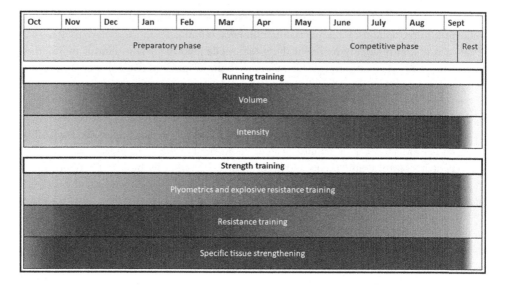

FIGURE 14.2 A generalised annual plan for a runner targeted a competitive track season in the Northern Hemisphere. The plan could also apply to a runner aiming for an early autumn road event, although the competitive phase could be shortened or removed. Darker shading indicates a higher relative emphasis on the type of training or activity category

avoided initially, low-level plyometrics (e.g. skipping, mini-hops, multi-directional jumps) can also be used concurrently alongside resistance training, which has been shown to be effective for enhancing running economy (Ache-Dias et al., 2017).

Although it is clear that significant gains in strength capabilities are possible when distance runners embark upon a strength training programme for the first time (Trowell et al., 2020), it is well-recognised that high volumes of aerobic running training attenuate strength-adaptation (Blagrove, 2013). Specifically, endurance training appears to compromise gains in explosive strength (or power) and may also interfere with the cellular signalling pathways that underpin an increase in muscle mass (Wilson et al., 2012). Despite this blunted adaptation, in the medium term (2–6 months), improvements in running economy, maximal speed, and performance are certainly possible by adding 2–3 sessions per week of strength training exercise (Blagrove, Howatson et al., 2018a). It is likely that higher volumes of running training (≥5 hours per week) are associated with interference in explosive force-related adaptations, but less so maximal strength (Vikmoen et al., 2020). As runners increase their training volume over long periods of time (>6 months), interference with strength-adaptation therefore becomes more likely (Coffey and Hawley, 2017). Similarly, in terms of organisation of training, an emphasis on explosive resistance training and plyometrics during periods of high running mileage seems unwise. Instead, heavier resistance training exercises should be prioritised when running volumes are high, with emphasis switched to explosive strength training when running volume decreases and intensity rises (Blagrove, 2014).

Short-Term Planning

The positioning of strength training within a training week is an important consideration for a runner. It is vital that key sessions each week are not compromised by high levels of fatigue and that strength training can be integrated effectively around a runner's lifestyle commitments. As discussed, high volumes of running can negatively affect the quality of strength work and interfere with adaptive processes; however, the reverse is also true. The residual fatigue from a bout of resistance or plyometric training impairs performance during subsequent running sessions if recovery is inadequate (Doma et al., 2017). Therefore, it is recommended that at least 24 hours separates a strength training session from a high-intensity running session.

For runners who are limited for time due to work, family and/or social commitments, it may only be possible to combine running training and strength work within the same session. In this scenario, as improvements in running are the priority, this should come first. It is also recommended that the bout of running is followed by a high carbohydrate and protein snack before any strength exercises are performed. There is also evidence in physically active individuals that adaptations to aerobic-based training are enhanced when resistance exercise is performed immediately after (Wang et al., 2011). Wherever possible, at least 3 hours should separate a running and a strength training session to allow fatigue to dissipate and minimise interference with strength adaptations (Baar, 2014). If running and strength training can remain as separate sessions on a given day, for recreational-level runners it is recommended that easy running is performed in the morning and strength training in the afternoon. For well-trained runners accustomed to strength training, performing strength work in the morning when less fatigued may be preferable, as they are likely to be sufficiently recovered for an afternoon/evening run. In highly trained runners, it is common for strength training sessions (involving mainly resistance training exercises) to be positioned on the same day, and within a few hours, of a hard interval training session. This polarised design to a training week means all high-intensity physical work (running and strength training) takes place on the same day, allowing days in between to be dedicated (active) recovery days.

One option to avoid the fatigue associated with sessions (~1 hour) of strength training is to divide traditional training sessions into smaller 'bite-size' training units (Blagrove, Howe et al., 2020). This approach, known as 'micro-dosing', may also appeal to those runners with busy lifestyles who struggle to find additional time in their schedules to add strength training sessions. Each training unit takes <20 minutes to complete, thus making it easy to integrate some purposeful strength training before or after running sessions. As previously highlighted, there may also be merit in using this strategy to reduce the risk of overuse injury long-term, although the efficacy for improving running economy and performance is currently uninvestigated. An example of how micro-dosing could be used across a training week is shown in Table 14.1, and an exercise routine is shown in Figure 14.3a. A common issue for non-elite runners is the lack of access to a suitable facility to perform resistance training. To some extent, the mini strength and conditioning routine shown in Figure 14.3a is also designed to address this issue.

A 'micro-dose' (1–6 sets at <10 sec per set) of high-intensity strength exercise (high load resistance or plyometrics) following a low-intensity run warm-up, and performed 5–10 min prior to a running session, may also be effective for enhancing subsequent performance in well-trained distance runners (Blagrove, Howatson et al., 2019c). A high-load exercise can elicit several physiological mechanisms that acutely augment neuromuscular performance in activities requiring sub-maximal or explosive force production, such as fast running (Blazevich and Babault, 2019). Indeed, a single set (5–6 repetitions) of a plyometric exercise (e.g. depth jumps or repeated maximal jumps) appears to acutely enhance running economy (Blagrove, Holding

TABLE 14.1 Example of a training week for a non-elite distance runner and organisation of strength training using a 'micro-dosing' approach, which includes two short resistance training sessions

`Day	Running training	Strength training
Monday	Easy moderate duration run	Resistance training exercises
Tuesday	Hard interval session	Mini S&C routine
Wednesday	Easy moderate duration run	Resistance training exercises
Thursday	Tempo run	Mini S&C routine
Friday	Rest	Rest
Saturday	Hill interval session	Mini S&C routine
Sunday	Easy long run	Mini S&C routine

Note: S&C = strength and conditioning. Alternatively, a lower frequency of strength training could be used, with 2–3 main sessions spread through the training week. Ideally, running training sessions and strength training should be separated by > 3 hours.

et al., 2019c; Wei et al., 2020), and band-resisted squat jumps (4 sets × 5 repetitions) have been shown to improve performance in a session of 5 × 1 km runs (Low et al., 2019). Moreover, a series of pre-session 'strides' (6 × 10 sec at 1500 m pace) wearing a weighted vest (20% of body mass) has also elicited an acute benefit to running economy and time to exhaustion in well-trained distance runners (Barnes et al., 2015).

Tapering and Peaking

As the competitive racing season begins or a targeted event approaches, running training will tend to reduce in volume to accommodate an increase in intensity at race pace or faster (see Figure 14.1 and Chapter 9). During this period, there may be a temptation to exclude strength training activities, especially if they are deemed too fatiguing to enable adequate freshness for races or key training sessions. It is likely that cessation of strength training will lead to noticeable deteriorations in maximal strength, submaximal strength and power after ~15 days (Bosquet et al., 2013). Excluding strength training following a successful intervention period has also been shown to result in a detraining effect, which is likely to cause improvements in performance to return to baseline levels within 6 weeks (Karsten et al., 2016). Reducing strength training frequency from two sessions per week during preparatory phases, to one session per week (and maintaining or slightly increasing intensity) during competitive or peaking phases seems enough to maintain previous strength and physiological improvements (Beattie et al., 2017). A single session of explosive squat training or plyometrics (3–6 sets × 8 repetitions) may also be sufficient to achieve improvements in running economy within 8 weeks (Berryman et al., 2010). Alternatively, the micro-dosing approach (described previously) to organising strength training through a training week offers an alternative strategy to preserve strength adaptations whilst minimising fatigue.

Exercise Selection

In studies that have shown a benefit of resistance training on running economy and/or performance, exercises with free weights have tended to be utilised (Johnston et al., 1997; Millet et al., 2002; Piacentini et al., 2013; Skovgaard et al., 2014; Beattie et al., 2017; Giovanelli et al., 2017). Studies that have used only resistance machines (Ferrauti et al., 2010; Vikmoen

Lateral lying leg raise		
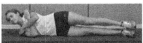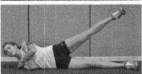	• Lie on your side with hips square to the ground • Attach a mini band around your ankles • Raise your leg upwards and slightly backwards in a controlled manner • Pause briefly in the top position before returning to the start position under control	Prescription: Perform 12 repetitions on each leg before moving onto the next exercise Progression and variation: • Change to a stiffer band • Perform in a standing position with hand against a wall
Drop landing		
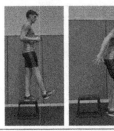	• Stand on a low (~30 cm high) box, step or sturdy chair • Step off the box with the toes of the free leg pulled towards your shin and the support leg straight • Land in a balanced position with knees slightly bent and pointing forward in alignment with toes	Prescription: Perform 12 repetitions before moving onto the next exercise Progression and variation: • Increase box height • Maximal jumps for height • Single-leg hop forward (for distance), sticking the landing • Zig-zag jumps
Elevated single leg bridge		
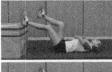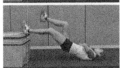	• Place the heel of one foot on a box (~45 cm high) or a sturdy chair • Place arms across chest • Hinging from the hips (with no bending in the spine), push hips upwards until there is a straight line between knee, hips and shoulders • Return to start position under control	Prescription: Perform 8-12 repetitions on each leg before moving onto the next exercise Progression and variation: • Nordic hamstring curl (with partner) • Place a weight across hips • Hold in top position (20 sec) and swing free leg
Single leg calf raise		
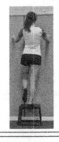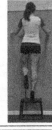	• Stand on one leg on a low step • Shuffle backwards so only the ball of the foot is in contact with the step and the heel drops below the level of the step • Using only finger tips for balance and maintaining a straight leg, raise up to tip-toes • Return to start position under control	Prescription: Perform 8-12 repetitions on each leg before moving onto the next exercise Progression and variation: • Perform with a bent leg • Wear a ruck sack with books or heavy objects in • Perform in-place mini hops
Side plank		
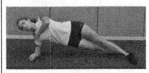	• Lying on side, place elbow directly under shoulder and the hand of the top arm on the opposite shoulder • Place the top foot in front of the bottom foot • Raise hips off ground until there is a straight line from ankle to shoulder • Hold this position	Prescription: Hold for 30 sec on each leg before moving back to the first exercise Progression and variation: • Front plank • Hold a weight on the top hip • Flex the top leg towards the chest whilst maintaining position

FIGURE 14.3a An example of a mini (home-based) strength and conditioning training routine that could be performed on most days of the week around running training

Back squat 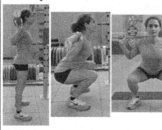	• Un-rack a barbell comfortably positioned across the upper back with an even overhand closed grip • Stand with feet shoulder wider apart with toes pointing outwards • With heels remaining in contact with the ground and remaining as upright as possible, flex at the ankle, knees and hips • Descend under control with knees aligned to toes, until hips are lower than knees • Leading with the chest, return explosively to the start position • Prescription: 3 sets of 8 repetitions (2-3 min recovery)
Romanian deadlift 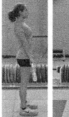 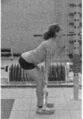	• Un-rack a barbell with an overhand closed grip and elbows straight • Flex the knees slightly • Maintaining a neutral back position with shoulder blades pulled together, flex from the hip and allow bar to slide down the thighs • When bar reaches the knee caps, return to start position Prescription: Perform 3 sets of 8 repetitions (2-3 min recovery between sets) Progression: • Increase load • Deadlift from the ground • Jump explosively from the bottom position (hang clean pull)
Dead-leg step-up 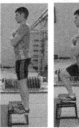	• Stand on a low box (~30 cm) or step with one foot overhanging the edge • Place hands across chest or straight out in front of you • With the free leg straight and toes pulled tight to shin, flex at the ankle, knee and hip on the standing leg • Maintain ankle, knee and hip alignment on the standing leg • Touch the ground lightly with the heel of the free leg and push down on the box to return to the start position Prescription: Perform 3 sets of 8 repetitions on each leg (2 min recovery between sets) Progression: • Increase box height • Perform with a barbell • Perform a single leg squat (without outside heel touch)
Reverse lunge 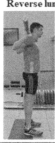 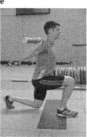	• Un-rack a barbell with an overhand closed grip • Take an exaggerated step backwards so the back foot lands with heel off the ground, and the front leg flexes so hips drop lower than the front knee • Weight should shift to the rear of front foot • Explosively drive off front leg back to standing position Prescription: Perform 3 sets of 8 repetitions on each leg (2 min recovery between sets) Progression: • Increase load • Finish with trail leg raised in front of you • Forward lunge
Press-up 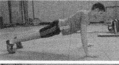 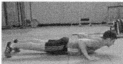	• Place hands directly underneath shoulders and feet hip width part • Raise hips and knees off the floor so there is alignment from heels to shoulders • Maintaining a straight torso position, bend the elbows so they remain close to the body until chest reaches the floor • Push aggressively against the floor to return to start position Prescription: Perform 3 sets of 8-12 repetitions (2-3 min recovery between sets) Upper body alternatives: • Inverted rows • Single arm dumbbell row • Pull-ups • Overhead press

FIGURE 14.3b An example of a basic resistance training session for a runner

et al., 2016) or single-joint exercises (Fletcher et al., 2010) have failed to show a positive effect of resistance training in runners. Multi-joint exercises using free weights are likely to provide a superior neuromuscular stimulus compared to machine-based or single-joint exercises as they demand greater levels of co-ordination, multi-planar control and activation of synergistic muscle groups (Schwanbeck et al., 2009) and they usually require force to be produced from closed-kinetic chain positions. These types of exercise also have a greater biomechanical similarity to the running action and so are therefore likely to provide a greater level of specificity and hence transfer of training effect. An example of a resistance training session is shown in Figure 14.3b.

It is advisable to include a mixture of bilateral and unilateral lower limb exercises in a strength training programme. Bilateral exercises require high levels of absolute force production and place a high demand on the central nervous system to recruit muscle fibres to produce force. Structurally loaded bilateral exercises (e.g. barbell back squat and deadlift) also cause sheering forces to the shaft of bones, resulting in improvements in strength of cortical bone (Lambert et al., 2020), which may lower the risk of bone-stress injury. Due to a phenomenon known as the 'bilateral deficit', most individuals are capable of generating more force, per leg (or the sum of forces on each leg), during single-leg exercises compared to a bilateral equivalent exercise (Dieën et al., 2003). Unilateral exercises therefore provide significant benefits to improving strength via this mechanism (Howe et al., 2014). Depending upon the exercise, single-leg dominant movements also tend to provide a higher level of movement specificity for runners (e.g. step-up, hopping, bounding), which makes them appealing. Specifically, greater activation of key stabilising muscles is required to resist unwanted movements in the frontal and transverse planes (McCurdy et al., 2010; Lubahn et al., 2011), which may provide a greater carryover to running.

An intuitive reason to use unilateral strength exercises is to correct an inter-limb asymmetry that may exist (Howe et al., 2014). Although a large strength imbalance (>15%) between legs has been associated with a higher risk of injury in female games players (Knapik et al., 1991), there is currently no evidence that strength asymmetry is a risk factor for overuse injury in runners. Recent data shows that inter-limb hip abduction (gluteal) strength differences of >9% in adolescent female distance runners are associated with poorer running economy (Blagrove, Bishop et al., 2020). To correct pronounced strength asymmetry, the approach is unlikely to be as simple as using a unilateral dominant programme of strength training exercises. It is possible that an inter-limb asymmetry is caused by mobility or motor control issues, rather than being a neuromuscular recruitment deficiency (Howe et al., 2014); therefore, these should also be assessed so compensatory movement strategies don't exacerbate the issue. Improving maximal strength on two legs has also been shown to reduce inter-limb strength asymmetry (Bazyler et al., 2014), so it is uncertain whether a pure unilateral programme would provide greater benefits in reducing the imbalance.

Summary

Distance running performance is principally limited by the cardiovascular and metabolic systems; however, neuromuscular factors contribute to running economy and maximal sprint speed, which can be enhanced using strength training activities. Overuse injuries in runners are common and can be the reason for quitting the sport. Of concern, low BMD is relatively common in runners, and running alone can be insufficient to stimulate improvements in

BMD. There is currently a lack of direct evidence that a long-term strength training intervention can reduce the likelihood of runners suffering an overuse injury. Despite this, it seems plausible that short bouts of frequent high-intensity strength exercise may lower the risk of developing bony, tendon- or ligament-related overuse injury. Furthermore, stronger gluteal muscles appear to be important for decreasing the chances of some types of overuse injuries, particularly in women. Initially, it is important that runners develop competency in a wide range of fundamental movement skills that can then be progressively loaded. Resistance training using multi-joint exercises should be performed at least twice per week and prioritised over plyometrics and explosive resistance training when the volume of running training is relatively high. Both bilateral and single-leg exercises offer benefits to runners; therefore, a combination of both should be incorporated into strength sessions. As part of a concurrent approach to the prescription of strength training, plyometric exercises should also be performed alongside resistance training, but initially in low volumes. As the competitive season or a targeted event approaches, resistance training volumes can be reduced and more explosive work prioritised on at least one occasion per week. The timing of strength training around running sessions is dependent upon the training status of the runner and their other lifestyle commitments. Wherever possible, runners should separate running and strength training by >3 hours within the same day, and leave > 24 hours after a strength training session before a high-intensity running session is attempted.

15

SPECIFIC CONDITIONING TO REDUCE INJURY RISK

Stuart Butler

Highlights

- Improving the strength of a muscle or specific structure is unlikely to alter running biomechanics but may enable tissues to withstand greater volumes of loading, thereby reducing injury risk.
- Conditioning exercises should be prescribed with a specific adaptation in mind that considers the primary function of biological tissues that are injured or vulnerable to injury.
- For the injured runner, conditioning programmes should aim to load the athlete using alternative 'off feet' methods and re-condition the injured tissues for a successful return to running training.
- Running drills, low-level plyometrics and mobility exercises (e.g. hurdle walkovers) should form an important part of a runner's conditioning routine and can be incorporated into pre-session warm-up routines.
- Targeted conditioning exercises should aim to develop the capacity and strength of structures around the foot and ankle, knee, hip and trunk using a volume-driven approach initially that progressively increases in intensity (load) over time.

Introduction

Prevention is said to be better than cure; however, the skill and art of running and load management within a technical framework are complex. Injury prevention is the panacea, but it may be better to view injury avoidance as a 'risk management strategy', with athletes and coaches agreeing on a shared plan to manage the risk. Based upon an initial screening and assessment of load capacity (see Chapter 7), a priority list of objectives and goals should be agreed within a training cycle/race plan. Identifying 'must do's', 'should do's' and 'could do's' provides a simple system to organise a program at any given time based upon the results of screening and an athlete's injury history. It is also worth considering what an athlete would do if they are unable to run for a period of time, i.e. a list of areas that could be developed if the opportunity arises.

It is apparent that increasing tissue strength does not alter the biomechanics of an athlete, but it may provide the tissue with more tolerance to load, thereby decreasing risk of injury. Loading specific structures and tissues is key; however, it is important to be aware that any additional (and possibly unnecessary) training designed to decrease injury risk is also adding to the total load the athlete experiences and may therefore inadvertently increase the risk of injury! It is also imperative that the global 'health' of an athlete is considered. If an athlete is not sleeping well, is highly stressed, and their performance markers are down, it might not be the appropriate time to add injury minimisation exercises. It is also important to consider the age of a runner: younger athletes tend to get more knee and bone injuries, whereas older runners experience a higher number of tendon and calf pathologies (McKean et al., 2006). This research in combination with data obtained from screening and assessments can help to guide specific exercise selection.

In Chapter 14 (Figure 14.1), it was explained that exercises can be placed on a movement specificity continuum with various running training sessions at one end and resistance training and conditioning exercises at the other. Based upon the principle of training specificity, it is therefore important that the wide variety of single joint isolated exercises designed to increase tissue capacity are also channelled into loaded movements and plyometric training. The aim of this chapter is to examine some of the global exercises that can be undertaken to reduce injury risk and how they can be coached. The chapter will also provide examples of isolation exercises that aim to increase tissue capacity.

Specific Tissue Considerations

Before appropriate exercises can be selected with the aim of improving a runner's performance and lowering risk of injury, it is important to remember the primary function of various tissues and structures (see Table 15.1). Muscles are responsible for the generation of force; tendons connect muscle to bone and are capable of storing and returning large amounts of elastic energy; bones provide the skeletal integrity and structure for the muscles and tendons to generate force; and ligaments connecting bone to bone are responsible for maintaining stability and providing proprioceptive feedback. This is a perhaps a slightly simplistic view as none of these structures work in isolation; however, when selecting an exercise stimulus to generate an adaptive response, it is important to recall the function of the specific tissue. For example, if a runner has a history of 'rolling' their ankle, targeting the ligamentous tissues around the ankle that provide passive restriction and proprioception must be considered, but also the strength of the musculature around the ankle and hips.

There is no such thing as a bad exercise for an athlete. The key is in the rationale and thought process behind each exercise, which changes depending upon the goal of the athlete and the available time. The principles of variety and progression, like any training programme, must also be applied. Often athletes will try to focus on their specific weaknesses and challenge themselves with tasks they have previously not excelled at; however, care must be taken to ensure that goals are achievable as persistent failure can lead to de-motivation. It is therefore sensible to include some exercises that an athlete is good at, as well as those they are trying to improve, which is far more likely to keep them engaged with a plan. It can also be highly motivating to provide an athlete with the knowledge to progress (advance) and regress an exercise to empower them to adapt within a session in response to their global health.

TABLE 15.1 Summary of the primary function of specific biological tissues and the focus of exercise activities to achieve adaptation

	Primary role	*Exercise activities*
Muscle	Force production	Specific loading
		Endurance to strength
Tendon	Elastic energy storage and release	Eccentrics/plyometrics
Bone	Structural integrity	Resistance training (high load)/plyometrics
Ligament	Balance/control	Proprioception

The Injured Runner

Even when injured, the main aim of a rehabilitation plan should always be to keep runners running. Therefore, wherever possible, running load should be modified before using the option to take an athlete 'off their feet'. If it is not possible for a runner to continue some light running, in addition to specific rehabilitation, it is important to 're-condition' tissues for the demands of running by providing a suitable stimulus to the structures that will be loaded during gait. Moreover, continuing to maintain the total training load during periods of injury using alternative exercise (i.e. other aerobic exercise modalities and conditioning work) will continue to provide some load to maintain tissue homeostasis. Specifically, it has been shown that during running the plantar flexors produce forces equivalent to eight times body weight, the quadriceps five times body weight and the hamstrings and hip flexors two times body weight (Dorn et al., 2012). These data suggest that even if an athlete is not running, they need to sufficiently load these muscle groups with more than body weight exercises to adequately prepare their tissues for the stresses they will encounter during running. In the case of severe injuries (e.g. grade 3 strains and sprains, bone fractures), where limbs are immobilised, significant muscle atrophy and strength occurs within a few days of complete rest (Gao et al., 2018). Compared to skeletal muscle, tendons are notoriously slow to adapt (Kjær et al., 2009) and respond more favourably to consistent cycles of loading. Therefore, wherever possible, it is important to continue to load tendons (with external resistance) whilst not running to adequately prepare the tissues for when the athlete returns to running.

Flexibility and Mobility

Whether runners should stretch regularly or not has been debated and discussed by coaches and athletes for decades. For every activity, joint, and individual there is likely to be an 'optimal' level of flexibility for performance and function. For distance running the optimal joint range of motion for most individuals is likely to be at the stiffer end of the stiffness–compliance continuum. In general, there appears to be an inverse relationship between flexibility and running economy (Gleim et al., 1990; Craib et al., 1996; Jones, 2002; Trehearn and Buresh, 2009; Hunter et al., 2011), suggesting that being less flexible (up to a point) is beneficial for running economy. Furthermore, chronic regular static stretching has little effect upon running economy (Shrier, 2004) and does not appear to reduce the risk of overuse injuries (Baxter et al., 2017).

Short term (as part of a warm-up), the scientific evidence indicates that a passive stretch, held for > 60 sec, allows an individual to achieve a greater range of motion at that joint, however the effect is short-lived and lasts only a few minutes (Behm, 2018). It also appears that long-duration (> 60 sec) static stretching decreases explosive power output for a short period of time (Behm et al., 2016). The reality is that runners are highly unlikely to hold a stretch for long enough, or with significant force to induce an effect, and passive stretching is therefore simply a part of their routine and psychological preparation. Moreover, recent findings demonstrate that when included as part of a warm-up routine, short duration (< 60 sec) static stretching does not impair strength and power performance (Blazevich et al., 2018) or running economy (Allison et al., 2008). Short duration static stretching can therefore be included as part of a warm-up routine in recreational-level runners, due to the positive impact of regular stretching on long-term flexibility; however, in high-performing runners, static stretching should be avoided due to the negative effects that have been reported on subsequent physical performance (Chaabene et al., 2019).

There is a strong argument that runners should utilise a more dynamic mobility (e.g. leg swings, walking lunge, squats, hurdle walkovers, etc.) and specific running drills to best prepare the body for running. Dynamic mobilisations exercise not only improves mobility through movement patterns akin to running, but can also improve posture, enhance intermuscular co-ordination and activate key muscle groups. Eccentric loading through wide ranges of movement can also increase mobility, so resistance training exercises can be used as a 'two-for-one' in terms of exercise prescription. There are several areas where specific joint restrictions or loss of mobility can be a risk factor of injury, and these will be highlighted within their respective anatomical locations later in the chapter.

Balance (Proprioception)

Balance is a highly complicated task-specific skill that can be developed but must be appropriate to the desired outcome. Better results have been shown by utilising postural tasks rather than an athlete on an unstable surface (Brachman et al., 2017); therefore, it is recommended that balance should be considered dynamic postural control, and hence must be trained accordingly. During periods of rapid growth around puberty, or injury, balance may deteriorate and need to be re-trained. It may be wise to try to keep the training exercises similar to running movement patterns, such as high knee holds or hurdle walkover drills with a medicine ball overhead. Ball throwing exercises can also be utilised and should progress from simple tasks (e.g. catching a ball whilst standing on one leg), to more complex (e.g. varying the height of the catch), and then to tasks with multiple stimuli (e.g. catch turn, land, receive a different ball). The balance challenges should be progressive by moving from slower to faster speeds, and with increasing reliance on decision-making.

How to Load

The principles of strength training were outlined in Chapter 14 and enable criticality around the specificity, overload and progression of any exercise that an athlete undertakes for the purposes of reducing injury risk. Running drills that are prescribed for specific adaptations can also form an important part of an athlete's remedial work by providing a specific loading stimulus and improving the skill of running. Drills can be used to increase the number of low-intensity plyometric foot contacts in a session or by slowing the running action down to challenge an individual's balance and coordination. Each category of running drills can be prescribed for multiple different reasons, but the way they are coached, and the specific focus

TABLE 15.2 Muscle contraction types, their common use in injury risk reduction and exercise prescription

Contraction type	Muscle action	Tempo	Sets and reps	Common use
Concentric	Muscle shortens	3 sec up, 3 sec down	3–5 sets 4–12 reps	Muscular strength Muscular endurance
Eccentric	Muscle lengthens under tension	10 sec down (lower phase)	3 sets 4–20 reps	Tendon loading
Isometric	Muscle static	30–45 sec holds	5 sets	Tendon pain inhibition/ building high-load tolerance

of each drill, drives the adaptation. The exercises described later in this chapter move from global exercises to more specific exercises, which may suit those runners with limited time and/or provide greater focus.

When prescribing exercises, the mode of muscular contraction also needs to be considered and how this influences the outcome of a specific exercise in the context of prehabilitation/ rehabilitation (see Table 15.2). It is also wise to discuss pain during and after exercise, especially in runners with a history of injury or a present pathology. Low levels of pain (0–3 out of 10) during exercises are acceptable; however, this should settle to baseline levels within 24 hours and changes can be examined over time.

The Lower Limb

Specific global loading of the entire lower limb may be best achieved by utilising running drills to create specific adaptations and provide technical feedback. Common running drills include A and B drills; A drills largely focus on the early-swing phase leg recovery action and stability during mid-stance; and B drills emphasise the late swing phase recovery action with correct 'paw back' and positioning of the foot strike relative to the hips. A-skips mimic the high knee drive and dorsiflexed ankle position associated with recovery of the swing leg, landing on the same foot before 'skipping' onto the other foot. B-skips again emphasise the high knee drive but add more knee extension before pulling the ankle rapidly back towards the ground under the hips, before skipping onto the opposite foot. Dribbling drills involve taking normal running steps through a reduced range of movement and more pronounced ankle dorsiflexion (flat foot ground contacts). Dribbles are often described as being ankle, calf or knee focused depending on the specific goals. Ankle dribbling drills involve taking very small steps, with the ankles dorsiflexed, minimal knee lift (stepping over ankles), and emphasis on ground contact. Ankle dribbles are a great drill for conditioning the foot for ground impact. Calf dribbling drills incorporate more knee lift (stepping over mid-calf) and should encourage the exchange (switch) of legs whilst maintaining ankle dorsiflexion. Again, this is great for conditioning the foot and ankle to be elastically stiff and strong. Knee dribbling drills have a higher knee lift (stepping over knees) and encourage hip and glute strength to maintain postural control and push through the floor. Straight legged running (or scissors drill) are also a useful way to reduce the braking forces using a long lever as an athlete's foot touches down at ground contact.

Figure 15.1 displays the main technical points for the A-skip, which can each be modified or emphasised using different variations of the drill to achieve a desired adaptation. By slowing the drill down and turning it into an A-walk, balance is challenged, which will likely improve the ligamentous stability at the ankle. If the drill is sped up with shorter ground contacts,

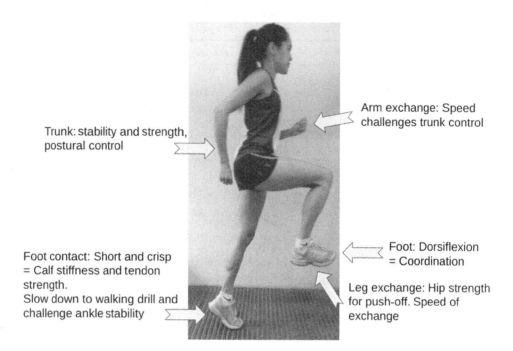

Arm exchange: Speed challenges trunk control

Trunk: stability and strength, postural control

Foot: Dorsiflexion = Coordination

Foot contact: Short and crisp = Calf stiffness and tendon strength.
Slow down to walking drill and challenge ankle stability

Leg exchange: Hip strength for push-off. Speed of exchange

FIGURE 15.1   Main technical points for coaching the A-skip drill

elastic energy storage capacity in the Achilles tendon is challenged, which can be progressed further by turning the exercise into plyometric bounding.

Hurdle walkovers provide another opportunity to develop coordination and balance whilst challenging the lumbopelvic complex. Simply stepping forwards and sideways over a hurdle (adapted to an athlete's height and mobility) encourages postural control and hip mobility, and it develops specific muscular strength around the hips. As with many of the drills, by slowing hurdle walkovers down to emphasis control, stability will be challenged. Moving from a running arm action to positioning arms overhead will provide a greater challenge to the trunk musculature, and speeding up the drill will develop rhythm and add a plyometric component. Modifying the drill so a runner spends more time on one leg before switching (e.g. forward two hurdles, back one hurdle) increases time under tension, so it overloads strength endurance to a greater extent. Finally, raising the height of the hurdles if it becomes too easy will challenge an athlete's hip mobility.

As previously discussed, global running skills can be used to develop adaptations; however, specific exercises provide the overload required for tissue adaptation based upon the required needs of the athlete. A key point that is often overlooked is the timing of prehabilitation/ rehabilitation sessions within a training week. Bone, ligament and tendon tissue responds best to brief bouts of high-intensity activity performed at high frequency (Bailey and Brooke-Wavell, 2010; Bohm et al., 2015; Baar, 2017). This does not mean athletes cannot train between bouts of loading, but it is important to consider how exercise sits alongside the programme of specific exercises. Ideally, any tendon loading exercise should be undertaken 4 hours before running, and hard runs/sessions should be on the same day as tendon loading. The exception to this is when tendon loading is introduced to a programme and a lower weight and higher repetition range is used initially (see the case study in Box 15.1). It usually takes at least a month for a tendon to display noticeable adaptation (Bohm et al., 2015) and they may require 3–4 months to settle after an injury.

For each key area we will provide coaches with a key exercise, a regression (easier) and a progression of the exercise. This is not an exclusive list; there are many exercise variants, and a great deal of this will depend on the individual athlete and their needs. The key question should always be, what tissue(s) do we need to load, and how are we going to achieve this?

The Growing Athlete

As discussed in Chapter 19, the young growing athlete needs special consideration. During puberty, adolescent athletes are likely to develop traction apophysitis (also known as 'growing pains') during growth spurts. These may limit performance and, in terms of developing a long-term athletic development strategy, need to be handled appropriately (with the guidance of a suitably qualified professional) to allow a child to continue participating in sport. Clinically, these can be described as the muscle and tendon pulling at the bone (usually illustrated by a tug on a jumper – no damage to the jumper, but the wearer of the jumper will be aware the jumper is being pulled). As a normal process, there is uncertainty around why some young athletes suffer more than others, but this is not a self-resolving condition and needs appropriate management/ guidance. These pains often occur in the heels (Severs) or knees (Osgood Slatters or Sinding Larsen Johansson syndrome) but can also occur at the hip (proximal rectus femoris), adductor or hamstring insertion. These issues require careful management as pain will inhibit strength and gradual/progressive loading is required through the structures to enable the athlete to perform their expected training loading. It may be wise to use isometric (static) versions of appropriate exercises for pain reduction and to apply some loading, before progressing to eccentric contractions. This should then further be progressed into landing drills and plyometrics before a return to running. It should be noted that during this time athletes may become slightly less coordinated, and balance will suffer. This is an ideal time to develop good running mechanics using walking drills and hurdle walkovers. This should be overseen by a suitably qualified practitioner and should include reassurance, education and empowerment (Esculier et al., 2018).

Bone-Related Injuries

Bony injuries exist on a continuum from periosteal inflammation to stress fractures (Table 15.3). However, it is important to recognise that not all bony pain leads to a stress fracture. Bone

TABLE 15.3 Stages of bony injury and common symptoms associated with each stage

Stage of bony injury	Common symptoms
Periosteal inflammation	
Inflammation of the outside of the bone	Diffuse pain, usually along the surface of a bone. Tends to settle with rest.
Bone marrow oedema	Worsening pain, may be present at rest or during activity (+/− swelling).
Stress fracture	Localised pain present with any weight bearing. Aggravated by impact and may include night and pain at rest.

stress injuries are caused by the load applied to the bone, exceeding the bone's ability to tolerate that load. Bones are constantly adapting, with cells that build bone and cells that remove bone working concurrently to respond to the demand placed upon the bone. In a colloquial sense it is logical to think of bone cells as a building crew who build bone, and a demolition crew who take the old bone away. In simple terms, any bony reaction is due to either the builders not working quickly enough or the demolition crew working too quickly, and this balance can be influenced by numerous factors. If a bone struggles to remodel at the required rate, then a 'stress reaction' may develop.

Whilst Table 15.3 does not provide an exhaustive list of signs and symptoms, diagnosis of a bony injury needs to reflect the context of each individual athlete and their training load. If an athlete has rapidly increased their running load and it is suspected that they may not be fuelling appropriately, a cautious approach is required and the bone pain should be fully investigated. The relative energy deficiency in sport (RED-S) syndrome is covered in Chapter 18, and whilst not every athlete who gets bony pain has RED-S, it is worthwhile to think holistically about the individual. Warden and colleagues (2014) provide a clinical commentary on the *Management and Prevention of Bone Stress Injuries in Long-Distance Runners*, which is an excellent resource for those wishing to better understand this area. It also provides some guidance that not all bone stress injuries are equal, and there are specific areas that may be deemed more high risk compared to others (Table 15.4). All bone stress injuries should be followed up by an appropriately qualified professional, especially in the young and developing athlete.

The best strategy to prevent bone stress injuries is to have a well-conditioned, well-fuelled, well-loaded athlete. An adolescent athlete who does not sleep at least 8 hours per night has a 1.7 times greater risk of injury (Milewski et al., 2014) and improving sleep quantity may help to decrease the risk of bone stress injury (Finestone and Milgrom, 2008). Dye (2005) coined the phrase 'envelope of function' to describe the homeostatic balance that exists between loading and tissue capacity. If the load (either in sudden and high magnitude or low and repetitive) exceeds the capacity of a tissue, then injury is likely to occur, leading to a decreased capacity in that tissue (Dye, 2005). Athletes tend to try to return to their previous load too rapidly, which again, causes them to break down with the same injury. In order to build an athlete's capacity and lower injury risk, there is a need to gradually increase the envelope of function using supramaximal overload that is sufficient for each individual athlete. Strength training can help to increase tissue capacity and has been shown to decrease injury rates compared to other types of low-level conditioning, e.g. stretching and proprioceptive balance training (Lauersen et al., 2014). As runners tend to possess higher bone mineral density than endurance athletes from non-weight-bearing sports and non-active individuals, it is important that the magnitude of loading is high and exposures brief (20–40 reps per day) to drive further bone adaptation (Umemura et al., 1997; Turner, 1998).

TABLE 15.4 Areas considered high and low risk for bone stress injuries in long-distance runners

High risk for bone stress injuries	*Lower risk for bone stress injuries*
Femoral neck	Medial shin
Foot (navicular/5th metatarsal)	Fibula
Tibia	Pelvis
Talus (ankle bone)	Heel (calcaneus)

Source: Adapted from Warden, Davis and Fredericson (2014).

Where to Focus Conditioning Efforts

Perhaps the most frequent reason given for injury is not stretching enough, and yet there is little evidence to support this theory (Yeung et al., 2011; Lauersen et al., 2014). Clinically, asymmetries in flexibility around the calves (knee to wall test – see Chapter 7), anterior hips (Thomas test), and glutes (medial rotation) are certainly worth monitoring. Individual variation in muscle recruitment patterns has been observed during running gait. However, it is clear that the gluteals, quadriceps and calves are active during stance (Chumanov et al., 2012; Dorn et al., 2012). The quadriceps appear to be the muscle that provides the largest contribution to the stance phase of gait, and the calf complex provides the greatest contribution to propulsion (Hamner et al., 2010; Dorn et al., 2012). Gait assessment (Chapter 13) may also help guide coaches and athletes towards where their key conditioning focus should be.

Individual Anatomical Sites and How to Optimally Condition

Calf Complex

Collectively known as the plantar flexors, the calf complex is responsible for large force generation during the propulsive phase of running. As running speed increases, stride length and frequency also increase, and ground contact time decreases. Therefore, the faster we run, the stiffer and stronger the plantar flexors need to be. Up to 7 m.s^{-1} (25.2 km.h^{-1}), the plantar flexors play an important role in generating vertical force to increase stride length (Dorn et al., 2012). At running speeds faster than 7 m.s^{-1}, the plantar flexors still have high levels of force generation but are not able to shorten quickly enough, so the hips and glutes act to increase stride frequency. Furthermore, when running at 4.45 min.km^{-1}, the plantar flexors produce forces in excess of eight times body weight, quadriceps approximately five times body weight and hips and hamstrings two times body weight (Lenhart et al., 2014). For most runners, the calf complex is therefore an obvious area to target for both performance and reduce of injury risk.

Plantar Flexor Assessment

The following tests are commonly used to assess function and capacity in the calf complex:

- Mobility – Knee to wall (lunge) test: see Chapter 7. Measure the distance from the big toe to the wall when the foot is flat on the floor and the knee is touching the wall. Check for asymmetry of no greater than 1 cm and distance should be greater than one third of foot length.
- Capacity failure – calf capacity test (straight leg and bent knee): see Chapter 7. At a rate of 1 second up, 1 second down, perform as many calf raises, first with a straight knee and then with a bent knee. Aim for within 10% of the opposite leg.
- Plyometric capacity test – side hop test: hopping side to side over two markers (tape) 30 cm apart, aiming for as many as possible in 30 sec. Males should target >55 reps; females >43 reps (Gustavsson et al., 2006). Compare side-to-side symmetry.
- Single leg explosive strength – hop height: standing on one leg with hands placed on hips; hop as high as possible. Use *My Jump* smartphone application to assess height.

Complete Calf Exercise: Skipping or Hopping

Can be utilised by using double or single leg variants aiming to increase duration for endurance and/or hop height for power.

> Gastrocnemius: Single leg calf raise (Figure 15.2)
> Regression: Double leg calf raise/static single leg hold.
> Progression: Weighted single leg calf raise.
> Add variety with: Double leg mini bounces progressing to single leg, skipping.

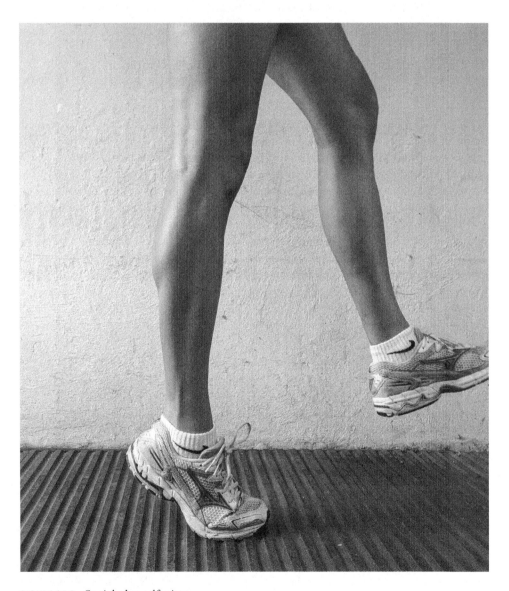

FIGURE 15.2 Straight leg calf raises

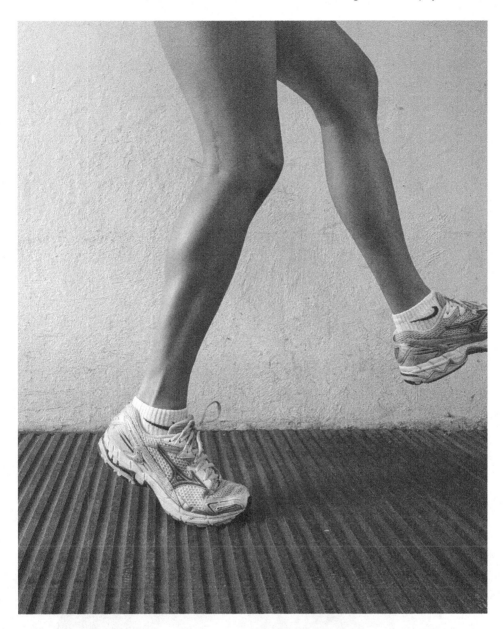

FIGURE 15.3 Bent knee calf raises

Soleus: Single leg bent knee calf raise (Figure 15.3)
Regression: Double leg bent knee calf raise/static single leg hold.
Progression: Weighted single leg bent knee calf raise.
Add variety with: Bent knee mini bounces progressing to single, skipping.

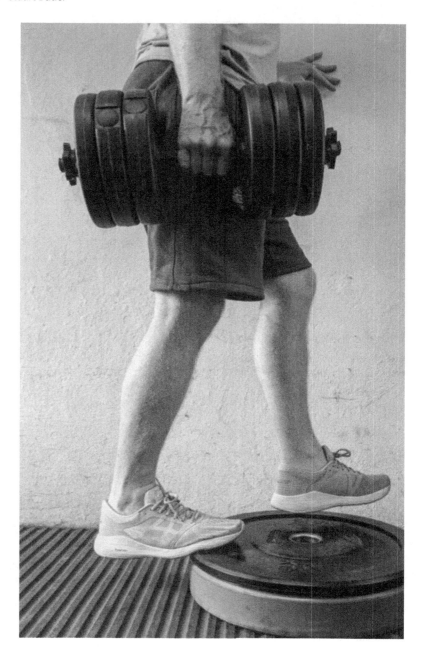

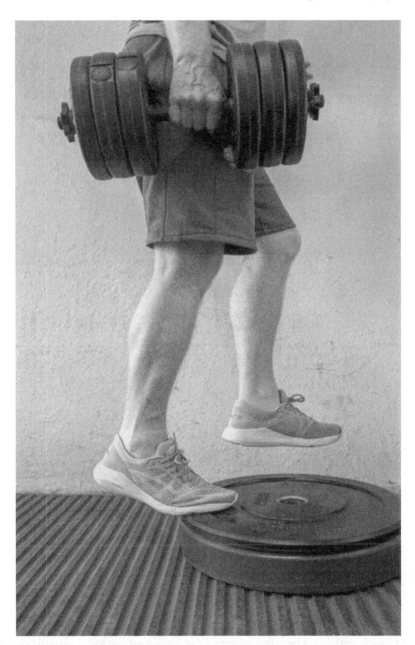

FIGURE 15.4 Weighted calf and Achilles tendon loading. Athletes may wish to consider only going to parallel, and going full range of motion should be used as a progression

Source: Adapted from Warden, Davis and Fredericson, 2014.

Achilles tendon loading: Calf raise on step (Figure 15.4)

Action: Eccentric (slow 3–10 sec lowering) loading going from tip toes to heel hanging below the level of the step. Progress from double leg to single leg.

Regression: Remove step to perform eccentric lowers to floor to decrease Achilles load or isometric (static) holds (>30 sec).

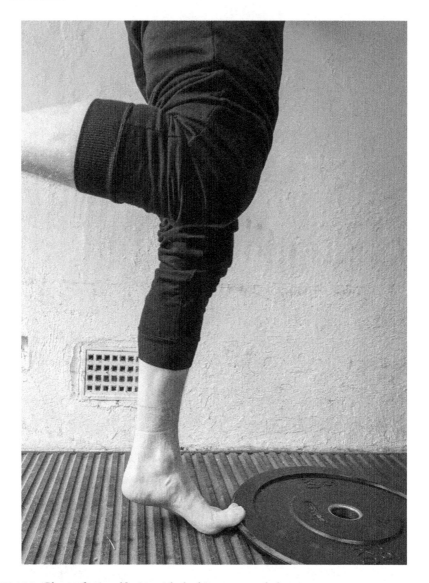

FIGURE 15.5 Plantar fascia calf raise with the big toe extended

Progression: Add weight (e.g. backpack, hold dumbbell) and slowly lower.
Add variety with: mini hopping, bilateral progressing to single leg, walking/running drills.
Plantar fascia: toe extended calf raise (Figure 15.5)

This connective tissue extends across the sole of the foot, and often causes pain towards the heel. The plantar fascia helps to propel the foot forward during ground contact and toe-off. It should be considered a tendon and developed accordingly.

Action: Eccentric lowering with big toe pulled up (usually supported by a rolled towel).
Regression: Isometric holds with toe pulled back and heel off the floor (approximately one inch) and held for >30 sec.

Progression: Add weight or perform off a step to increase range of motion.
Anterior shin (Tibialis Anterior): seated toe raises (Figure 15.6a)

The tibialis anterior muscle decelerates the foot prior to ground contact and therefore is best trained eccentrically.

Action: Seated on a chair or bench with weight plate positioned on the foot; pull toes upwards.
Regression: Perform seated on floor with band anchored away from body.
Progression: Increase weight, decrease repetitions.
Add variety with: Walking on heels progressing to running drills with emphasis on ankle dorsiflexion.
Medial shin (tibialis posterior): Eccentric calf raises on a decline board (Figure 15.6b)

The tibialis posterior eccentrically resists pronation (arch lowering) of the foot and is commonly associated with 'shin splints' (medial tibial stress syndrome).

Action: Same as calf raise with emphasis on eccentric slow lower phase on a decline board (with the inside of the shin facing down the slope).
Regression: Isometric/eccentric lowers to floor squeezing a ball between heels.
Progression: Add weight to decline board lowers.
Add variety with: Emphasise turning the foot in, and slowly (eccentrically) turning back out.
Lateral calf (peroneals): Eccentric calf raises on a decline board (Figure 15.6c)

The peroneals are responsible for everting (turning out) the foot but also have an eccentric role in stabilising the foot.

Action: Eccentric lowers on a decline board (with the inside of the shin facing up the slope).
Regression: Isometric/eccentric lowers to floor with slight duck feet.

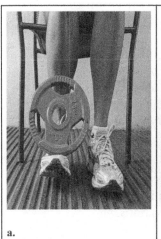 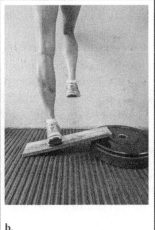 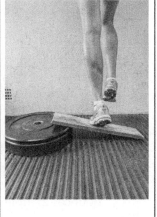

a.   b.   c.

FIGURE 15.6a-c Exercises for conditioning the anterior shin (a), medial shin (b) and lateral shin muscles (c)

Progression: Add weight to decline board lowers.

Add variety with: Emphasise turning the foot out, and slowly (eccentrically) turning back in.

Proprioception (Balance)

Action: Challenge postural stability by standing on one leg and performing a ball throw-catch drill or transfer weight from side-to-side.

Regression: Double leg postural challenge.

Progression: Plyometric (jumps) with change of direction and/or unexpected nudge.

Add variety with: Depth jumps and twists and turns; running change of direction drills.

BOX 15.1   CASE STUDY: 40-YEAR-OLD MALE RUNNER WITH RIGHT ACHILLES TENDINOPATHY HISTORY*

Present symptoms: Mild morning stiffness, slightly stiff at the start of a run but eases off. Full training and undertaking all sessions. No other changes to established training plan.

Outcome: Single leg calf raises to failure at a rate of 1 per second. Right 36 reps/Left 50 reps.

Goals: Pain-free running.

Tendon-specific rehabilitation plan ('Must do'):

If sore, perform 5 sets × 45 sec holds with heel approximately 2" from floor (+/– weight).

3 sets × 20 reps slow eccentric lowers (10 sec) from tip toe to floor daily (>4 hours before running) for 2–4 weeks with the aim to build capacity.

Progress to 3 sets × 20 reps (10 sec lower) eccentrically off a step daily.

Progress to weighted lowers (i.e. 5 kg in a backpack). As weight goes up, decrease the reps. 3 sets × 15 reps, 3 sets × 10 reps, 4 sets × 6 reps, etc and allow extra rest, i.e.: exercises on alternate days.

Aim for 2 sets of 4 reps with heavy weight every 72 hours.

General lower limb ('Should do'):

Plantar flexor strength – Calf raises and soleus raises.

Plyometric progressions from double leg mini bounces, single leg mini bounces, double leg high bounces, single leg hops, etc.

Supporting rehab ('Could do'):

Glute strengthening plan including but not exclusively – side plank, bridges, crab walks, single leg RDL, clams.

Add on to sessions:

A-skips – emphasising ground contact and to provide side-to-side comparison.

Hurdle walkovers – postural and lumbopelvic control.

Review Outcomes: Single leg calf capacity test Right vs. Left. Hopping side to side (as many as possible in 30 sec) comparison right vs. left.

*Diagnosis from suitably qualified professionals with all other potential causes excluded and the athlete having a clear understanding of the pathology. Rehabilitation plans are uniquely specific and should be a collaboration of all those supporting an athlete.

Foot

The foot works primarily to transfer force. The Achilles functions as a spring to store and return elastic energy, and the plantar fascia on the sole of the foot acts with the big toe to work as another spring. Much debate exists over the role of foot type, and whilst little consensus exists, it may be better to acknowledge that there is little that can be done to change it. Orthotics and shoe type only act to shift the focus of loading; however, this approach may be required only in some runners at specific times. High arched rigid feet are very stiff springs and the force gets pushed up into the Achilles and shin bone. A flatter foot may be more flexible and place more demand on the supporting musculature (calf, medial and lateral shin muscle groups) and will need a slower increase in loading or extra support through the running shoe.

Rotation on the Spot (Barefoot)

Action: In standing on one leg, rotate in a full circle by slightly rocking from heel to toe and across the arch of the foot.

Regression: Toe curling on the spot.

Progression: Low-grade plyometrics.

Add variety with: Performing in sand.

Knee

The following tests are commonly used to assess function and capacity around the knee:

- Single leg squat test: perform as many single leg squats to and from a chair continuously.
- Vertical jump testing (see Chapter 7).

Quadriceps strength is known to be a risk factor for knee-related pathology; therefore any gain in force producing capability will likely reduce injury risk and improve running economy.

Squat exercise (see Chapter 14).

Regression: Wall squat (pain-free position) trying to use a duration of > 30 sec holds.

Progression: Single leg squat

Add variety with: Step-ups (concentric), step downs (eccentric), hops and skips, box jumps.

Hips (Anterior)

The front (anterior) of hips and the ability to flex the hip are often overlooked and are a common site of injury in adolescent runners.

Reverse Nordic exercise (Figure 15.7)

> Action: From a kneeling position and pivoting from the knees, move slowly (10 sec) backwards towards the heels, keeping shoulders, hips and knees aligned (no lower back hyperextension).
>
> Regression: Slow squat to a chair with minimal ankle bend, taking 10 seconds to lower to chair.

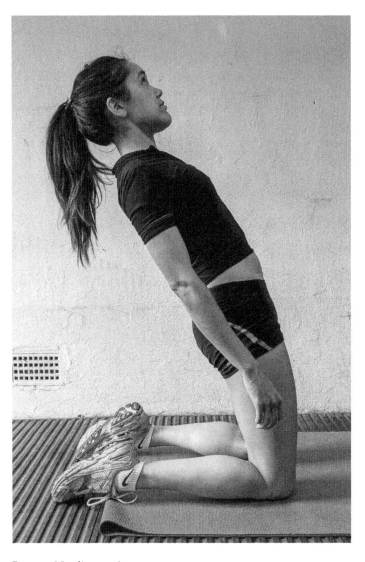

FIGURE 15.7   Reverse Nordic exercise

Progression: Weighted reverse Nordic (holding weight to chest).

Add variety with: Single leg step-up, step downs, single leg squats.

Abdominals

The 'core' has received a great deal of attention over the past decade, and it might be wise to just think about it as two sets of muscles: deep muscles that have a stability role and more superficial muscles that act as the prime movers. Most multi-joint general exercises (e.g. squats, step-ups, lunging, jumping, etc) will always involve the abdominals. Based upon this, it is questionable whether isolation exercises for developing specific muscles within the trunk are necessary for non-injured runners. Three categories of exercises tend to be used for this purpose, and may have utility in runners who suffer from low back pain: deep stability exercises (i.e. Pilates), contraction moving exercises (e.g. sit-ups) and anti-rotational exercises (i.e. stiff trunk with weight moving side to side or resisted perturbations). No one type of exercise is superior to another, and it is always good to evaluate function and build an athlete's individual program based upon their needs.

Side plank with dynamic hip flexion (Figure 15.8)

> Action: Lie on your side supporting your body weight with forearm (elbow directly under shoulder) and feet. There should be alignment between shoulders, hips, knees and ankles. Flex top leg towards chest, maintaining a stiff trunk and bottom leg position.
> Regression: Side plank on knees (Figure 15.8).
> Progression: Single leg stand moving a resistance band across the body.
> Add variety with: Pilates, variety of standard sit-ups and leg lowers, dynamic wood chops with weight.

Gluteals

A great deal of focus has been placed on the role of 'glutes', whether the deep intrinsic gluteal muscles that stabilise the hip, or the gluteus maximus which acts to propel an athlete

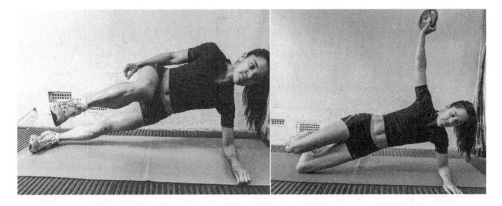

FIGURE 15.8 Long lever side plank with dynamic knee flexion (left) and short lever side plank (from knees) with upper body stimulus (right)

forward during late stance phase. Research suggests that improving glute strength may not influence running mechanics (this potentially needs gait retraining) but may offer some injury resistance due to increased muscle capacity (Willy and Davis, 2011, 2013; Baggaley et al., 2015) and improve running economy (Blagrove et al., 2018a). Multi-joint single leg exercises such as step-up, single leg glute bridges and lunging patterns produce the highest levels of muscle activation in both the gluteus maximus and intrinsic gluteal muscles (Reiman et al., 2012; Neto et al., 2020) and so should be prioritised in exercise selection. Even bilateral multi-joint exercises such as glute bridge, squats, deadlifts and hip thrusts develop very high levels of activation in the gluteal muscles compared to isolation-type exercises such as clams, side lying leg raises and prone (face down) position leg raises (Reiman et al., 2012; Neto et al., 2020).

Iliotibial band (ITB) pain/syndrome is often thought to be a knee pathology. It is painful around the knee, but the force is transferred by the ITB from the gluteals. The ITB itself has a high tensile strength and can't be stretched, but it has pain receptors, which is why pressing or rolling it hurts but does little to change the length. To alter the load around the knee (via ITB) careful evaluation of the hip mobility (especially medial rotation) and pelvic drop (Trendelenburg's sign) should be undertaken to prescribe mobility or strengthening exercises. Bulgarian split lunges (foot on bench behind) should be in a program as they condition both the front leg (strength) and the rear leg to the shearing forces of the ITB. The exercise can be advanced by bringing the rear foot closer to the glutes (increased knee flexion), adding weights or progressing to staggered stance plyometric jumps.

> Gluteus maximus: Hip thrust (Figure 15.9)
> Action: Position shoulders across a chair or bench and knees at a right angle. Place a plate or bar across the hips. Starting with knees, hips and shoulders aligned, lower the hips down until they reach just above the ground and return to the start position.
> Regression: Glute bridge with resistance band (Figure 15.9)
> Progression: Step-up
> Add variety with: Adding weight, single leg deadlift, single leg squat.
> Intrinsic gluteal muscles (gluteus medius/minimus/piriformis, etc.): Side plank (Figure 15.8)

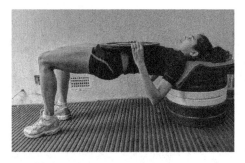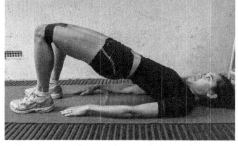

FIGURE 15.9 Start position of the hip thrust exercise (left) and top position of the glute bridge with resistance band (right)

Regression: Side lying abduction (leg raise).
Progression: Side plank with weight.
Add variety with: Hip drops/hitches (off of a step), clams, deadlifts.

Adductors

The adductors are used to stabilise the hips during the stance phase of running and act as a hip extensor during late stance (push-off).

Copenhagen adductor bridge exercise

Action: Same as the side plank exercise but with top foot only positioned on a low bench, with bottom leg hanging free.
Regression: Adductor bridge from knee off bench/chair/box.
Progression: Weighted adductor bridge.
Add variety with: Squats, sumo squats, lunges, lateral lunges.

Hamstrings

Higher levels of hamstring muscle strength have been associated with decreased injury rates and increased force production during locomotion. Runners need to build capacity and subsequently develop specific strength required for their own needs/deficits. Proximal hamstring tendinopathy is a common pathology in distance runners, with a similar aetiology as Achilles tendinopathy. The tendon attaching the hamstrings to the pelvis becomes thicker and stiff, sometimes limiting performance. Whilst little scientific research presently exists outlining how to manage this injury, the use of eccentric loading appears to be beneficial.

Nordic hamstring exercise (Figure 15.10)

Action: Kneel down with ankles anchored by a partner or fixed object. Maintaining alignment between knees, hips and shoulders, lower hips and torso forward slowly towards the ground. Avoid any flexion at the hips or through the spine.
Regression: Band-assisted Nordic hamstring exercise.
Progression: Weighted Nordic hamstring exercise.
Add variety with: Arabesques, long lever hamstring bridges, Romanian deadlifts.

Upper Body

The upper body should not be neglected as the running arm action counter-balances rotations through the trunk caused by forces generated by the legs. The upper limb can be conditioned specifically by practicing running drills and performing hurdle walk-overs. It may also be prudent to add some upper limb exercises to general conditioning routines. For example, during a step-up, a shoulder press could be added, or a side plank could include holding a weight in the top arm (Figure 15.8).

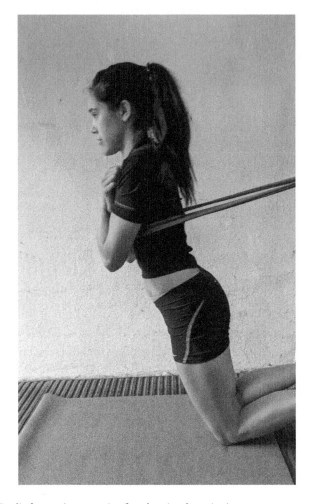

FIGURE 15.10   Nordic hamstring exercise (band–assisted version)

BOX 15.2   EXAMPLE CIRCUIT FOR DISTANCE RUNNERS WITH A MUSCULAR CAPACITY FOCUS

Conditioning Circuit (2x Per Week)

> Calf raises (Straight and bent knee)
> Squats
> Hip hitches
> Step-ups
> Plank
> Side plank
> Banded Nordic hamstring exercise
> Skipping

Start with body-weight resistance and 3 sets of 20 reps on each exercise. Over time, lower the repetitions but add resistance (e.g. 3 sets of 12 reps plus 5 kg; 3 sets of 6 repetitions plus 12 kg, etc).

Warm Up Drills (at the Start of Interval Training Sessions, 2x Per Week)

Hurdle walkovers (forwards and sideways) 6–8 hurdles
A-Skips 30 m
B-Skips 30 m
Scissor runs 30 m

Focus on building up the volume and skill initially (2–4 sets per exercise), progressing to increasing the speed and force of contraction.

Summary

Improving muscle strength and capacity does not necessarily affect gait or running movement patterns. It is more commonly thought that these adaptations provide the tissues with an increased tolerance to the load experienced during running, and runners are therefore less likely to be injured. Runners should think carefully about the holistic total load they experience before high volumes of 'extra' work are introduced. An under-fuelled and stressed athlete with a poor sleep pattern is significantly more likely to get injured and recover poorly. This chapter has offered sensible start points for a runner to start conditioning exercises; however, it is important that athletes 'buy in' and understand the benefits so they can be empowered to make sensible decisions around their loading and progressions. When a runner develops an injury and is off their feet, adapting exercises to maintain loading and muscle strength (and maybe even gain strength) is important so they can return to the sport without re-injury. This chapter is not a definitive list, and there are many ways to achieve the same results, but conditioning exercise prescription needs to consider an athlete's training age and injury history to provide the best plan for each individual. The plan should be athlete-centred, focusing on long-term athletic development, and decisions should involve all parties. Prescription of exercises should use an adaptation-led approach that targets key tissues and utilises the best stimulus to achieve positive changes to the integrity of that tissue.

PART III

Specific Issues and Populations

16

TRAINING MONITORING

Mark R. Homer and Charles R. Pedlar

Highlights

- Monitoring tools allow runners to estimate the point on the fatigue-recovery-compensation curve that they are on, and therefore determine whether long-term training stimulus is inadequate, appropriate or potentially damaging.
- Basic tracking of training load (volume, intensity, frequency) with metrics such as distances/durations, training impulse, rating of perceived exertion, blood lactate and heart rate should form the basis of consistent monitoring.
- Subjective monitoring tools, such as a strong coach-athlete relationship, mood profiling and perceived stress, can be as effective as objective physiological measures at detecting changes in acute and chronic training load; however, it is important responses are accurate, honest and recorded consistently.
- Female non-hormonal contraceptive users are encouraged to track their menstrual cycle length to provide an indication of adequate energy intake.
- Blood and saliva biomarkers offer an objective means of monitoring the physiological response to training load and recovery; however, these should be taken regularly and interpreted with suitable expertise to ascertain 'normal' variation for individual athletes.
- Decisions on when to use monitoring tools should consider factors such as the point in the training programme when measures are taken, the degree of disruption caused, cost and whether measurements can be taken reliably.

Introduction

Following the First World War, running training underwent an accelerated evolution. Pioneers like Paavo Nurmi and his Finnish colleagues blended increasing volumes with interval training on their way to dominating middle- and long-distance running at the Antwerp and Paris Olympics of the early 1920s. Nurmi trained and raced with a stopwatch in his hand in order to pace his running and distribute his effort equally. No doubt this also helped him to monitor the short- and long-term effects of his training as he prepared for performance. This is arguably one of the first instances of athletes using an external variable to inform their running. Now, the handheld-stopwatch has been replaced with a powerful wrist-borne computer with more processing power than the Apollo 11 control room that successfully guided men to the moon and back. We now have the ability to monitor both internal and external metrics of training load and health to comprehensively quantify the responses to discrete and extended phases of training.

This chapter will initially discuss *why* monitoring is important, and the principles that can be followed in order to use monitoring effectively in a running context. It will then delve into the various types of monitoring tools available to athletes and coaches including heart rate monitoring, blood lactate, rate of perceived exertion, sleep, menstrual cycle, blood biomarker and questionnaires. It will provide advice on how to include them in a periodised programme. Finally, it will explain the potential pitfalls in a now-crowded running technology market and what the future may hold as hardware/software applications, sports science techniques and data analysis continually evolve. We will focus on markers of health, training and physiological adaptation. It is beyond the scope of this chapter to discuss more technical running components such as gait analysis.

Why Monitor?

The benefit of a training stimulus is related to its dose. Too little and there will be little-to-no effect, too large and the influence may be damaging rather than beneficial (Figure 16.1a). Athletes must train in the 'Goldilocks zone' where volume (duration and intensity) must be 'just right'. This is dependent on several factors, including the aim of the training session, the level of athlete fatigue and psychological factors, to name a few. Borrowing a term from the world of toxicology, the theory of hormesis explains how the benefit of a substance (i.e. training) is related to its dose (reviewed by Calabrese, 2018). In theory, administering the optimal dose appears simple, but the variables that affect an athlete's responses to training are individual, varied and constantly changing – making hormesis a moving target (Peake et al., 2015; Pingitore et al., 2015).

The primary goal of any training programme is to improve performance while protecting (and potentially enhancing) the physiological and psychological well-being of an athlete. Responses and adaptations follow the well-reported (if oversimplified) general adaptation model (Figure 16.1b) where a training stimulus is followed by a period of fatigue and adaptation to allow the body to better cope with the demands of subsequent exercise. Through progressive overload, adaptation leads to improvements in the determinants of running performance (Figure 16.1b, example A). Conversely, a weak stimulus that fails to cause adequate fatigue, coupled with excessive recovery, will not provide sufficient overload and result in a stagnation or regression in performance (Figure 16.1b, example B). An excessive stimulus, with insufficient rest, will not allow supercompensation and result in under-recovery and further complications in time, if not addressed (Figure 16.1b, example C). There are several ways in which monitoring tools can be utilised to assist decision-making in this process, described here.

Record Keeping

Fundamentally, tracking training load (duration, intensity and frequency) provides quantification of what an athlete has actually done. This is the starting point for any analysis or discussion before any detail or nuance is added. It allows for simple comparisons to be made

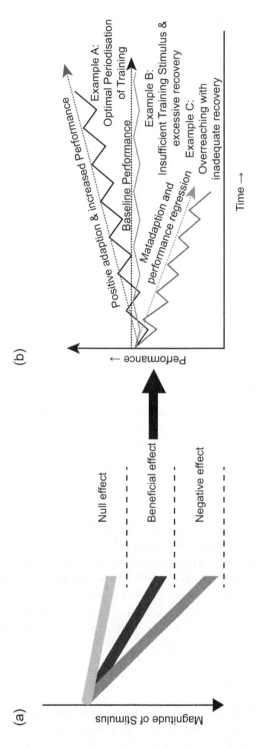

FIGURE 16.1 The acute and chronic hormetic response to exercise training. Monitoring can help identify which trajectory the athlete is following

between phases of a programme for different individuals or season-to-season changes. Data collection should be consistent and accurate to facilitate analysis. Incomplete data sets can render comparisons useless, and any changes made should align with historical information.

Accurate Delivery of a Prescribed Programme

By adding additional metrics such as zone distribution (via speed, heart rate, rating of perceived exertion [RPE], etc. detailed later in this chapter) the coach or athlete can compare planned training with executed training. This is an important distinction that should not be taken for granted – regardless of whether a programme is considered to be working or not. A major predictor of athlete success is the completion of the planned training programme (Raysmith and Drew, 2016). If a programme has not been followed with some degree of completeness, it is difficult to make evidence-based changes to future iterations of a programme.

Reducing Guesswork and Bias

Through consistent monitoring, coaches and athletes can reduce the risk of confirmation bias, the tendency to look for information that supports previously held beliefs. Considering all potentially confounding variables allows for changes in performance to be explained accurately. For example, wind conditions may have a significant effect on a training effort and should be incorporated into the analysis of split times. Ignoring such information could result in misjudging progress (positively or negatively).

Avoiding Injury and Illness

Much of the recent focus of training load monitoring, particularly in team sports, is related to minimising the training that is lost to injury and illness, with the ultimate goal of predicting such incidences in order to manipulate programmes to avoid them. In a group of 33 international track and field athletes, monitored over a 5-year period, (Raysmith and Drew, 2016) demonstrated that completing 80% of planned training weeks led to a seven-times higher probability of achieving a performance goal, and training availability accounted for 86% of successful seasons.

Calculation of acute and chronic workload ratio (ACWR; Gabbett, 2016) in order to balance training-phase to training-phase changes in volume and intensity have become popular in some sports; however, this has yet to be rigorously tested in a distance running setting. The ACWR can be applied to running training with relative ease due to the reduced variables at play in comparison to sports with a larger range of training modalities. It is widely accepted that sudden or abrupt changes in training load should be avoided, and this metric may provide an objective means of avoiding large step changes that may increase the risk of injury (Gabbett, 2020).

Research and Development

The effectiveness of novel interventions is difficult to quantify in an athletic environment. The number of confounding variables that can affect performance, such as current training load, sleep, mental fatigue, etc., make attributing the effect of different variables difficult. A routine training monitoring approach can be used to isolate the impact of a new piece of equipment or performance supplement. For example, a reduced heart rate and rate of perceived exertion at a given running speed, with a new intervention applied, would provide evidence of efficacy.

How to Monitor

Having discussed *why* we monitor factors affecting running performance and some principles that should underpin the process (see Table 16.1), we now consider the tools available to a coach or athlete to collect relevant information related to running performance.

Subjective vs. Objective

Monitoring can be subjective (e.g. a reflection of an individual's feelings or opinions), objective (quantifiable data) or a combination of the two. Subjective data have long been a tool of

TABLE 16.1 Principles of monitoring

Principle	Considerations	For example
Accuracy	How close to the actual value is the measurement you have made?	A GPS watch will not always record the length of a 400 m running track accurately.
Validity	How does the monitoring tool relate to performance? Is what you are monitoring a determinant of performance?	A lower heart rate at a given running speed suggests improved running economy, a variable known to be a determinant of endurance running performance.
Reliability	How repeatable is the result of the measurement you have made?	If you measure blood lactate in the same way several times, you will expect a certain variability in the result. This variability needs to be acceptable for the measurement device to be deployed.
Consistency	Are you controlling related variables to isolate what you want to measure and attribute change to it?	Time of day. Running surface and footwear. Weather conditions (temperature, humidity, wind).
Discretion	Athletes may react differently if they are being 'tested'.	Heart rate may increase if an athlete is anxious about being tested.
Time frame	What is the time frame for the period of monitoring? Set a time frame for a monitoring intervention. Stop and review.	Monitoring an athlete through several microcycles of training will likely yield improvements in the variables measured, but these cannot go on improving forever. Planning monitoring over a set number of microcycles avoids stagnation. A variable such as sleep quality need not be measured continuously if sleep quality is good.
Targeted	Can you isolate key variables that are determinants of health and performance?	A routine blood test provided by a general practitioner might not measure variables related to athlete performance.
Analysis	How you are interpreting the information you are collecting? Are you using appropriate statistical analysis? Are changes in your data meaningful?	If the change in blood lactate measured on two separate occasions is not greater than the measurement error of the device, it may not be a meaningful change.

the coach whether consciously or not. An understanding of individual athletes' behavioural responses to a stimulus can be used effectively to monitor and adjust training load. Examples can range from a coach using their relationship with the athlete and their experience to assess mood and asking 'How do you feel?' to structured, more formal questioning. At the risk of stereotyping, sport scientists are more comfortable at the more quantifiable end of the subjective-objective data continuum, where reassurance is found in numbers and facts rather than in feelings and emotional responses.

Objective data are generally more straightforward. The collection of quantifiable data allows for a more 'black and white' approach to analysing progress and change. In the academic world, statistical measures of 'significance' have traditionally been used to assess the likelihood that a change or difference is due to chance, rather than a true difference in outcome between groups or interventions. While useful for large groups in clinical conditions to report 'trends', such tests are reliant on average data and can be misleading in their clear-cut 'difference or no difference' reporting methods.

Cross-over exists between subjective and objective monitoring. The use of objective questionnaires requires athletes to provide quantifiable scores for markers of health and recovery. In a systematic review of objective and subjective measures of athlete well-being, changes to acute and chronic training load were detected by markers including mood disturbance and perceived stress more sensitively than immunity, inflammation and muscle damage measures with little consistent association between the two types of assessment (Saw et al., 2016). The following section highlights some key objective and subjective markers and their strengths and limitations.

Individual Variation and Statistical Considerations

In athletic performance (and many other fields), individuals respond differently to stimuli. A programme that works well for one runner may be less effective for another and be detrimental for somebody else. The same goes for recovery, elements of nutrition and the myriad of related interventions available to athletes. Therefore, it is important to look beyond the average response and examine the variation within it.

When scrutinising athlete data, it is important to consider what the smallest meaningful or worthwhile change in a variable is, and account for the measurement error of a monitoring tool alongside it. Some equipment has a higher test-to-test variability than what would be considered a worthwhile change in a metric, suggesting that differences in results cannot be attributed to improved performance.

For example, a handheld blood lactate monitor (discussed in the next section) with an overall measurement error of 3% could report an actual value of 4 $mMol.L^{-1}$ as anywhere between 3.88–4.12 $mMol.L^{-1}$, with this range growing as the lactate value increases (e.g. at 10 $mMol.L^{-1}$ the range could be 9.7–10.3 $mMol.L^{-1}$). Such variation could mask a meaningful change in the blood lactate response to exercise and affect the identification of thresholds used to prescribe training intensity and track adaptation. More 'reliable' errors do exist that lead to equipment consistently over or under reporting a result.

Specific Monitoring Methods

This section covers specific monitoring tools that can be used to quantify training, recovery and general athlete health. A range of objective and subjective markers are discussed.

Volume and Intensity

The total training load experienced by runners comprises volume (duration or distance) and intensity. The physiological impact of a given training mileage (volume) at a high intensity will be markedly different to the same mileage at a lower intensity. Ground reaction forces increase linearly with running speed, resulting in greater musculoskeletal damage, and metabolic rate is higher at faster speeds, resulting in greater substrate use. The increase in substrate use is non-linear and causes an exponential rise in blood lactate with a linear increase in exercise intensity. Attempts have been made to derive a single summary statistic that captures total load, and the most well established is the TRaining IMPulse (TRIMP), which is the product of time and intensity (typically measured with heart rate). The original TRIMP formula accounts for the non-linear increase in blood lactate (Banister et al., 1991) by using intensity zones, to avoid a disproportionate weighting from lower intensity exercise, using the following formula.

$$\text{TRIMP} = \text{duration (mins)} \times \frac{\left(Exercise\ HR - resting\ HR \right)}{\left(Maximum\ HR - resting\ HR \right)}$$
$$\times \text{weighting factor based on blood lactate}$$

An individualized TRIMP (iTRIMP) that was specifically validated in runners (Manzi et al., 2009) moved away from using average heart rate and fixed constants in the calculation, replacing them with values derived from an individual runner's plotted lactate curve (see section below) to create a more precise iTRIMP value. Greater weekly iTRIMP values were related to greater improvements in running speed at fixed blood lactate values, 5,000 m and 10,000 m running performance (Manzi et al., 2009).

Rating of Perceived Exertion (RPE)

The runner's perception of effort is perhaps one of the most informative data points possible, since the brain is adept at bringing together myriad internal signals to judge effort. A scale of Rating of Perceived Exertion (RPE) is a well-established tool for quantifying effort at any point in time. Typically two versions are used: the 6–20 scale (Figure 16.2) or the 0–10 scale (Borg, 1982). The RPE scale has been comprehensively validated. It predicts time to exhaustion well across a range of environmental conditions (Crewe et al., 2008).

To summarise complete training sessions with a single RPE rating, the 'Session RPE' (sRPE) provides a useful single value to summarise the overall effort required. However, it is important to note that sRPE can vary between individuals, and several factors can influence this score including the time after the session that sRPE was recorded, the method of recording (paper vs. electronic tool), and the gender of the runners (Roos et al., 2018). Therefore, applying the principle of consistency (see Table 16.1) is critical.

Global Positioning Systems (GPS)

GPS integrated into wrist watches and smartphones, combined with tracking apps, have revolutionised monitoring of running distance and speed over the past decade, with 90% of regular runners reported to use GPS in the USA (Moore and Willy, 2019). Devices have been shown

```
         6
         7    Very, very light
         8
         9       Very light
        10
        11      Fairly light
        12
        13    Somewhat hard
        14
        15         Hard
        16
        17      Very hard
        18
        19    Very, very hard
        20
```

FIGURE 16.2   Borg's 6–20 Rating of Perceived Exertion scale

Source: Borg (1982).

to be accurate when tested over half-marathon and marathon distances, with greater accuracy reported for wrist-worn devices as opposed to smartphone devices (Pobiruchin et al., 2017). GPS devices facilitate the assimilation of data into software platforms and have revolutionised the ease with which runners can monitor a host of metrics and easily share them with others.

Heart Rate

As a determinant of cardiac output, heart rate monitoring provides an indicator of cardiovascular workload. With successful adaptation to training, a lower heart rate will be evident at a comparable speed (or a faster speed for a comparable heart rate), as a clear indicator of improved running economy. Heart rate is also increased in the presence of several other stressors, including psychological stress, thermal stress and the presence of illness. Additionally, there may be some fluctuation in heart rate according to circadian rhythm (time of day) or stage of the menstrual cycle. Therefore, heart rate provides a global physiological 'stress' marker.

Chest strap heart rate monitors are well established as an accurate means of measuring heart rate during running. A word of caution: the interval between heart beats (the R-R interval) varies continuously, and the heart rate displayed by a device is a calculated value that may vary by device and according to settings; for example, a 5 sec average vs. a 30 sec average. When monitoring an athlete and comparing data across time, the same devices should be used and the settings kept consistent. Recently, wrist-worn heart rate sensors have become popular as they provide a convenient alternative to the chest strap; however, this comes with a loss of consistency (Pasadyn et al., 2019).

Some key terms to be aware of in heart rate monitoring:

- *Resting heart rate*: the number of heart beats per minute at rest, not affected by recent exercise. This is commonly measured upon waking.
- *Maximum heart rate*: the highest heart rate achieved by an individual during an incremental exercise test, typically lasting between 12 and 20 minutes.
- *Heart rate reserve*: the maximum heart rate minus the resting heart rate.

The variability in heart beats per unit of time as a measure of autonomic nervous system function is used to assess the response and adaptation to training stimulus (among other stimuli). In simple terms, *Heart Rate Variability* (HRV) is a measure of the balance between sympathetic (stress or 'fight or flight') and parasympathetic (relaxation or 'rest and digest') nervous system control. Chronically increased HRV is indicative of parasympathetic tone and associated with increased recovery, while chronically decreased HRV suggests increased stress and potential maladaptation.

Research suggests that HRV can be used to monitor and predict training adaptation in runners (Vesterinen et al., 2013). This can subsequently be used to inform the training process in order to maximise adaptation if interpreted correctly. However, the use of HRV as a marker of overreaching is less well supported (Bellenger et al., 2016). Once restricted to electrocardiogram (ECG) measurement, HRV monitoring is now a standard feature of heart rate monitors and available via smartphone applications, although care should be taken to ensure that tools have been validated before incorporating their use into daily practice.

Blood Lactate

The concentration of lactate in the blood has been used to assess the physiological responses to exercise since the 1970s. Previously reserved for exercise physiology laboratories, advances in technology have led to field-based tests using relatively inexpensive handheld lactate analysers. Blood lactate is an essential by-product of carbohydrate breakdown to produce energy within muscle cells. Far from being a waste product, lactate plays a key role in recycling glucose and regulating substrate utilisation (Brooks, 2018).

Lactate production increases with exercise intensity as muscle fibre recruitment increases – particularly the carbohydrate hungry fast-twitch fibres. This accumulation is actually *in response* to an increase in muscle cell acidosis caused by the build-up of hydrogen ions resulting from the splitting of large amounts of adenosine triphosphate (ATP) to produce energy, rather than the cause. Therefore, concentrations of blood lactate are an 'indirect' marker of energy system contribution and the associated muscle cell acidosis. Directly measuring hydrogen ions in the muscle is invasive and time consuming, requiring a muscle biopsy, and is therefore not suitable for routine athlete monitoring. Blood lactate can be assessed in seconds by the analysis of a pin-prick capillary blood sample and offers a practical surrogate solution.

Lactate can be used to inform training in two major ways. Traditionally, the curvilinear response of blood lactate (as with ventilatory markers) to increasing exercise intensity is used to identify thresholds that signify the transition between exercise intensity domains with different physiological responses (moderate, heavy and severe). These are used to prescribe training intensities, monitor adaptation and predict performance (Newell et al., 2015). A wide range of lactate indices are commonly used to test athletes (see Chapter 6). As a monitoring tool, blood lactate testing has been incorporated into regular training sessions as a means of monitoring the responses to different training intensities. This allows coaches and athletes to make 'in session' interventions to maximise the responses to individual sessions and monitor adaptation over time.

Various tools are available to collect, analyse and process blood lactate information. For a coach in the field, handheld analysers provide almost immediate feedback. Note that data derived from handheld lactate analysers can differ considerably from benchtop analysers, so the data should not be used interchangeably (van Someren et al., 2005). Calculation of exercise thresholds such as the lactate turnpoint can be complex and open to interpretation. However, several tools are now available that calculate parameters using established algorithms based on raw speed, lactate, heart rate and oxygen consumption (if available) data. As with all capillary blood sampling, it is essential that proper procedures are followed to ensure safety, and therefore, it is recommended that a sport scientist qualified to work with blood samples oversees this process.

Critical Speed

As discussed, training intensities derived from laboratory-derived oxygen consumption and blood lactate thresholds are widely used to prescribe and monitor load in runners. The concept of critical speed has more recently been utilised to identify the highest sustainable oxidative metabolic rate using the relationship between running speed and the duration for which it can be sustained (Jones et al., 2019). As a monitoring tool, critical speed can be used to assess changes in endurance and high-intensity exercise capacity (Pettitt and Dicks, 2017). See Chapter 6 for more details on measurement and interpretation of a runner's critical speed.

Body Composition

Body mass and body composition are important determinants of endurance running performance. In a longitudinal analysis of marathon performance, Marc et al. (2014) identified a decrease in morphological indicators such as body mass and body mass index (BMI) associated with faster marathon times over a 10-year period. This is primarily attributable to the influence of body mass on running economy and the influence of body fat on thermoregulation. However, it is important to note that a lower body mass and BMI increase the risk of relative energy deficiency in sport (RED-S), where the balance of dietary energy intake and energy expenditure is compromised and physiological function is diminished – causing disruption to metabolic rate, bone health, immunity and menstrual function (amongst other systems) (Mountjoy et al., 2014). Chapter 18 explores the RED-S syndrome in further depth.

Monitoring body composition is therefore important, but the implications of timing, interpretation, feedback and interventions must be carefully considered. To increase the accuracy and reliability of data, measurements should be consistently taken on waking, fasted and following a toilet visit. Several tools exist to monitor the composition and distribution of body tissue that vary in their practicability, expense and accuracy (Ackland et al., 2012).

Sleep

Sleep is a fundamental process for the maintenance of health and has been widely recognised as a priority for optimum recovery in athletes. The sleep state is characterised by cyclical hormonal and antioxidant variations that facilitate recovery. Endurance athletes may require slightly more sleep than non-athletes; however, there is wide individual variation and no magic number for sleep requirement (Gupta et al., 2017), and some studies have reported poor sleep in athletes compared to healthy controls (Leeder et al., 2012a).

Monitoring sleep is something of a minefield. In order to measure sleep accurately, the gold standard method is polysomnography measured in a sleep laboratory. Various sleep monitoring devices exist that attempt to derive similar information by less cumbersome methods, but at the expense of accuracy and precision. Wearable sleep devices tend to underestimate sleep disruptions and overestimate total sleep time and sleep efficiency. Halson (2019) comprehensively reviewed approaches to sleep monitoring in athletes.

For the distance runner, sleep can be disrupted by travel schedules, altitude, physiological and psychological stress. Monitoring sleep can help to identify a clinical sleep disorder, in which case the athlete should be referred to an appropriate health care professional. There is a risk with sleep monitoring that the athlete becomes worried about the data, and this impacts upon sleep quality! A prudent approach, therefore, might be to establish if sleep is broadly sufficient over a single micro-cycle, then cease the routine monitoring.

Menstrual Cycle

The female menstrual cycle is characterised by significant fluctuations in female hormones, and the most well-known of these are oestrogen, progesterone, luteinizing hormone and follicle stimulating hormone. It has been known for decades that the distinct phases of the cycle can have a significant impact upon aspects of sports performance (Reilly, 2000). The menstrual cycle is strongly influenced by energy availability, such that during phases of heavy training where an energy deficit is more likely, the normal fluctuation in hormones becomes lost. Extended periods with an absence of menstruation are associated with poor bone health (increased stress fracture risk) and a host of other negative outcomes, encapsulated in the RED-S framework (Mountjoy et al., 2018a). It is desirable, therefore, for a female athlete to maintain a regular menstrual cycle, since it is a strong indicator that energy availability is adequate to support training and adaptation. Thus, monitoring the menstrual cycle gives an indication of adequate energy availability to support adaptation to training (see Chapter 18).

Approximately half of all female athletes have a 'normal' menstrual cycle with wide individual variability in the magnitude and impact of fluctuating hormones. Several physiological systems are influenced by these fluctuating hormones. Menstrual cycle symptoms can vary according to the phase of the menstrual cycle and can vary in severity and frequency. In some cases, symptoms can be debilitating and lead to athletes missing training. Tracking symptoms and seeking advice on how to combat these symptoms may therefore be a valuable exercise to help athletes complete their training. Chapter 20 discusses these issues in further detail.

Blood and Saliva Biomarkers of Health

Certain biomarkers lend themselves to monitoring recovery status in athletes, offering an objective tool to help inform training decisions. Identifying short- and long-term trends in biomarker data can help athletes and coaches to balance training load with recovery, maintaining an appropriate hormetic stimulus (see theory of hormesis, described earlier in this chapter), i.e. when to push on and increase training load versus dialling back and focusing on recovery.

Several biomarkers are available for point-of-care testing, using either a small capillary blood sample or saliva sample. These include creatine kinase as a marker of acute muscle damage; c-reactive protein as a marker of inflammation; urea as a marker of protein catabolism, redox biomarkers such as hydroperoxides; and hormones such as testosterone and cortisol. It is important that these biomarkers are measured consistently with an appropriate degree of scientific rigour, for example, standardising the time of day when the samples are collected and ensuring the samples are drawn and processed by a competent technician. An exhaustive list of considerations is beyond the scope of this chapter, but these are covered in some detail by Pedlar et al. (2019).

A word of caution with blood biomarker monitoring: biomarkers should be considered alongside subjective, behavioural and performance information to assist with decision-making. Athletes are often outliers, and we expect to see different data from the general population. For example, with endurance training, fluctuations in plasma volume according to training volume are likely, which influences the haematocrit and haemoglobin results. Establishing what is 'normal' for each athlete is important; see Pedlar, Newell and Lewis (Pedlar et al., 2019), in order to establish individual thresholds. This is the same theory applied in the Athlete Biological Passport, where an individual 'normal' range is established over several observations.

Psychological Status

The value of subjective markers either in unison or in contrast with objective monitoring has been discussed. The Profile of Mood States (POMS) and the Recovery-Stress Questionnaire for Athletes (RESTQ) are two of the more established tools in this field, although others such as the Multi-Component Training Distress Scale (MTDS) and Daily Analyses of Life Demands of Athletes (DALDA) do exist. Also, much simpler methods are often used in the field that have the advantage of brevity but lack depth.

The POMS questionnaire (McNair et al., 1971) requires athletes to respond to a list of words using a Likert scale based on their current feelings. Words are associated with six main emotional states: tension, depression, anger, vigour, fatigue and confusion. A profile is produced to assess changes to the mood state over time. Since its development in 1971, POMS has been used extensively in sport and adapted for length and age of participant in recent years. Several studies have demonstrated a relationship between training load or performance and mood disturbance scores (Beedie et al., 2000). Online tools are available for athletes to self-monitor their mood (Lane and Terry, 2016).

The RESTQ-36-R-Sport is a shortened version of the original RESTQ-Sport questionnaire (Kellmann and Kallus, 2001). It is divided into 12 subscales with 3 'Likert scale' questions for each. Three sub-scales relate to general stress, three to sport-related stress, three to general recovery and three to sport-related recovery covering physical, emotional, behavioural and social factors. These divisions allow for a detailed analysis of an athlete's psychological status, and the questionnaire has been effective in monitoring individuals and teams. A comprehensive analysis (Saw et al., 2016) suggested that the questionnaire was responsive to changes in both acute and chronic training load.

When contemplating a measure of psychological status, a coach or athlete must consider whether a particular tool has been designed for use with athletic populations. Saw et al. (2016) suggest that tools designed for such use are more effective than generic questionnaires. Also, it is worth considering the timing of administration and any burden this places on an athlete. It may be appropriate to use short and simple tools daily that can assess acute changes in status. Anecdotally, the authors have had have found it useful to use daily changes in the response to Likert scale questions including 'readiness to train', 'perceived shape' and 'recovery from previous day's training' administered as part of a morning monitoring test battery in order to assess recovery. Longer more detailed questionnaires such as POMS or RESTQ can be used less frequently, e.g. at the end of training cycles to assess the responses to chronic training.

Monitoring Distribution

Having discussed the *why*, *how* and *what* of useful monitoring for running, it is now worth considering the *when*. Figure 16.3 provides an example of the previously discussed methods of monitoring and how they could be distributed during an example training programme. This timing of monitoring tools depends on several factors, and monitoring should be organised around key milestones in a training programme. Baseline data should be collected and repeated around key interventions including training camps and competitions. The degree of disruption caused by interventions is a necessary consideration. For example, a full laboratory testing profile or haematological analysis can be informative and influential. However, they can also be expensive, time consuming and disruptive to training. A balance must be struck, and such tools used sparingly to avoid impacting on competition preparation.

The sensitivity of a measure influences how often it should be used. For example, as discussed, waking heart rate is a sensitive measure of the accurate response to training which can vary daily. Daily monitoring can encourage acute changes to training in response to fluctuations. In contrast, some measurements can vary due to the influence of extraneous variables. Body weight, for example, can differ by approximately 1 kg on consecutive days due to variations in diet, hydration, menstrual cycle and travel. Monitoring body weight daily and calculating a rolling 5-day average can account for such variation and allow coaches and athletes to account for the 'noise' of misleading individual changes.

ATHLETE CASE STUDY PERSPECTIVE

Andy Baddeley: Olympic finalist (1500 m) and parkrun world record holder

Training monitoring formed a crucial part of my programme when I was competing at my peak. I was lucky enough to have access to top-class physiology support, and my coach and I integrated this into our plan. There were two elements of monitoring that were the most useful for me, namely outdoor lactate testing during my threshold runs, and routine blood testing.

I used the data from lab-based lactate profiling to guide my heart rate zones for my threshold runs, but owing to my gait, I always found that treadmill running didn't accurately reflect my true physiological response to 'real' outdoor training. To this end, my outdoor threshold runs were monitored by taking blood samples before, during (every 2 miles) and after my 6-mile threshold runs. These weekly runs are one of the things that I feel contributed most to my success. I learnt to effectively 'feel' my threshold, and there were periods where I could accurately gauge intensity to within a single BPM without looking at my HR monitor.

This monitoring allowed me to push right up to, but crucially not beyond, my lactate threshold – maximising the benefit I was able to take from those sessions. To compound this benefit, they gave me the confidence to know with certainty that I was optimising my training in a way that I knew it was unlikely my rivals were. As a 1500 m runner, I was able to run a 30-minute 10 km at threshold effort by perfectly fine-tuning this process.

> *My coach and I also used regular blood testing to inform our monthly training plan. I usu-*
> *ally worked off a routine with three hard weeks followed by an easier week, but the blood tests*
> *helped us to avoid pushing too hard if I was run down, and to bring easier weeks in earlier*
> *than we might otherwise have done. There's a very fine line between maximising training*
> *benefit and overdoing it, and as an athlete it can be hard to psychologically justify easing*
> *back. My coach knew me so well, and honesty was such a huge part of our relationship that*
> *he could usually read the signs, but the testing added an extra layer or knowledge to work*
> *from.*
>
> *It's worth saying that I was selective with my monitoring methods, and throughout my*
> *career the only runs I did with a GPS watch were those threshold runs. The rest of my easy*
> *and steady runs were all run to feel, allowing my body to govern how fast I felt like running.*
> *Similarly, on reflection, because I had such extensive data, there were periods where I knew*
> *categorically that I was less fit than I had been previously – something that can be tough to*
> *deal with psychologically. I would advise all coaches and athletes to bear that in mind, and*
> *to use testing selectively, and always with a clear goal. When I knew why we were doing*
> *something, I could handle the results and work out a plan to get to where I needed to be. As*
> *an example, testing simply to confirm that someone is in good shape, at a critical point in a*
> *racing season, runs the unnecessary risk of showing someone they're not quite where they*
> *need to be, without the time to do anything about it.*

Further Considerations

If any monitoring programme is to be successful, the *why, how* and *when* factors discussed earlier must be considered in unison. Through working with athletes and coaches at different competitive levels, the authors have experienced some additional factors that have provided the opportunity for further reflection. In the author's experience, the usefulness of a monitoring programme is dependent on the athlete's perception of how (and if) the data collected are used. Failure to see change based on responses can lead to a reduction in the value an athlete sees in accurately recording information. Poor communication between coach and athlete that fails to explain why, for example, volume or intensity are increased despite fatigue may affect future adherence. It may be that this is what the coach feels is required from a particular block of training, and the athlete must push on to get it done – this must be discussed openly.

Athletes not being honest, accurate or consistent with their subjective ratings can also affect the usefulness of monitoring information. Not wishing to show weakness in a competitive environment where selection is at stake, the misremembering of information and simply forgetting to record information are all possible scenarios for athletes under extreme pressure for long periods of time. The inability to rely on athlete-generated information can lead some coaches to seek additional objective markers at the expense of their athlete's subjective feelings, and a damaging cycle ensues.

The lack of agreement that Saw et al. (2016) identified between certain objective and subjective measures can be interpreted as a positive finding. Athletes will not always be able to accurately report the response that leads to the most effective manipulation of their training programme. Fatigue, life-stress and many other external factors could contribute to ratings of perception that may not influence their responses to a training stimulus. This is where objective markers can be useful. If accurate, reliable and valid, physiological markers may not be

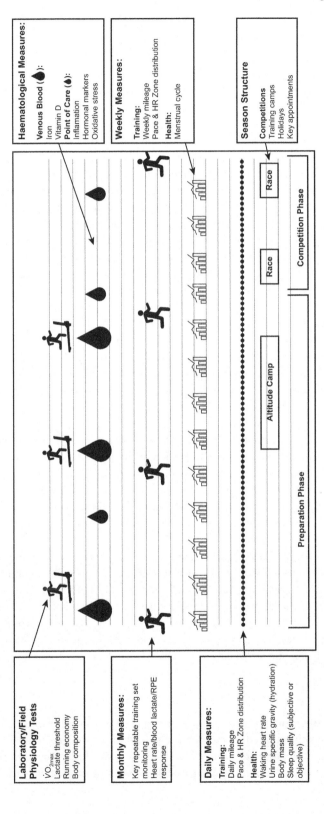

FIGURE 16.3 Distribution of monitoring tools

influenced by the same psychological variables (although they may be affected by different ones) and allow for an isolated look at individual components of performance.

Objective monitoring brings a different set of threats and opportunities. There are clear benefits of using the quantifiable data that have already been discussed; increased insight, visualisation and granular detail. However, such information also increases the chances of confirmation bias where isolated information is used (either consciously or unconsciously) to support an opinion or viewpoint. The risk of 'cherry picking' information that supports a particular narrative is not a new concept, or one that is limited to sports performance.

As technology develops and monitoring tools improve, there comes a point where it may be possible to switch sampling methods or replace a metric altogether. This can lead to difficult decisions for the coach or athlete. Changing the way a particular variable is monitored can make it difficult to use historical data for comparison. It can therefore be tempting to resist change, even though it may improve the usefulness of improved methods. This decision should be based on the risk vs. reward of any potential conversion.

As the amount and quality of incoming data feeds increase, the education provided for those attempting to use it has inevitably fallen behind. While the potential for improved performance through detailed monitoring is clear, the pitfalls of more and more information should not be ignored. Coaches need education to help them interpret the data they are now collecting and communicate its relevance to their athletes. The interaction of different variables must be considered, as using metrics independent of each other can be misleading. With this in mind, numerous platforms are available that attempt to provide a single point of contact for athletes and coaches to summarise training and performance. The cost-benefit balance of such systems should be considered, alongside their flexibility. Platforms are rarely sports-specific and may not cater for all monitoring tools that a coach or athlete wishes to incorporate.

Advances in data management techniques allow numerous data sources to be combined and analysed with relative autonomy. This has led to the production of algorithms that calculate multifactorial models of training adaptation and recovery that have become standard features of health and fitness products in recent years. The reliability and validity of these metrics are not fully supported in the literature, but this has not stopped investigation into the next stage of development – the use of machine learning or artificial intelligence to further improve global athletic performance.

The biological nature of athletic data and the inability to incorporate all the variables that affect a result can limit the usefulness of such modelling. This may be a good thing, as the human ability to make decisions should not be lost. Data should be used to inform decisions, not make them. An all-encompassing objective marker that adheres to all the principles of monitoring listed in Table 16.1 does not exist. Therefore, a culture of trust and honesty between athlete and coach is vital to provide as complete a picture of physiological and psychological performance and well-being as possible.

Summary

In the pursuit of continual improvement, runners require a physiological overload (i.e. a training stimulus), which is followed by an adequate period of recovery to allow for adaptations to take place. Judging appropriate training workloads for individual runners, particularly over long periods of time, can be problematic, particularly when other lifestyle 'stressors' that also cause physiological perturbations are considered. Monitoring tools provide a means of estimating whether a training dosage has been sufficient to cause a fatigue response (acutely), an improvement (in medium–long term) or a negative overreaching response (in medium–long term). Simply recording training load using the distance/duration of sessions, training impulse and potentially heart rate and blood lactate during sessions should form the basis of monitoring for runners. Subjective monitoring tools can be used alongside these to detect whether an athlete is sufficiently recovered or beginning to show signs of overreaching, assuming that reflections are honest, accurate and recorded consistently. In this regard, the importance of a strong coach–athlete relationship cannot be understated. Objective physiological markers taken from blood and saliva samples also provide an accurate way of monitoring stress and recovery, if measures are taken regularly, and profiles for individual runner are generated. Female non-hormonal contraceptive users are encouraged to track their menstrual cycle as this can provide supplementary information alongside energy intake to support training and lifestyle demands.

17

RECOVERY STRATEGIES

Glyn Howatson and Tom Clifford

Highlights

- Ensure the basics of hydration, nutrition and sleep are adequately catered for – no recovery intervention can hope to succeed unless these pillars are adequately met.
- Determine if a strategy is necessary or whether adequate recovery can be attained without intervention.
- Understand the training and competition stressors causing reductions in performance and the delayed recovery before applying the intervention – this will help you choose the right intervention.
- Contemplate the relative importance of short-term recovery and long-term adaptation; consider how the idea of hormesis could be applied.
- The importance of athlete belief in the intervention should not be underestimated.

Introduction

The concept of recovery has been an established ideology of medicine that dates to Hippocrates (c. 460 BC). This idea is based on the premise that the maintenance of physiological balance through rest was central to healing. As years have advanced, the pursuit of improved athletic performance has led to athletes engaging in higher training volume and intensity, leading to the growing interest in exercise recovery strategies. This is particularly important when demanding training and competition schedules make the appropriate balance between physiological stress, recovery and subsequent adaptation difficult to optimise. A successful recovery regimen could lead to: (1) improved physiological adaptation; (2) reduced training- or competition-induced stress; (3) improve recovery times to allow for additional training stimulus; and (4) optimised recovery in periods of competition congestion.

Runners can adopt a huge range of strategies to help improve recovery, such as cryotherapy, compression garments and nutrition. Interestingly, there are many interventions that lack a solid evidence-base and their use is largely stooped in anecdote and hearsay. Importantly, many interventions are only likely to yield modest, but potentially meaningful changes in recovery. However, these can only be realised if the fundamental principles of recovery are well executed; namely, adequate hydration, fuel restoration (with adequate carbohydrate, protein and fat) and good quality and quantity of sleep. This chapter aims to provide a combination of evidence for the fundamentals of exercise recovery, and to further explore some traditional and more contemporary strategies that might be of value to runners.

Principles and Approach to Recovery

Observations of amateur and professional athletic environments show an extensive use of recovery strategies but without a clear need or rationale. For example, it is critical to understand whether insufficient recovery is the cause of a reduction in the capacity to train or compete. Very often, with sufficient time, the body will recover without the need for additional interventions above and beyond the fundamentals of hydration, adequate nutrition and sleep. By having a good understanding of the physiological stress that is induced by training and competition, it is possible to discern what interventions might be of use. Distance running is characterised by a high metabolic demand that is coupled with a high degree of mechanical loading from the constant eccentric loaded contractions (where the muscle lengthens under tension) from repetitive ground contacts. When coupled, these challenges can produce muscle damage and inflammation and can increase the production of reactive oxygen and nitrogen species that cause oxidative stress. In the runner, this can manifest itself as reduced muscle function, greater muscle stiffness that leads to a loss of flexibility, and muscle soreness. If athletes train or compete whilst experiencing these symptoms, it is highly likely their performance will be below par. In addition to competing in a less-than-optimal state, there is an increased potential risk for injury (Howatson and Van Someren, 2008) because of the reduction in joint position sense and reaction time. In circumstances such as these, inadequate recovery is the underlying issue, and therefore identification of a recovery strategy to accelerate and restore function might be necessary. In a conceptual model of exercise recovery (Figure 17.1), the restoration of function will occur over time, but the application of a recovery strategy has the potential to accelerate the return of function to the basal state sooner. This is particularly important during intensified training, and competition schedules where performance at the highest level is required frequently within short time periods.

Getting the Basics Right

Re-Hydration

Most athletes will finish exercise with some degree of fluid deficit, also known as hypohydration (Evans et al., 2017). If hypohydration exceeds 2–3% loss in body mass, aerobic capacity, cognitive function and motor learning can be impaired (Funnell et al., 2019; James, Funnell, et al., 2019a) Thus, if the fluid deficit is not restored following exercise, subsequent performance could be compromised (Evans et al., 2017).

For optimal rehydration, it is currently recommended that 125–150% of fluid lost during exercise (estimated via body mass losses) is consumed in the subsequent hours (Evans et al., 2017). As an example, a 60 kg athlete, who weighs 1.5 kg less following a 90-minute run, should consume 1.75–2.00 litres of fluid in the hours following. This volume should not only restore hydration status but also cover additional losses from sweating and urination during the recovery period (Thomas et al., 2016). However, it is not always practical to weigh yourself

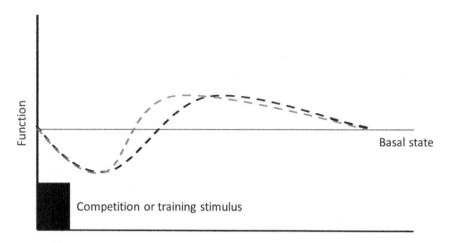

FIGURE 17.1 Conceptual timeline of the recovery process. The dashed black line indicates the timeline of unassisted recovery following training, where in the fullness of time, function is restored to the basal state. If a positive adaptive response is achieved, the basal state will be exceeded, and the target adaptive response can be achieved. If a further stimulus is not introduced to the system, the function will return to the basal state. The dashed grey line illustrates the conceptual introduction of a successful recovery strategy where the return of function is accelerated with no loss in any adaptive response

before and after training or competition to determine your fluid needs. One way to overcome this is to work out your sweat rate (e.g. litres lost per hour) for a given intensity, duration and environment, and then use these data to estimate your body mass losses in future events/sessions in similar conditions (Evans et al., 2017). This is probably necessary only if training or competition is ≤8 hours apart, if you have a high sweat rate (≥1.2 litres per hour) and if the preceding exercise was ≥2 hours. Where possible, fluid should be consumed with electrolytes such as sodium or alongside sodium-containing foods, as this promotes fluid absorption, retention and hence ensures faster re-hydration (Thomas et al., 2016).

Nutrition for Recovery From Endurance Exercise

Carbohydrates

Restoration of muscle and liver glycogen stores is of principal importance to the recovery process. This can be achieved by consuming carbohydrate-rich foods such as pasta, bread, rice and cereals. The volume and timing of carbohydrate intake is largely dictated by the duration and intensity of the completed exercise.

With regards to timing, when recovery between moderate to hard training sessions is limited to ≤8 hours, carbohydrates should be consumed immediately upon the cessation of exercise (Ivy et al., 1988; Moore, 2015). This is to take advantage of the muscle contraction-induced increase in muscle and liver glycogen enzymes that are active immediately in the hours following exercise (Ivy et al., 1988). Glycogen re-synthesis can be optimised further by consuming carbohydrates at a rate of ≥1.2 $g \cdot hour^{-1}$ within the first 4 hours after exercise (Burke et al., 2004; Burke et al., 2017a). If such amounts (e.g., 72 g for a 60 kg athlete) are not available or not tolerable, consuming carbohydrates at a lower rate (0.8 g·hour^{-1}), but alongside dietary protein (0.3 g·hour^{-1}) will have similar effects on glycogen re-synthesis (Van Loon et al., 2000; Burke et al., 2004). After ~4 hours, normal eating patterns can be resumed, as long as sufficient amounts of carbohydrates are consumed for the rest of the day (Burke et al., 2017a). However, what is deemed 'sufficient' depends highly on context, with contemporary recommendations highlighting the importance of periodising carbohydrate intake to match daily training demands (Stellingwerff, 2012; Jeukendrup, 2017). As outlined in Chapter 4, it is currently recommended that for low-intensity or short-duration activities (e.g. technical drills sessions or recovery runs ≤ 60 min) athletes should aim to consume 3–5 g·day^{-1} of carbohydrate, increasing this to 5–7 g·day^{-1} for moderate-intensity training (e.g., 60 min per day), 6–10 g·day^{-1} for longer-duration training (e.g. 1–3 hours of activity over the day) or 10–12 g·day^{-1} in the longest (e.g. 4–5 hours activity over the day) sessions (Thomas et al., 2016).

The glycaemic index (GI) of carbohydrate foods is another important consideration for maximising glycogen re-synthesis following exercise (see Chapter 4). Generally, high GI foods like white bread and jellied sweets are thought to be more effective than low GI foods like wholegrain rice and wholemeal bread at stimulating glycogen-re-synthesis following exercise, owing to the fact they are absorbed more quickly (Moore, 2015). However, if ≥ 8 hours of recovery time is available between sessions, this is less important, as will be discussed.

Glycogen re-synthesis, specifically in the liver, might be further accelerated by consuming carbohydrates that contain a mixture of glucose and fructose (sucrose) post-exercise. Indeed, recent research has shown that post-exercise liver (but not muscle) glycogen repletion is much greater when ≥1.5 g·hour^{-1} of carbohydrates are consumed as sucrose, instead of glucose, following exercise (Fuchs et al., 2016). Most foods contain a mixture of glucose and fructose (amongst other sugars); however, fruit juice and fruits (e.g. apples) contain higher amounts of fructose than other carbohydrates like bread and pasta and therefore should be consumed alongside these foods when glycogen repletion is a priority.

The immediate (≤8 hours) carbohydrate feeding strategies outlined earlier might not be necessary if: (1) the preceding exercise bout was of low duration (≤60 min) and intensity (e.g. recovery run), resulting in minimal glycogen depletion; and/or (2) there are ≥8 hours recovery time available between training sessions or competition (Parkin et al., 1997; Thomas et al., 2016). In either scenario, if, for example, carbohydrates are not consumed until 2 hours post-exercise, and at 0.6 g·hour^{-1}, glycogen repletion rates should not be compromised before the next session (assuming this is ≥8 hours away) as long as the overall amount is commensurate with the per-training load recommendations (e.g. 10–12 g·day^{-1}) previously mentioned (Parkin et al., 1997; Moore, 2015).

Protein

It is well established that endurance exercise is a potent stimulator of muscle protein turnover. This process is the balance between (1) removal or remodelling of structural proteins, a catabolic process typically referred to as muscle protein breakdown (MPB); and (2) the synthesis and accretion of new proteins; an anabolic process typically referred to as muscle protein synthesis (MPS) (Mascher et al., 2007; Moore et al., 2014a; Rowlands et al., 2014). While the net balance between MPB and MPS is critical for muscle repair and remodelling following exercise, it is specifically the increase in MPS (as opposed to decrease in MPB) that is thought to be most fundamental to the repair, remodelling and synthesis of functional muscle proteins

(Tipton and Wolfe, 2001; Tipton et al., 2018). As such, maximising MPS in the post-exercise period should be a priority for all endurance athletes.

Dietary protein can augment MPS and the post-exercise anabolic response (Tipton and Wolfe, 2001; Moore et al., 2014a; Macnaughton et al., 2016). The amino acids that make up protein can be used to repair various structures in skeletal muscle, as well as connective tissue like ligaments and tendons (Beelen et al., 2010; Moore, 2015). In addition, recent research (Townsend et al., 2017) has shown that ingesting whey protein (0.5 g·kg of body mass^{-1}; BM) following exhaustive treadmill running exercise (75% of maximal oxygen uptake) attenuates markers of bone resorption, which could have important implications for improving bone health and ultimately reducing stress fracture risk in endurance athletes.

Current recommendations for optimal post-exercise protein intake are individualised to body weight. In the immediate hours post-exercise, 0.25–0.30 g·kg BM^{-1} of dietary protein (15–18 g for a 60 kg athlete) is likely sufficient to maximise MPS in younger adults (Moore, 2015). In older adults (≥50 years), 24 g for a 60 kg athlete might be required for the same effects due to age-related anabolic resistance (Phillips et al., 2016). Ideally, this first feed would be immediately upon finishing exercise; subsequent feeds, of similar quantities (~0.25–0.30 g·kg BM^{-1}, or 0.40 g·kg BM^{-1} for older adults), should then be repeated every 2–4 hours (Moore et al., 2012a; Areta et al., 2013; Moore, 2015). This pattern of protein intake should aim to equate to ~1.2–1.7 g·kg BM·day^{-1} per day (depending on the number of feeds) and is thought to optimise daily MPS and subsequent tissue remodelling in athletes (Moore, 2015).

Different protein sources have different absorption rates and effects on MPS, and therefore the type of protein ingested post-exercise is an important consideration. Animal and dairy proteins tend to be digested faster and stimulate MPS to a greater extent than non-animal sources (Tang et al., 2009; van Vliet et al., 2015). As such, animal protein such as beef, fish and dairy proteins like whey and casein are preferred to non-animal sources like soy and wheat for maximising post-prandial MPS (van Vliet et al., 2015; Gorissen and Witard, 2018). In the immediate hours post-exercise, whey protein supplements are popular amongst athletes, owing to the rapid absorption and the fact whey contains high amounts of the essential amino acids, especially leucine, that is a potent trigger of MPS (Burd et al., 2012, 2019; Rowlands et al., 2014). However, athletes might be wary that supplements are contaminated with substances banned by the World Anti-Doping Authority. One way to avoid consuming a contaminated supplement is to ensure any supplements are sourced from a trusted manufacturer who can ratify that their product has been batch tested to not contain banned substances. An informed athlete should buy only from manufacturers that are listed on these databases (e.g. 'Informed Sport') and ideally would consult an appropriately qualified sports nutrition professional before purchasing. However, arguably the best way to circumvent these issues is to have a balanced diet that contains the macro-nutrients required to support recovery (see Chapter 4).

Cow's milk is an excellent option for a convenient and very cheap post-exercise recovery drink. Cow's milk is a mixture of whey (~20%) and casein (~80%) protein that has been shown to increase MPS to a greater extent than non-animal sources (Wilkinson et al., 2007). Milk has the added benefit of containing carbohydrates and electrolytes that support re-fuelling and re-hydration goals, respectively (James, Stevenson, et al., 2019b). Furthermore, the current recommended intake of 0.25–0.30 g·kg BM^{-1} of protein post-exercise can be met with ~400–600 ml of semi-skimmed milk. The wide availability of cow's milk, its low cost and its high protein content make it an ideal and efficacious choice for maximising post-exercise MPS and recovery (James, Stevenson, et al., 2019b).

Sleep and Recovery

Sleep is considered integral to psychological and physiological health (Halson, 2014; Watson, 2017). It is widely accepted that part of the function of sleep is to help restore biological homeostasis and central nervous system function. Failure to get sufficient sleep (7–9 hours per night; Watson, 2017) can impair endocrine function, emotion regulation and next-day performance of cognitive and motor tasks, and therefore it plays an important role in optimising function in the next wakeful period (Halson, 2013). Specific to endurance athletes, partial sleep can affect well-being and health and can compromise exercise performance (Halson, 2014; Watson, 2017; Kölling et al., 2019). There is also growing concern that athletes in sleep debt are at an increased risk of musculoskeletal injury (Freitas et al., 2020) that could be attributable to modified immunological responses, where sleep deprivation has been linked to rises in pro-inflammatory biomarkers (Dáttilo et al., 2020). In addition, longitudinal research in athletes indicates that poor sleep is inversely correlated with winning competitions (Brandt et al., 2017; Juliff et al., 2018); thus, it is vitally important that athletes get sufficient sleep to optimise recovery, adaptations and subsequent performance.

Sufficient sleep might be of greater importance to endurance athletes than strength and power athletes as partial sleep loss, in which a few hours are lost per night, seems to have a more pronounced negative effect on aerobic performance than muscle strength. In one example, Chase et al. (2017) examined how sleep restriction affected performance in the day following a heavy training session. A group of well-trained male cyclists (VO_{2max}: ≥60 mL·kg^{-1}·min^{-1}) performed ≥60 min of high-intensity cycling, and resistance exercise followed by a night of normal sleep (~7 hours) or a night of restricted sleep (~2.5 hours). The following morning, muscle soreness and isometric muscle strength were unaffected by the sleep restriction, but 3 km cycling time trial performance was much slower than baseline in the sleep restriction than the control condition (−4% vs. −0.5% slower, respectively). In a further similar example (Rae et al., 2017), power output during a cycling test was impaired in the 24 hours following ~55 min of high-intensity exercise and a night of half normal sleep quantity (3.8 vs. 7.5 hours). The mechanisms behind these negative effects on endurance performance are not entirely clear, but reduced motivation and increased perception of effort has been suggested as likely candidates (Watson, 2017; Halson, 2013; Rae et al., 2017).

Overall, sleep restriction or disturbance will not have a positive effect on performance and recovery, but of course there is likely a high inter-individual variability between athletes (Kölling et al., 2019). Consequently, general recommendations need to be tailored to the individual to determine optimal sleeping patterns (Kölling et al., 2019). Notwithstanding, sleep is undoubtedly important for well-being and health, and thus the most prudent approach, and the one most likely to avoid compromising recovery and exercise performance, is to ensure athletes get 7–9 hours of quality sleep per night and that they feel relatively fresh and ready to perform, especially around competition. For further information on sleep for athletes, the reader is directed to some excellent reviews (Halson, 2014, 2019; Gupta et al., 2017; Kölling et al., 2019).

Contemporary Recovery Strategies

Cryotherapy

Cryotherapy reduces tissue temperature and blood flow with the goal to reduce the inflammation and oxidative stress associated with strenuous exercise, and hence further damage

(Merrick, 2002). Consequently, it has attracted a great deal of attention from athletes to facilitate recovery following challenging training and competition (Versey et al., 2013). It can be administered in a number of ways following exercise; typically for athletes, the most common modes are cold water immersion (CWI) and whole-body cryotherapy (WBC). More recent emerging research has investigated the use of phase change material (PCM) that provides a simpler and cheaper method of cooling than more traditional methods.

Cold Water Immersion

CWI is the most commonly used form of cryotherapy and has also been the most researched intervention. Despite this, the body of evidence is far from conclusive, mostly because of confounding issues that make the picture difficult to decipher. This is largely due to the different exercise modes used, the depth and temperature of the water and the duration and frequency of the immersion (White et al., 2014; Vieira et al., 2016). Most CWI interventions are delivered immediately after exercise at 8–15°C. The CWI intervention can often result in reduced soreness and in some cases recovery of dynamic muscle function (Leeder et al., 2012b), although the data from individual studies are quite mixed, with some showing some a positive effect and others showing no effect. Importantly, for runners, there is a general trend to CWI being more beneficial for metabolically challenging exercise like running, and most studies do not show a negative effect, which is an important consideration when applying any intervention (Leeder et al., 2012b).

Water immersions that are colder than 15°C increase discomfort, decrease the time that can be tolerated (Versey et al., 2011) and do not seem to confer any additional benefits (Poppendieck et al., 2013). This is worth considering, because the magnitude and duration of cooling (particularly for deeper muscles) will depend on the duration of the immersion. As a general guide, 1 minute for every degree of temperature is a good rule of thumb; for example, a 10 min immersion for 10°C and 15 min for 15°C, and so on. Even for longer immersions, it is not clear if the duration of immersion is sufficient to truly influence recovery in a meaningful way, so if feasible, repeated immersions might have additional benefit. Additionally, it is common to see athletes in rubbish bins as opposed to a seated tub; this is because the pressure can be manipulated depending on the water depth and provide the potential added benefit of hydrostatic pressure (Wilcock et al., 2006). The deeper the water, the greater the pressure, which has been argued to enhance vasoconstriction (Gregson et al., 2011; Mawhinney et al., 2013). This was investigated by Leeder et al. (2015) who showed no additional benefit of seated (30 cm depth) versus standing (120 cm) positions in recovery following a muscle-damaging running activity.

It is also worth noting that CWI can be well tolerated by some athletes, but others find it incredibly difficult to deal with, and it can cause undue stress and anxiety. If the latter is the case, the balance between what you hope to achieve from the intervention and the additional stress it causes the athlete needs to be carefully considered. In general, if an athlete believes the intervention to be of little or no benefit coupled with high stress, it is likely to outweigh any potential benefit that might be achieved.

Whole Body Cryotherapy

WBC involves exposing the whole body to very cold air (−110°C to −160°C) for durations of 2–4 min in a chamber that resembles a sauna. Historically, it has been used in Eastern

Europe for treating pathological conditions that display pain, oedema and inflammation. In recent years WBC has gained traction as a recovery tool following strenuous exercise by proposing to reduce inflammation (Banfi et al., 2010; Ziemann et al., 2012), muscle damage (Banfi et al., 2009; Hausswirth et al., 2011; Ferreira-Junior et al., 2015) and soreness (Ziemann et al., 2012). The return of function is not clear, although the evidence suggests that immediate exposure to WBC will likely provide a better chance of a positive effect on function (Hausswirth et al., 2011; Ziemann et al., 2012; Ferreira-Junior et al., 2015), while others have shown no difference compared delayed exposure after the exercise (Costello et al., 2012).

A relevant piece of research for runners evaluated the efficacy of CWI and WBC on performance following a marathon run and showed that WBC negatively impacted the recovery of muscle function compared to CWI, but neither intervention was more or less effective than a placebo (Wilson et al., 2018). In a follow-up study, WBC was found to be more effective than CWI at attenuating soreness and strength following resistance training, but again, neither intervention was more effective than the placebo (Wilson et al., 2019). These studies illustrate that WBC might be less beneficial for running recovery than damaging resistance-type training and therefore the relevance for runners could be questionable. In addition, although there is some promise, the use of WBC is very much for the elite, given that there are very few *in situ*, they are expensive to use and maintain and they require large spaces to deliver the intervention, making it very difficult to administer. Furthermore, studies indicating that WBC might help to reduce soreness could be attributable to an athlete's belief and placebo effects; therefore, the cost-benefit to the athlete should be considered when delivering these sorts of interventions.

Phase Change Material

PCM was developed by NASA in 1975, based on prototype work using liquid cooling garments as a method of passively controlling spacesuit temperature when severe temperatures are encountered. Since then, much of the previous human research on PCM cooling has focused on the temperature-regulating effect (Gao et al., 2010) and cooling effect to elicit thermal comfort from heat strain (Barwood et al., 2009; House et al., 2013). In appearance, PCM looks like a standard ice pack but contains a combination of salt and oils that can be altered to change the freeze point. It can be applied directly to the skin surface and easily accommodated under garments for extended periods to treat large muscle masses in a way that is simple to apply, logistically easier and more tolerable for the athlete. The added advantage is that little additional kit is required; it is portable and practicable.

In a novel application of PCM, researchers at Northumbria University, UK, in collaboration with the Nicholas Institute of Sports Medicine and Athletic Trauma in New York, applied PCM to extend the duration of treatment of cryotherapy in exercise recovery. The research has shown that PCM application, with a freeze/thaw temperature of 15°C, can be applied for prolonged durations (3–6 hours) and have a beneficial effect on recovery from damaging exercise (Clifford et al., 2018; Kwiecien et al., 2018; McHugh et al., 2019). Specifically, dynamic muscle function is returned at an accelerated rate and muscle soreness in the days following the exercise is lower. In a very applied study, where professional footballers utilised the intervention after a football match whilst travelling on a bus from away fixtures, there was improved return of muscle function and reduced soreness (Clifford et al., 2018). In addition, the players reported the intervention to be tolerable, and they believed the PCM to be of benefit. The positive influence of the PCM has been attributable to the extended period of cooling that is possible. Whilst the intramuscular temperature at deeper and superficial levels is comparable to CWI, the ability to cool for longer is vastly extended with PCM (Kwiecien et al., 2019). Although further research into recovery from endurance running exercise is required, PCM does hold some promise and is already being used by many elite athletes with some reported success.

Compression Garments

Compression garments are a category of clothing used to provide mechanical support to limbs. These garments are often graduated, with the greatest pressure exerted at the distal aspect of the limb, reducing in pressure towards the proximal aspect; this creates a pressure gradient. The graduated pressure is suggested to improve venous hemodynamics (Ibegbuna et al., 2003) and assist in the maintenance of fluid homeostasis; therefore, these mechanisms could be helpful for managing swelling and inflammation, thereby enhancing exercise recovery. Manufacturers claim that the garments can improve circulation, attenuate swelling and oedema and, in some cases, enhance performance and improve recovery (Trenell et al., 2006; Kraemer et al., 2010; Bottaro et al., 2011).

The use of compression garments in sport has become increasingly popular due to various claims surrounding their benefits (Hill et al., 2014). However, evidence for the efficacy of compression garments in alleviating symptoms of muscle damage is equivocal with studies both supporting (Jakeman et al., 2010; MacRae et al., 2011) and refuting the use of garments. MacRae et al. (2011), in their descriptive review on compression garments, indicated that discrepancies in findings might be due to differences between studies in the populations, modality of exercise, degree of compression, type of compression garment and duration of treatment. However, a more recent and comprehensive meta-analysis showed that compression garments can reduce muscle damage indices such as soreness and accelerate recovery of muscle function (Hill et al., 2014), but the most positive effects were following resistance-type exercise. A subsequent meta-analysis (Brown et al., 2017) was able to break down all types of exercise and delineate between cycling, running and resistance training. This work showed some benefit in performance from endurance activity like running and improved recovery from running-based activities.

Despite the widespread use of compression garments, the evidence is not overwhelming, but on balance they certainly do not have a negative effect. A question that has arisen from the recovery literature is the discrepancy between study design, compression of the garments and length of administration. This was systematically researched by Dr Jess Hill who showed that commercially available compression garments in general do not exert sufficient pressure, and often fall some distance short of the recommended compression needed for a physiological effect (Hill et al., 2015). This highlighted that many of the previous studies might be invalid because the compression from the garments worn might have been insufficient. In a recent study, custom-fitted garments were used to examine recovery after repeated sprint running and were shown to reduce muscle soreness and improve muscle function in comparison to a control group and 'off the shelf' garments (Brown et al., 2020). Collectively, it seems that the use of compression garments used immediately after running might be of benefit to support recovery, but care should be exercised to ensure the garments are appropriately fitted and provide sufficient compression.

Stretching

Stretching is normally used to increase flexibility and joint range of motion (Weerapong et al., 2005) and is a common practice in sporting environments due to the belief that it can reduce the risk of injury and improve performance (LaRoche and Connolly, 2006; Behm and Chaouachi, 2011). Whilst there is good evidence that stretching can help increase flexibility and joint range of motion, it has also been proposed to be effective in the recovery process to reduce muscle soreness and muscle stiffness (Torres et al., 2007). Several review articles suggest stretching can bring about changes in muscle-tendon length and stiffness and hence improve flexibility (Reisman et al., 2005; Weerapong et al., 2005; Behm and Chaouachi, 2011). These changes could then assist in reducing the negative effects of strenuous training and competition. Some support for this was shown by LaRoche and Connolly (2006) who showed that a 4-week stretching programme was able to maintain flexibility following damaging exercise, although no change in muscle soreness was seen. Likewise, others have observed that an 8-day stretching protocol consisting of three, 30 sec passive stretches of the quadriceps muscle group did not affect markers of recovery; but conceptually, the stretch duration could be insufficient to provide a benefit (Lund et al., 2007). Collectively, the research findings suggest that stretching before or after exercise provides little or no benefit for recovery (Henschke, 2011). Although there is a good rationale for the use of stretching for runners in developing some physical attributes (flexibility) and injury prevention (Barnett, 2006), it is probably of little use in assisting in recovery beyond being part of habitual warm-up, cool-down or stand-alone session activities.

Massage

Massage is a very popular intervention to help support exercise recovery. In fact, there are few athletes at the elite level that do not have a massage therapist to utilise massage as a recovery tool. Despite the obvious widespread use of massage, the supporting evidence is thin in the extreme. Massage has been used in an attempt to reduce muscle soreness from strenuous exercise, although studies have found little or no benefit in post-exercise massage therapies compared to rest only. In a well-controlled study, Smith et al. (1994) showed a significant reduction in soreness when massage was administered 2 hours post-exercise. These significant observations were attributed to a disruption in inflammatory cell accumulation and hence a reduction in pain (Smith et al., 1994). Conversely, Gulick et al. (1996) found the signs and symptoms of delayed onset of muscle soreness were not abated when massage was applied after a damaging bout of eccentric exercise.

It is very difficult to draw comparisons between investigations due to methodological discrepancies in treatment time and the techniques used. Perhaps by examining specific techniques, an effective massage method and duration for reducing symptoms of exercise induced muscle damage (EIMD) might be achieved. In a recent addition to the literature, Monteiro Rodrigues et al. (2020) showed that a short bout of effleurage massage increased blood perfusion and hence showed evidence of improved microcirculation. However, realising these potential physiological changes in athletes is not easy to detect. For example, in a randomised trial of 78 runners, massage was shown to have a small positive effect on thigh pain after training, but there were no performance changes (Bender et al., 2019). There are numerous examples of modest changes in soreness in the literature, but clear physiological benefit is not evident. What is certainly true of massage is that many athletes 'feel' better, which cannot be underestimated. The simple therapeutic armamentarium of 'laying on of hands' can be of benefit to the athlete in supporting recovery.

Foam Rolling

Over the last decade or so, foam rolling has gained enormous popularity in athletic arenas. It is difficult not to trip over foam rollers in strength and conditioning (S&C) facilities, and athletes are often armed with a foam roller during training. There are suggestions, particularly within the S&C community, that foam rolling might increase training efficiency, competition preparation and accelerate exercise recovery. But is there any evidence to support their use, or are they just the Emperor's new clothes? Foam rolling is predominantly used as tool for self-massage where body weight is used to apply pressure to different parts of the body (often muscle and other soft tissue; Pearcey et al., 2015). It certainly is time-efficient and provides an easy and cost-effective intervention that is akin to massage and hence is attractive to athletes; however, the athlete belief in the benefits of foam rollers might actually exceed any physiological benefit. This is not necessarily a bad thing, as long as there is certainty (like all recovery strategies) that it is not having a detrimental effect.

The supporting evidence for the use of foam rolling for recovery is very thin, and there is no consensus on the efficacy of this intervention (Cheatham et al., 2015; Pearcey et al., 2015). The possible benefits are attributed to mechanical, neurological, physiological and psychophysiological underpinnings (Wiewelhove et al., 2019). Collectively, these factors are thought to be influenced by the manipulation of tissue, an analgesic effect, altering blood flow, an increase overall well-being and a potential placebo effect (Phillips et al., 2018). In a recent systematic review with meta-analysis, Wiewelhove et al. (2019) explored the effect of foam rolling on performance and recovery. Only a few studies were identified, some of which were considered of limited quality, which led the authors to suggesting there is no consensus on the optimal duration, pressure and frequency for foam rolling. They showed some benefit of foam rolling conducted before exercise on sprint performance and flexibility. However, with the exception of modest changes in muscle pain, there were no benefits on post-exercise recovery (Wiewelhove et al., 2019). Based on these data, foam rolling does not seem to have any negative effects, but any real benefits in exercise recovery might also be limited.

Dietary Supplements

If recovery time between important training sessions or competition is limited (e.g. ≤72 hours), runners might consider additional dietary supplements to help alleviate some of the symptoms of EIMD. Of the research conducted to date, the category of supplements showing the most promise are the so-called 'functional foods'. These foods typically refer to plant foods that are naturally rich in anti-inflammatory and antioxidant phytonutrients. Because strenuous exercise evokes a transient but robust inflammatory response, which involves the release of reactive oxygen and nitrogen species (also known as free radicals), these cellular processes are thought to contribute, at least in part, to the symptoms of EIMD. Thus, the rationale for consuming these supplements is that they might mitigate some of free radical or inflammatory related damage to structures involved in muscle force production during high intensity exercise (Paulsen et al., 2014a; Reid, 2016).

To date, functional food supplements have shown more promise than the traditional agents (vitamin C and E or non-steroidal anti-inflammatory drugs) purported to aid recovery via these mechanisms (Myburgh, 2014; Lundberg and Howatson, 2018; Marika et al., 2019). Indeed, cherry juice (Howatson et al., 2010; Bell et al., 2015, 2016; Brown et al., 2019), blueberry juice (McLeay et al., 2012), pomegranate juice (Trombold et al., 2010, 2011; Machin et al., 2014) and turmeric (Drobnic et al., 2014; Nicol et al., 2015) have all been shown to help alleviate some of the symptoms of EIMD. For a detailed overview of all the functional foods that have been examined for their potential to attenuate EIMD, the interested reader should consult a recent article on the topic (Bowtell and Kelly, 2019). The rest of this section will discuss only dietary supplements with the most evidence to support their effects as recovery aids following strenuous exercise.

To date, cherry juice has probably shown the most promise for aiding recovery from endurance-type exercise. The benefits of cherries are thought to stem from their high concentrations of phytochemicals, especially anthocyanins, which have potent antioxidant anti-inflammatory effects (Bell et al., 2014; Keane et al., 2016). In a study by Howatson et al. (2010), cherry juice ingestion before and after the London Marathon attenuated markers of inflammation and accelerated the recovery of isometric muscle strength in the 2 days following the race. Subsequent studies confirmed these beneficial effects in endurance cyclists (Bell et al., 2015, 2016). In the latter of these studies, cherry juice ingestion enhanced muscle function recovery in the three days following 110 min of high-intensity cycling exercise. Thus, cherry juice might be a useful supplement to expedite recovery following high-intensity training sessions or long duration races that evoke symptoms of EIMD.

Curcumin, a phytochemical from the turmeric root, has also shown promise as a recovery aid following strenuous exercise. Like cherries, curcumin is thought to aid recovery via anti-inflammatory and antioxidant mechanisms (Drobnic et al., 2014; Fernández-Lázaro et al., 2020). Several studies have shown that curcumin reduces the activity of nuclear factor kappa B, a transcription factor that upregulates pro-inflammatory mediators associated with muscle damage (Thaloor et al., 1999; Sahin et al., 2016). Drobnic et al. (2014) were the first to examine the effects of curcumin supplementation on markers of EIMD. They showed that taking curcumin (200 mg·day^{-1}) 2 days before and 4 days after 45 min of downhill running, which evoked significant muscle damage, reduced delayed onset of muscle soreness, systemic levels of inflammation and structural damage to the thigh musculature. Since this study, there have been several others suggesting that curcumin supplementation reduces markers of muscle damage following strenuous exercise, ostensibly by reducing inflammation and free radical-mediated damage, also known as oxidative stress (Nicol et al., 2015; Tanabe et al., 2015; Basham et al., 2019). Although not all studies report beneficial effects, a recent systematic review of the literature suggested that on the balance of available evidence, curcumin appears to be a safe and efficacious supplement for attenuating symptoms of muscle damage (Fernández-Lázaro et al., 2020). Runners who often suffer from symptoms of damage (muscle soreness, stiffness, loss of muscle function) might consider supplementing with curcumin a few days before and after key training sessions and events in which rapid recovery is a priority.

Not all dietary interventions shown to alleviate symptoms of EIMD are rich in phytochemicals. There is emerging evidence that omega-3 polyunsaturated fatty acids, enriched in fish oils, have an important role in the regulation of muscle tissue and recovery from exercise (Tachtsis et al., 2018). The major mechanism by which fish oils could influence recovery is via modulation of the acute inflammatory response following strenuous exercise (Philpott et al., 2019). Indeed, studies have found that lipid mediators derived from fish oil, collectively known as resolvins and protectins, reduce inflammatory responses, which helps to facilitate homeostasis (Seki et al., 2010; Serhan and Petasis, 2011).

In clinical populations, omega-3-rich fish oils and their derivatives have long been known to reduce symptoms of muscle and joint pain and are considered useful adjuvant analgesics (Goldberg and Katz, 2007; Lee et al., 2012). However, only in the last decade have studies emerged suggesting that they can reduce muscle soreness, inflammation, and other deleterious symptoms associated with muscle damaging exercise (Philpott et al., 2019). For example, DiLorenzo et al. (2014) found that taking fish oil (2 g·day^{-1}) for 28 days prior to and 2 days following eccentric exercise with the elbow flexors reduced blood markers of inflammation and damage but did not benefit soreness or recovery of muscle function. More recently, Philpott et al. (2018) examined if 6 weeks of daily fish oil (1100 mg) and whey protein supplementation would enhance recovery following eccentric exercise of the knee extensors. They found that creatine kinase and soreness were lower in the 72 hours following exercise in subjects taking the fish oil-whey protein beverage. However, like in the study of Di Lorenzo et al. (2014), strength was unaffected, suggesting that fish oil might expedite the recovery of some but not all markers of muscle damage.

A recent review acknowledged that fish oil holds promise as a recovery aid but cautioned that the overall evidence to support these effects in athletes is moderate at present (Philpott et al., 2019). They did point out that consuming large amounts of omega-3 in the diet or via a fish oil supplement does not appear to be detrimental to recovery or adaptation. This is important because ≥ 2 weeks of supplementation is required to detect a marked increase in omega-3 fatty acid levels and, thus, anti-inflammatory effects might not be realised with lower doses (Philpott et al., 2019). Another important yet unresolved issue is the optimal daily dose required. Benefits have been seen with 1–4 g·day^{-1} which might not be achievable via diet alone; hence, fish oil supplements are often used in research and are recommended for optimal effects (Philpott et al., 2019). Thus, from a practical point of view, if planning to use fish oil to expedite recovery, a supplement might be required, and it should be consumed several weeks in advance for optimal effects.

Exercise Adaptations

It is important to note that some scientists caution against the use of recovery interventions that interfere with exercise-induced inflammation or free radical production (Paulsen et al., 2014a). This is due to the emerging role of inflammatory processes and free radicals such as hydrogen peroxide in stimulating exercise adaptations. Indeed, some have observed that supplements with antioxidant functions interfere with mitochondrial biogenesis (Paulsen et al., 2014b; Morrison et al., 2015), raising the possibility that these supplements could blunt training-induced adaptations important for endurance performance, like an enhanced $\dot{V}O_{2max}$. At present, the vast majority of studies have been conducted with vitamin C and E as opposed to non-steroidal anti-inflammatory drugs or functional foods. Although there is evidence that vitamin C and E might blunt training-induced changes in aerobic capacity of rats (Gomez-Cabrera et al., 2008b), there is currently a lack of evidence supporting similar impairments with antioxidant-like supplements in humans (Yfanti et al., 2011; Paulsen et al., 2014b; Peake et al., 2015). A review by Peake et al. (2015) concluded that while vitamins C and E appear to blunt some molecular changes induced by endurance type exercise, the evidence that this translates to changes at the performance level is lacking. This position was supported by a recent meta-analysis that found there was no effect of long-term vitamin C and E supplementation on training adaptations associated with endurance performance (Clifford et al., 2019). Therefore, there is currently insufficient evidence to suggest that dietary supplements with antioxidant functions will blunt training adaptations. Importantly, these interventions do not extinguish inflammation and oxidative stress, but rather reduce the magnitude. This calls into question whether high levels of inflammation and oxidative stress are necessary, and perhaps only small increases are required to get the requisite adaptative signalling response.

The approach recommended here is to view the usefulness of antioxidant and functional food supplements, particularly with regards to recovery, as highly context dependent. For instance, their chronic use throughout a preparatory phase of season might interfere with molecular signalling processes and possibly hinder longer-term training adaptations. However, the acute use of these supplements, when the need to minimise the adverse effects of performance (i.e. soreness and losses in muscle function) far outweigh the need for adaptation, could form part of a recovery strategy to restore optimal performance and/or reduce any lingering discomfort. One way to conceptualise this is the use of hormesis (Figure 17.2). In simple terms, the exercise stress imposed by training is relatively linear, insofar as the more you do, the better you are likely to get. However there comes a point when further increases in intensity or volume can become maladaptive because the level of inflammation and oxidative stress is very high, for example. This is the conceptual point when additional help in the form of recovery strategies can support athletes to reduce the potential for maladaptation or performance decreases. The other time to implement recovery strategies is when baseline cannot be naturally achieved in the requisite time. A good example might be when there is competition congestion and several rounds or races must be completed in a short period of time when there is insufficient time to completely recover.

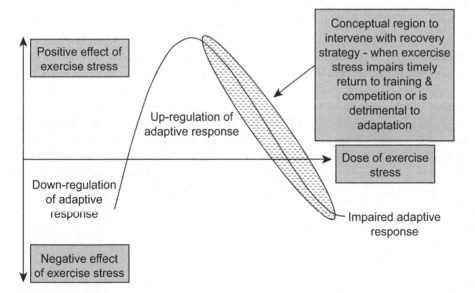

FIGURE 17.2   Theoretical hormesis curve. As the dose of exercise increases, so too does the positive effect from exercise. There comes a point where exercise dose can induce maladaptive effects, and this is the conceptual point where recovery interventions might be of benefit

Athlete Belief and the Power of Placebo

As alluded to throughout this chapter, an important consideration in the application of interventions is athlete belief. This is particularly pertinent given that a growing body of evidence indicates that recovery is related to individual preference and perceptions of the intervention. Practitioners must recognise and manage the influence of the belief and placebo effects if the application of recovery strategies is to be successful. Given the need to achieve coach and athlete buy-in to any intervention, there is an obvious challenge to balance an evidence-based approach with the beliefs and expectations of coaches and athletes (Halson and Martin, 2013). In cases where an athlete believes in a particular recovery strategy despite a lack of supporting scientific evidence, the demand on resource (financial, time, effort), the cost (i.e. what is sacrificed by engaging in a particular strategy) and critically, the potential for harm or a negative performance effect, must be evaluated. On balance, if there is no negative effect and the athlete believes in the intervention, then, even in light of little supporting evidence, the intervention could actually be beneficial. It is therefore important to use recovery strategies on a very individualised basis to ensure the most benefit can be gained from an intervention.

Summary

Training sessions and competitions cause transient impairments to performance that results from a variety of physiological disturbances. During the recovery process that ensues following exercise, a range of interventions could be utilised with the aim of improving physiological adaptation, reducing physiological stress and/or enhancing recovery time. Addressing the basics – hydration, sound nutrition and adequate sleep – should form the priority of any runner's recovery routine. It is highly unlikely that any other recovery strategy will be beneficial unless these three pillars of recovery are adequately met. Beyond these important macro-strategies, other recovery interventions (i.e. cryotherapy, compression garments, 'functional foods') may also offer some benefits. These recovery strategies can make a positive influence on returning athletes to the basal state but should be used judiciously depending on the focus of the individual, the training volume, time available for recovery and the focus of the training stress. Many practitioners and elite runners currently implement recovery strategies during championship situations or after specific training sessions when performance in the subsequent rounds of competition or training sessions is of paramount importance. In contrast, the use of recovery strategies could be limited or avoided when long-term physiological adaptation to the training-induced stress is the priority. Finally, the importance of athlete belief in the intervention should not be underestimated, because despite limited evidence for physiological benefit in some recovery techniques (e.g. stretching, foam rolling, massage), these interventions can still be beneficial due to the power of placebo.

18

LOW ENERGY AVAILABILITY

Identification, Management and Treatment

Jessica Piasecki

Highlights

- When runners fail to consume enough calories in their diet to support their training, daily living tasks, and normal physical functioning, a state of low energy availability can arise.
- The Female Athlete Triad describes a medical condition containing three inter-related conditions: low energy availability, menstrual cycle dysfunction and low bone mineral density.
- The relative energy deficiency in sport (RED-S) syndrome was developed to reflect the broad range of potentially serious health and performance consequences that can result from prolonged periods of low energy availability in both male and female athletes.
- Several tools are available to identify athletes who may be at risk of developing the Triad and RED-S.
- Governing bodies and coaches have a duty of care towards their athletes; therefore, an understanding of RED-S is of paramount importance.

Introduction

Energy is a necessity for all bodily functions. In the case of runners, energy availability is the energy that is left over for daily functioning of the body after the energy expended during exercise is taken away from the energy consumed in food. Low energy availability occurs when there is insufficient energy left to fuel other life processes such as those needed to maintain health and daily activity. This may arise if the runner is unaware of the amount of energy expended throughout their training, or if they fail to match energy intake when increasing physical training. Alternatively, runners may purposefully restrict dietary intakes, due to the perception that being 'lighter' is beneficial for their performance. If a state of low energy availability persists over a prolonged period of time, a syndrome known as 'relative energy deficiency in sport' (RED-S) can arise, which results in impaired physiological function affecting a range of systems within the body, including metabolism, bone health, tissue repair, cardiovascular health, immunity and reproductive function (Mountjoy et al., 2014).

This chapter aims to describe how low energy availability develops and can be assessed in an applied setting. Sections also cover relevant and current research that may help readers gain a better understanding of the importance of the RED-S syndrome to allow informed decisions to be made with regards to themselves or the athletes they support.

Key Definitions of Energy Balance

Energy balance is defined by the First Law of Thermodynamics (Kondepudi, 2008), as the amount of dietary energy added to or lost from the body's own energy stores following the completion all physiological processes within a day (Loucks et al., 2011; Loucks, 2004). Energy balance can be calculated as energy intake minus total energy expenditure. The concept of energy balance can be difficult to manage within an athlete's diet and training programme due to the issues with collecting accurate information on energy intake and expenditure (Loucks, 2004; Loucks et al., 2011). Energy deficiency is a negative discrepancy in energy balance whereby energy intake is less than total energy expenditure. This deficit creates a loss in stored energy and causes compensatory mechanisms to maintain homeostasis in vital physiological systems but reduce the functioning of others, e.g. reproductive function causing menstrual cycle irregularity (Otis et al., 1997). Adjustments are also common within endocrine, metabolic and functional systems, although more research is needed to assess other systemic changes following a prolonged energy deficit (Mountjoy et al., 2014).

Energy availability is the remaining energy for the body's metabolic systems following the deduction of energy costs required to carry out normal physiological systems. For a runner, this is the remaining energy available for maintaining normal bodily function following the energy cost of exercise. Energy availability is equal to energy intake minus energy expended from exercise (Wade and Jones, 2004). Low energy availability occurs when an individual's energy intake is inadequate for maintaining the energy costs required for normal physiological functions as well as for sporting performance (Mountjoy et al., 2014). Healthy energy availability has been categorised in adult populations as a value of ~45 kcal.kg fat free mass $(FFM)^{-1}.day^{-1}$, and low energy availability has been categorised as below ~ 30 kcal.kg FFM^{-1}. day^{-1} (Nattiv et al., 1994).

Assessing Energy Expenditure

Assessing the components of an athlete's energy balance is difficult due to the complexity of its two components (Loucks et al., 2011). Total energy expenditure is comprised of various factors including physical activity, basal metabolic rate (BMR) and the thermic effect of food. Collectively, these three components encompass all energy outputs of one individual system, illustrating the difficulties in obtaining an of accurate value (Hills et al., 2014; Schoeller et al., 1995). To add to the complications, BMR can be altered by a range of environmental factors such as food consumption, drug intake, genetics and physical activity. Given this complexity, it can be very hard to accurately research and monitor precise energy intake within athlete populations.

Self-report diaries are often utilised in research and applied settings to monitor and measure energy intake. This method tends to involve questionnaires and food diaries that are kept by athletes, allowing large populations to be monitored effectively (Stone et al., 1999). However, this method can also be unreliable, due to athletes not accurately defining their food and/or amounts, as well as being time-consuming for the athlete to complete. Additionally, self-reporting energy intake can exude some level of bias as athletes may be attempting to 'eat better' for the time period they are under observation to avoid judgement. There are similar issues with the measurement of total energy expenditure; therefore, without constant observations and direct calorimetry (to measure resting metabolic rate), the validity of data is questionable. Self-report is frequently used in scientific research as it requires fewer financial resources than other, more valid, methods (Stone et al., 1999).

Self-reporting food intake can be considered the best field method for collecting a large amount of data for analysis and is the most easily integrated within runners. Dual methods using equipment in conjunction with self-reporting can be considered more appropriate in defining total energy expenditure. Most athletes now employ the use of global positioning systems (GPS) and heart rate devices, which makes the monitoring of training more accurate than previously (Melin et al., 2014) and improves the validity of screening for athletes at risk of RED-S. The Low Energy Availability in Females Questionnaire (LEAF-Q) is also a validated tool that can identify female athletes at risk of RED-S.

The Female Athlete Triad

The Female Athlete Triad (Triad) was first coined in 1992 by the American College of Sports Medicine encompassing the interrelated phenomena of disordered eating, amenorrhea and osteoporosis (Otis et al., 1997). This triad identifies how low energy availability can have an impact on the menstrual cycle of females (tending to become absent or irregular). Menstrual cycle dysfunction is caused by low levels of oestrogen, which is a key regulator of bone formation. Consequently, low oestrogen results in a decline in bone health, and in most severe cases osteoporosis (the third dimension of the Triad). The Female Athlete Coalition (De Souza et al., 2014b) subsequently published a consensus statement on the Triad, in response to the high volume of emerging research on poor bone health in female athletes, particularly in endurance events and sports requiring a lean body physique. The consensus statement offers expert guidance on identifying and treating this condition and provides help for coaches and practitioners with return-to-play decisions. Several revisions of the Triad have developed the concept into a three-dimensional triangular model (Figure 18.1) displaying each of the three components on a continuum, with optimal energy availability, regular menstruation and optimal bone health lying on one side of the spectrum, and low energy availability, amenorrhoea and osteoporosis lying at the opposite end (De Souza et al., 2014b; Nattiv et al., 1994).

Critics of the Triad highlight that this excludes male athletes and does not identify reasons for an energy deficit (Manore et al., 2007). It is important to recognise that eating disorders cannot be defined as the aetiology of low energy availability. This was demonstrated in a study on 40 female athletes, which showed that while 63% of the sample were identified as having low energy availability, only 25% were categorised as positive for having an eating disorder (Melin et al., 2014). Eating disorders or disordered eating is therefore not the only reason that low energy availability may arise.

Development of Relative Energy Deficiency in Sport

RED-S is a new term, originally put forward by the International Olympic Committee (IOC), to encompass the numerous physiological implications that may arise as a result of prolonged low energy availability (Figure 18.2. Mountjoy et al., 2014). The intention of using

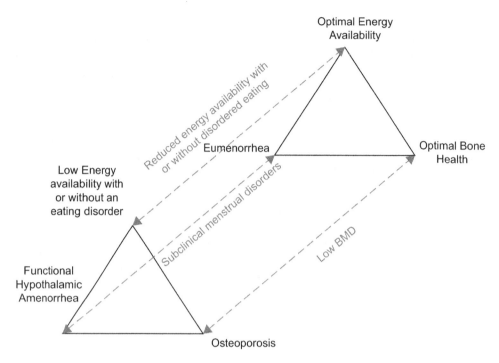

FIGURE 18.1 The Female Athlete Triad showing the spectrums of energy availability, menstrual function and bone mineral density (BMD). An athlete's condition may move along each spectrum at a different rate, in either direction, depending on their diet and training habits. Energy availability may affect bone mineral density both directly via metabolic hormones and indirectly via menstrual dysfunctions, leading to changes in oestrogen

Source: Taken from Nattiv et al. (2007).

RED-S was to extend beyond the Triad to include a greater number of physiological and health-related implications that are associated with low energy availability. Ultimately, as with the Triad, low energy availability may be either intentional or unintentional, and if sustained over a long period of time, an athlete's health and performance will be negatively affected.

If a runner is exposed to long periods of low energy availability in which they, intentionally or unintentionally, do not meet the energy demands of their training and day-to-day life, then they are at a heightened risk of developing RED-S. Specifically, RED-S increases the likelihood of illness and infection, alters circulating hormonal levels, increases susceptibility for injury and lengthens the time taken to grow and repair damaged muscles (Ackerman et al., 2018; Barrack et al., 2013; Shimizu et al., 2012; Petkus et al., 2017; Loucks et al., 1992; Elliott-Sale et al., 2018). If the athlete has one, many or all of these alterations due to low energy availability, then their performance will also be affected as a consequence of decreased glycogen stores, endurance performance, concentration, coordination, adaptability and impaired judgement (Melin et al., 2019).

The term RED-S not only broadens the potential impact of low energy availability compared to the Triad, but it also allows the syndrome to be applied to male athletes who may also experience a number of the same physiological consequences. It has been suggested that males experience similar monthly fluctuations in hormones to that of females, but this is widely

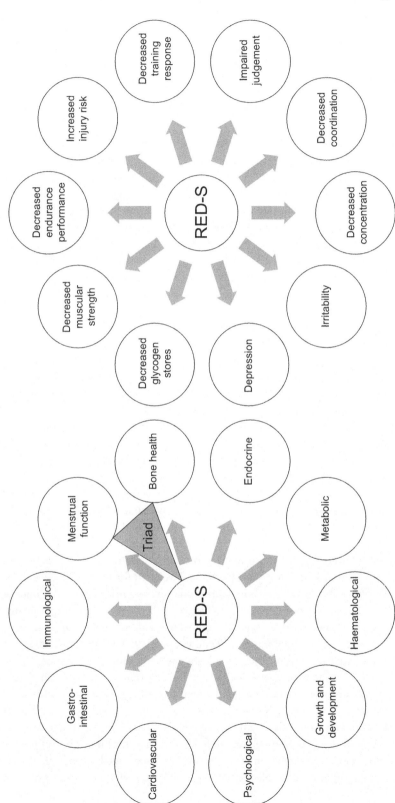

FIGURE 18.2 The left image denotes the health consequences of relative energy deficiency in sport (RED–S), and the right image shows the performance consequences of RED–S. ★ Psychological consequences can either precede RED-S or be the results of RED-S

Source: Taken from Mountjoy et al. (2014).

under-researched due to inadequacy and consistency of methods (Tenforde et al., 2016). A recent update on the RED-S paradigm suggested that future research should be directed towards the inclusion of male athletes (Mountjoy et al., 2018a) as well as increasing awareness and education to athletes, coaches, parents and other practitioners.

Research on RED-S

Most research that is available on RED-S has been drawn from studies with small sample sizes and a limited number of variables. In 2016 only a handful of publications were available on RED-S; however, in recent years there have been a plethora of publications, with over 20 original research studies published in 2019 and 2020 investigating the implications of low energy availability. Using validated questionnaires (Brief Eating Disorder in Athletes Questionnaire, Eating Disorder Screen for Primary Care and self-reported history of eating disorders or disordered eating), Ackerman et al. (2018) assessed energy availability, and the health and performance consequences of RED-S in a group of around 1000 female athletes. Data revealed that approximately half of the athletes surveyed had experienced low energy availability, which was clearly associated with health and performance consequences. These data reaffirm the high prevalence of female athletes that experience both these health and performance consequences as a result of low energy availability.

One of the main reasons for the development of the RED-S framework is to ensure that research in males at risk or with low energy availability is increased. The inclusion of males in RED-S related research is currently limited, and only since the definition of RED-S have males begun to be included, or deemed at risk for low energy availability, alongside females. Studies have demonstrated a high prevalence of males at risk of RED-S within endurance sports. Of 108 non-elite competitive endurance athletes ~80% were deemed to be at risk for low energy availability; in particular, cyclists had a very low energy intake at around 29 kcal/kg FFM/day compared to runners at 34 kcal/kg FFM/day (Lane et al., 2019).

A six-point assessment has been validated to determine the risk of developing the Triad and suffering a bone stress-related injury (see Table 18.1). The factors identified in the model for being at risk of developing the Triad are: a low energy availability (with or without disordered eating/eating disorder), low body mass index (BMI), delayed age of menarche (onset of periods), oligomenorrhea (longer menstrual cycles) and/or amenorrhea, and low bone mineral density and/or stress reaction/fracture (De Souza et al., 2020; Joy et al., 2014). An adapted version of the risk assessment system has been developed for male athletes, including low energy availability, low BMI, low bone mineral density and prior bone stress injuries (Kraus et al., 2019). These factors are strongly predictive with the prospective injuries sustained by male athletes, suggesting that males are at a similar risk as females for bone stress injuries in low energy availability environments (Kraus et al., 2019; Tenforde et al., 2016).

In male athletes, compared to females, there is no obvious indication that may suggest an athlete is at risk of RED-S that may warrant further investigation. In contrast, in female athletes who are non-hormonal contraceptive users, regularity of the menstrual cycle can be used as a barometer to indicate when RED-S may be developing. Specific menstrual cycle dysfunctions such as anovulatory cycle (seemingly normal menstrual pattern but absence of ovulation) or luteal phase defect (low progesterone levels and/or a short luteal phase) require more detailed testing. However, female runners are strongly encouraged to track their own cycle, behaviours, and symptoms to enable them to recognise and respond to changes quickly.

TABLE 18.1 Female Athlete Triad cumulative risk assessment

Risk factors	Low risk = 0 points each	Moderate risk = 1 point each	High risk = 2 points each
Low EA with or without DE/ED	No dietary restriction	Some restriction; current/past history of DE	Meets DSM-V criteria for ED
Low BMI	BMI greater or equal to 18.5 or 90% EW★★ or weight stable	BMI between 17.5 and 18.5 or less than 90% EW or 5–10% weight loss/month	BMI less than or equal to 17.5, or less than 85% EW or 10% or greater weight loss per month
Delayed menarche	Menarche before 15 years	Menarche 15–16 years	Menarche greater or equal to 16 years
Oligomenorrhea and/or amenorrhea	More than 9 menses in 12 months	6–9 menses in 12 months ★	Fewer than 6 menses in 12 months
Low BMD	Z score less than or equal to −1.0	Z score between −1.0★★★ and −2.0	Z score less than or equal to −2.0
Stress reaction and/or fracture	None	1	Greater than or equal to 2 or more than or equal to 1 at a high risk site+
Cumulative risk (total each column then add for total score)	Points +	Points +	Points = Total Score

Source: Kraus *et al.* (2019); De Souza *et al.* (2020, 2014a)

Note: This assessment provides an objective method of determining an athlete's risk using risk stratification and evidence-based risk factors for the Female Athlete Triad. BMD, bone mineral density; BMI, body mass index; DE, disordered eating; DSM-V, *Diagnostic and Statistical Manual of Mental Disorders*, 5th edition; EA, energy availability; ED, eating disorder; EW, expected weight.

‡ Some dietary restriction as evidenced by self-report or low/inadequate energy intake on diet logs.
★ History/current history.
★★ ≥90% EW; absolute BMI cut-offs should not be used for adolescents.
★★★ Weight-bearing sport. †High-risk skeletal sites associated with low BMD and delay in return to play in athletes with one or more components of the Triad include stress reaction/fracture of trabecular sites (femoral neck, sacrum, pelvis).

For males a similar score as detailed previously is now available without the necessity to include the delayed menarche and oligomenorrhea/amenorrhea risk.

Changes to the male reproductive system as a result of low energy availability require more intricate assessment, some of which may necessitate sperm and fertility analysis. However, a few studies have been performed to evidence changes in metabolism and reproduction in males with low energy availability (McColl et al., 1989; Hackney et al., 1988) but more studies are required to evaluate dietary and endocrine function over a longer time period.

In studies that have included male athletes, it can be concluded that testosterone is affected by low energy availability, in a similar manner to the alterations of the hypothalamic-pituitary-axis that influences oestrogen levels in females. Testosterone is an important anabolic hormone that regulates sex drive, contributes to production of red blood cells and is responsible for re-building damaged tissues (e.g. bone and muscle) following exercise bouts. A small number of studies have demonstrated 10–30% lower levels of testosterone amongst male endurance runners training at a high volume (over 100 km per week). Moreover, even male athletes on a lower volume of endurance training have still demonstrated lower levels of testosterone in comparison to sedentary or less active males (Tenforde et al., 2016). Some studies have shown that as mileage of endurance runners increases, testosterone levels decrease at a similar rate (Wheeler et al., 1986); however, these studies do reiterate that the lower levels of testosterone that tend to be observed are still considered to be within a 'normal' range. However, the long-term implications of low testosterone in male athletes is currently unknown.

RED-S 'at Risk' Assessment Tool

A proposed clinical assessment tool is available for medical practitioners that enables athletes to be screened for RED-S and categorised at different levels of risk (Mountjoy et al., 2015a; Mountjoy et al., 2015b). The tool provides a traffic light system, which uses specific behaviours and symptoms associated with RED-S to categorise athletes (see Table 18.2). The assessment tool also details specific guidance for return to training and performance. Diagnosing RED-S can be difficult due to the subtle and sometimes unrecognisable symptoms. Therefore, it is necessary to focus on those athletes most at risk for developing RED-S, which includes athletes in endurance sports such as distance running. If early detection is possible, then improvements in performances are still achievable, as is the prevention of long-term health consequences. It is recommended that screening is undertaken as part of a periodic health exam/routine check-up when an athlete presents with one of some of the following symptoms; disordered eating/eating disorders, weight loss, lack of normal growth and development, endocrine dysfunction, recurrent injuries and illnesses, decreased performance/performance variability or mood changes.

Any athletes who are in the red and yellow risk categories should receive medical treatment, preferably undertaken by a team of health professionals, which would include a sports medical doctor, a sports dietician, an exercise physiologist, coaches and sports psychologists, as and when appropriate. Treatment should focus on correcting the energy deficit through increasing energy intake and/or decreasing the energy expended. Prior to the athlete returning to sport a full assessment of the athlete's heath and nutritional requirements are necessary (detailed in the steps that follow).

> *Step 1*: Evaluations of health status; this should be conducted by a medical practitioner taking into account the demographics, medical symptoms history and seriousness of their current status.
>
> *Step 2*: Evaluation of participation risk; taking into account the type of sport played and completion level.
>
> *Step 3*: Decision modification; return to training may be adjusted according to time of the season, pressure from the athlete and external pressures and any fears of litigation.

Preventing RED-S

The cornerstone of RED-S prevention is education, with runners themselves, plus parents, coaches, teachers and practitioners that provide support to athletes. It is currently concerning that less than half of practitioners working with athletes and runners can accurately identify the Triad components (see: Mountjoy et al., 2018a). More worryingly, many female runners have been informed by their coaches or medical professionals that an absence of menstrual

TABLE 18.2 Risk assessment model for RED-S

High risk; no start	Moderate risk; caution	Low risk; go
Serious eating disorders	Prolonged low % body fat	Healthy eating habits
Other serious psychological and physiological conditions associated with low EA	Substantial weight loss within short time frame	with appropriate energy availability
Extreme weight loss techniques	Attenuation of expected growth and development	Normal hormonal and metabolic function
	Abnormal menstrual cycle	Healthy BMD
	Menarche after age 16	Healthy musculoskeletal
	Abnormal hormone profile in males	system
	Reduced BMD	
	History of stress fractures	
	Lack of progress	
	Energy deficiency	

Source: Taken from Mountjoy *et al.* (2015a).

Note: EA, energy availability; BMD, bone mineral density

High risk – Red Light; this is a very serious situation for the athlete and any sport participation would pose serious risk to the athlete's health (male or female).

Moderate risk – Yellow Light; supervised sports participation is suitable with an adequate treatment plan in place. Evaluation of the athlete's progression and risk should be carried out at regular intervals to detect changes in clinical status.

Low risk – Green Light; full sport participation is appropriate.

cycles is 'normal' for exercising females, despite clear scientific evidence that menstrual dysfunction is a risk factor for bone stress injury.

The following recommendations are largely for coaches, but should be used by runners themselves and sports medicine professionals working with athletes:

- Coaches and practitioners are responsible for enhancing their knowledge of this concept.
- Coaches should aim to build strong relationships with their athletes and families to enable open conversations and discussions around the issue of eating disorders and RED-S.
- Coaches should reduce emphasis on body weight being an important determinant of performance in distance running. Instead, focus should be placed upon nutrition and health as the most important means of enhancing performance.
- Coaches should never be critical of an athlete's body shape or weight.
- Coaches should be aware (and educate their athletes) that exceptional performances by an athlete does not necessarily mean the athlete is healthy.
- If weight loss is part of a distance runner's objectives, goals should be long-term, realistic and health-promoting.
- Coaches can relay the importance of a healthy balanced diet and emphasise that any increases in training volume should be met with increases in energy intake.
- When presented with an athlete whose performance has deteriorated despite a period of uninterrupted training, coaches should consider that it may be related to low energy availability. If coaches suspect that this is the case, they should consult with a qualified nutritionist or dietician to investigate further.

- For younger runners who may be competing in other school and extracurricular sports, monitoring the volume of physical exercise and adjusting for the needs of the individual athlete is crucial.
- Wherever possible, athletes should undergo an annual health examination to screen for eating disorders, weight loss, growth (in the case of young athletes), menstrual dysfunction, injury history, illnesses and performance changes. Governing bodies should include adequate education within coaching qualifications and ensure that athletes at elite through to beginner level have the relevant knowledge of RED-S to support their training needs,

Summary and Reflections

Energy deficiency occurs when the balance between energy intake from the diet is exceeded by the energy required for physical training, daily living activities and normal physiological functions. Chronic periods of low energy availability are common in distance runners, either because they unintentionally do not consume enough calories to support the energy they expend in training, or intentionally as they believe that weight loss will provide them with a performance advantage. The Female Athlete Triad provides a medical framework that describes three inter-related conditions (low energy availability with or without disordered eating or an eating disorder, menstrual dysfunction and low bone mineral density) that each exist on a continuum from normal/optimal to serious endpoints. More recently, the term RED-S was developed by the IOC to describe a syndrome caused by low energy availability that negatively impacts a broader range of physiological systems in both males and females. These physiological consequences can manifest in poor health, injury and deteriorations in running performance. Despite there being a lack of research around RED-S, the concept has most certainly raised awareness in the running and coaching community of the health and performance consequences of low energy availability. Several assessment tools are available for those at risk of the Triad and RED-S, including the Female Athlete Triad cumulative risk assessment, LEAF-Q, and risk assessment model for RED-S. Coaches should endeavour to educate themselves and their runners about RED-S, be vigilant for signs of disordered eating, and downplay the importance of weight loss as a performance enhancement strategy. Further research is required to better understand the mechanisms of RED-S and its prevalence amongst sub-populations of athletes, including male runners, para-athletes and different ethnicities.

As many well-established names in the endurance running world have now begun to share their own experiences of RED-S, there seems to be an increasing awareness of the serious health-related issues than can arise as a result of chronic low energy availability. Raising awareness in this manner gives the younger generation of athletes a relatable 'role model' and a better sense of these issues, re-iterating the importance of adequate energy intake. For older athletes, this information and insight was not readily available when they were at their peak, even at the elite level. For the current generation there is now an opportunity to reduce the number of negative consequences that young athletes have suffered in the past. It should be noted that RED-S does not exclusively occur in elite populations, those at the 'sub-elite level', compete and train to a high level but often without additional support. As such, these groups should also be made aware of the consequences of RED-S and how to avoid the syndrome. Governing bodies and those involved with the design of coach education curricula across all sports have a duty of care to protect their current and prospective athletes of the future. The more athletes that can make it through their careers with adequate energy intake, the higher calibre of athlete populations we are likely to have in years to come.

19

NURTURING YOUNG DISTANCE RUNNERS

Richard C. Blagrove, Philip E. Kearney and Karla L. Drew

Highlights

- Young athletes (<16 years old) are frequently pressurised into specialising in distance running from an early age in the belief that this is the best long-term approach to achieve success as a senior athlete.
- Success as a junior distance runner is a poor indicator of adult potential.
- Early specialisation in distance running is strongly associated with a high prevalence of overuse injury, drop-out, poor bone health, psychological burnout, overtraining and delayed menarche.
- The most common pathway to senior success as a runner involves participating in several sports during childhood and teenage years, and specialising in a single sport only during late adolescence (16 years+)
- Effective long-term development of young athletes should encompass a well-rounded programme of physical activities and sports, including strength training.

Introduction

Recent data from Sport England's active people survey indicate that childhood participation in athletics and distance running is increasing. Athletics is the sixth most popular sport amongst 11- to 14-year-olds in the UK, and 18% of this age group regularly participate in cross-country or road running (*Statista*, 2018). Junior *parkrun* also sees approximately twenty thousand 4- to 14-year-olds participating in distance running events around the UK every Sunday morning. Some of these youngsters will enjoy their early experiences of the sport and decide to join their local Athletics Club. Many will subsequently choose to focus their training efforts on reaching the highest level as a senior runner. For junior runners that excel at a young age, research shows that very few transition into successful senior runners, and a high proportion drop out of the sport altogether (Bussmann and Alfermann, 1994; Enoksen, 2011; Shibli and Barrett, 2011).

Nurturing a talented young distance runner into a successful senior is a challenging task. Given the current popularity of the sport and the plethora of long-term health benefits associated with running, it is important that parents, coaches and teachers are aware of the factors and training practices that are likely to lessen the risk of drop-out and maximise the likelihood of young runners achieving their long-term potential. Clearly a genuine passion and involvement in the sport of distance running from a relatively young age is important if an athlete wishes to succeed at the highest level as a senior. However, the timing of specialisation in the sport and the volume of specific running training utilised at various stages of growth and maturation is more controversial.

Growth, Maturation and Development Considerations

The tempo (rate) and timing (chronological age) of biological growth and maturation varies considerably between physiological systems, sexes and individuals. *Development* is a more general qualitative concept that is behavioural as well as biological (Stratton and Oliver, 2014). Development of physiological systems affects a range of biomotor qualities that have important physical performance consequences; however, development of cognitive (knowledge, problem solving, understanding) and affective (social, relationships) domains are also important for performance, and these factors may mature at different times. During childhood (from age 2 to the start of adolescence), growth and maturation of biological systems are relatively steady and similar between sexes. Adolescence commences at the onset of puberty, which is problematic to define, but typically occurs around 10 years of age in girls and 11 years of age in boys. Changes in the hormonal system during adolescence stimulate the development of secondary sexual characteristics, as well as a rapid change in stature, known as 'peak height velocity', or more colloquially, the 'growth spurt'. The timing of these changes is difficult to predict and assess, however, due to the large inter-individual variability that exists.

Radiographic skeletal age assessment perhaps represents the gold standard in measurement of maturity status, but it is costly, is time-consuming and requires specialist equipment. Sexual age can be assessed by a trained medical professional but is invasive; however, the onset of menstruation (menarche) in girls provides a useful marker of maturation in the reproductive system. Tracking of stature and body mass by taking measurements every three months after childhood offers a cheap strategy to detect when the growth spurt is occurring with reasonable confidence. When this strategy is not practical, several equations that utilise anthropometric ratios have been developed using sitting height and leg length or stature (Mirwald et al., 2002; Moore et al., 2015). The most straightforward of these equations for practitioners to use is shown in Box 19.1 (Moore et al., 2015). This equation is most accurate for circa-pubertal young performers, i.e. boys age 12–14 years and girls age 11–13 years (Koziel and Malina, 2018). When error is accounted for in these somatic estimations of maturity, it is recommended that young athletes are at least 6 months post peak-height velocity before they are considered 'post-pubertal'. Although these equations provide important insight into biological maturation status, cognitive and affective maturation may not occur in synchrony with physical development; therefore, judgements concerning readiness to engage in higher volumes of training should not be made purely on the basis of the values generated from these equations.

Determinants of Performance in Young Runners

In studies that have assessed the physiological factors that determine performance in young runners, participants have typically been similar for age but may differ markedly in their

---

BOX 19.1 CALCULATING MATURITY OFFSET (MOORE ET AL., 2015):

Boys = −7.999994 + [0.0036124 × (age × stature)]
Girls = −7.709133 + [0.0042232 × (age × stature)]

Age is measured in decimal years and stature is taken as standing height in centimetres.

Example

For a 13.5-year-old girl who is 168 cm tall.

Maturity offset (years) = −7.709133 + [0.0042232 × (13.5 × 168)] = 1.9 years post peak-height velocity.

---

maturation status and level of training. This is likely to influence the extent to which physiological parameters correlate with performance measures compared to groups of well-trained adult runners, who generally have similar characteristics with respect to these confounding variables. Moreover, the method used to partition groups of young participants for differences in body size for variables such as maximal oxygen uptake ($\dot{V}O_{2max}$) and running economy is also likely to influence findings (Eisenmann et al., 2001).

In general, the physiological determinants of performance for adolescents appears to be similar to those of adult runners. A number of investigations have confirmed that $\dot{V}O_{2max}$ is a significant predictor (r = 0.5–0.9) of performance for 1500 m (Abe et al., 1998; Almarwaey et al., 2003; Blagrove et al., 2019c), 3 km (Abe et al., 1998; Blagrove et al., 2019c; Mahon et al., 1996; Unnithan et al., 1995), 5 km (Abe et al., 1998; Cunningham, 1990) and cross-country (Cole et al., 2006; Fernhall et al., 1996) in young (10–18 years) groups of runners. Running economy (or oxygen uptake at ventilatory threshold or lactate threshold) also appears to be related to middle- (Almarwaey et al., 2003; Blagrove et al., 2019c; Mayers and Gutin, 1979; Unnithan et al., 1995) and long-distance performance (Cole et al., 2006; Fernhall et al., 1996), although this is not always the case (Abe et al., 1998; Cunningham, 1990). The discrepancy in findings in these studies is likely due to the small inter-individual variability in running economy despite differences in running performance compared to other studies. Additionally, speed at $\dot{V}O_{2max}$ (Abe et al., 1998; Almarwaey et al., 2003; Blagrove et al., 2019c; Cole et al., 2006; Cunningham, 1990) and fractional utilisation (Mahon et al., 1996; Unnithan et al., 1995) have also been shown to significantly correlate with distance running performance in adolescents.

'Trainability' of Aerobic Capabilities

During running tasks, prepubertal children exhibit poor mechanical efficiency and a high oxygen cost, thus have a lower overall work capacity compared to post-pubertal adolescents and adults (Frost et al., 1997; Moritani et al., 1989). As a result of changes in anatomical, metabolic and thermoregulatory factors during the adolescent growth spurt, efficiency improves, and aerobic exercise performance is enhanced. Despite possessing a lower work capacity compared to adults, surprisingly, children have similar $\dot{V}O_{2max}$ values (when scaled for body mass) to young adults (Vinet et al., 2002). Prior to puberty, children have underdeveloped anaerobic metabolic pathways and therefore rely heavily upon energy contribution from oxidative metabolism during exercise. During puberty, when muscle mass increases and anaerobic energy pathways develop, the relative energy contribution from oxidative metabolism decreases (Fleischman et al., 2010). It has been speculated that endurance-based training may become more important during early adulthood to offset the reduction brought about during puberty (Ratel and Blazevich, 2017); however, this has not yet been scientifically verified.

The changes that occur in $\dot{V}O_{2max}$ during adolescence are highly complex and are influenced by numerous factors. Appropriate scaling for body mass is one important ongoing area of controversy (Armstrong, 2017). In both sexes during childhood, $\dot{V}O_{2max}$ increases linearly with age; however, there is a divergence in the rate of improvement after around 8 years of age. Post-puberty, females experience little change in absolute $\dot{V}O_{2max}$ values, whereas male scores continue to rise until adulthood. Expressed relative to body mass, differences between sexes are even more pronounced. Once puberty has commenced, $\dot{V}O_{2max}$ ($mL \cdot kg^{-1} \cdot min^{-1}$) decreases gradually each year (8–18 years) for females into early adulthood but remains relatively unchanged in males (Armstrong and Barker, 2011).

The extent to which aerobic capabilities are trainable during childhood and adolescence is an area of ongoing debate (McNarry et al., 2014; Armstrong, 2017). Due to the naturally high aerobic capacities possessed by children, compared to adults, it has been suggested that prepubertal children are less adaptable to endurance training or that a 'maturational threshold' exists where endurance training starts to become more effective (Mercier et al., 1987; Payne and Morrow, 1993; Rowland, 1985). However, this does not appear to be the case, as a large number of studies have shown that aerobic capabilities and performance can be improved in children, and these improvements are similar in those <11 years and >11 years of age (Armstrong and Barker, 2011; McNarry and Jones, 2014). It is likely that previous speculations around a potential period of enhanced aerobic trainability during adolescence are heavily influenced by methodological limitations, most notably a lack of consideration for baseline fitness in participants. Constraining young athletes to specific types of training during 'windows of opportunity' lacks evidence and has potential risks such as overtraining and burnout (McNarry et al., 2014).

A close relationship exists between many measures of physical performance and maturity; therefore, during early adolescence, the runners labelled as the most 'talented' are usually the most biologically mature, despite being of the same chronological age as the rest of their comparator group. This is almost certainly the case with young male distance runners who excel within their peer group between the ages of 11 and 15 years (under-13 and under-15 age groups; Kearney et al., 2018). The increase in androgenic hormones during early puberty provides natural increases in explosive power, sprint speed and anaerobic capacity, as well as the aforementioned changes to aerobic capabilities. A more physically mature adolescent competing against a field of largely less-developed boys, despite being of the same chronological age, will therefore possess a significant advantage during a race. Performance during early-adolescent years is typically a poor predictor of a young runner's future potential (see the next section). Thus, maturation status should be considered, and the importance of psychosocial behaviours should not be overlooked.

It may also be the case that over longer distances (i.e. cross-country), the best female runners in younger age groups (under-15) are late-developers with less mature physical features. Distance runners are typically lighter and have lower body fat than swimmers and other track and field athletes (Housch et al., 1984). The physically under-developed appearance of many high-performing adolescent female distance runners suggests they may excel due to their physically immature musculoskeletal structure. A narrower pelvic girdle, lower body fat percentage and lighter mass are all likely to provide a benefit to physiological qualities such as maximal oxygen uptake and running economy (Anderson, 1996). Late maturation of the female reproductive system (i.e. delayed menarche) could be a natural occurrence (Malina, 1994) but could also be caused by insufficient energy intake and/or excessive training.

Early Sport Specialisation

It is understandable how a coach or parent seeking to maximise a young athlete's performance potential might encourage intensive training in a single sport on a year-round basis from an early age (i.e., early specialisation). For this reason, young athletes are sometimes pressured into focusing their training on a single sport at a young age from their club or school coaches, fervent parents or to obtain a collegiate athletic scholarship (Bell et al., 2018; Brooks et al., 2018; Gould et al., 2009; Post et al., 2018). For example, a survey of parents and coaches involved in track and field within the United Kingdom revealed that 29% of parents and 7% of coaches advocated that athletes should train year-round at 12 years of age (Kearney et al., 2020). Furthermore, 31% of parents and 8% of coaches advocated athletes specialising in in track and field by 14 years of age, while 28% of parents and 13% of coaches advocated specialising in a single athletic discipline by 14 years of age (Kearney et al., 2020). There are several well-publicised accounts of highly successful runners who report training very hard during their early adolescent years and who competed exclusively in the sport (Denison, 2004; Miller, 1981; Tjelta, 2019), which naturally inspires youth runners and their parents/coaches to copy this approach. Extreme examples can be found at the opposite end of the spectrum too, such as Australian athlete Sinead Divers, who started running aged 33, and at the time of writing holds the IAAF over-40s 10,000 m world record and is ranked 19th in the world over the marathon. However, these stories are the exceptions (Bahenský, 2019), and the most common pathway to senior success involves participating in several sports during the childhood and teenage years and specialising only during late adolescence (Bergeron et al., 2015; Güllich, 2018; Huxley et al., 2017).

Arguments for early specialisation are typically based on economic reasons; as organisations have limited resources (e.g., limited places on development squads), then athletes who are performing at a higher level relative to their peers will have an advantage in gaining access to those resources (Ericsson et al., 1993). However, middle-distance runners typically peak during a 2.5- to 3-year window centred around age 25 years for men and 27 for women (Haugen et al., 2018; Hollings et al., 2014), with marathon runners peaking slightly later (~28–29 years; Haugen et al., 2018). Thus, there is plenty of time for an individual to develop without engaging in intensive training during early adolescence. Furthermore, early engagement in intensive training brings considerable risks (Blagrove et al., 2017; Myer et al., 2011). For example, Huxley et al. (2014) tracked the training profiles and injuries of Australian track and field athletes who were members of a regional emerging talent squad. Athletes who suffered a serious injury (defined as time off training ≥ 3 weeks) had trained at a higher intensity and had a greater yearly training load at age 13–14 years, and reported more high-intensity training sessions at age 13–14 and 15–16 years than their uninjured peers. 17.3% of athletes in the sample had to retire due to injuries prior to turning 18 years. These results clearly highlight the dangers inherent in engaging in adult-like training practices too early in a young runner's development.

The value in adopting a 'slow and steady' approach to athlete development is further supported by research examining the relationship between performances at differing age grades in youth track and field. Kearney and Hayes (2018) identified all athletes ranked in the top 20 of youth track and field in the United Kingdom between 2005 and 2015 and examined the extent to which athletes retained their top ranking in subsequent age grades. The results for middle-distance runners are given in Table 19.1. The table clearly shows that only a minority of top performing 12- and 14-year-olds retain their top-ranked status by Under 20 (male, 9.3%; female, 14.8%). Even between the two oldest age categories examined, only 40% of athletes who were top ranked at U17 retained their top 20 ranking at U20. The dropout from athletics amongst these high-performing individuals is also stark; for example, at most 50% of Under 15 middle distance runners who were ranked in the Top 20 were still competing as 19-year-olds (see also Shibli and Barrett, 2011).

While Kearney and Hayes (2018) primarily focused on the relationship between performances at different stages of youth development, other researchers have further examined the relationship between youth and senior success. For example, Bahenský (2019) investigated historical data on female distance runners from the Czech Republic. The majority of the best female distance runners in the U16 (85%) and U18 (65%) age grades ran their personal best before the age of 20. Athletes who were successful from U16 through to adulthood were rare exceptions. In an investigation of Spanish middle- and long-distance runners, Latorre-Román et al. (2018) reported that of 270 individuals ranked in the top 10 in long- or middle-distance events as a Cadet (U15), Youth (U17) and Junior (U20) in 2004, only 12 (10 male, 2 female) were also listed as top 10 seniors in 2014. Similarly, Weippert et al. (2020) analysed individual performance trajectories of German international-level middle-distance runners from the age of 14 until their top performance. Forty percent of male middle-distance runners who would progress to represent Germany internationally as seniors had not run fast enough at age 16 to meet the national association standard to earmark them as having potential for the future; this

TABLE 19.1 The extent to which athletes ranked in the top 20 at an age grade (a) remain participating in athletics and (b) retain their top 20 ranking across age grades

Age Grade Comparison	Male		Female	
	% Still Competing	% Retained Top 20 Ranking	% Still Competing	% Retained Top 20 Ranking
U13–U15	79	31	84	39
U13–U17	59	22	56	25
U13–U20	40	9	32	15
U15–U17	80	38	78	47
U15–U20	50	18	46	25
U17–U20	73	40	60	42

Note: N = number of athletes ranked in the top 20 identified within the sample.

group included a future Olympic champion. In contrast to the male athletes, and to the results from both Bahenský (2019) and Latorre-Román et al. (2018), only two runners out of the 32 cases examined from the female sample had not reach the standard set for 16-year-olds. Taken together, these results for distance runners are consistent with investigations of a broader range of track and field events (e.g., Foss et al., 2019; Kearney and Hayes, 2018) and clearly illustrate that youth success is a poor indicator of adult potential.

Rather than focusing on performances, other research has investigated the practice activities undertaken by successful track and field athletes using a variety of survey and interview-based approaches (Güllich, 2018; Huxley et al., 2017; Huxley et al., 2018). Güllich (2018) matched pairs of athletes from German national squads based on sex, discipline (including middle-distance events) and baseline performance in competitions when they were aged either 13 (junior sample) or 19 years (senior sample). Participants completed a detailed survey on the types of activities engaged in across all sports and all ages. Their unequal subsequent performance development during junior (13–17 years; n = 138) and senior (19–23+ years; n = 80) age ranges defined 'strong responders' and 'weak responders'. Junior-age strong responders were found to have accumulated more organised practice in athletics than weak responders (e.g., age 14–15 years, weak responders had 636 hours organized athletics training versus 792 hours for strong responders; age 16–17 years, 946 for weak responders and 1194 for strong responders), while there were no differences between the groups in the amounts of all other types of activities or starting ages. That is, early investment in athletics training can facilitate junior success. However, the results were very different when senior performances were examined. In contrast to those who responded favourably to training up to age 17, senior-age strong responders did not accumulate a greater amount of organised or nonorganized practice in athletics. However, they had engaged in more organised practice and competitions in other sports over more years (9 vs. 2 years) and specialised in athletics at a later age than weak responders (16 vs. 11 years). Thus, rather than specialising in athletics, it appears that the interplay of childhood/adolescent practice in other sports alongside gradually increasing practice in athletics maximises an athlete's potential for long-term performance improvement into adulthood.

These results from Güllich (2018) are consistent with research by Huxley and colleagues (Huxley et al., 2017, 2018) on Australian Olympic and World Championships track and field athletes. These studies reported that while many participants were involved in track and field from a young age, the majority were late specialisers. These high-performing athletes were not ready to fully invest in intense training in a single discipline until late adolescence (on average, 17.7 years old). Interviews with 14 elite Australian junior track and field athletes who had successfully transitioned into elite senior careers revealed that parents' understanding that some athletes were not ready to specialise before 16 years of age, and in some cases even by age 18–19, was particularly important (Huxley et al., 2018). This delay enabled athletes to make a full commitment when they were physically, mentally and socially ready, rather than giving up because of pressure, expectations and unsupportive behaviours by parents and coaches (see also MacPhail and Kirk, 2006). In relation to middle-distance running in particular, Tjelta's (2019) account of three brothers who all won European Championships over 1500 m illustrates the diverse and individual nature of pathways to expertise; while one brother (the youngest) specialised in distance running at 12 years of age, Tjelta (2019) reports that the others participated in football and cross-country skiing throughout their adolescence. Thus, in addition to an openness to engage with other sporting activities, it is important to recognise that there is considerable variability in the pathways to specialisation undertaken by high- performance athletes.

Relatively little research has focused on the specific training activities undertaken by successful distance runners during their development. In a comparison of elite standard long-distance runners from Kenya and Spain, and national standard Spanish athletes, Casado et al. (2019a) showed no evidence that starting systematic training at a younger age was advantageous. Furthermore, elite and national standard distance runners showed no differences in the accumulated distance in tempo runs, long interval training or short interval training. Indeed, the only variable that consistently differentiated elite and national standard Spanish runners was accumulated distance in easy runs. These findings are relatively consistent with those of Young and Salmela (2010), who found no differences between Canadian national, provincial and club level runners in terms of the average age at which they began running (National: 12.9 ± 2.4 years; Provincial: 11.5 ± 2.4 years; Club: 11.5 ± 2.9 years), or the average age at which they began year-round full-time training (National: 16.1 ± 1.9 years; Provincial: 14.8 ± 1.8 years; Club: 16.3 ± 2.4 years). Similarly, national, provincial and club athletes did not differ in terms of the total volume of training that they had accumulated, or the volume of distance-specific training (e.g., interval training). However, national runners could be distinguished from the other groups on the basis of the amount of weight training and technique-focused practice that they had accumulated at various points in their development. Thus it appears that coaches wishing to ensuring effective long-term development of their charges should emphasise training practices that supplement endurance development (e.g., technique, weight training, easy runs) rather than intensive race-specific training that produces short-term benefits at the cost of long-term risk (Güllich, 2018; Huxley et al., 2014).

Psychosocial Factors

Drew (2020) qualitatively explored the psychosocial factors associated with the junior-to-senior transition in the context of British track and field athletes. Figure 19.1 outlines the internal and external factors athletes perceived to impact their transition and compares the findings from those who experienced a successful transition outcome to those who did not.

The results from the study demonstrate that the process of transition from junior to senior level is unique to each athlete and involves various factors that have the potential to aid or hinder athletes' progress. Athletes perceived that the transition is an ever-changing dynamic process and the factors associated with the transition are not fixed, with some factors becoming more salient than others at various points of the transition, and vice versa. Consistent with existing literature, the study highlights a number of psychosocial factors that can facilitate the junior-to-senior transition (e.g., patience, understanding of the transition process, sport-specific knowledge; Mills et al., 2012; Pummell and Lavallee, 2019), in addition to a number of debilitative factors (e.g., increase in pressure, injuries, over-trained as a junior/burnout; Jones et al., 2014; Pummell et al., 2008). For example, athletes believed it was important to view the transition as a long-term process and perceived patience to be a crucial psychological resource during the transition period. As one 1500 m Olympic finalist reflected, "I didn't over-train as a young athlete. I didn't try and do too much too soon, I was patient". Furthermore, the study highlighted the complex nature of the transition as the factors perceived to influence the transition vary amongst individuals. For example, a factor that one athlete perceives as particularly challenging (e.g., increase in pressure to perform) may not be identified by another athlete or may even be perceived as a motivator to the transition.

Nurturing Young Distance Runners

A SUCCESSFUL TRANSITION

Individual Facilitators (6)	External Facilitators (6)
Psychological factors (6) – Determination and commitment, Resilience, Work-ethic, Patience, Confidence, Intrinsic Motivation	World Junior Championship experiences (2) – Motivated them to pursue athletics career, Prepared them for senior championships
Achieving a life balance	Social support (8) – Parents, Coach, Training partners, Peers, Physiotherapist, Medical support, Family members, Sport psychologist
Championship learning experiences	The Coach (2) – Trust in coach, Coach planned for the long-term
Clearly defined goals and progression	Early exposure to senior environment
Sport-specific knowledge	Early senior success
Competition coping strategies	Financial support

Individual Debilitators (1)	External Debilitators (3)
Psychological factors – Increase in Pressure	World Junior Championship experiences – increase in pressure to perform as a senior
	Financial pressure
	Injuries

AN UNSUCCESSFUL TRANSITION

Individual Facilitators (2)	External Facilitators (4)
Psychological factors (2) – Patience, Resourcefulness	World Junior Championship experiences (3) – Increased confidence, prepared them for senior championships, fun
Natural ability	Social support (3) – Parents, Partner, University
	Financial support
	Positive training environment (2) – modelling successful senior athletes/training partners, developed technical proficiency

Individual Debilitators (7)	External Debilitators (7)
Psychological factors (2) – Increase in pressure, Loss of motivation	World Junior Championship experiences – increase in pressure to perform as a senior
Competition behaviours (3) – Negative mindset, Unprepared for senior competition, did not cope well with losing after junior success	Financial pressure
Sacrifices did not seem worth it	Injuries
Sport is more serious as a senior	Over-trained as a junior/ Burnout
Exclusive athletic identity	Increase in qualification standards from junior-to-senior
Unrealistic expectations of the transition period and progression	The coach (3) – Relationship changed during transition, Change of coach did not work, Lack of quality coaches
Mental health concerns	Lack of facilities

FIGURE 19.1 Individual and external factors perceived to impact the junior-to-senior transition in British track-and-field athletes

Source: Drew (2020).

Risks Associated With Early Specialisation in Distance Running

Early specialisation in a single sport is often characterised by high volumes of physical training that over a prolonged period can cause serious health consequences. These issues are also likely to contribute to the high drop-out rates observed during late-adolescence (Enoksen, 2011; Konittinen et al., 2013; Shibli and Barrett, 2011). It is probable that an optimal volume of sport-specific training exists for each individual performer at various stages of their development, which provides sufficient overload to adequately prepare musculoskeletal structures and physiological systems for higher volumes of specific training in the future, but does not expose the individual to high levels of risk. These risks can be summarised as follows (Blagrove et al., 2017; Myer et al., 2015; Côté et al., 2009).

Relative Energy Deficiency in Sport (RED-S)

The RED-S syndrome describes a range of negative physiological and psychological symptoms that affect metabolism, reproductive function, bone health, immunity, protein synthesis and cardiovascular health as a consequence of chronic low energy availability (Mountjoy et al., 2014). When intensive training regimens are combined with insufficient energy intake and recovery to support the exercise being undertaken, young athletes are at risk of developing RED-S (Hoch et al., 2009). Athletes who specialise in disciplines that demand high levels of leanness and endurance, such as distance running events, are particularly vulnerable (Nichols et al., 2006). Several important consequences associated with developing RED-S at a young age are summarised in the following and discussed in detail in Chapter 18.

Menstrual Cycle Dysfunction

The menstrual cycle is highly sensitive to physiological stress; therefore, female athletes engaged in intensive physical training programs are susceptible to developing menstrual cycle dysfunctions. High amounts of physical training and lifestyle stress can cause a negative energy balance, which first affects the female reproductive system as it is non-vital for survival (Horn et al., 2014). Primary amenorrhea is the absence of menstrual cycles at age 15 despite normal growth and signs of secondary sexual characteristics. A lack of menarche 3 years after initial development of secondary sexual characteristics, or no sign of these characteristics by the age of 14, is also a cause for concern (Weiss Kelly et al., 2016). Secondary amenorrhea is the absence of menses for more than 3 consecutive months or 6 months in females who have previously had regular menses. Oligomenorrhea is defined as menstrual cycles that occur >35 days apart (Horn et al., 2014). For active girls, the timing of menarche relative to peak height velocity is generally similar to non-athletic girls (Geithner et al., 1998). However, there is a high prevalence of menstrual dysfunctions during adolescence, particularly in athletes involved in intensive sports training (Hoch et al., 2009).

Poor Bone Health

The female sex hormone oestrogen, which contributes to regulating the menstrual cycle, plays an important role in bone formation. It is therefore unsurprising that adolescent athletes who present with amenorrhea possess significantly lower bone mineral density compared to eumenorrheic (regular menses) young athletes and non-athletic controls (Barrack et al., 2008). A relationship between age at menarche and likelihood of stress fractures has also been reported (Bennell et al., 1996b). This is particularly worrying, as adolescence represents an important window of opportunity for formation of bone density. By adulthood, approximately 90% of bone mass has been accrued (Sabatier et al., 1996); therefore, young female athletes who experience primary amenorrhea and fail to maximise bone mass during their development years are unlikely to compensate at a later age, even following resumption of menses (Baxter-Jones et al., 2011). A low bone mineral density increases the risk of stress fracture injuries, but also osteoporosis and sustaining fractures from falls in later life.

Overuse Injury

Early specialisation and maturation status have both been identified as independent risk factors for overuse injury in young athletes (Myer et al., 2015). High volumes of training are generally associated with a higher risk of injury in adolescent athletes (Emery, 2003; Maffulli et al., 2005), particularly those who participate in a single sport, as opposed to a range of sports (Hall et al., 2015; Jayanthi et al., 2015). During adolescence, the connective tissues, muscles and bones develop in a non-linear manner and are not fully developed until late adolescence. Following the adolescent growth spurt, there is often a lag in the development of the neuromuscular system, which can affect strength and coordination (Quatman-Yates et al., 2012). Rapid changes in stature, strength and limb lengths can contribute to poor movement patterns, and inappropriate attenuation of forces may exacerbate risk of injury when combined with high-volume regimens of physical work (Hawkins and Metheny, 2001). Moreover, female athletes with menstrual cycle abnormalities are also three times more likely to sustain a musculoskeletal injury compared to eumenorrheic adolescents (Barrack et al., 2014; Rauh et al., 2010). Although the association between menstrual disturbances and injury is not causative, a low energy state alters the profile of thyroid and stress hormones, which directly affects bone metabolism and the health of muscle and connective tissue (Lindholm et al., 1995; Loucks et al., 1989).

Mental Health Issues

A decision to specialise and compete year-round in a single sport brings an inevitable pressure to achieve pre-determined goals and continually progress. This pressure is often further compounded by the pressures placed on young athletes by coaches and parents. Chronic exposures to highly stressful and professionalised sporting environments at a young age are unlikely to be effective at nurturing talented performers into future elite athletes (Moesch et al., 2011; Waldron et al., 2019). Intrinsic motivation factors, such as enjoyment of practice, are most important in retaining young athletes and achieving long-term ambitions (Le Bars et al., 2009). Appropriate psychological challenges during an athlete's development stimulate a positive response to promote long-term attainment of goals (Collins et al., 2016). However, excessive psychological overload resulting from unrealistic expectations can be detrimental, causing depression, anxiety and ultimately burnout (Waldron et al., 2019). From a psychosocial perspective, concern has also been raised that placing high training demands on a young athlete limits their opportunity to develop a normal, multifaceted identity (Coakley, 1992). Young athletes who specialise in a single sport report they become consumed by their training and feel a sense of isolation (Coakley, 1992). When fitted around school timetables, intensive training programmes severely restrict the time young athletes can dedicate to other activities. Therefore, young athletes develop a unidimensional identity and feel defined by their sport, which can lead to stress and anxiety if they fail to reach their goals.

Overtraining

Overtraining is caused by an accumulation of training and non-training stress, which results in chronic under-performance, taking several weeks or months to recover from (Meeusen et al., 2013). Approximately one-third of competitive athletes (13–18 years) across a range of sports in various countries have suffered from overtraining-related symptoms or burnout at least once (Gustafsson et al., 2007; Matos et al., 2011; Raglin et al., 2000). Overtraining is characterised by a plethora of signs and symptoms, which are derived from several different physiological systems including: increased perception of effort during exercise, frequent upper respiratory tract infections, sleep disruption, excessive muscular fatigue and a loss of appetite. Many of these symptoms are also likely to impact other aspects of a young athlete's lifestyle, including their academic work and social life.

Limited Skills and Experiences

Early sport-specialisation, particularly in activities involving repetitive actions like distance running, limits the acquisition of a wide range of motor skills. This may seem beneficial in the short term, for the child athlete aspiring to greatness in their chosen event; however, it drastically limits opportunities to participate in other sports, which the performer may enjoy or excel in (Stodden et al., 2013). Equally, a reduction in motor skills could adversely affect life-long participation in physical activity as the athlete feels limited to the sport they have always competed in. Furthermore, participation in a single sport limits the opportunities for human interaction in other social spheres (Coakley, 1992). It has been hypothesised that these lost opportunities for development of a diverse range of sports skills may in part contribute to the current high levels of physical inactivity and obesity in adulthood (Mostafavifar et al., 2013).

Long-Term Development of Youth Athletes

Unlike many game sports in European and Western countries, high-performing young distance runners are rarely placed into highly structured talent development systems that are controlled by professional clubs or governing bodies. In many respects this is likely to provide several advantages, such as less pressure to travel and compete, and a greater flexibility to participate in other sports at a young age. However, a lack of specialist support in this scenario can also mean that guidance on training and competition schedules at various stages of a young athlete's development is left to parents and inexperienced club coaches.

Contemporary approaches to long-term athlete development suggest children and adolescents should avoid training routines that focus on intensive training in a single sport (for >8 months per year), or a total weekly training volume which exceeds the athlete's age in years, until late adolescence (Lloyd and Oliver, 2012; Myer et al., 2016). Figure 19.2 provides a visual representation of a long-term development model for a youth athlete. The pie charts on the right-hand side of Figure 19.2 represent a theoretical distribution of activities for a

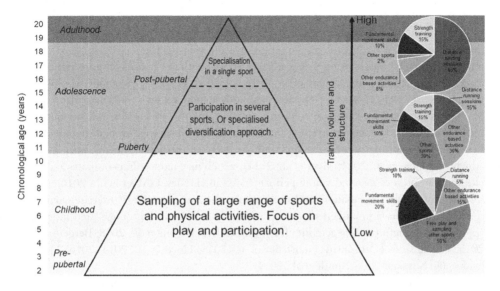

FIGURE 19.2 Suggested performance pyramid and model for long-term development of a youth performer who displays talent and/or motivation to succeed as a distance runner. The width of the pyramid represents the number of sports/activities that the performer should aim to participate in. The pie charts represent a theoretical example from three different time points (~8, ~13, ~17 years old) of a young athlete's development to illustrate how various physical activities and sports could be distributed

fictional young athlete who displays talent and/or a high level of motivation for distance running during their development. Whilst some degree of sport specialisation is necessary during adolescence to reach elite status, the timing of single-sport specialisation is more contentious. Evidence across a range of sports shows elite senior athletes tend to specialise at a later age and to participate in a diverse range of sports during their childhood (Côté et al., 2009; Moesch et al., 2011). Young athletes who adopt an early-diversification, late-specialisation approach to their development have fewer injuries, are at less risk of overtraining and play sports longer than those who specialise in one sport before puberty (Brenner and Council of Sports Medicine and Fitness, 2016; DiFiori et al., 2014). A recent reconceptualised approach to the idea of sampling before late adolescence, is a domain-specific approach termed 'specialised diversification' (Côté and Erickson, 2015). Using this method, it is recommended that a young performer who enjoys participating in endurance-based sports could specialise in this sport-specific domain, and sample through different experiences within this domain during adolescence. For example, a young athlete who enjoys and excels in distance running events could participate in cross-country, road and track running, swimming, cycling and orienteering. Emphasis should remain on free play and sampling of activities within these contexts, rather than high volumes of deliberate practice and structured training.

Strength Training for Young Athletes

The long-term health and fitness benefits of participating in a well-rounded programme of physical activities and sports during childhood and adolescence, which promotes physical literacy and develops a breadth of physical qualities, has been recognised by the International Olympic Committee (Bergeron et al., 2015). A key component of a systematic approach to the development of young athletes is a progressive and well-managed programme of strength training, which enables aspiring young athletes to cope with the rigours of sports training and reach their potential (Faigenbaum et al., 2016; Lloyd et al., 2014). Strength training techniques develop a broad range of physical capacities such as agility, speed, muscular strength, balance, co-ordination, and motor control, which underpin performance across numerous sports and everyday living tasks (Lloyd and Oliver, 2012). Moreover, strength training activities which develop neuromuscular function are likely to offset the risk of injury in youth athletes (DiFiori et al., 2014; Myer et al., 2011), which may reduce drop-out rates and facilitate the transition of talented young performers to an elite level (Myer et al., 2016). Several leading professional organisations and authorities in the area of paediatric exercise science and sports medicine have published statements advocating the inclusion of age- and individual-appropriate strength training activities for young athletes (Behm et al., 2008; Bergeron et al., 2015; Faigenbaum et al., 2016; Granacher et al., 2016; Lloyd et al., 2014, 2016; McCambridge and Stricker, 2008; Smith et al., 2014).

A large body of literature exists that demonstrates strength training activities are a safe and effective way of enhancing proxy measures of athletic performance in children and adolescents of both sexes (Behringer et al., 2010, 2011; Blagrove et al., 2020; Harries et al., 2012; Lesinski et al., 2016). Specifically, in post-pubertal adolescents, compared to sport-only training, various forms of strength training augment improvements in muscular strength, explosive power, muscular endurance, sprint speed, agility test time and general motor skills.

The safety of resistance training (i.e. lifting weights) in young athletes has previously been questioned with concerns centred around epiphyseal plate injury and growth abnormalities the most commonly cited (Benton, 1982; Gumbs et al., 1982; Legwold and Kummant, 1982). However, any isolated observations associated with damage to growth cartilage appear to be related to poor lifting technique or inappropriate training volumes. Providing training is supervised and prescribed by a qualified practitioner, the current consensus in the field of pediatric sports medicine indicates that strength training is not inherently harmful and does not pose a risk to epiphyseal plates or normal growth (Lloyd et al., 2014; Milone et al., 2013; Myers et al., 2017). Indeed, prospective investigations that have included appropriate levels of supervision and coaching have demonstrated no increased incidence of physeal-related injury (Ramsay et al., 1990) and overall low injury rates (Lillegard et al., 1997).

Research investigating the impact of strength training techniques on performance-related measures in young athletes has tended to use participants from field-based sports, martial arts, court sports, aquatic sports, gymnastics and strength-based sports (Granacher et al., 2016; Lesinski et al., 2016). Two studies have used middle- or long-distance runners between the ages of 15 and 18 years old (Blagrove et al., 2018b; Mikkola et al., 2007). Mikkola et al. (2007) took a group of trained male and female distance runners (17.3 years, $\dot{V}O_{2max}$: 62.5 ml·kg^{-1}·min^{-1}) and, following 8 weeks of heavy- and explosive-strength training, observed improvements in anaerobic capabilities (speed during a maximal anaerobic running test and 30 m sprint time). Similarly, Blagrove and colleagues (2018b) also found significant improvements in sprint speed and a 'possibly beneficial' effect on RE following 10 weeks of strength training. Importantly, this study reduced the overall volume of running by around a third (29%) to accommodate the addition of two weekly strength training sessions (Blagrove et al., 2018b). This demonstrates that, at least for a period of several months in this age group, greater gains can be achieved in important determinants of performance when two running sessions per week are replaced with strength training.

Summary

Young athletes represent a vulnerable population, and participation in sport provides an important vehicle to facilitate their physical, social and psychological development. Distance running is becoming increasingly popular amongst adolescents; therefore, coaches, parents, teachers and practitioners have an obligation to ensure the long-term well-being and development of this group. The tempo and timing of growth, development and maturation varies considerably in a group of young athletes of the same chronological age, therefore the runners who excel at a young age tend to be the most physically mature relative to their peer group. Unfortunately, for those athletes who specialise in middle- or long-distance events at a young age (≤15 years old), and rank highly in their age group, achieving the same level of success as a senior runner is rare. Specialisation in the sport of distance running at the exclusion of all other sports before the age of 16 years old tends to be associated with a range of negative health implications that result in drop-out during late adolescence. These include overuse injury, poor bone health, psychological burnout, overtraining and delayed menarche. The transition from junior- to senior-level competition should be viewed as a long-term process, and elite senior athletes perceive patience to be a crucial psychological resource. Although there is considerable variability in the routes that high-performing distance runners take to reach an elite status, the most common pathway to senior success involves participating in several sports during childhood and teenage years, and specialising in a single sport only during late adolescence. Adopting an early-diversification, late-specialisation approach to long-term athlete development tends to result in fewer injuries, reduces the risk of overtraining and lowers rates of drop-out compared to those who specialise in one sport before puberty. Strength training also represents a safe and effective form of exercise that young athletes should engage with from an early age to offset the risk of injury as training volume progressively increases.

20

CONSIDERATIONS FOR THE FEMALE RUNNER

Georgie Bruinvels, Esther Goldsmith and Nicola Brown

Highlights

- From pre-puberty through to post-menopause, distinct variation occurs in hormonal profiles that can affect a whole range of different physiological systems and can influence health and performance.
- These hormonal changes are likely to be highly individual and can affect readiness to train.
- There are a number of menstrual dysfunctions and disorders that runners may be susceptible to and should be screened for.
- The use of hormonal contraception can alter hormonal profile; therefore, it is essential to educate athletes on the mechanisms of action prior to use.
- Tracking menstrual symptoms and cycles helps athletes to best understand their individual cycle and enables them to be proactive and prepared. Understanding potential risk factors for symptoms is also key.
- Breast pain is common in female athletes and level of breast support worn can influence biomechanical and physiological variables; therefore, particular care and attention should be applied to finding the most appropriate and well-fitted sports bra to reduce long-term health issues and negative performance implications.

Introduction

Many physiological differences exist between men and women, yet it is often assumed that research findings from studies conducted in males can be directly applied to women. Although this may be the case for some of the recommendations provided in the sport and exercise science literature, there are important sex differences in the physiology of men and women that must be considered when designing physical training and nutrition interventions. From puberty through to menopause, women's bodies experience a number of natural physiological changes and events, which the male body does not. These can have a large impact upon health, participation in exercise and performance-related outcomes. It is important that coaches and runners are aware of these and can respond appropriately to minimise any negative impacts. The menstrual cycle describes the hormonal process that a woman's body experiences approximately once per month to prepare for the possibility of pregnancy. The female sex hormones associated with the menstrual cycle influence a multitude of different physiological systems and processes; therefore, fluctuations in these hormones may impact a runner's emotions, physical readiness and adaptative processes. Further, as addressed in Chapter 18, exercise training is known to increase the likelihood of menstrual cycle irregularities and dysfunctions. A high proportion of women also use a hormonal contraceptive, which can help manage menstrual-cycle-related symptoms but have several important training and performance implications that runners and coaches should be aware of. Breast-related issues such as exercise-induced breast pain and embarrassment can also affect a high number of female runners and represent a topical area of research in sports medicine. The aims of this chapter are to explore the science underpinning these female-related physiological issues and provide recommendations to runners and coaches around how best to manage these issues.

Sex Hormones Across the Female Lifespan

Throughout the female lifespan, there are ongoing fluctuations in the reproductive hormonal milieu, with significant changes marking key developments or stages in life. These transitions may cause changes to exercise training programmes and alter requirements for maintaining health and, where relevant, performance. Reproductive hormonal release is a tightly regulated process, primarily controlled by the hypothalamic pituitary gonadal (HPG) axis. Aberration to the process, when not caused by an obvious change in life stage e.g. pregnancy or menopause, can result in a need to seek medical advice, and a subsequent multi-disciplinary medical approach may be necessary, including a nutritionist or psychologist, for example.

The HPG axis controls the secretion of gonadatrophin releasing hormone (GnRH), which is released in a pulsatile manner in response to a complex feedback system. GnRH regulates the release of the gonadotrophins, luteinizing hormone (LH) and follicle stimulating hormone (FSH). In women, LH and FSH act on the ovaries to trigger the reproduction pathway through the two primary female sex hormones, oestrogen and progesterone. In the absence of hormonal contraception use, menstrual dysfunction and pregnancy, from menarche until perimenopause, release of LH and FSH is tightly controlled by the HPG axis, resulting in ovarian activity. Marked by significant changes to the hormonal profile, the female lifecycle can be broken down into infancy, puberty, the reproductive years, pregnancy, perimenopause, and post-menopause. This chapter will primarily focus on the reproductive years; however, the physiology underpinning the other life stages will also be outlined.

Puberty

Typically, between the ages of 7 and 10, girls start to experience a surge in activity of GnRH, resulting in an increase in the secretion of gonadotrophins (Wood et al., 2019). This causes an increase in the release of the ovarian hormones, oestrogen and progesterone. As a result, girls start to develop secondary sex characteristics (e.g. breast budding, pubic and underarm hair), and typically towards the end of puberty, menarche (the onset of menstruation) occurs. On average, puberty lasts 2–5 years, and girls usually go through this approximately 2 years earlier than boys. Increased GnRH production also controls puberty in boys, and through this process testosterone release is increased (Wood et al., 2019). Testosterone is an anabolic hormone, which, in a sporting context largely explains the sex-specific differences in strength, power and endurance. There is a disproportionately greater risk of girls dropping out from sport when compared to boys, and one of the primary causes for this is the body changes that accompany puberty. It is also important to have awareness that some of the anatomical changes that occur during puberty, which can also negatively affect performance and can be a cause of embarrassment. There are numerous benefits to pursuing regular exercise throughout puberty (Hasselstrøm et al., 2002); therefore, it is essential to support girls through this process; having an appreciation for the substantial anatomical and physiological differences that arise during puberty to keep girls engaged and physically active. Caution should be applied to specialising in a particular sport pre-puberty or during puberty, as has been discussed elsewhere (Blagrove et al., 2017).

Perimenopause and Menopause

The perimenopausal period can be characterised by a reduction in pulsatility of GnRH. In early perimenopause, LH levels tend to remain stable, and FSH levels increase and continue to increase through the menopausal period. Oestrogen levels initially increase but then sharply decline alongside progesterone towards the end of this phase. Menopause is the ceasing of menstruation and is characterised by cessation of progesterone production and very low oestrogen concentrations. Low concentrations of oestrogen can have negative health consequences for some (e.g. reduced bone mineral density, increased risk of cardiovascular disease, and depressive symptoms), and hormone replacement therapy can sometimes be offered as a management strategy for post-menopausal women (Lobo, 2017). There are numerous benefits to participating in physical activity both during and after the menopausal transition (Grindler and Santoro, 2015). However, optimal exercise requirements alter alongside the transition in hormonal profile from that of eumenorrheic women, so specific and tailored training programmes are warranted (Zhao et al., 2017).

Pregnancy

Pregnancy can be characterised by a dramatic change in hormonal profile; the first trimester is dominated by human chorionic gonadotrophin hormone, with an initial spike of progesterone. During the second trimester, progesterone steadily increases alongside oestrogen and prolactin, and finally, in the third trimester there is a sharp oxytocin spike. Relaxin levels are at their highest in the first trimester but remain relatively high throughout all three trimesters. Oxytocin and prolactin are of relevance during the initial post-partum phase, and the length of time of lactation will specifically impact prolactin production. While specific research and recommendations are beyond the scope of this chapter, it is important to note that exercise pre- and post-partum needs to be managed very carefully, and individuals should seek specific advice from qualified practitioners. For example, while one of the primary roles of relaxin is to facilitate the anatomical changes that occur as a result of the developing foetus, it can also increase joint laxity, therefore increase risk of certain injury types. A set of guidelines have recently been published aiding practitioners with the management of this time period (Donnelly et al., 2020).

The Menstrual Cycle

The menstrual cycle is part of a tightly regulated feedback process involving the release of FSH and LH from the pituitary gland in response to the pulsatile secretions of GnRH from the hypothalamus. FSH and LH then act on the ovaries to control the release of oestrogen (primarily 17-b oestradiol) and progesterone. This is a highly sensitive process, and there are a number of factors which can result in perturbation.

A 'eumenorrheic' menstrual cycle typically lasts 22–35 days (Fehring et al., 2006). As shown in Figure 20.1, it can be split into two phases, the follicular phase (days 1–14 in a 28-day cycle) and the luteal phase (days 15–28 in a 28-day cycle), with ovulation occurring between these. Oestrogen and progesterone fluctuate in a cyclical manner throughout the whole cycle. The follicular phase begins with the shedding of the uterus lining (menstruation), which typically lasts 3–7 days. Menstruation is characterised by low levels of oestrogen and progesterone, and these low levels enable the hypothalamic derived GnRH to start stimulating FSH and LH release from the anterior pituitary gland. FSH specifically stimulates growth and development of a group of ovarian follicles. The maturation and growth of these follicles triggers oestrogen secretion; oestrogen levels steadily increase through the follicular phase. This causes thickening of the endometrial lining, while also inhibiting FSH secretion. A dominant follicle emerges, now secreting increasing amounts of oestrogen. As oestrogen levels reach a peak, LH surges, pausing oestrogen release from the dominant follicle, driving rupture of the ovarian follicle, causing ovum release and triggering the formation of the corpus luteum. This is termed ovulation. During the luteal phase, the corpus luteum is stimulated to secrete oestrogen and progesterone; however, in the absence of fertilisation, these will start to decline and the luteolysis of the corpus luteum will occur. The fall in these hormones triggers endometrium shedding (menstruation), as the cycle starts again on day one (Maybin and Critchley,

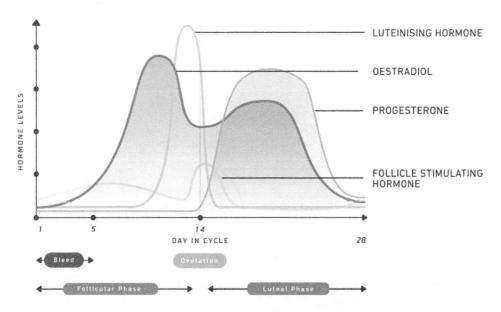

FIGURE 20.1 The hormonal fluctuations that occur throughout the menstrual cycle

2015; Critchley et al., 2020). Many factors are involved in the control of FSH and LH including stress, metabolic status (including energy availability), psychological elements and exercise.

While the primary function of oestrogen and progesterone is to drive reproduction, they also impact physiological non-reproductive systems and are vital for the maintenance of homeostasis (see Figure 20.2). Circulating in the blood, they have been shown to affect cardiovascular, immune, skeletal and central nervous systems, in addition to acting on cells in the kidneys, hypothalamus (Heritage et al., 1980), bone marrow, skin, and liver (Heritage et al., 1980; Smith et al., 1995; Dubey and Jackson, 2001; Gustafsson, 2003; Khan and Ahmed, 2016). It is clear that both oestrogen and progesterone can have profound effects on female physiology, having the potential to influence a myriad of processes which, in turn, could impact wellness, exercise training and performance.

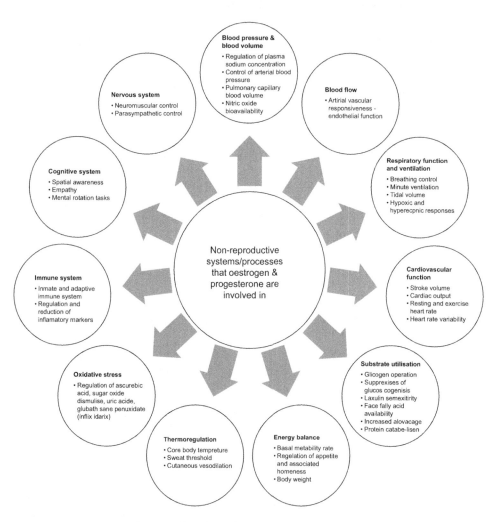

FIGURE 20.2 Non-reproductive physiological systems/processes in which ovarian hormones, oestrogen and progesterone, are involved

Source: Oosthuyse and Bosch (2010); Lebrun et al. (2013).

While it must be acknowledged that, until recently, there has been a sparsity of research specifically focusing on female exercise physiology, both how this differs to that in males and how this changes at different times in the menstrual cycle, over the last 20–30 years some emerging research has highlighted the potential non-reproductive effects of the ovarian hormones, which warrant consideration when working with female athletes. It is, however, important to consider the individual nature of these effects; not only how they may differ between women, but also at different stages of a woman's life.

Whilst understanding the individual effects that oestrogen and progesterone may have throughout a menstrual cycle is beneficial, it can be helpful to consider these effects in regard to the different phases of the menstrual cycle.

Menstruation (Approximately, Days 1–5 of a 28-Day Cycle)

Physiology. The premenstrual decline in ovarian hormones causes an inflammatory response, which triggers the breakdown of the uterus lining and menstrual blood loss (Maybin and Critchley, 2015). There is an associated increased expression of inflammatory mediators such as C-reactive protein (CRP) (Gaskins et al., 2012). This is one of the causes of symptoms and has the potential to influence recovery from training. White cell count may also be lower during this phase, altering risk of certain types of illness and necessitating best practice around fuelling and sleep (Nowak et al., 2016).

Exercise training and performance. Due to the significant likelihood for menstrual cycle-related symptoms at this time, athletes often cite that their training and performance is negatively affected during menstruation (Armour et al., 2020). However, recent reviews concluded there to be a trivial performance decline at this time (McNulty et al., 2020; Blagrove et al., 2020c). Common reasons for a perceived negative impact upon physical performance during this period include fatigue and altered energy levels. These may arise due to: altered metabolic rate/energy expenditure, increased disturbed sleep and changes in dietary choices, as well as the previously mentioned increases in inflammation. One study found self-reported muscle soreness to increase in this window (Romero-Parra et al., 2020). Symptoms should therefore be tracked and monitored on an individual basis. Some research has specifically found motor control and myofascial force transmission patterns to be affected by the low concentrations of ovarian hormones (Dedrick et al., 2008). This could result in impaired neuromuscular control and therefore necessitates an emphasis on activation exercises and drills, particularly before any intense exercise.

Nutrition. A focus should be applied to the inclusion of foods with anti-inflammatory properties and those containing antioxidants to aid with managing the increased concentration of inflammatory mediators during this phase. Nutrients such as fish oils and specific antioxidants have been shown to reduce inflammation (Lewis et al., 2020) and oxidative stress (Serafini and Peluso, 2017).

Mid-Late Follicular Phase (Approximately Days 6–14 of a 28-Day Cycle)

Physiology. After menstruation, there is a steady increase in oestrogen until it reaches a threshold, just prior to ovulation. Increases in oestrogen during the follicular phase are often linked with decreased symptoms, and increased energy and positivity.

Specifically, increased oestrogen production is associated with increased serotonin and catecholamine release which can positively affect mood and sleep quality (Wihlbäck et al., 2004).

Exercise training and performance. Some research suggests that strength training during the follicular phase may result in great increases in muscular strength compared to training in the luteal phase (Sung et al., 2014; Julian et al., 2017). The specific mechanism for this is unclear, but it is hypothesised to be linked to an oestrogen-mediated faster recovery, potentially through membrane stabilisation, increased antioxidant capacity, or the increased catabolic effects of progesterone seen in the luteal phase (Isacco and Boisseau, 2017; Faustmann et al., 2018). Although a slight bias towards strength training may be prudent during this phase compared to others, it must also be acknowledged that oestrogen is often associated with altered stability and laxity of joints, as well as a reduction in proprioception and altered general muscle activation patterns (Eiling et al., 2007; Bryant et al., 2011; Casey et al., 2014). It is well evidenced that women are two to eight times more likely than men to experience non-contact anterior cruciate ligament (ACL) injuries, and emerging research suggests that the incidence of such injuries may be elevated just prior to ovulation (Herzberg et al., 2017). Both increases in joint laxity and decreased neuromuscular control are thought to contribute to this, and therefore, whilst prevalence of ACL injury risk is relatively low in runners when compared to team sports, these hormone-driven changes are under-researched in relation to other injuries. Therefore, consideration for best practice and risk reduction is needed, specifically around warm-up, cool down and recovery practices. It is also important to appreciate that risk of such injuries is likely to be greater in certain individuals more so than others.

Nutrition. As noted in Figure 20.2, oestrogen and progesterone may affect glycogen storage. During the follicular phase, the influence of increased oestrogen concentrations may result in reduced glycogen storage (Oosthuyse and Bosch, 2010). However, this can be offset by increased carbohydrate intake (moderate carbohydrate loading; see Chapter 4) prior to endurance training of more than 1hour (McLay et al., 2007).

Energy balance and availability are crucial to maintain health and performance as an athlete, to which the menstrual cycle is particularly sensitive. Research shows that energy manipulation in the follicular phase results in severe energy deficits and causes disruptions in LH pulsatility, ovarian function and menstrual cycle characteristics (Loucks and Thuma, 2003). Therefore, whilst appetite may be slightly suppressed in the follicular phase, sufficient energy intake throughout the day is vital in order to maintain a regular menstrual cycle and healthy hormonal profile.

Luteal Phase (Early- to Mid-Luteal; Approximately Days 15–23 of a 28-Day Cycle)

Physiology. Just after ovulation there is an increase in both oestrogen and progesterone. These hormones typically remain high for around a week in a eumenorrheic cycle. The increase in progesterone is often detected by an increase in core/basal body temperature (BBT). BBT typically increases by 0.3–0.5 °C (Marshall, 1963) and is often accompanied by elevations in resting heart rate (by two to eight beats per minute)

(Jonge et al., 2012; Julian et al., 2017), which may also be sustained during sub-maximal exercise (Jonge et al., 2012). The increase in BBT may be of importance (and may impact performance) when exercising in hot and humid conditions, and this should be taken into individual consideration (Jonge et al., 2012).

Exercise training and performance. Elevations in BBT and resting heart rate are also important to consider when conducting daily monitoring and/or when training in specific heart rate zones. Increases in progesterone may also cause increases in ventilation rate and exhaled nitric oxide during the luteal phase. Whilst, for many athletes, this doesn't appear to impact training and performance (McNulty et al., 2020), those with existing ventilatory conditions (e.g. asthma) may experience symptoms during this time (Mandhane et al., 2009). Recent research suggests that aerobic performance may be inhibited in the mid-luteal phase as a result of increased ratings of fatigue and a more negative mood state (Freemas et al., 2020). Therefore, strategies to enhance sleep, improve mood and reduce stress should be implemented with athletes affected by these changes in emotional state during the luteal phase.

Nutrition. High concentrations of progesterone are associated with increased insulin resistance and decreased insulin sensitivity, thereby often causing unstable blood sugar levels (Yeung et al., 2010). Basal metabolic rate is also thought to be higher as a result of increased energy expenditure in this phase when compared to the follicular phase (Zhang et al., 2020). As a result, female athletes may need to pay attention to diet, potentially increasing frequency and amount of food intake in order to avoid dips in energy, focusing on complex carbohydrates and good-quality protein sources (see Chapter 4). Whilst cravings may result in decreased energy levels at this time, sleep disturbances and decreased sleep quality are also more common in the luteal phase, and therefore best practices around sleep and/or taking naps may be encouraged (Baker and Driver, 2007; Baker and Lee, 2018). Finally, breakdown of muscle protein may be increased in the luteal phase, as progesterone is linked to increased turnover of amino acids (Wallace et al., 2010; Faustmann et al., 2018). This may be offset by increasing/ensuring sufficient intake of protein before and after training (see Chapter 4 and Chapter 17).

Premenstrual Phase (Approximately Days 24–28 of a 28-Day Cycle)

Physiology. This phase is characterised by a dramatic decline in hormones, triggering the onset of menstruation. Similar to the menstrual phase, this is accompanied by a release of inflammatory mediators and increased oxidative stress (Gaskins et al., 2012).

Training. As a result of the increased inflammatory profile and other effects of the withdrawal of hormones, optimal recovery windows between training can be extended. Therefore, attention is required to applying best practice with regard to recovery strategies (see Chapter 17). It is also important to appreciate that many women experience a range of symptoms during this phase, and these can affect their readiness to train (Armour et al., 2020; Findlay et al., 2020). Mood disturbances are particularly common and often occur concomitantly with changes in motivation. Both psychological and physical symptoms (such as stomach cramps and lower back pain) may be improved by light-to-moderate aerobic exercise and yoga practice (Vaghela et al., 2019). Psychological stress also has the potential to exacerbate symptoms, so where possible this should be managed. There is also evidence to suggest that sleep quality and duration may be reduced pre-menstruation (Baker and Driver, 2004), and this may exaggerate the severity of certain pre-menstrual syndrome (PMS) symptoms. This may contribute to elongated recovery windows and increase risk of other factors such as illness and injury that are often associated with sleep deprivation.

Nutrition. Due to the inflammatory nature of this phase, intake of fruits, vegetables, Omega-3 fatty acids, and food/drink with known anti-inflammatory properties (e.g. green tea) should be encouraged (Yamada and Takeda, 2018; MoradiFili et al., 2020). Inadequate intakes of micronutrients such as calcium, vitamin D, B vitamins, and magnesium have been proposed to be risk factors for symptoms (Girman et al., 2002). The luteal phase observations of increased muscle breakdown are also sustained here, meaning protein intake around training is important.

The Menstrual Cycle and Exercise Performance

It should be acknowledged that, despite the potential effects of the menstrual cycle on exercise and training, most of the sports science research has not found that menstrual cycle phase impacts objective measures of performance (e.g. in time-to-exhaustion tests, maximal strength or time trials) (Blagrove et al., 2020c; McNulty et al., 2020). This suggests that female athletes can perform to their potential regardless of menstrual cycle phase (McNulty et al., 2020). However, it is important to consider the potential for this to be influenced by observation bias, the training status of participants and methodological limitations, such as considering only certain time points in the menstrual cycle. Recent subjective testimonials from athletes citing the negative impact of their menstrual cycle on performance displays that further work must be done to manage symptoms effectively and reduce the likelihood of this occurring (Armour et al., 2020; Findlay et al., 2020). There is also a high amount of inter- and intra-individual variation in hormonal changes across the menstrual cycle, and therefore a personalised/individual approach is imperative.

Key Points

- The hormonal fluctuations throughout the menstrual cycle warrant consideration regarding nutrition, sleep, recovery and physiological monitoring.
- An individualised approach is essential; everyone is unique, and athletes should be encouraged to understand and work with their individual physiology.
- Menstrual cycle-related symptoms can perceptually negatively affect athletic performance, individual strategies should be put in place to address these.

Menstrual Cycle Patterns in Athletes

Athletes are more likely to have an irregular menstrual cycle than non-athletes (Nazem and Ackerman, 2012). Pre-pubertal participation in intense exercise typically delays onset of menarche by around a year, and also increases likelihood of future menstrual disorders (Nazem and Ackerman, 2012; Blagrove et al., 2017). The prevalence of oligomenorrhea (infrequent menstruation) and amenorrhea (absent menstruation) is increased in athletes, particularly in those competing in endurance running (Nazem and Ackerman, 2012), where there is a perception that a low body mass is desirable for performance. Susceptibility to secondary amenorrhea (see the section on dysfunctional cycle length for a definition) is also increased in those who undertake exercise, while also common in those with delayed circadian rhythm due to alterations in melatonin release, e.g. in-flight attendants (Radowicka et al., 2013). This is hypothesised to be caused by the impact of melatonin on LH and could have implications for athletes undergoing long-haul travel. However, further research is required to investigate this.

Menstrual Dysfunction and Disorders

A wide range of different menstrual irregularities and disorders can occur, and female runners may be more susceptible to some of these. These can be broadly broken down into those which are structural or functional in nature, and those which are circumstantial; however, there may be crossover between the two. Where a dysfunction or disorder is suspected, medical follow-up is essential. Where there is no underlying medical pathology, other factors that may exert stress on the HPG axis should be considered. This stress can manifest in several ways: increasing or decreasing cycle length, increasing or decreasing blood loss and/or exacerbating symptoms.

Potential factors that may impart excess stress on the HPG axis include:

- Nutritional intake:

    - Quantity – not consuming the correct quantity of macronutrients to fuel the requirements of the body, and to keep it in an 'adaptive' state.
    - Type – it is important to consume enough food from all macronutrient groups and to include a wide array of micronutrients.
    - Timing – extended periods of fasting place extra stress on the body and can result in dysfunctions.

- Psychological stress:

    - Periods of increased anxiety or worry can cause HPG dysregulation, either suppressing GnRH activity or heightening symptoms

- Travel:

    - Whilst the mechanism is still not completely identified, periods of frequent travel, particularly across time zones, can result in more irregular and erratic cycles.

- Sleep:

    - Disruptions to sleep can increase cortisol (a stress hormone), which can then disrupt the HPG axis.

- Exercise:

    - Sudden increases in exercise volume and/or intensity without sufficient recovery can place extra stress on the HPG axis.

The most prevalent dysfunctions and disorders are outlined next.

Dysfunctional Cycle Length

Cycle length can be extended (amenorrhoea or oligomenorrhoea) or shortened (polymenorrhoea) from a eumenorrheic cycle length of 22–35 days for a number of different reasons, usually as a result of excess stress on the HPG axis, as outlined earlier. Some menstrual dysfunctions can increase likelihood of these atypical aberrations.

Amenorrhoea – used to describe the absence of or cessation of menstruation. There are two types of amenorrhoea. Primary amenorrhoea is the absence of menses at age 15 years in the presence of normal growth and secondary sexual characteristics. Despite the likelihood of this scenario being greater in female runners, medical input should always be sought if menarche has not commenced by 15 years of age. Secondary amenorrhoea is the absence of menstruation for more than 3 months where cycles had previously been established.

Oligomenorrhoea – used to describe infrequent menstrual periods; typically fewer than 6–8 menstrual periods each year, or gaps of 35 days or more between menstrual periods.

Polymenorrhoea – used to describe a shorter than 'normal' menstrual cycle, where total menstrual cycle length is 21 days or less.

Heavy Menstrual Bleeding

Heavy menstrual bleeding (HMB) is very common, with ~20–45% of menstruating women having a history of the condition (El-Hemaidi et al., 2007; Marret et al., 2010; Santos et al., 2011). Research suggests that athletes are as likely to have HMB as non-athletes, with over a third of marathon runners reporting a history of HMB (Bruinvels et al., 2016). Diagnosis of HMB is challenging; historically, a total blood loss volume was used to identify whether a woman was a heavy bleeder. However, this is problematic to measure due to (a) hygiene concerns, (b) the total blood volume from woman to woman varies significantly, meaning that the relative amount of blood loss is much more relevant, (c) not all menstrual fluid is blood, (d) additional blood can be lost when passing urine, defecating, or through flooding into clothing or bedding. More recently, a more subjective definition of HMB has been created and utilised by the National Institute for Care Excellence. This includes "excessive menstrual blood loss which interferes with a woman's physical, social, emotional and/or material quality of life" (Davies and Kadir, 2017). Other research has also used a diagnostic series including: (1) flooding through clothes or onto bedding, (2) a need for frequent changes of sanitary towels or tampons (every 2 hours or less, or 12 sanitary items per day), (3) need for double sanitary protection (tampons and towels) and (4) passing of large blood clots. Where two or more of the outlined criteria are reported, HMB is identified.

HMB can be caused by an underlying structural or non-structural gynaecological problem, so where HMB is suspected, medical investigation to check for any underlying cause is warranted. The impacts of HMB can be vast, affecting quality of life, mood, energy levels and productivity amongst other aspects. It is also a condition that frequently goes unnoticed and undiscussed, especially amongst certain cultures.

In sport, the potential psychological implications must be considered, particularly where sports kit may reveal flooding. Research has shown that those with a history of HMB are more likely to self-report negative effects of the menstrual cycle on exercise training and performance (Bruinvels et al., 2016). Those with HMB can often have more severe menstrual symptoms such as menstrual cramps, which could, in part, be attributed to the inflammatory nature of this condition (Maybin et al., 2011). As a result, recovery windows between intense exercise may need to be elongated in the menstrual phase. HMB also has clinical repercussions, increasing susceptibility to iron deficiency and, if left untreated, iron deficiency anaemia (IDA). Regardless of menstrual blood loss, those who exercise are already at an increased risk of iron deficiency and IDA (Siegel et al., 1979; Telford et al., 2003; Peeling et al., 2008), so monitoring iron status is recommended. Where HMB is present, this need is clearly enhanced, so iron status should regularly be monitored.

Actions:

- Screen for HMB.
- Where HMB is thought present, underlying medical conditions should be screened for.
- Iron status should regularly be checked.
- Cycles should be tracked, and symptoms should be logged.
- Consideration should be applied to the use of white sports kit.

Endometriosis

Endometriosis occurs when the lining of the uterus (endometrium) grows in other parts of the body (Bulun et al., 2019). This is an inflammatory condition that can be debilitating and result in severe symptoms and heavy bleeding. While research suggests that 10% of women have endometriosis, diagnosis takes on average 7.5 years, suggesting that prevalence may in fact be greater (Bulun et al., 2019). There is currently no evidence to suggest that prevalence of endometriosis may be different in those who exercise, and anecdotally a number of high-profile athletes have highlighted diagnosis with this condition. Given the inflammatory nature of endometriosis (Bulun et al., 2019), recovery times from exercise may be increased, and dietary modification may be necessary.

Polycystic Ovarian Syndrome (PCOS)

Sufferers of PCOS have altered ovarian function, often resulting in a reduced ability of the ovarian follicles to release an egg (ovulation). PCOS is typically characterised by the presence of fluid-filled cysts in the ovaries, higher levels of male hormones (androgens) in the body, and irregular or absent menstrual cycles. The potential metabolic consequences of PCOS warrant consideration, and medical input should be sought for management. PCOS is thought to affect 8–13% of women (Stepto et al., 2019); however, around half of these women will not experience symptoms. Amongst athletes, prevalence is unsure, although despite a need for more research, exercise is believed to be a good form of management (Stepto et al., 2019).

Ovarian Cysts

Ovarian cysts are fluid-filled sacs that develop on the ovaries. Typically, these are asymptomatic, disappearing naturally after a few months. However, they may burst, causing significant pain and requiring professional medical treatment.

Other Menstrual Dysfunctions

There are also a number of other hormonal perturbations that can be common in exercising women, such as anovulation, and there are some less common menstrual dysfunctions, such as polyps and adenomyosis. While these are beyond the scope of this chapter, where any of these dysfunctions are thought present, medical input should be sought.

Menstrual Cycle Symptoms

It is widely evidenced that symptoms associated with the menstrual cycle are common, and up to 93% of athletes self-report performance detriments, or negative experiences broadly associated with their menstrual cycle (Martin et al., 2018; Findlay et al., 2020). This is most likely caused by symptoms that occur as a result of the hormonal fluctuations (as detailed previously). Typically, symptoms occur either just before the onset of menstruation or during menstruation, in association with the premenstrual decline in hormones.

Premenstrual Syndrome and Primary Dysmenorrhoea

PMS involves a range of physical and/or psychological symptoms in the days prior to menstruation (Green et al., 2017). Primary dysmenorrhoea refers to chronic and cyclic pain just before and/or during menstruation, where there is no underlying pathology evident (Dawood, 1987). Some women can also experience pain around ovulation (Faust et al., 2019). There are several different mechanisms attributed to the development of symptoms, but symptoms primarily occur where there are dramatic changes in hormone levels. It is likely that the manifestation of symptoms varies by individual, and some women are more sensitive to one or other of the ovarian hormones, or a ratio of the hormones.

Depending on the nature of the symptoms, these may affect readiness to train and recovery. If symptoms are mood related, recent studies have shown exercise can help with management (Freemas et al., 2020), potentially through the release of endorphins. Where symptoms are inflammatory in nature, ability to recover from exercise may be increased. It is advisable to monitor symptoms to ensure that this has been considered. It would also be beneficial to utilise recovery strategies, evaluate nutrition and factor in enough sleep to help mitigate any negative effects.

Premenstrual Dysphoric Disorder

Premenstrual dysphoric disorder (PMDD) is thought to affect around 12% of women (Hofmeister and Bodden, 2016). It is often referred to as a severe form of PMS. Typically, both psychological/emotional and physical symptoms can be experienced during the luteal phase, often ceasing soon after the onset of menstruation (Hofmeister and Bodden, 2016). The primary cause is thought to be increased sensitivity to the ovarian hormones, but there is also likely to be a genetic component (Hofmeister and Bodden, 2016). A number of different management strategies have been discussed elsewhere, but regardless, it is particularly important to track symptoms and identify factors that can exacerbate or help symptoms.

Symptom Management

While research is still identifying specific management strategies and causes for these symptoms, there are several known dietary and lifestyle factors that can increase risk. There are also a number of management strategies that have been found to be effective for symptom relief. For example, physical activity, aerobic exercise and yoga demonstrably reduce menstrual cycle-related pain (Vaghela et al., 2019).

Due to the individual nature of menstrual cycles and symptoms, it is important for athletes to track their own cycle so they can learn more about their individual characteristics, amongst a plethora of other benefits. In some cases, hormonal contraception may be advised as a form of medical management for menstrual dysfunction. Prior to use it is important to ensure full understanding regarding the systemic impact of this type of hormonal intervention.

Key Points

- There are a plethora of menstrual dysfunctions, some of which are more common in athletes.
- Some dysfunctions are a result of dysfunctional structure or function (e.g. endometriosis, PCOS), while others occur as a result of lifestyle and circumstance (e.g. amenorrhea) and some are influenced by both (e.g. HMB, menstrual cycle symptoms).
- For any suspected dysfunction, medical advice should be sought.

Hormonal Contraception

Around 50% of elite athletes in the UK are reported to use hormonal contraception (Martin et al., 2018). There are a number of different types of hormonal contraception that all have the primary aim of preventing pregnancy. They partly do this by controlling release of the natural, endogenous hormones, oestrogen and/or progesterone (Hickey and Kaunitz, 2011). The mechanisms of action and the impact that they may have both at a localised and systemic level vary and may also be specific to an individual. Hormonal contraception can be broadly broken down into two categories; those containing a combination of exogenous oestrogen and a progestin (referred to as 'combined'), and those only containing progestin (referred to as 'progestin-only'). There are a wide range of reasons for using an hormonal contraceptive, including: a means to regulate cycles, reduce the impact of the menstrual cycle on performance, or to help manage symptoms, although some also experience unwanted symptoms as a result of use (Martin et al., 2018).

Combined Hormonal Contraception

There are three different types of combined hormonal contraception; the oral contraceptive pill (OCP), the transdermal patch and the transvaginal ring.

Oral Contraceptive Pill (OCP)

OCPs are historically the most common type of hormonal contraception and contain the exogenous hormones oestrogen and a progestin, and typically users follow a 28-day pattern of pill use (Hickey and Kaunitz, 2011). These exogenous hormones work by acting on the hypothalamus to prevent gonadotrophin release and inhibit ovulation. As a result, release of endogenous hormones is consistently and significantly reduced. There are a wide range of different types of OCP, containing different doses of exogenous hormones. Most formulations contain the exogenous hormones ethinyl oestradiol or oestradiol valerate, and a progestin such as levonorgestrel, norethisterone, gestodene or desogestrel (Hickey and Kaunitz, 2011). Typical regimens include either taking 21 active pills that contain these exogenous hormones, followed by 7 hormone-free days where a placebo pill is taken, or 24 active pills followed by 4 hormone-free placebo days. OCP regimens can, however, vary; some varieties have a lower dose of oestrogen, and others contain different doses of hormone throughout the pill cycle (Hickey and Kaunitz, 2011). Some newer formulations also have more active days over a longer cycle. More recently some have advocated back-to-back OCP use to ensure no bleed, but more research is required to fully appreciate the potential physiological consequences of this regimen.

Taking an active pill results in a daily surge of exogenous hormone, thus creating a different hormonal profile to a eumenorrheic cycle. It is common to have a bleed during the exogenous hormone withdrawal phase. This is, however, not to be confused with a menstrual period, as this is just a side effect of stopping the taking of a daily hormone dose.

While the OCP is often taken for many reasons, there are some additional non-reproductive implications to consider prior to use. Some formulations have been found to result in: systemic low-grade inflammation (Cauci et al., 2017); increased oxidative stress (Cauci et al., 2016); an enhanced risk of pulmonary embolism (Stegeman et al., 2013), and other thromboembolic events (Urrutia et al., 2013); an increased risk of depression (Anderl et al., 2019); an altered metabolic profile (Wang et al., 2016) and negative repercussions on bone health (Allaway et al., 2020). Therefore, the potential advantages of OCP use need to be balanced against potential negative implications, and it is important to fully understand potential implications prior to use. There also appears to be significant variation in how women respond to different formulations.

Contraceptive Patch and Vaginal Ring

These forms of hormonal contraception provide regular delivery of endogenous oestrogen and progestin, without the need to take a daily pill. The primary mechanism of action for these types of hormonal contraception is the same as the OCP; through the suppression of GnRH activity, which prevents ovulation. The contraceptive patch needs to be replaced weekly, and the ring every 4 weeks. In both instances, users have 3 weeks of active endogenous hormone, followed by a non-hormonal week, where a 'withdrawal bleed' is likely. Again, symptoms can be common in users, with breast pain, cramps, nausea and vomiting often cited in patch users (Creinin et al., 2008).

Progestin-Only Hormonal Contraception

There are several different mechanisms by which progestin-only forms of hormonal contraception act, including the suppression of ovulation, thickening of the cervical mucus and thinning of the endometrial lining. There are four primary types of progestin-only options, including the progestin-only pill, the intrauterine device (or system), the hormonal implant and the Depot Medroxyprogesterone Acetate (DMPA) injection. Women who have other underlying health implications or who are particularly sensitive to oestrogen may particularly be encouraged to use progestin-only options.

Progestin-Only Pill

This works by providing a daily exogenous dose of progestin. The dose of progestin is typically lower than that in combined OCPs, and here active pills are continually taken. Progestin-only pills work through all three of the mechanisms outlined earlier; suppression of ovulation, thickening of cervical mucus and thinning of the endometrial lining. However, it is important to note that ovulation is not always suppressed. The most common side effect of the progestin-only pill is unpredictable bleeding patterns.

Depot Medroxyprogesterone Acetate (DMPA)

The DMPA progestin-only injection can either be inserted into muscle (intramuscular) or under the skin (subcutaneous). This works by downregulating GnRH secretion, and therefore inhibiting ovulation. As a result, oestrogen levels are typically low. Users of this form of contraception require injections every three months. From an athletic perspective, some research has found the DMPA injection to have a degree of viral immunosuppression (Bull et al., 2019), and based on this it would be advisable to carefully monitor any potential increase in infection rate in athletes. Research has also found bone mineral density (BMD) to be reduced with DMPA use (Lopez et al., 2015), likely due to the suppression of oestrogen. However, this may be restored in the long term, after discontinuation. Caution should be applied to DMPA use in athletes, particularly where risk of low BMD is already increased.

Intrauterine System/Device

The levonorgestrel-releasing intrauterine system (IUS; sometimes termed intrauterine device or IUD, depending on geographical colloquialism) delivers a small amount of progestin daily, with an effective contraceptive lifespan of 5 years. The IUS/IUD primarily works by thickening the cervical mucus and by thinning the endometrial lining. Most women using this form of hormonal contraception still ovulate, despite some experiencing no menstrual blood loss. A reduction in menstrual blood loss is a common outcome from hormonal IUS/IUD use, so it is often used as a form of HMB management. Unpredictable bleeding may also occur with use.

Hormonal Implant

The progestin-only implant is injected subdermally and provides a steady daily release of progestin, with the dose gradually decreasing over its 3-year lifespan. This contains a higher dose of progestin when compared to the IUS/IUD. The primary mechanism of action is to inhibit ovulation, but cervical mucus thickening is also likely. The most common side effect of use is unpredictable bleeding.

Combined Hormonal Contraception and Exercise

A number of studies have investigated how the use of combined HC may affect adaptation to exercise training, exercise performance, adaptation to environmental conditions, metabolism and injury risk. As with all elements of this chapter, there is a need to appreciate the likelihood for responses to differ between individuals. A recent review concluded there to be a trivial reduction in performance in OCP users when compared to non-users (Elliott-Sale et al., 2020). However, as highlighted in the review, use of the OCP should be considered on an individual basis; for example, where an underlying menstrual dysfunction is present, the benefits of OCP use could vastly outweigh the trivial potential to affect performance. The potential for a degree of low-grade inflammation to be present with some types of HC could also affect adaptation to training (Cauci et al., 2017), and recovery, particularly after damaging exercise (Mackay et al., 2019). This should be monitored from the onset of HC use, and attention should be paid to if recovery times appear elongated in users. A small detrimental effect of OCP use on heat tolerance during exercise has also been shown when comparing OCP users and non-users (Minahan et al., 2017). As a result, when preparing to exercise in hot and humid conditions, extra emphasis should be placed on heat acclimation.

While the potential impact of the DMPA injection and the combined OCP on BMD has been outlined, some studies have evaluated the use of the OCP for reduction in ACL injury risk (Herzberg et al., 2017). It appears that OCPs could be used 'in season' to mitigate the oestrogen peak that is associated with increased ligament laxity, potentially causing risk of ACL rupture to be enhanced. There is, however, a significant need for further research regarding use of hormonal contraception, training and injury risk before conclusive guidance can be provided.

Key Points

- There are many different types and formulations of hormonal contraceptives, and athletes should be fully informed about their effects prior to use.
- Some hormonal contraceptives may affect aspects of athletic training and performance. However, where avoidance of pregnancy or treatment of underlying dysfunctions are sought, they may be the best option.
- Use of hormonal contraceptives should be done on a case-by-case approach.

Breast Health Considerations

Being unique to the female, the breast is an evolving area of research in sports science and medicine (Brown et al., 2014a). The breast has limited intrinsic support, and consequently excessive breast movement can occur during physical activity (Page and Steele, 1999; Scurr et al., 2009, 2010, 2011). A number of negative consequences are linked to breast movement. These include: exercise-induced breast pain, reported in up to 72% of exercising females (Gehlsen and Albohm, 1980); potential breast sag, hypothesised to occur as a result of damage to the weak supporting structures of the breast (Mason et al., 1999; Page and Steele, 1999); and embarrassment (Burnett et al., 2015; Starr et al., 2005; Scurr et al., 2016). These breast-related issues can deter women from exercising, with one in five adult women (Burnett et al., 2015) and over half of adolescent girls (Scurr et al., 2016) reporting the breast as a barrier to exercise.

For distance runners specifically, breast motion is an important consideration. The breasts are estimated to bounce ~10,000 times during 1 hour of slow running (McGhee et al., 2013).

Over a third of 1285 female London Marathon runners surveyed reported experiencing breast pain during training, with one in five of these reporting that it impacted their training (Brown et al., 2014a). In another sample of 540 female athletes competing nationally or internationally across 49 different sports, 44% reported experiencing exercise-induced breast pain (Brisbine et al., 2020). Additionally, research during running has suggested that improvements in breast support can reduce or eliminate breast pain, influence ground reaction forces, alter gait kinematics (see Chapter 13), and improve perceptions of comfort and exertion (Brown and Scurr, 2016; Milligan et al., 2014; Milligan et al., 2015; White et al., 2009, 2011b, 2015; Risius et al., 2016; Shivitz, 2001). The following sections will provide a brief overview of breast anatomy to aid understanding of why and how the breast moves during exercise, outline the types of breast support available on the market for exercising females and the importance of correct bra fit, and finally, provide a summary of how breast support can impact sporting performance.

Breast Anatomy and Breast Movement

The adult female breast sits over the pectoralis major muscle and usually extends anteriorly from the second to sixth rib, while spreading laterally from the sternum to the midaxillary line (Gefen and Dilmoney, 2007; Page and Steele, 1999). Each breast weighs approximately 200 g (small breasts, e.g. A and B cups) to 1000 g (large breasts, e.g. ≥ D cup), with the left breast often being larger than the right breast (Gefen and Dilmoney, 2007; Page and Steele, 1999). The breast contains fatty, fibrous and glandular tissue, with the proportion of these tissues varying between females (Hassiotou and Geddes, 2013; Parmar et al., 2011). Most women experience changes in the size and shape of their breasts at different stages of their life, affected by hormonal changes during the menstrual cycle, pregnancy and menopause, as well as the use of oral contraception or hormone therapy (Gefen and Dilmoney, 2007).

The breast skin and the fibrous tissue in the breast (referred to as "Cooper's ligaments") provide the breast's only natural support. The breast skin is reported to provide the most support to limit breast movement (Hindle, 1991); however, it is recognised that both breast skin thickness and breast skin elasticity decrease with increasing age, with skin thickness starting to significantly decline when a women is in her mid-40s (Coltman et al., 2017; Ulger et al., 2003) and skin elasticity reducing after the age of 25 years (Coltman et al., 2017). Furthermore, the Cooper's ligaments are not comparable to ligaments that attach muscles to bone or support joints (Gefen and Dilmoney, 2007; McGhee and Steele, 2020a). The primary function of these ligaments, located in the superficial fascia of the breast, are to separate the breast's lobules, and the limited support offered by these structures is thought to be due to their attachment to the deep fascia, which overlays the pectoralis major muscle (Page and Steele, 1999).

Due to the limited anatomical support provided by the breast skin and Cooper's ligaments, the breasts can move excessively over the chest wall in three-dimensions: vertically, forwards and sideways (Bowles et al., 2008; Scurr et al., 2011). Around half (56%) of the multidirectional breast movement observed during walking and running occurs in the vertical direction, with the remainder occurring in the mediolateral (side to side) direction and the anterior-posterior (forwards and backwards) direction (Scurr et al., 2009). During unsupported (bare-breasted) treadmill running, breasts have been reported to move, relative to the torso, from 1 cm vertically in walking (Mason et al., 1999) up to 15.2 cm during running (Scurr et al.,

2011). Mediolateral movement has been reported to reach up to 6.2 cm, with anterior-posterior movement reaching 5.9 cm (Wood et al., 2012). Although research has identified that breast displacement increases as cup size increases (Wood et al., 2012), breast motion is not an issue that is exclusive to women with larger breasts. More than 7 cm of vertical breast displacement has been observed in unsupported (bare-breasted) A and B cup participants (Lorentzen and Lawson, 1987). Therefore, it is important that all females, regardless of breast size, are educated about the importance of wearing appropriate breast support during exercise.

Breast Support and Bra Fit

Over the past decade increased understanding of how the breast moves during exercise has been used to determine the effectiveness of different bras at reducing breast motion and inform sports bra design. Numerous studies have consistently shown that well-designed sports bras are more effective in limiting breast motion during running, compared to when a woman is not wearing any external breast support, or is wearing a standard-fashion bra or crop top (Chen et al., 2016; Gehlsen and Albohm, 1980; Lawson and Lorentzen, 1990; Lorentzen and Lawson, 1987; McGhee and Steele, 2010a; McGhee et al., 2013; Milligan et al., 2015; Risius et al., 2015; Scurr et al., 2010; White et al., 2009; Wood et al., 2012). However, sports bra use among adult females is relatively low. In the UK only 32% of adult females are reported to wear a sports bra during exercise. Among adult populations in China and Australia, sports bra use has been reported to be around 40% (Bowles et al., 2008; Chen et al., 2019). Education on the types of breast support available and how to obtain the correct bra fit is important to improve sports bra use and allow women to exercise in greater comfort.

Currently, there are three distinct sports bra designs on the market: compression, encapsulation and combination. Compression sports bras typically pull over the head, do not have cups and restrict breast motion by compressing the breast to distribute their mass across the chest wall (Page and Steele, 1999; Starr et al., 2005). Encapsulation sports bras support each breast individually in separate, structured cups to limit breast movement (Page and Steele, 1999; Starr et al., 2005). Compression bras both encapsulate and compress the breasts, although in varying degrees they are dependent on the sports bra design. Some research has suggested that encapsulation sports bras are more effective than compression bras in reducing vertical breast motion, particularly for larger-breasted women (cups sizes D and above) (Lorentzen and Lawson, 1987; McGhee and Steele, 2010; Starr et al., 2005). However, these claims have been challenged, with other research reporting no difference in the performance of these bra types in reducing breast movement (White et al., 2009). The lack of consensus on the success of these bra types is likely influenced by the wide variation in sports bras features such as closure methods, back designs, cup styling, fabric elasticity and adjustability options (Page and Steele, 1999; Zhou et al., 2013; Yu and Zhou, 2016). It is also important to recognise that no one sports bra will suit all women. Many factors, including age, breast size and the type of physical activity being undertaken, may influence the type of sports bra features that are most effective or comfortable (McGhee and Steele, 2020b).

There are various back designs for sports bras including crossover back, racer back, vertical centre, T-back, U-back and straight back. For distance runners, who experience repetitive vertical breast movement, sports bras with a straight back, or U-back design, are thought to be more effective due to the direction of the force acting on these should straps be more aligned with the direction of breast gravity (Yu and Zhou, 2016). Additionally, straight back designs with a wide strap width (4.5 cm) are reportedly more comfortable and reduce bra-strap pressure on the shoulders (Coltman et al., 2015). Other desirable design features may include a high neckline (i.e. the neckline reaches the upper boundary of the breast tissue) to prevent upward movement of the breast, adjustable shoulder straps to accommodate for varying torso lengths and breast positions (Zhou et al., 2013; Coltman et al., 2015), and a bra made from material that can wick sweat away from the body to help maintain a comfortable breast temperature and avoid skin irritation (McGhee and Steele, 2020b; Ayres et al., 2013).

The bra market offers a wide choice of brands, styles and sizes, making the selection of appropriate, well-fitted bras difficult (Brown et al., 2018). Not only do bras produced by different manufacturers have inconsistent sizing; breasts change size, shape and position through the menstrual cycle and throughout life. Furthermore, most women are not trained in bra sizing and fitting, nor do they have enough knowledge to make bra purchasing decisions (Wood et al., 2008). This may explain the high percentage of women wearing incorrectly fitting bras, which is reported to range from 70% to 100% (Greenbaum et al., 2003; McGhee and Steele, 2010b; Pechter, 1998; Wood et al., 2008). A bra must fit correctly to provide comfort and adequate breast support. If the bra size is wrong, it will not provide effective support, regardless of how good the design of the bra (Page and Steele, 1999). The most common bra fit mistakes women make are wearing band sizes that are too big and wearing cup sizes that are too small (White and Scurr, 2012). Research has found the traditional method of a tape measurement to establish bra size to be unreliable, with this method overestimating the underband size in 76% of cases and underestimating the cup size in 84% of cases. Literature suggests that females should be educated on professional bra fitting criteria to improve their ability to independently choose a well-fitted bra, thus reducing the negative health outcomes associated with wearing ill-fitting bras and allowing them to exercise in greater comfort. (Brown et al., 2018; Boschma et al., 1996; Chen et al., 2019; McGhee and Steele, 2010b). The key things to check when trying on a bra are:

1. *The underband*: this should be level all around the body. It should not be so tight that it is uncomfortable, affects breathing or makes flesh bulge over the band, but the band should fit firmly around the chest.
2. *The cups*: people often wear cups that are too small, causing the breasts to spill out. Too big and the cup hangs away from the breasts. The breasts should be enclosed within the cups, with no bulging or gaping at the top or sides.
3. *The shoulder straps*: these should be adjusted to comfortably provide breast support without being too tight (digging into the skin), or too loose that they slip off the shoulders. Ideally, two stacked fingers should fit comfortably between the shoulder and the strap.
4. *The centre front*: this should sit flat against the chest. If it doesn't, the cup might be too small.
5. *The underwire*: the underwire (if the bra has one) should follow the natural crease of the breasts and not rest on any breast tissue, including under the arms.

Whether it's a sports bra, or an everyday bra, considering these fit principles will help to select the bra that fits best. For females participating in high volumes of exercise, it is also important to consider sports bra replacement, although there is a lack of evidence to quantify how often a sports bra should be replaced. Anecdotally, it is recommended that a sports bra should be replaced after 100 workouts or 8 to 10 months of regular use (whichever comes first), or as frequently as footwear is replaced (Brown et al., 2014b). It is also worth noting that whilst it is common to see sports bras categorised as low-, medium-, and high-impact, dependent on the level of support they provide, evidence-based standards to inform these categories have yet to be established.

Breast Support and Sporting Performance

It is well established that wearing a well-designed, well-fitted sports bra can limit breast motion and consequently eliminate or reduce the negative consequences associated with this breast motion. However, the impact of breast support on sporting performance is less understood. Although in its infancy, research has begun to explore how wearing varying levels of breast support can impact biomechanical and physiological measures. Findings have indicated possible performance effects when wearing 'high-level' breast support (such as a sports bra) versus 'low-level' breast support (such as an 'everyday' bra). For example, increased ground reaction forces have been observed when assessing participants running in lower levels of breast support compared to higher levels (Shivitz, 2001; White et al., 2009) This may have implications for runners due to exposure to a higher intensity of stress, which could lead to increased injury risk over time. Additionally, when examining movement patterns over a 5 km treadmill run, Milligan et al. (2015) identified less economical upper-body running profiles when participants ran in low-level breast support. These findings agree with those of Boschma (1994) who also reported that torso movement decreased with low-level breast support and that this decrease was more pronounced in larger-breasted (size C and D cup) participants compared to smaller-breasted. Stride length, and distance covered have also been reported to reduce when running in low-level support compared to high level support, with stride length decreasing by 4 cm in low-level support. Furthermore, although limited research has explored the effect of breast support on upper-body muscle activity, increases in pectoralis major, anterior and medial deltoid activity have been observed when exercising in high-level breast support, which may lead to fatigue (Milligan et al., 2014). These findings suggest that running in low-level breast support may have important implications for performance.

Perceptual differences in level of exertion were also noted in the 5 km running study by Milligan et al. (2015), with participants reporting a higher rate of perceived exertion at every kilometre interval when running in low-level support compared to high-level support. This indicates that not only does exercising in high-level breast support result in more economical movement patterns, but that it may psychologically have a positive effect during running. Similar perceptual findings were identified by White et al. (2009) when examining breathing mechanics, with participants reporting that it felt 'harder' and 'more uncomfortable' to run in lower-level support (White et al., 2011a). It is a common perception that sports bras restrict breathing; however, Bowles et al. (2005) reported no difference in spirometry measures during submaximal treadmill running between no bra, everyday bra or sports bra conditions. In contrast, some research has identified no decline in movement patterns, ground reaction forces or muscle activity when wearing lower levels of breast support (Risius et al., 2016; White et al., 2015), and further research is needed to firmly establish the impact of breast support level. However, given the volume of research that has consistently shown that breast motion decreases and level of breast support increases, exercising females should engage in sports bra use for both health and, potential performance benefits.

Summary

To ensure health and to aspire to optimal performance, it is advised that female runners and practitioners working with female athletes should gain an understanding about how hormones fluctuate throughout different life stages, and the potential associated implications. This should facilitate more discussion in this area. Given the individual nature of hormonal changes and the response to them, it is important for athletes to track their own menstrual cycle, and their associated wellness. The menstrual cycle can be used as a 'vital sign'; where symptoms are severe, cycle length is irregular or bleeding is excessive, medical advice should be sought. Exercise induced breast pain is common in female runners, and level of breast support worn can influence biomechanical and physiological variables; therefore, particular care and attention should be applied to finding the most appropriate and well-fitted sports bra to reduce long-term health issues and negative performance implications. Athletes should not accept symptoms and suffer in silence; coaches and practitioners should work together to manage symptoms and any perceived performance detriments.

21

PERFORMANCE DECLINE IN MASTER ENDURANCE RUNNERS

Ceri E. Diss and Arran Parmar

Highlights

- Ageing is an inevitable fact that affects all runners, and their performance.
- From the age of approximately 45 years there is a linear decrease in performance until approximately 65–70 years of age, when the rate of decline increases.
- The key changes that take place are a decline in aerobic capability and a loss of muscle mass.
- Declines in aerobic fitness affects maximal oxygen uptake ($\dot{V}O_{2max}$) and the speed at maximum metabolic steady state but not the $\%\dot{V}O_{2max}$ it occurs at, while running economy does not seem to be affected.
- A loss of muscle mass reduces maximum speed and is likely related to changes in running gait seen in older runners.
- Gait changes in older runners include reduced stride length but not stride frequency, reduced ankle joint moments and a reduced ability to tolerate impact force.
- Training can help to off-set the rate of decline.

Introduction

Performance in endurance running events is relatively stable throughout an athlete's career, with fluctuations owing primarily to physiological adaptations to training. As a result of the natural ageing process, however, performance declines across all event distances irrespective of the competitive level of athlete or the training methods engaged in (Baker et al., 2003; Trappe, 2007; Willy and Paquette, 2019; Young and Starkes, 2005). The decline in performance as a result of ageing can initially be seen from the age of approximately 45, with a relatively linear rate of decline thereafter for both middle- (800 m to 3000 m) and long-distance (5000 m to marathon) events. This rate of decline, however, increases exponentially from the age of approximately 70 for middle-distance events (Figure 21.1), and approximately 65 years of age for long-distance events (Figure 21.2). Clearly, a downward trend between running performance and age is evident, indicating negative age-related changes in metabolic and

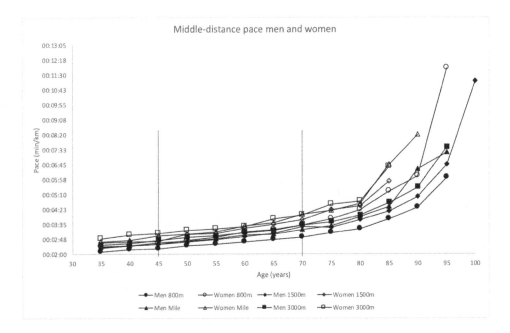

FIGURE 21.1 Middle-distance men's and women's master records by age group presented as pace. The first vertical line represents the initial linear rate of decline of performance with age. The second vertical line represents the start of the exponential rate of decline of performance with age

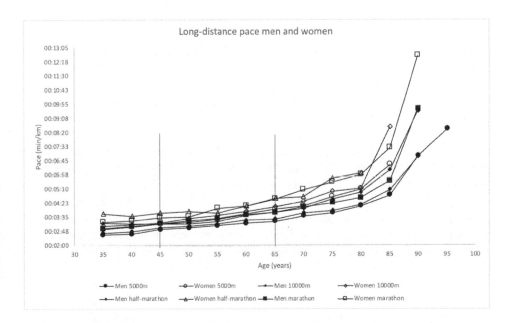

FIGURE 21.2 Long-distance men's and women's master records by age group presented as pace. The first vertical line represents the initial linear rate of decline of performance with age. The second vertical line represents the start of the exponential rate of decline of performance with age

mechanical determinants of endurance performance. This chapter will provide an overview of how the metabolic determinants of endurance performance (outlined in Chapter 1) are affected by age and why this results in a decline in performance.

Research into the declines in performance in masters age-group endurance runners remains limited, with much of the evidence in this area being cross-sectional rather than longitudinal. Cross-sectional studies are able only to provide comparisons between younger and older populations at a certain point in time, whereas longitudinal studies provide evidence for the rate of decline in performance over time. As such, the evidence presented, and conclusions drawn, should be interpreted with this in mind.

Maximal Aerobic Power

Maximal aerobic power ($\dot{V}O_{2max}$) is considered a fundamental determinant of endurance running performance (Bassett and Howley, 2000). The $\dot{V}O_{2max}$ of an athlete represents the maximum rate of oxygen able to utilised by the body and is directly linked to the rate of ATP generation that can be maintained during endurance exercise (Astrand et al., 1964; Bassett and Howley, 2000; Joyner, 1991). In comparisons of recreational and elite endurance runners, elite populations consistently show significantly higher $\dot{V}O_{2max}$ values than their recreational counterparts; with further evidence showing elite runners commonly maintain a $\dot{V}O_2 \geq$ 60 mL·kg^{-1}·min^{-1} throughout an endurance race (Bassett and Howley, 2000; Joyner, 1991; Midgley et al., 2007). The ability to sustain such a high $\dot{V}O_2$ throughout the duration of a race requires an athlete to possess a $\dot{V}O_{2max} > 70$ mL·kg^{-1}·min^{-1}, as endurance races such as the marathon are typically performed at 80–90% $\dot{V}O_{2max}$ (Bassett and Howley, 2000; Billat, 2001; Midgley et al., 2007). As an endurance athlete ages, however, sustaining such a high absolute $\dot{V}O_2$ is compromised due to age-related declines in $\dot{V}O_{2max}$, contributing to the observed decline in endurance performance (Baker et al., 2003; Trappe, 2007; Willy and Paquette, 2019). Numerous studies have reported age-related declines in $\dot{V}O_{2max}$ due to decreases in both central and peripheral physiological factors known to mediate $\dot{V}O_{2max}$ (Everman et al., 2018; Reaburn and Dascombe, 2008; Tanaka and Seals, 2008; Trappe et al., 1996; Valenzuela et al., 2020; Willy and Paquette, 2019). Specifically, a 22-year longitudinal study of endurance runners reported declines in $\dot{V}O_{2max}$ of 13–34%, equating to approximately 6–15% per decade (Trappe et al., 1996). Similarly, a later longitudinal study reported a 22% decline in $\dot{V}O_{2max}$ over approximately 8.2 years equating to an average rate of 2.9% per year, with the rate of decline being 1.8%, 2.8%, and 3.7% for runners in their 50s, 60s, and 70s, respectively, indicating a greater rate of decline with age (Katzel et al., 2001).

The declines in $\dot{V}O_{2max}$ could potentially be due to declines in either central (O_2 delivery) or peripheral (O_2 extraction) factors; the evidence for each of these will now be considered. Central factors relate to the delivery of oxygen to the working muscle and are split into two main systems: the pulmonary system – responsible for the uptake of oxygen from the atmosphere into the body, and the cardiovascular system – responsible for the transport of oxygen to tissue cells via the blood (Astorino et al., 2017; Baker et al., 2003; Bassett and Howley, 2000; Joyner, 1991; Reaburn and Dascombe, 2008; Tanaka and Seals, 2008). As age increases, pulmonary function is impaired as a result of reductions in maximal ventilatory capacity and pulmonary gas exchange (Everman et al., 2018; Valenzuela et al., 2020). Age-related decreases in ventilatory capacity occur due to increases in chest wall thickness and reductions in ventilatory muscle strength, resulting in a reduced dynamic lung volume (Knudson et al., 1983;

Lowery et al., 2013). Reductions in dynamic lung volume have been reported to decrease by 12–20% in trained older adults over a 6-year period, with the rate of decline increasing with age, similar to that displayed previously in healthy individuals (McClaran et al., 1995; Ware et al., 1990). Impairments in pulmonary gas exchange are a result of age-induced ventilation-perfusion mismatch, leading to a progressive decline in the arterial partial pressure of oxygen, along with changes in lung internal geometry reducing alveolar surface area (Sorbini et al., 1968; Thurlbeck and Angus, 1975). These reductions in pulmonary function contribute to the associated declines in $\dot{V}O_{2max}$, albeit comparatively less than the associated age-related changes that occur in cardiovascular function.

Maximal cardiac output ($\dot{Q}_{max}$), is commonly referred to as a primary factor mediating changes in $\dot{V}O_{2max}$ (Astorino et al., 2017; Bassett and Howley, 2000; Laursen and Jenkins, 2002; Levine, 2008). $\dot{Q}_{max}$ is a product of maximal stroke volume (SV_{max}) and heart rate (HR_{max}), with changes in SV_{max} viewed as the main limiting factor of $\dot{V}O_{2max}$ due to HR_{max} remaining relatively unchanged as a result of training (Bassett and Howley, 2000; Buchheit and Laursen, 2013a; Laursen and Jenkins, 2002). As age increases, changes in cardiac structure occur due to increases in left ventricular (LV) wall thickness resulting from an accumulation of interstitial connective tissue and amyloid deposits (degraded proteins forming fibrous deposits as plaques) (Lye and Donnellan, 2000; Reaburn and Dascombe, 2008; Willy and Paquette, 2019). Such changes reduce LV compliance and in turn end diastolic filling, thereby reducing SV_{max} at reported rates of 0.4–0.5% per year (Arbab-Zadeh et al., 2004; Fujimoto et al., 2012; Kasch et al., 1993; Rivera et al., 1989). Furthermore, HR_{max} decreases with increasing age at a rate of 3–5% per decade as a consequence of neurodegeneration and impaired responsiveness (De Marnefffe et al., 1986; Marti and Howald, 1990; Reaburn and Dascombe, 2008; Stuart et al., 2018). While HR_{max} may not be considered a major limiting factor mediating $\dot{V}O_{2max}$, reductions in HR_{max} contribute to declines in $\dot{Q}_{max}$. These age-related declines in SV_{max} and HR_{max} lead to decreases in $\dot{Q}_{max}$, ultimately causing a decline in $\dot{V}O_{2max}$. In addition to the declines in SV_{max} and HR_{max}, the ageing process results in an increased stiffness of cardiac valves and central arteries. This results in a decreased laminar blood flow, reducing the ability to supply the working muscles with oxygen (Lye and Donnellan, 2000; Vaitkevicius et al., 1993). Along with this, older adults exhibit decreased vasodilatory capacity and impaired functional sympatholysis (vasoconstriction stimulated by neural sympathetic activity) during exercise (Christou and Seals, 2008; Reaburn and Dascombe, 2008). These further contribute to the compromised supply of oxygen, impaired cardiovascular function, and ultimately the age-related decline in $\dot{V}O_{2max}$ (Mortensen et al., 2012; Tschakovsky et al., 2002). The combined declines in the function of the pulmonary and cardiovascular systems indicate age-related impairments in these central factors are inevitable, consequently contributing to the decline in $\dot{V}O_{2max}$ and in turn compromising endurance performance.

Peripheral factors relate to the utilisation of oxygen by tissue cells, which in this context are the muscles active during running (Bassett and Howley, 2000; Carrick-Ranson et al., 2012; Rivera et al., 1989; Tanaka and Seals, 2003). The peripheral factors contributing to the utilisation of inspired oxygen can be reduced to the capacity of the blood to transport oxygen to the muscle, and the capacity of the muscle cells to extract and utilise the supplied oxygen (Bassett and Howley, 2000; Tanaka and Seals, 2003, 2008). The oxygen-carrying capacity of the blood is primarily mediated by the concentration of haemoglobin in the blood, as oxygen binds to haemoglobin so that it can be transported to tissue cells (Schmidt and Prommer, 2010). $\dot{V}O_{2max}$ has been shown to change proportionally with changes in total haemoglobin concentration; however, total haemoglobin concentration decreases with age at a rate of approximately 5.5 g·L^{-1} (-3.7%) per decade (Calbet et al., 2006; Salive et al., 1992; Schmidt and Prommer, 2010). Such age-related declines in haemoglobin concentration impair the oxygen-carrying capacity of the blood, compromising the supply of oxygen to the working muscle and thereby reducing $\dot{V}O_{2max}$. Extraction of oxygen at the muscle is determined by the diffusion rate of oxygen into skeletal muscle from the capillaries, and the concentration and function of mitochondria within skeletal muscle cells (Coggan et al., 1993; di Prampero, 1985; Gifford et al., 2016). The diffusion rate of oxygen into the muscle is dependent upon muscle capillary density and the mean capillary transit time, with an increased density allowing a greater rate and volume of oxygen to diffuse into the muscle cells (Bassett and Howley, 2000; Gifford et al., 2016; Laursen and Jenkins, 2002). As age increases, muscle capillary density decreases, compromising the ability to offload oxygen from the haemoglobin into skeletal muscle (Esposito et al., 2011; Gates et al., 2009; Groen et al., 2014; Van der Zwaard et al., 2016). Similarly, mitochondrial concentration and function decrease with age, resulting in a decreased capacity to utilise the supplied oxygen to generate ATP via the electron transport chain at a reported rate of 5–10% per decade (Chistiakov et al., 2014; Lanza and Sreekumaran Nair, 2010; Proctor and Parker, 2006). These age-related decrements in peripheral factors mediating oxygen utilisation at the skeletal muscle reduce the arteriovenous oxygen difference (a-$\bar{v}$ O$_2$ diff), impairing the rate of oxygen availability for ATP resynthesis and reducing $\dot{V}O_{2max}$ (Baker et al., 2003; Carrick-Ranson et al., 2012; Willy and Paquette, 2019).

Training Offsets Ageing Effects

The age-related impairments in central and peripheral factors leading to a decline in $\dot{V}O_{2max}$ are inevitable. Fortunately, however, the evidence from masters age-group endurance runners shows this can be attenuated by training. Higher levels of vigorous physical activity are associated with a lower annual relative decline in pulmonary function (Tanaka and Seals, 2003, 2008; Trappe et al., 1996; Young and Starkes, 2005). Similarly, although increases in age led to declines in pulmonary function in both masters age-group endurance athletes and age-matched inactive controls, masters athletes exhibited a 9% higher dynamic lung volume (Degens et al., 2013).

Such benefits of regular physical activity have also been documented for cardiovascular function. Specifically, masters age-group endurance athletes commonly display significantly higher $\dot{Q}_{max}$ values than their sedentary counterparts, and even similar, if not higher values than sedentary younger populations (Montero and Díaz-Cañestro, 2015; Reaburn and Dascombe, 2008; Tanaka and Seals, 2008). The age-related declines in LV function have also been shown to be attenuated as a result of continued participation in vigorous physical activity. In comparison to age-matched inactive populations and young healthy controls, master athletes had preserved LV function, reduced stiffness of the cardiac valves and arteries. Collectively, this can reduce end diastolic filling, and to a lesser degree blood flow is impaired, thereby reducing SV$_{max}$, $\dot{Q}_{max}$, and ultimately $\dot{V}O_{2max}$ (Arbab-Zadeh et al., 2004; Bhella et al., 2014; Howden et al., 2018; Prasad et al., 2007). Masters age-group athletes have also shown that irrespective of training volume and intensity, HR$_{max}$ continues to decline with age, resulting in a proportional decline in SV$_{max}$, $\dot{Q}_{max}$, and $\dot{V}O_{2max}$; albeit to a lesser rate of approximately 5% per decade (Carrick-Ranson et al., 2012; Hagberg et al., 1985; Hawkins et al., 2001; Marti and Howald, 1990).

The rate of decline as a result of ageing in peripheral factors mediating $\dot{V}O_{2max}$ have also been shown to be attenuated in masters age-group athletes in comparison to age-matched sedentary populations. Mitochondrial density and function along with capillary density have been reported to be 30–60% greater in these athletes in comparison to their untrained counterparts, with training volume being positively associated with capillary density and mitochondrial biogenesis (Andersen and Henriksson, 1977; Gries et al., 2018; Iversen et al., 2011; Trappe et al., 1995). As a result, master athletes present with a significantly higher arteriovenous oxygen difference (a-$\bar{v}$ O_2 diff) than their inactive counterparts, attenuating the declines in $\dot{V}O_{2max}$ associated with age.

Clearly, lifelong physical activity has a preserving effect upon the function of central and peripheral factors mediating $\dot{V}O_{2max}$. The maintenance of high-volume training and high-intensity training as age increases appear to be effective methods to attenuate age-related declines in $\dot{V}O_{2max}$, and in turn endurance performance in masters athletes. However, the decline in $\dot{V}O_{2max}$ as a result of the ageing process is inevitable, irrespective of training status, with only the rate of decline appearing to be reduced with physical activity. Consequently, masters age group endurance athletes still suffer the same decline in $\dot{V}O_{2max}$, albeit at a slower rate, ultimately contributing to the decline in endurance running performance associated with age.

Maximum Metabolic Steady State

The speed at maximum steady state or percentage of $\dot{V}O_{2max}$ at this intensity (%$\dot{V}O_{2max}$) is a stronger predictor of endurance running performance than $\dot{V}O_{2max}$ in young (< aged 35) endurance runners with similar $\dot{V}O_{2max}$ values (Bassett and Howley, 2000; Coyle, 1995; Fay et al., 1989; Nicholson and Sleivert, 2001). In runners aged over 35, both $\dot{V}O_{2max}$ and the maximum metabolic steady state have been shown to be equally strong predictors of endurance performance, with higher values in both physiological markers associated with better performances (Evans et al., 1995; Iwaoka et al., 1988; Tanaka et al., 1990; Wiswell et al., 2001). As a result of the ageing process, contrasting findings have been reported as they relate to changes in maximum metabolic steady state.

Endurance performance clearly declines with age due to an overall lower performance velocity (Tanaka and Seals, 2008; Trappe, 2007; Trappe et al., 1996; Willy and Paquette, 2019). This is mirrored in masters age runners who display decreases in the running speed at maximum metabolic steady state as age increases, and unsurprisingly a lower speed when compared to younger runners (Baker et al., 2003; Evans et al., 1995; Iwaoka et al., 1988; Wiswell et al., 2001).

When expressed as a %$\dot{V}O_{2max}$, however, maximum steady state appears to increase with age with cross-sectional comparisons of masters age-group runners to performance matched younger runners displaying increases in %$\dot{V}O_{2max}$ (Allen et al., 1985; Evans et al., 1995; Trappe et al., 1996; Wiswell et al., 2000). It should be noted, however, that in all cross-sectional comparisons, master age-group runners displayed lower $\dot{V}O_{2max}$ values with increasing age compared to their younger counterparts. Such decreases in $\dot{V}O_{2max}$ may contribute to the higher %$\dot{V}O_{2max}$ observed despite a lower speed at maximum steady state. Supporting this, in competitive cyclists and triathletes classified as young (25.9 ± 1.0 years), middle-aged (43.2 ± 1.0 years), and older (64.6 ± 2.7 years), declines in $\dot{V}O_{2max}$ were observed as age increased (young: 67.7 ± 1.2 mL·kg^{-1}·min^{-1}, middle-aged: 56.0 ± 2.6 mL·kg^{-1}·min^{-1}, older: 47.0 ± 2.6 mL·kg^{-1}·min^{-1}) (Mattern et al., 2003). Similarly, the speed at maximum metabolic steady state followed the same trend as the decline in $\dot{V}O_{2max}$ when expressed as a $\%\dot{V}O_{2max}$: 80.8 ± 0.9%, 76.1 ± 1.4%, 69.9% ± 1.5% in the young, middle-aged, and older athlete groups, respectively.

Age-related reductions in race performance appear to be attributable, at least in part, to declines in the maximum metabolic steady state. It can therefore be surmised from the available evidence that when expressed as a performance velocity or intensity, the maximum metabolic steady state decreases as a result of the ageing process (Marcell et al., 2003; Mattern et al., 2003; Wiswell et al., 2000). Missing from the research on masters aged runners are studies using muscle biopsy to examine the metabolic capacity of the ageing muscle in trained and age-matched sedentary controls.

Running Economy

Economy during running is measured as the oxygen, or energetic, cost to perform at a given intensity, typically determined at a sub-maximal intensity below the maximum metabolic steady state (Morgan et al., 1989b). Similar to maximum metabolic steady state, running economy (RE) has been shown to be a stronger predictor of endurance running performance in athletes homogenous in $\dot{V}O_{2max}$ (Allen et al., 1985; Conley and Krahenbuhl, 1980; Daniels and Daniels, 1992; Morgan et al., 1989b). A lower RE indicates a lower energy expenditure to run at a given intensity (Morgan et al., 1989b). If all other aspects were equal, this would enable a given running speed to be sustained for a longer duration than an athlete with a worse RE. In contrast to the age-related declines in $\dot{V}O_{2max}$ and maximum metabolic steady state, studies on masters aged endurance runners indicate RE does not suffer the same fate. A cross-sectional comparison of young (25 ± 3 years) and masters aged runners (56 ± 5 years) showed no differences in RE during a 10 km race when matched for performance, despite master athletes displaying a 9% lower $\dot{V}O_{2max}$ (Allen et al., 1985). Likewise, a cross-sectional comparison of young (18–39 years), middle-aged (40–59 years), and older (60+ years) endurance runners reported similar RE values of 30–45 mL·kg^{-1}·min^{-1} at 9–15 km·h^{-1} between all age groups, despite the middle-aged and older runners displaying an 11.2% and a 31.2% lower $\dot{V}O_{2max}$ than the young runners (Quinn et al., 2011).

Several longitudinal studies have reported similar observations in RE as age increases, further indicating age-related declines in endurance performance are not associated with changes in RE in masters aged endurance runners (Evans et al., 1995; Trappe et al., 1995; Trappe et al., 1996). In studies investigating muscle-fibre type distribution in masters aged runners, the percentage of type 1 fibres has been reported to be similar to younger runners when matched for performance (Coggan et al., 1990; Trappe et al., 1995). The percentage of type 1 muscle fibres is positively associated with RE and endurance performance (Horowitz et al., 1994; Trappe, 2007). The similar percentage distribution of type 1 muscle fibres irrespective of age in endurance runners is suggested to be indicative of the lack of decline in RE. Age-related declines in endurance running performance appear to not be associated with RE (Reaburn and Dascombe, 2008; Tanaka and Seals, 2008).

Anaerobic and Neuromuscular Factors

The anaerobic speed reserve (ASR) is a physiological phenomenon commonly identified as the difference between the speed at $\dot{V}O_{2max}$ (s$\dot{V}O_{2max}$) and the maximal sprint speed (MSS)

(Buchheit and Laursen, 2013a). This provides a speed range available to an athlete that can be utilised with an increasing proportion of energy supplied via the anaerobic system up to MSS (Buchheit and Laursen, 2013a; Buchheit and Mendez-Villanueva, 2014). The ASR is therefore indicative of a finite work capacity, with the duration that work within this speed reserve can be sustained for diminishing as MSS is approached (Buchheit and Mendez-Villanueva, 2014). In endurance runners, the ASR is commonly reported to be relatively small due to the $s\dot{V}O_{2max}$ being close to the MSS (Billat, 2001; Julio et al., 2020). The high $s\dot{V}O_{2max}$ and small ASR have been suggested to be an optimal physiological profile in endurance runners, enabling running speeds closer to the MSS to be sustained with a lower contribution from the anaerobic energy system. This would reduce the accumulation of fatigue-related metabolites and thereby increase exercise tolerance (Buchheit and Mendez-Villanueva, 2014; Bundle et al., 2003; Weyand and Davis, 2005).

With increasing age, reductions in MSS and anaerobic performance have commonly been reported in masters age group track and field runners (100 m–400 m), cyclists, and triathletes (Baker et al., 2003; Gent and Norton, 2013; Reaburn and Dascombe, 2009). Such declines have not been investigated in masters aged endurance runners, although these findings suggest similar age-related declines might occur. These decreases in MSS and anaerobic are associated with declines in muscle mass, muscle fibre size, and a redistribution of muscle fibre type associated with age-related declines in performance (Baker et al., 2003; Fair, 2007; Gent and Norton, 2013; Korhonen et al., 2003; Reaburn and Dascombe, 2009). Age-related declines in muscle mass have been reported in older non-athletic individuals, endurance-trained, and sprint-trained masters aged athletes (Chambers et al., 2020; Harridge et al., 1997; Janssen et al., 2000; Korhonen et al., 2006). An attenuated rate of decline of muscle mass in resistance-trained masters aged sprinters, who displayed similar active muscle mass and muscle fibre size to young sedentary controls (Klitgaard et al., 1990; Korhonen et al., 2006). In contrast, masters aged endurance runners presented with near identical declines in muscle mass and muscle fibre size to age-matched sedentary individuals, despite lifelong participation in strenuous endurance exercise (Trappe et al., 1995; Trappe et al., 1996).

High-level endurance runners have been reported to perform more regular strength training than their lower-level counterparts (Blagrove et al., 2020b), perhaps indicating that masters aged runners should engage in more strength training to attenuate declines in muscle mass and fibre size. In addition, a redistribution of muscle fibre type has been reported, with needle biopsy studies indicating higher ratios of type 1 to type 2 muscle fibre areas with increasing age in both healthy, inactive individuals and national and international sprint runners (Essen-Gustavsson and Borges, 1986; Evans and Lexell, 1995; Korhonen et al., 2006). Increases in the proportion of type 1 fibres at the expense of type 2 fibres with age reduces the ability to produce maximal force and in turn likely contributes to decreases in MSS (Blazevich, 2006; Evans and Lexell, 1995; Korhonen et al., 2006; Trappe et al., 1995). The age-related reductions in MSS and $\dot{V}O_{2max}$ will probably reduce the ASR, along with the absolute velocities associated with these physiological markers. This translates to decrements in race pace with increasing age, as faster paces require a greater anaerobic contribution and utilisation of type 2 fibres leading to a greater accumulation of fatigue-related metabolites, which is unsustainable during an endurance performance (Buchheit and Laursen, 2013a, 2013b; Bundle et al., 2003; Weyand and Davis, 2005). The presented evidence indicates that age-related declines in skeletal muscle architecture and anaerobic capacity contribute to reductions in endurance performance, irrespective of training volume and intensity in master endurance runners (Brisswalter and Nosaka, 2013; Reaburn and Dascombe, 2009).

Age-Based Biomechanics of Running Gait

Running Performance

Masters age group athletes have a high level of fitness throughout their life span with minor changes in their aerobic capacity and body composition (Knechtle et al., 2012). There are, however, many factors that potentially contribute to age-based performance decline, but $\dot{V}O_{2max}$ and the loss of skeletal muscle mass are considered the prime components (Trappe et al., 2009). A gradual loss in skeletal muscle mass is inevitable and starts at around 50 years of age, but it is dependent on the individual's level of activity. The loss of muscle mass could negatively affect force-generating capability, which could in turn influence running gait. Despite the high rates of participation in masters age-group running, particularly long distance, little research has been conducted on this population.

The running gaits of three different age groups of experienced runners, all of whom had run sub-40 minute 10 km and finished in the top 20 in their county cross-country championships, were compared (Diss et al., 2015). The age groups were 26–32 years old (Senior), 50–54 years (Master 50) and 60–64 years (Master 60). Not only was there the inevitable ageing-based decline in running speed, there were also changes in gait. Table 21.1 illustrates the running speed, step length, and step frequency for each age group, when running at 90% of their current time for 10 km. Although, the masters' groups shorter step length was a contributing factor to the decline in their running speed, they were able to slightly increase their step frequency by 2.18% (Master 50) and 7.27% (Master 60) compared to the Senior athletes.

A slower running speed demonstrated by masters aged athletes results in a lower trajectory in the flight phase and consequentially a reduction in vertical and horizontal velocity at initial foot-ground contact. The reduced velocities are a result of a reduction in impulse generation, the product of force and time, during the whole of foot-ground contact (stance phase). This may be desirable due to the reduction in muscle fibres and strength associated with age (Grabiner and Enoka, 1995). However, the length of time Masters aged runners spend in the stance phase is longer compared to Seniors. Despite this, the impulse generated is lower and must therefore be a result of a reduction in vertical and horizontal ground reaction forces (GRF) throughout stance.

TABLE 21.1 The mean ± standard deviation of running speed, step length, step frequency, and the athletes' current 10 km time for each group

	Senior	Masters 50	Masters 60
Testing running speed (m·s⁻¹) @ 90% of 10 km time	4.13 ± 0.54	3.75 ± 0.46	3.34 ± 0.04
Step length (m)	1.52 ± 0.22	1.35 ± 0.21	1.14 ± 0.13
Step frequency (Hz)	2.75 ± 0.20	2.81 ± 0.27	2.95 ± 0.24
Current 10 km time (minutes:seconds)	36:31	40:00	44:55

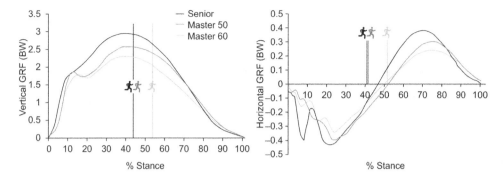

FIGURE 21.3   The mean vertical and horizontal ground reaction forces during the stance phase for all groups. The vertical line and stick figure illustrate the time of amortisation

Source: From Diss et al. (2015).

Baltzopoulos and Maganaris (2009) reported that changes on the myofilament overlap occur with age, and that these affect not only the muscle force production but also the rate of force production and transmission through the tendons to the skeletal muscle. To reduce the potential effect of this on age-based decline in running speed, specific training should be aimed at increasing force production during both the eccentric (when the centre of mass is moving downwards) and the concentric (when the centre of mass is moving upwards) phases of stance. In their review on age, locomotion, and physical training, Mian et al. (2007) reported benefits from high-load strength training. They also reported that the training should be multifaceted if an improvement in dynamic motion were to be seen with age. Improvements in locomotion of healthy, independent elderly individuals have been found with strength training using light loads e.g. body weight, resistance bands in conjunction with aerobic, balance and flexibility training. The extent to which this would transfer to masters aged runners has yet to be established, but it seems plausible.

Figure 21.3 depicts the maximal vertical ground reaction force (GRF) during the stance phase, with values ranging from 2–3 times body weight across all three age groups. The GRF contributes to running performance and should be as large as possible. The amortisation phase, which is the transition from eccentric to concentric phase of the stretch-shortening cycle, is marked for each age-group of runners. Ideally, the amortisation phase should occur at the same time as the maximal vertical GRF to allow a quick transition from a downward to an upward motion. For the Senior and Master 50 athletes, amortisation occurred at 44% and 45% of the stance phase, approximately in line with the maximal vertical GRF, whereas it occurs later for the oldest age group. The Master 60 athlete's amortisation occurs at 53% of the stance phase and was after the maximal vertical GRF. It appears that the maximal vertical GRF is a mechanism for controlling the lowering of the centre of mass in the eccentric phase (possibly enhancing stability) rather than the transition between the two phases for the older runners. Therefore, the training for the master athlete, particularly over the age of 55 years, should not only be targeted at increasing force during stance but also the transitioning from a downward motion to an upwards one.

The requirement for specific strength training (see Chapter 14) to reduce the rate of decline in force production with age is also supported by the outcomes of the vertical

TABLE 21.2 The mean ± standard deviation of the sagittal plane lower body joint angles for each age group to the nearest degree. The range of motion (ROM) is from initial foot-ground contact to amortisation. A negative ankle angle indicates plantarflexion, and a negative hip angle indicates extension

	Senior	Master 50	Master 60
Ankle ROM	28 ± 5	15 ± 5	17 ± 7
Knee ROM	26 ± 5	30 ± 6	24 ± 4
Hip ROM	9 ± 2	10 ± 3	11 ± 3
Ankle at toe-off	−4 ± 11	−5 ± 6	8 ± 11
Knee at toe-off	8 ± 4	11 ± 7	13 ± 7
Hip at toe-off	−11 ± 3	−9 ± 4	−8 ± 4

(maximum vertical GRF) and horizontal (peak horizontal GRF) propulsive forces. When running at 90% of their current 10 km pace, Diss et al. (2015) found that the maximum vertical GRF (mean ± standard deviation) was 3.02 ± 0.36, 2.61 ± 0.25, and 2.31 ± 0.20 BW for senior, master 50, and master 60 runners respectively. Furthermore, the maximum horizontal propulsive GRF (mean ± standard deviation) was 0.41 ± 0.08, 0.31 ± 0.05, and 0.25 ± 0.07 BW for senior, master 50, and master 60 athletes respectively. These propulsive forces are the active part of the GRF production, primarily generated by activated leg extensor muscles. It is these muscles that should therefore be the focus of strength training. Using a complex 3-D simulation of 92 variables, Hamner et al. (2010) reported that during late stance, the ankle plantar flexor muscles (soleus and gastrocnemius) along with the gluteus medius and maximus, were the main contributors. Table 21.2 reports the sagittal plane lower body joint angles at toe-off (Diss et al., 2015). The Master 60 group remained in dorsiflexion at toe-off; this could be a function of both reduced strength in the ankle plantar flexors and/or flexibility at the ankle joint. Both have specific, local, training implications for the ankle joint with age. Also, hip extension was reduced at toe-off for both Master 50 and Master 60 groups, which has been attributed to a reduction in the flexibility of the iliopsoas (Souza et al., 2015).

Injury and Impact

Running is an injury-prone sport, with annual injury rates reportedly as high as 75% (Willson et al., 2014). Figure 21.3 illustrates the first peak vertical GRF, which occurs as the foot first collides with the ground. It is a passive force, where the body does not have time to respond to its magnitude, often referred to as the impact force. The gradient of the impact force defines the rate at which the impact force occurs and is mainly by the muscles of the lower body. Whilst both the absolute and rate of impact force are low compared to other sports (i.e. triple jump, gymnastics) it is the repetitive, cumulative, nature of the impact force which eventually overloads the musculoskeletal system and contributes towards injury. Research on the passive impact force remains inconclusive (Winter, 1990; Derrick et al., 2000) and runners demonstrate high-impact force variability and extensive adaptive capability. In support of this notion, no significant change in impact force with age occurs (mean ± standard deviation: Senior = 2.21 ± 0.71, Master 50 = 2.18 ± 0.56, Master 60 = 1.94 ± 0.41 BW) (Diss et al., 2015). However, the rate of impact force was found to be significantly negatively correlated with age

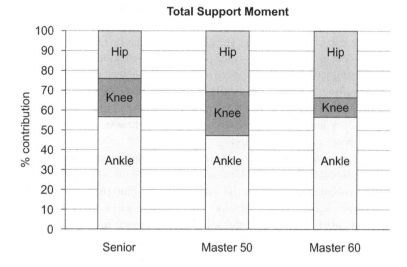

FIGURE 21.4 The total sagittal plane support moment and the contribution of each lower body joint at amortisation for each group

TABLE 21.3 The mean ± standard deviation for the sagittal plane lower joint moments at amortisation and the total support moment for each age group. The moments were normalised to body weight and leg length and hence are dimensionless

	Senior	Master 50	Master 60
Ankle	0.38 ± 0.05	0.26 ± 0.06	0.22 ± 0.05
Knee	0.13 ± 0.11	0.12 ± 0.06	0.04 ± 0.04
Hip	0.16 ± 0.06	0.17 ± 0.06	0.13 ± 0.03
Total Support Moment	0.67	0.55	0.39

(mean ± standard deviation: Senior = 101.52 ± 45.82, Master 50 = 66.69 ± 18.60, Master 60 = 67.45 ± 24.75 BW/s). A reduced capacity to absorb high rates of impact force may be a mechanism to reduce the likelihood of injury in the older athletes.

At the beginning of the stance phase, the body is required to decelerate, and in the horizontal direction, braking forces occur. Braking forces occur when the body's centre of mass is behind the point of force application. Figure 21.3 illustrates two peak braking forces which are significantly greater for the Senior athletes compared to the Masters (mean ± standard deviation: Senior = 0.71 ± 0.30, Master 50 = 0.47 ± 0.11, Master 60 = 0.41 ± 0.11 BW). The greater braking force could be attributed to the greater horizontal running velocity demonstrated by the younger athletes, but it also shows an inability by the Master athletes to create high braking forces to decrease the horizontal velocity of the body. Overall, these findings show that the Master athletes have an inability to attenuate high vertical rates of GRF and generate high horizontal braking forces. Both of these factors have been attributed to the loss of skeletal muscle mass, the function of the remaining muscle mass and the eccentric stretch.

During the stance phase, the lower body joints create moments, causing them to either flex or extend. The lower body joints' move through a range of motion during the stance phase. If an athlete's joint moments are higher compared to another, then the muscles have to work harder to move the joint. This has potential implications for running economy and also increases the risk of injury. Winter (1980) suggested that by examining the total support moment at a specific time during the stance phase (i.e. amortisation) the contribution of each joint can be determined. Table 21.3 illustrates the joint moments at amortisation (Diss et al., 2015) with a significant reduction ($P < 0.01$) in the ankle and total support moment between Senior and both Master groups. The total support moment at amortisation decreases with age, and Figure 21.4 illustrates the relative contribution, where in the Master 60s, knee joint provides a small percentage contribution.

The reasons for a reduction in the ankle moment at amortisation and in the total support moment can be twofold. Firstly, the older runners appear to minimise the load placed on the musculoskeletal system, particularly at the ankle and knee joints, to reduce the risk of injury. Secondly, the lower body joints in the older runners have a reduced ability to generate the joint forces, particularly at the knee and ankle in comparison to the young runners. Such findings further support the need for strength training with age and that it should be targeted at the proximal (knee) and distal (ankle) joints of the shank.

Compared to Senior runners, the ankle joint ROM was significantly lower ($P < 0.05$) in both Master groups. Additionally, the ankle joint at toe-off was significantly ($P < 0.05$) different greater for the Master 60 compared to both the Senior and Master 50 groups. The ROM of the lower body joints provides an insight about their contribution to the attenuation of impact forces up to amortisation. The significant reduction at the ankle joint could possibly be explained, again, by the reduced flexibility at this joint and provides evidence for the change in the mechanical loading response with age. The longer eccentric phase and reduced ankle ROM for the Master 60 group may be a desire to slowly move the foot to a flat position at mid-stance, improving stability. The knee joint ROM was similar between each group and has been reported to have a relationship with the passive impact vertical GRF (Derrick et al., 2000). Since this force has been found to be athlete dependent, this would explain the lack of difference in the knee joint dissipation of force between the groups.

Summary

Declines in endurance performance with increasing age appear inevitable. However, the rate of decline can at least be attenuated by maintaining a consistent, high training volume and including high training intensities (Everman et al., 2018; Reaburn and Dascombe, 2008, 2009; Tanaka and Seals, 2008; Willy and Paquette, 2019). Similarly, incorporating regular strength training can aid in the maintenance of lean muscle mass and muscle strength, as endurance training alone does not provide the stimulus for such adaptations (Blagrove et al., 2020b; Hawkins and Wiswell, 2003; Reaburn and Dascombe, 2009). Maintaining such practices within the training regime could potentially reduce the rate of performance decline associated with increasing age. Nevertheless, the age-related declines in the metabolic factors outlined clearly contribute to the reductions in endurance performance; however, mechanical factors also play a fundamental role in determining endurance performance.

A change in age-based running gait biomechanics is inevitable and is mostly affected by the changes in musculoskeletal mass. Master athletes' running performance declines with age which is a function of a shorter step length whilst maintaining the ability to achieve a high step frequency. Although the vertical and horizontal GRF attenuation requirements are lower with age, the inhibited ankle joint compliancy and extensor moments are potential contributors to changes in running gait. Whilst the knee joint showed continued compliancy with age, the relative contribution to the support moment in the elderly runner was very low. To minimise the detrimental effects of ageing on running performance and injury, an enhanced execution of the ankle and knee joint biomechanical function would be beneficial.

REFERENCES

Abbiss, C. R. and Laursen, P. B. (2008) Describing and understanding pacing strategies during athletic competition. *Sports Medicine*, 38(3), pp. 239–252.

Abe, D., Muraki, S., Yanagawa, K., Fukuoka, Y. and Niihata, S. (2007) Changes in EMG characteristics and metabolic energy cost during 90-min prolonged running. *Gait Posture*, 26(4), pp. 607–610.

Abe, D., Yanagawa, K., Yamanobe, K. and Tamura, K. (1998) Assessment of middle-distance running performance in sub-elite young runners using energy cost of running. *European Journal of Applied Physiology and Occupational Physiology*, 77(4), pp. 320–325.

Abidi, M. (2012) Behind the victory prostration. www.the-platform.org.uk/2012/09/06/the-meaning-behind-the-victory-prostration/. Accessed on 08/09/2020.

Ache-Dias, J. et al. (2017) Effect of jump interval training on kinematics of the lower limbs and running economy. *Journal of Strength and Conditioning Research*, 32(2), pp. 416–422. doi: 10.1519/JSC.0000000000002332.

Achten, J. and Jeukendrup, A. E. (2004) Optimizing fat oxidation through exercise and diet. *Nutrition*, 20(7), pp. 716–727. doi: 10.1016/J.NUT.2004.04.005.

Ackerman, K. E., Holtzman, B., Cooper, K. M. et al. (2018) Low energy availability surrogates correlate with health and performance consequences of relative energy deficiency in sport. *British Journal of Sports Medicine*, 53(10), pp. 628–633.

Ackland, T. R., Lohman, T. G., Sundgot-Borgen, J., Maughan, R. J., Meyer, N. L., Stewart, A. D. and Müller, W. (2012) Current status of body composition assessment in sport. *Sports Medicine*, 42, pp. 227–249.

Adams, D., Pozzi, F., Willy, R. W., Carrol, A. and Zeni, J. (2018) Altering cadence or vertical oscillation during running: Effects on running related injury factors. *International Journal of Sports Physical Therapy*, 13, pp. 633–642.

Aitchison, C., Turner, L. A., Ansley, L., Thompson, K. G., Micklewright, D. and Gibson, A. S. C. (2013) Inner dialogue and its relationship to perceived exertion during different running intensities. *Perceptual and Motor Skills*, 117(1), pp. 11–30.

Albracht, K. and Arampatzis, A. (2013) Exercise-induced changes in triceps surae tendon stiffness and muscle strength affect running economy in humans. *European Journal of Applied Physiology*, 113(6), pp. 1605–1615. doi: 10.1007/s00421-012-2585-4.

Alenezi, F., Herrington, L., Jones, P. and Jones, R. (2014) Relationships between lower limb biomechanics during single leg squat with running and cutting tasks: A preliminary investigation. *British Journal of Sports Medicine*, 48(7), pp. 560–561.

Allaway, H. C. M., Misra, M., Southmayd, E. A., Stone, M. S., Weaver, C. M., Petkus, D. L. and Souza, M. J. D. (2020) Are the effects of oral and vaginal contraceptives on bone formation in young women mediated via the growth hormone-IGF-I axis? *Frontiers in Endocrinology*, 11, p. 334.

Allen, D. G., Lamb, G. D. and Westerblad, H. (2008) Skeletal muscle fatigue: Cellular mechanisms. *Physical Review*, 88(1), pp. 287–332. doi: 10.1152/PHYSREV.00015.2007.

Allen, W. K., Seals, D. R., Hurley, B. F., Ehsani, A. A. and Hagberg, J. M. (1985) Lactate threshold and distance-running performance in young and older endurance athletes. *Journal of Applied Physiology*, 58(4), pp. 1281–1284.

Allison, S. J., Bailey, D. M. and Folland, J. P. (2008) Prolonged static stretching does not influence running economy despite changes in neuromuscular function. *Journal of Sports Sciences*, 26(14), pp. 1489–1495.

Almarwaey, O. A., Jones, A. M. and Tolfrey, K. (2003) Physiological correlates with endurance running performance in trained adolescents. *Medicine and Science in Sports and Exercise*, 35(3), pp. 480–487.

Altman, A. R. and Davis, I. S. (2016) Prospective comparison of running injuries between shod and barefoot runners. *British Journal of Sports Medicine*, 50, pp. 476–480.

American College of Sports Medicine, American Dietetic Association and Dietitians of Canada (2000) Joint position statement: Nutrition and athletic performance: American College of Sports Medicine, American Dietetic Association, and Dietitians of Canada. *Medicine and Science in Sports and Exercise*, 32(12), pp. 2130–2145.

Anderl, C., Li, G. and Chen, F. S. (2019) Oral contraceptive use in adolescence predicts lasting vulnerability to depression in adulthood. *Journal of Child Psychology and Psychiatry, and Allied Disciplines*, 61(2), pp. 148–156.

Andersen, P. and Henriksson, J. (1977) Capillary supply of the quadriceps femoris muscle of man: Adaptive response to exercise. *The Journal of Physiology*, 270(3), pp. 677–690.

Anderson, T. (1996) Biomechanics and running economy. *Sports Medicine*, 22(2), pp. 76–89.

Angus, S. D. (2014) Did recent world record marathon runners employ optimal pacing strategies? *Journal of Sports Sciences*, 32(1), pp. 31–45.

Angus, S. D. and Waterhouse, B. J. (2011) Pacing strategy from high-frequency field data: More evidence for neural regulation? *Medicine and Science in Sports and Exercise*, 43(12), pp. 2405–2411.

Anstiss, P. A., Meijen, C. and Marcora, S. M. (2018) The sources of self-efficacy in experienced and competitive endurance athletes. *International Journal of Sport and Exercise Psychology*, published online. doi: 10.1080/1612197X.2018.1549584.

Antonini Philippe, R., Rochat, N., Vauthier, M. and Hauw, D. (2016) The story of withdrawals during an ultra-trail running race: A qualitative investigation of runners' courses of experience. *The Sport Psychologist*, 30, pp. 361–375.

Appell, H.-J., Soares, J. M. C. and Duarte, J. A. R. (1992) Exercise, muscle damage and fatigue. *Sports Medicine*, 13(2), pp. 108–115.

Aragón, S., Lapresa, D., Arana, J., Anguera, M. T. and Garzón, B. (2016) Tactical behaviour of winning athletes in major championship 1500-m and 5000-m track finals. *European Journal of Sport Science*, 16(3), pp. 279–286.

Arampatzis, A., De Monte, G., Karamanidis, K., Morley-Klapsing, G., Stafilidis, S. and Brüggemann, G.-P. (2006) Influence of the muscle-tendon unit's mechanical and morphological properties on running economy. *The Journal of Experimental Biology*, 209(17), pp. 3345–3357.

Arbab-Zadeh, A., Dijk, E., Prasad, A., Fu, Q., Torres, P., Zhang, R., Thomas, J. D., Palmer, D. and Levine, B. D. (2004) Effect of aging and physical activity on left ventricular compliance. *Circulation*, 110(13), pp. 1799–1805.

Arellano, C. J. and Kram, R. (2011) The effects of step width and arm swing on energetic cost and lateral balance during running. *Journal of Biomechanics*, 44, pp. 1291–1295.

Arellano, C. J. and Kram, R. (2014) Partitioning the metabolic cost of human running: A task-by-task approach. *Integrative and Comparative Biology*, 54, pp. 1084–1098.

Areta, J. L. et al. (2013) Timing and distribution of protein ingestion during prolonged recovery from resistance exercise alters myofibrillar protein synthesis. *The Journal of Physiology*, 591(9), pp. 2319–2331. doi: 10.1113/JPHYSIOL.2012.244897.

Armour, M., Parry, K. A., Steel, K. and Smith, C. A. (2020) Australian female athlete perceptions of the challenges associated with training and competing when menstrual symptoms are present. *International Journal of Sports Science & Coaching*, 15(3), pp. 316–323.

Armstrong, N. (2017) Top 10 research questions related to youth aerobic fitness. *Research Quarterly for Exercise and Sport*, 88(2), pp. 130–148.

Armstrong, N. and Barker, A. R. (2011) Endurance training and elite young athletes. *Medicine and Sports Science*, 56, pp. 59–83.

Askling, C., Saartok, T. and Thorstensson, A. (2006) Type of acute hamstring strain affects flexibility, strength, and time to return to pre-injury level. *British Journal of Sports Medicine*, 40(1), pp. 40–44.

Astorino, T. A., Edmunds, R. M., Clark, A., King, L., Gallant, R. A., Namm, S., Fischer, A. and Wood, K. M. (2017) High-intensity interval training increases cardiac output and VO2max. *Medicine & Science in Sports & Exercise*, 49(2), pp. 265–273.

Astrand, P. O., Cuddy, T. E., Ssltin, B. and Stenberg, J. (1964) Cardiac output during submaximal and maximal work. *Journal of Applied Physiology*, 19, pp. 268–274.

Astrup, A. et al. (2011) The role of reducing intakes of saturated fat in the prevention of cardiovascular disease: Where does the evidence stand in 2010? *The American Journal of Clinical Nutrition*, 93(4), pp. 684–688. doi: 10.3945/AJCN.110.004622.

Atkinson, F. S., Foster-Powell, K. and Brand-Miller, J. C. (2008) International tables of glycemic index and glycemic load values: 2008. *Diabetes Care*, 31(12), pp. 2281–2283. doi: 10.2337/DC08-1239.

Atkinson, G. and Nevill, A. M. (1998) Statistical methods for assessing measurement error (reliability) in variables relevant to sports medicine. *Sports Medicine*, 26(4), pp. 217–238.

Aubry, A., Hausswirth, C., Louis, J., Coutts, A. J. and Le Meur, Y. (2014) Functional overreaching: The key to peak performance during the taper? *Medicine and Science in Sports and Exercise*, 46(9), pp. 1769–1777. doi: 10.1249/MSS.0000000000000301.

Ayres, B., White, J., Hedger, W. and Scurr, J. (2013) Female upper body and breast skin temperature and thermal comfort following exercise. *Ergonomics*, 56(7), pp. 1194–1202.

Baar, K. (2014) Using molecular biology to maximize concurrent training. *Sports Medicine*, 44(Suppl. 2), pp. S117–S125. doi: 10.1007/s40279-014-0252-0.

Baar, K. (2017) Minimizing injury and maximizing return to play: Lessons from engineered ligaments. *Sports Medicine*, 47(1), pp. 5–11.

Baar, K. and McGee, S. L. (2008) Optimizing training adaptations by manipulating glycogen. *European Journal of Sport Science*, 8(2), pp. 97–106. doi: 10.1080/17461390801919094.

Bachero-Mena, B. et al. (2017) Relationships between sprint, jumping and strength abilities, and 800 m performance in male athletes of national and international levels. *Journal of Human Kinetics*, 58(1), pp. 187–195.

Bacon, A. P., Carter, R. E., Ogle, E. A. and Joyner, M. J. (2013) VO2max trainability and high intensity interval training in humans: A meta-analysis. *PLoS One*, 8(9), p. e73182.

Baggaley, M., Noehren, B., Clasey, J. L., Shapiro, R. and Pohl, M. B. (2015) Frontal plane kinematics of the hip during running: Are they related to hip anatomy and strength? *Gait & Posture*, 42(4), pp. 505–510.

Bahenský, P. (2019) Success of elite adolescent female runners in adulthood. *Studia Sportiva*, 13(1), pp. 6–16.

Bailey, C. A. and Brooke-Wavell, K. S. F. (2010) Optimum frequency of exercise for bone health: Randomised controlled trial of a high-impact unilateral intervention. *Bone*, 46(4), pp. 1043–1049.

Baker, A. B., Tang, Y. Q. and Turner, M. J. (2003) Percentage decline in masters superathlete track and field performance with aging. *Experimental Aging Research*, 29(1), pp. 47–65.

Baker, F. C. and Driver, H. S. (2004) Self-reported sleep across the menstrual cycle in young, healthy women. *Journal of Psychosomatic Research*, 56(2), pp. 239–243.

Baker, F. C. and Driver, H. S. (2007) Circadian rhythms, sleep, and the menstrual cycle. *Sleep Medicine*, 8(6), pp. 613–622.

Baker, F. C. and Lee, K. A. (2018) Menstrual cycle effects on sleep. *Sleep Medicine Clinics*, 13(3), pp. 283–294.

Balsalobre-Fernández, C., Glaister, M. and Lockey, R. A. (2015) The validity and reliability of an iPhone app for measuring vertical jump performance. *Journal of Sports Sciences*, 33(15), pp. 1574–1579.

Baltich, J. et al. (2017) Running injuries in novice runners enrolled in different training interventions: A pilot randomized controlled trial. *Scandinavian Journal of Medicine & Science in Sports*, 27(11), pp. 1372–1383. doi: 10.1111/SMS.12743.

Baltzopoulos, V. and Maganaris, C. (2009) Biomechanics of human movement and muscle-tendon function. In Maughan, R. (ed.) *The Olympic textbook of science in sport: Encyclopedia of sports medicine. An IOC Medical Commission Publication.* Oxford: Blackwell. (15), pp. 215–229.

Bandura, A. (1997) *Self-efficacy: The exercise of control.* New York, WH: Freeman and Company.

Banerjee, A. V. (1992) A simple model of herd behavior. *The Quarterly Journal of Economics*, 107(3), pp. 797–817.

Banfi, G. et al. (2009) Effects of whole-body cryotherapy on serum mediators of inflammation and serum muscle enzymes in athletes. *Journal of Thermal Biology.* doi: 10.1016/j.jtherbio.2008.10.003.

Banfi, G. et al. (2010) Whole-body cryotherapy in athletes. *Sports Medicine.* doi: 10.2165/11531940-000000000-00000.

Banister, E. W., Carter, J. B. and Zarkadas, P. C. (1999) Training theory and taper: Validation in triathlon athletes. *European Journal of Applied Physiology and Occupational Physiology*, 79(2), pp. 182–191. doi: 10.1007/s004210050493.

Banister, E. W., Green, H., McDougall, J. and Wenger, H. (1991) *Physiological testing of elite athletes.* Champaign, IL: Human Kinetics.

Barnes, K. R. and Kilding, A. E. (2015a) Running economy: Measurement, norms, and determining factors. *Sports Medicine-Open*, 1(1), p. 8.

Barnes, K. R. and Kilding, A. E. (2015b) Strategies to improve running economy. *Sports Medicine*, 45(1), pp. 37–56.

Barnes, K. R., McGuigan, M. R. and Kilding, A. E. (2014) Lower-body determinants of running economy in male and female distance runners. *Journal of Strength and Conditioning Research*, 16/10/2013, 28(5), pp. 1289–1297. doi: 10.1519/jsc.0000000000000267.

Barnes, K. R. et al. (2015) Warm-up with a weighted vest improves running performance via leg stiffness and running economy. *Journal of Science and Medicne in Sport*, 18(1), pp. 103–108. doi: 10.1016/j.jsams.2013.12.005.

Barnett, A. (2006) Using recovery modalities between training sessions in elite athletes: Does it help? *Sports Medicine.* doi: 10.2165/00007256-200636090-00005.

Barrack, M. T., Ackerman, K. E. and Gibbs, J. C. (2013) Update on the female athlete triad. *Current Reviews in Musculoskeletal Medicine*, 6(2), pp. 195–204.

Barrack, M. T., Fredericson, M., Tenforde, A. S. and Nattiv, A. (2017) Evidence of a cumulative effect for risk factors predicting low bone mass among male adolescent athletes. *British Journal of Sports Medicine*, 51(3), pp. 200–205. doi: 10.1136/BJSPORTS-2016-096698.

Barrack, M. T., Gibbs, J. C., De Souza, M. J. et al. (2014) Higher incidence of bone stress injuries with increasing female athlete triad-related risk factors: A prospective multisite study of exercising girls and women. *American Journal of Sports Medicine*, 42, pp. 949–958.

Barrack, M. T., Rauh, M. J. and Nichols, J. F. (2008) Prevalence of and traits associated with low BMD among female adolescent runners. *Medicine and Science in Sports and Exercise*, 40, pp. 2015–2021.

Barwood, M. J., Corbett, J., Wagstaff, C. R., McVeigh, D. and Thelwell, R. C. (2015) Improvement of 10-km time-trial cycling with motivational self-talk compared with neutral self-talk. *International Journal of Sports Physiology and Performance*, 10(2), pp. 166–171.

Barwood, M. J. et al. (2009) Post-exercise cooling techniques in hot, humid conditions. *European Journal of Applied Physiology.* doi: 10.1007/s00421-009-1135-1.

Basham, S. A. et al. (2019) Effect of curcumin supplementation on exercise-induced oxidative stress, inflammation, muscle damage, and muscle soreness. *Journal of Dietary Supplements.* doi: 10.1080/19390211.2019.1604604.

Bassett, D. R., Jr. and Howley, E. T. (1997) Maximal oxygen uptake: 'Classical' versus 'contemporary' viewpoints. *Medicine & Science in Sports & Exercise*, 29(5), pp. 591–603.

Bassett, D. R., Jr. and Howley, E. T. (2000) Limiting factors for maximum oxygen uptake and determinants of endurance performance. *Medicine and Science in Sports and Exercise*, 32(1), pp. 70–84.

Baumeister, R. F. (2016) Toward a general theory of motivation: Problems, challenges, opportunities, and the big picture. *Motivation and Emotion*, 40(1), pp. 1–10.

Baxter, C. et al. (2017) Impact of stretching on the performance and injury risk of long-distance runners. *Research in Sports Medicine*, 25(1), pp. 78–90.

Baxter-Jones, A. D., Faulkner, R. A., Forwood, M. R. et al. (2011) Bone mineral accrual from 8 to 30 years of age: An estimation of peak bone mass. *Journal of Bone Mineral Research*, 26, pp. 1729–1739.

Bazett-Jones, D. M., Cobb, S. C., Huddleston, W. E., O'Connor, K. M., Armstrong, B. S. R. and Earl-Boehm, J. E. (2013) Effect of patellofemoral pain on strength and mechanics after an exhaustive run. *Medicine and Science in Sports and Exercise*, 45(7), pp. 1331–1339.

Bazyler, C. D. et al. (2014) The effects of strength training on isometric force production symmetry in recreationally trained males. *Journal of Trainology*, pp. 6–10. doi: 10.17338/TRAINOLOGY.3.1_6.

Beattie, K. et al. (2014) The effect of strength training on performance in endurance athletes. *Sports Medicine*, 44(6), pp. 845–865. doi: 10.1007/s40279-014-0157-y.

Beattie, K., Carson, B. P., Lyons, M., Rossiter, A. and Kenny, I. C. (2017) The effect of strength training on performance indicators in distance runners. *Journal of Strength and Conditioning Research*, 03/05/2016, 31(1), pp. 9–23. doi: 10.1519/jsc.0000000000001464.

Beaver, W. L., Wasserman, K. and Whipp, B. J. (2016) A new method for detecting anaerobic threshold by gas exchange. *Journal of Applied Physiology*. https://doi.org/10.1152/jappl.1986.60.6.2020.

Beck, O. N., Kipp, S., Byrnes, W. C. and Kram, R. (2018) Use aerobic energy expenditure instead of oxygen uptake to quantify exercise intensity and predict endurance performance. *Journal of Applied Physiology, (1985)*, 125(2), pp. 672–674.

Becker, J., Nakajima, M. and Wu, W. F. W. (2018) Factors contributing to medial tibial stress syndrome in runners: A prospective study. *Medicine and Science in Sports and Exercise*, 50(10), pp. 2092–2100. doi: 10.1249/MSS.0000000000001674.

Beedie, C. J., Lane, A. M. and Wilson, M. G. (2012) A possible role for emotion and emotion regulation in physiological responses to false performance feedback in 10 mile laboratory cycling. *Applied Psychophysiology and Biofeedback*, 37(4), pp. 269–277.

Beedie, C. J., Terry, P. C. and Lane, A. M. (2000) The profile of mood states and athletic performance: Two meta-analyses. *Journal of Applied Sport Psychology*, 12(1), pp. 49–68.

Beelen, M. et al. (2010) Nutritional strategies to promote postexercise recovery. *International Journal of Sport Nutrition and Exercise Metabolism*. doi: 10.1123/ijsnem.20.6.515.

Behm, D. G. (2018) *The science and physiology of flexibility and stretching: Implications and applications in sport performance and health*. Oxon, UK: Routledge.

Behm, D. G. and Chaouachi, A. (2011) A review of the acute effects of static and dynamic stretching on performance. *European Journal of Applied Physiology*. doi: 10.1007/s00421-011-1879-2.

Behm, D. G., Faigenbaum, A. D., Falk, B. and Klentrou, P. (2008) Canadian society for exercise physiology position paper: Resistance training in children and adolescents. *Applied Physiology, Nutrition, and Metabolism*, 33(3), pp. 547–561.

Behm, D. G. et al. (2016) Acute effects of muscle stretching on physical performance, range of motion, and injury incidence in healthy active individuals: A systematic review. *Applied Physiology, Nutrition, and Metabolism*, 41(1), pp. 1–11.

Behringer, M., vom Heede, A. V., Matthews, M. and Mester, J. (2011) Effects of strength training on motor performance skills in children and adolescents: A meta-analysis. *Pediatric Exercise Science*, 23(2), pp. 186–206.

Behringer, M., vom Heede, A. V., Yue, Z. and Mester, J. (2010) Effects of resistance training in children and adolescents: A meta-analysis. *Pediatrics*, 126(5), pp. 1199–1210.

Bell, D. R., Post, E. G., Trigsted, S. M. et al. (2018) Parents' awareness and perceptions of sport specialization and injury prevention recommendations. *Clinical Journal of Sport Medicine*, published ahead of print. doi: 10.1097/JSM.0000000000000648.

Bell, P. G. et al. (2014) The role of cherries in exercise and health. *Scandinavian Journal of Medicine and Science in Sports*. doi: 10.1111/sms.12085.

Bell, P. G. et al. (2015) Recovery facilitation with montmorency cherries following high-intensity, metabolically challenging exercise. *Applied Physiology, Nutrition and Metabolism*. doi: 10.1139/apnm-2014-0244.

Bell, P. G. et al. (2016) The effects of montmorency tart cherry concentrate supplementation on recovery following prolonged, intermittent exercise. *Nutrients*. doi: 10.3390/nu8070441.

Bellenger, C. R., Fuller, J. T., Thomson, R. L., Davison, K., Robertson, E. Y. and Buckley, J. D. (2016) Monitoring athletic training status through autonomic heart rate regulation: A systematic review and meta-analysis. *Sports Medicine*, 46, pp. 1461–1486.

Bellinger, P., Arnold, B. and Minahan, C. (2019) Quantifying the training-intensity distribution in middle-distance runners: The influence of different methods of training-intensity quantification. *International Journal of Sports Physiology and Performance*. https://doi.org/10.1123/ijspp.2019-0298.

Belval, L. N. et al. (2019) Practical hydration solutions for sports. *Nutrients*, 11(7). doi: 10.3390/NU11071550.

Bender, P. U. et al. (2019) Massage therapy slightly decreased pain intensity after habitual running, but had no effect on fatigue, mood or physical performance: A randomised trial. *Journal of Physiotherapy*. doi: 10.1016/j.jphys.2019.02.006.

Benedetti, M. G. et al. (2018) The effectiveness of physical exercise on bone density in osteoporotic patients. *BioMed Research International*, 2018, p. 4840531. doi: 10.1155/2018/4840531.

Beneke, R. and Hütler, M. (2005) The effect of training on running economy and performance in recreational athletes. *Medicine & Science in Sports & Exercise*, 37(10), pp. 1794–1799.

Bennell, K. L., Malcolm, S. A., Thomas, S. A., Wark, J. D. and Brukner, P. D. (1996a) The incidence and distribution of stress fractures in competitive track and field athletes: A twelve-month prospective study. *American Journal of Sports Medicine*, 24, pp. 211–217.

Bennell, K. L., Malcolm, S. A., Thomas, S. A. et al. (1996b) Risk factors for stress fractures in track and field athletes: A twelve-month prospective study. *American Journal of Sports Medicine*, 24, pp. 810–818.

Bennett, H., Davison, K., Arnold, J., Martin, M., Wood, S. and Norton, K. (2019) Reliability of a movement quality assessment tool to guide exercise prescription (MovementSCREEN). *International Journal of Sports Physical Therapy*, 14(3), pp. 424–435.

Bennett, H., Davison, K., Arnold, J., Slattery, F., Martin, M. and Norton, K. (2017) Multicomponent musculoskeletal movement assessment tools: A systematic review and critical appraisal of their development and applicability to professional practice. *The Journal of Strength & Conditioning Research*, 31(10), pp. 2903–2919.

Benton, J. W. (1982) Epiphyseal fracture in sports. *The Physician and Sports Medicine*, 10(11), pp. 62–71.

Bergeron, M. F., Mountjoy, M., Armstrong, N. et al. (2015) International Olympic Committee consensus statement on youth athletic development. *British Journal of Sports Medicine*, 49(13), pp. 843–851.

Bergström, J., Hermansen, L., Hultman, E. and Saltin, B. (1967) Diet, muscle glycogen and physical performance. *Acta Physiologica Scandinavica*, 71(2–3), pp. 140–150. doi: 10.1111/j.1748-1716.1967.tb03720.x.

Berryman, N., Maurel, D. B. and Bosquet, L. (2010) Effect of plyometric vs. dynamic weight training on the energy cost of running. *Journal of Strength and Conditioning Research*, 15/06/2010, 24(7), pp. 1818–1825. doi: 10.1519/JSC.0b013e3181def1f5.

Berryman, N. et al. (2017) Strength training for middle- and long-distance performance: A meta-analysis. *International Journal of Sports Physiology and Performance*, pp. 1–27. doi: 10.1123/ijspp.2017-0032.

Berthoin, S., Baquet, G., Dupont, G. and Van Praagh, E. (2006) Critical velocity during continuous and intermittent exercises in children. *European Journal of Applied Physiology*, 98(2), pp. 132–138.

Besco, R., Sureda, A., Tur, J. A. And Pons, A. (2012) The effect of nitric-oxide-related supplements on human performance. *Sports Medicine*, 42(2), pp. 99–117.

Bhella, P. S., Hastings, J. L., Fujimoto, N., Shibata, S., Carrick-Ranson, G., Palmer, M. D., Boyd, K. N., Adams-Huet, B. and Levine, B. D. (2014) Impact of lifelong exercise 'dose' on left ventricular compliance and distensibility. *Journal of the American College of Cardiology*, 64(12), pp. 1257–1266.

Bigland-Ritchie, B. and Woods, J. J. (1984) Changes in muscle contractile properties and neural control during human muscular fatigue. *Muscle and Nerve*, 7(9), pp. 691–699.

Billat, V. L. (2001) Interval training for performance: A scientific and empirical practice: Special recommendations for middle- and long-distance running: Part I: Aerobic interval training. *Sports Medicine*, 31(1), pp. 13–31.

Billat, V. L., Demarle, A., Slawinski, J., Paiva, M. and Koralsztein, J. P. (2001) Physical and training characteristics of top-class marathon runners. *Medicine and Science in Sports and Exercise*. https://doi.org/10.1097/00005768-200112000-00018.

Billat, V. L., Flechet, B., Petit, B., Muriaux, G. and Koralsztein, J. P. (1999) Interval training at VO$_{2max}$: Effects on aerobic performance and overtraining markers. *Medicine and Science in Sports and Exercise*, 31(1), pp. 156–163.

Billat, V. L., Lepretre, P. M., Heugas, A. M., Laurence, M. H., Salim, D. and Koralsztein, J. P. (2003) Training and bioenergetic characteristics in elite male and female Kenyan runners. *Medicine and Science in Sports and Exercise*. https://doi.org/10.1249/01.MSS.0000053556.59992.A9.

Bird, S. and Barrington-Higgs, B. (2010) Exploring the deadlift. *Strength & Conditioning Journal*, 32(2), pp. 46–51.

Bishop, C., Turner, A. and Read, P. (2018) Training methods and considerations for practitioners to reduce interlimb asymmetries. *Strength & Conditioning Journal*, 40(2), pp. 40–46.

Bishop, D. J., Botella, J. and Granata, C. (2019) CrossTalk opposing view: Exercise training volume is more important than training intensity to promote increases in mitochondrial content. *The Journal of Physiology*, 597(16), pp. 4115–4118.

Bitchell, C. L., McCarthy-Ryan, M., Goom, T. and Moore, I. S. (2019) Spring-mass characteristics during human locomotion: Running experience and physiological considerations of blood lactate accumulation. *European Journal of Sport Science*, 19, pp. 1328–1335.

Black, M. I., Allen, S. J., Forrester, S. E. and Folland, J. P. (2020) The anthropometry of economical running. *Medicine & Science in Sports & Exercise*, 52(3), pp. 762–770.

Blagrove, R. (2013) Programmes of concurrent strength and endurance training: How to minimize the interference effect: Part 1: Evidence and mechanisms of interference. *Professional Strength and Conditioning*, 31, pp. 7–14.

Blagrove, R. (2014) Minimising the interference effect during programmes of concurrent strength and endurance training: Part 2: Programming recommendations. *Professional Strength and Conditioning*, 32, pp. 15–22.

Blagrove, R. (2015) *Strength and conditioning for endurance running*. Wiltshire, UK: The Crowood Press.

Blagrove, R. C., Bishop, C. et al. (2020a) Inter-limb strength asymmetry in adolescent distance runners: Test-retest reliability and relationships with performance and running economy. *Journal of Sports Sciences*, published online. doi: 10.1080/02640414.2020.1820183.

Blagrove, R. C., Brown, N., Howatson, G. and Hayes, P. (2020b) Strength and conditioning habits of competitive distance runners. *Journal of Strength and Conditioning Research*, 34(5), pp. 1392–1399. doi: 10.1519/JSC.0000000000002261.

Blagrove, R. C., Bruinvels, G. and Pedlar, C. R. (2020c) Variations in strength-related measures during the menstrual cycle in eumenorrheic women: A systematic review and meta-analysis. *Journal of Science and Medicine in Sport*, 23(12), pp. 1220–1227.

Blagrove, R. C., Bruinvels, G. and Read, P. (2017) Early sport specialization and intensive training in adolescent female athletes: Risks and recommendations. *Strength and Conditioning Journal*, 39(5), pp. 14–23.

Blagrove, R. C., Holding, K. M. et al. (2019a) Efficacy of depth jumps to elicit a post-activation performance enhancement in junior endurance runners. *Journal of Science and Medicine in Sport*, 22(2), pp. 239–244. doi: 10.1016/j.jsams.2018.07.023.

Blagrove, R. C., Howatson, G. and Hayes, P. R. (2019b) Use of loaded conditioning activities to potentiate middle- and long-distance performance: A narrative review and practical applications. *Journal of Strength and Conditioning Research*, 33(8), pp. 2288–2297. doi: 10.1519/JSC.0000000000002456.

Blagrove, R. C., Howatson, G., Pedlar, C. R. and Hayes, P. R. (2019c) Quantification of aerobic determinants of performance in post-pubertal adolescent middle-distance runners. *European Journal of Applied Physiology*, 119(8), pp. 1865–1874.

Blagrove, R. C., Howatson, G. and Hayes, P. R. (2018a) Effects of strength training on the physiological determinants of middle- and long-distance running performance: A systematic review. *Sports Medicine*, 48(5). doi: 10.1007/s40279-017-0835-7.

Blagrove, R. C., Howe, L. P., Cushion, E. J. (2018b) Effects of strength training on postpubertal adolescent distance runners. *Medicine and Science in Sports and Exercise*, 50(6), pp. 1224–1232. doi: 10.1249/MSS.0000000000001543.

Blagrove, R. C., Howe, L. P., Howatson, G. and Hayes, P. R. (2020) Strength and conditioning for adolescent endurance runners. *Strength and Conditioning Journal*, 42(1), pp. 2–11. doi: 10.1519/SSC.0000000000000425.

Blagrove, R. C. et al. (2019) Quantification of aerobic determinants of performance in post-pubertal adolescent middle-distance runners. *European Journal of Applied Physiology*, 119(8), pp. 1865–1874. doi: 10.1007/s00421-019-04175-w.

Blanchfield, A. W., Hardy, J., De Morree, H. M., Staiano, W. and Marcora, S. M. (2014) Talking yourself out of exhaustion: The effects of self-talk on endurance performance. *Medicine and Science in Sports and Exercise*, 46(5), pp. 998–1007.

Blazevich, A. J. (2006) Effects of physical training and detraining, immobilisation, growth and aging on human fascicle geometry. *Sports Medicine*, 36(12), pp. 1003–1017.

Blazevich, A. J. and Babault, N. (2019) Post-activation potentiation versus post-activation performance enhancement in humans: Historical perspective, underlying mechanisms, and current issues. *Frontiers in Physiology*, 10. doi: 10.3389/FPHYS.2019.01359.

Blazevich, A. J. et al. (2018) No effect of muscle stretching within a full, dynamic warm-up on athletic performance. *Medicine and Science in Sport and Exercise*, 50(6), pp. 1258–1266.

Boccia, G., Dardanello, D., Tarperi, C., Festa, L., La Torre, A., Pellegrini, B., Schena, F. and Rainoldi, A. (2017a) Fatigue-induced dissociation between rate of force development and maximal force across repeated rapid contractions. *Human Movement Science*, 54, pp. 267–275.

Boccia, G., Dardanello, D., Tarperi, C., Rosso, V., Festa, L., La Torre, A., Pellegrini, B., Schena, F. and Rainoldi, A. (2017b) Decrease of muscle fiber conduction velocity correlates with strength loss after an endurance run. *Physiological Measurement*, 38, pp. 233–240.

Bohl, C. H. and Volpe, S. L. (2002) Magnesium and exercise. *Critical Reviews in Food Science and Nutrition*, 42(6), pp. 533–563. doi: 10.1080/20024091054247.

Bohm, S., Mersmann, F. and Arampatzis, A. (2015) Human tendon adaptation in response to mechanical loading: A systematic review and meta-analysis of exercise intervention studies on healthy adults. *Sports Medicine-Open*, 1(1), p. 7.

Bohm, S. et al. (2019) The force-length-velocity potential of the human soleus muscle is related to the energetic cost of running. *Proceedings of the Royal Society–Biological Sciences*, 286(1917). doi: 10.1098/RSPB.2019.2560.

Bolger, R. et al. (2015) Sprinting performance and resistance-based training interventions: A systematic review. *The Journal of Strength & Conditioning Research*, 29(4), pp. 1146–1156.

Borg, G. A. V. (1982) Psychophysical bases of perceived exertion. *Medicine and Science in Sports and Exercise*, 14(5), pp. 377–381.

Borg, G. A. V. (1998) *Borg's perceived exertion and pain scales*. Champaign, IL: Human Kinetics.

Boschma, A. L. C. (1994) Breast support for the active woman: Relationship to 3D kinematics of running (Unpublished Master's Thesis). Oregon State University, Oregon.

Boschma, A. L. C., Smith, G. A. and Lawson, L. (1996) Breast support for the active woman: Relationship to 3D kinematics of running. *Medicine and Science in Sports and Exercise*, 26, p. S99.

Bosquet, L., Delhors, P., Duchene, A., Dupont, G. and Leger, L. (2007a) Anaerobic running capacity determined from a 3-parameter systems model: Relationship with other anaerobic indices and with running performance in the 800 m-run. *International Journal of Sports Medicine*, 28(6), pp. 495–500.

Bosquet, L., Montpetit, J., Arvisais, D. and Mujika, I. (2007b) Effects of tapering on performance: A meta-analysis. *Medicine and Science in Sports and Exercise*, 39(8), pp. 1358–1365. doi: 10.1249/mss.0b013e31806010e0.

Bosquet, L. et al. (2013) Effect of training cessation on muscular performance: A meta-analysis. *Scandinavian Journal of Medicine & Science in Sports*, 23(3). doi: 10.1111/SMS.12047.

Bottaro, M. et al. (2011) Neuromuscular compression garments: Effects on neuromuscular strength and recovery. *Journal of Human Kinetics*. doi: 10.2478/v10078-011-0055-4.

Boullosa, D., Esteve-Lanao, J., Casado, A., Peyré-Tartaruga, L. A., Gomes da Rosa, R. and Del Coso, J. (2020) Factors affecting training and physical performance in recreational endurance runners. *Sports*. https://doi.org/10.3390/sports8030035.

Bourdon, P. C., Cardinale, M., Murray, A., Gastin, P., Kellmann, M., Varley, M. C., Gabbett, T. J., Coutts, A. J., Burgess, D. J., Gregson, W. and Cable, N. T. (2017) Monitoring athlete training loads: Consensus statement. *International Journal of Sports Physiology and Performance*, 12, pp. S2161–S2170.

Bovens, A. M., Janssen, G. M., Vermeer, H. G., Hoeberigs, J. H., Janssen, M. P. and Verstappen, F. T. (1989) Occurrence of running injuries in adults following a supervised training program. *International Journal of Sports Medicine*, 10(Suppl. 3), pp. S186–S190.

Bowles, K. A., Steele, J. R. and Chaunchaiyakul, R. (2005) Do current sports brassiere designs impede respiratory function? *Medicine & Science in Sports & Exercise*, 37(9), pp.1633–1640.

Bowles, K. A., Steele, J. R. and Munro, B. (2008) What are the breast support choices of Australian women during physical activity? *British Journal of Sports Medicine*, 42(8), pp. 670–673.

Bowtell, J. and Kelly, V. (2019) Fruit-derived polyphenol supplementation for athlete recovery and performance. *Sports Medicine*, 49(Suppl. 1), pp. 3–23. doi: 10.1007/s40279-018-0998-x.

Brachman, A. et al. (2017) Balance training programs in athletes: A systematic review. *Journal of Human Kinetics*, 58(1), pp. 45–64.

Bragada, J. A., Santos, P. A., Maia, J. A., Colaco, P. J., Lopes, V. P. and Barbosa, T. M. (2010) Longitudinal study in 3,000 m male runners: Relationship between performance and selected physiological parameters. *Journal of Science and Medicine in Sport,* 9(3), pp. 439–444.

Brainyquote (2020) Paula Radcliffe quotes. www.brainyquote.com/quotes/paula_radcliffe_432016. Accessed on 08/09/2020.

Bramah, C., Preece, S. J., Gill, N. and Herrington, L. (2018) Is there a pathological gait associated with common soft tissue running injuries. *American Journal of Sports Medicine*, 46(12), pp. 3023–3031. doi: 10.1177/0363546518793657.

Bramah, C., Preece, S. J., Gill, N. and Herrington, L. (2019) A 10% Increase in step rate improves running kinematics and clinical outcomes in runners with patellofemoral pain at 4 weeks and 3 months. *American Journal of Sports Medicine*, 47, pp. 3406–3413.

Bramble, D. M. and Lieberman, D. E. (2004) Endurance running and the evolution of Homo. *Nature*, 432(7015), pp. 345–352.

Brandon, L. J. (1995) Physiological factors associated with middle distance running performance. *Sports Medicine*, 19(4), pp. 268–277.

Brandt, R., Bevilacqua, G. G. and Andrade, A. (2017) Perceived sleep quality, mood states, and their relationship with performance among brazilian elite athletes during a competitive period. *Journal of Strength and Conditioning Research*. doi: 10.1519/JSC.0000000000001551.

Brearley, S. and Bishop, C. (2019) Transfer of training: How specific should we be? *Strength & Conditioning Journal*, 41(3), pp. 97–109.

Bredeweg, S. W. et al. (2012) The effectiveness of a preconditioning programme on preventing running-related injuries in novice runners: A randomised controlled trial. *British Journal of Sports Medicine*, 46(12), pp. 865–870. doi: 10.1136/BJSPORTS-2012-091397.

Bredt, D. S. (1999) Endogenous nitric oxide synthesis: Biological functions and pathophysiology. *Free Radical Research*, 31(6), pp. 577–596.

Breen, D. T., Foster, J., Falvey, E. and Franklyn-Miller, A. (2015) Gait re-training to alleviate the symptoms of anterior exertional lower leg pain: A case series. *International Journal of Sports Physical Therapy*, 10, pp. 85–94.

Brenner, J. S. and Council of Sports Medicine and Fitness (2016) Sports specialization and intensive training in young athletes. *Pediatrics*, 138(3), p. e20162148.

Brewer, J., Williams, C. and Patton, A. (1988) The influence of high carbohydrate diets on endurance running performance. *European Journal of Applied Physiology*, 57(6), pp. 698–706. doi: 10.1007/BF01075991.

Brick, N. E., MacIntyre, T. and Campbell, M. (2014) Attentional focus in endurance activity: New paradigms and future directions. *International Review of Sport and Exercise Psychology*, 7(1), pp. 106–134.

Brick, N. E., MacIntyre, T. and Schücker, L. (2019) Attentional focus and cognitive strategies during endurance activity. In Meijen, C. (ed.) *Endurance performance in sport: Psychological theory and interventions*. Oxon, UK: Routledge, pp. 113–124.

Brick, N. E., McElhinney, M. J. and Metcalfe, R. S. (2018) The effects of facial expression and relaxation cues on movement economy, physiological, and perceptual responses during running. *Psychology of Sport and Exercise*, 34, pp. 20–28.

Brindle, R. A., Milner, C. E., Zhang, S. and Fitzhugh, E. C. (2014) Changing step width alters lower extremity biomechanics during running. *Gait & Posture*, 39, pp. 124–128.

Bring, B. V., Chan, M., Devine, R. C., Collins, C. L., Diehl, J. and Burkam, B. (2018) Functional movement screening and injury rates in high school and collegiate runners: A retrospective analysis of 3 prospective observational studies. *Clinical Journal of Sport Medicine*, 28(4), pp. 358–363.

Brisbine, B. R., Steele, J. R., Phillips, E. J. and McGhee, D. E. (2020) Breast pain affects the performance of elite female athletes. *Journal of Sports Sciences*, 38(5), pp. 528–553.

Brisswalter, J. and Hausswirth, C. (2008) Consequences of drafting on human locomotion: Benefits on sports performance. *International Journal of Sports Physiology and Performance*, 3(1), pp. 3–15.

Brisswalter, J. and Nosaka, K. (2013) Neuromuscular factors associated with decline in long-distance running performance in master athletes. *Sports Medicine*, 43(1), pp. 51–63.

Brook, N. (1992) *Endurance running events*. Birmingham, England: British Athletics Federation.

Brooks, G. A. (2001) Lactate doesn't necessarily cause fatigue: Why are we surprised? *The Journal of Physiology*, 536(1), p. 1. doi: 10.1111/J.1469-7793.2001.T01-1-00001.X.

Brooks, G. A. (2018) The science and translation of lactate shuttle theory. *Cell Metab*, 27, pp. 757–785.

Brooks, M. A., Post, E. G., Trigsted, S. M. et al. (2018) Knowledge, attitudes, and beliefs of youth club athletes toward sport specialization and sport participation. *Orthopaedic Journal of Sports Medicine*, 6(5), p. e2325967118769836.

Brown, F. et al. (2017) Compression garments and recovery from exercise: A meta-analysis. *Sports Medicine*. doi: 10.1007/s40279-017-0728-9.

Brown, F. et al. (2020) Custom-fitted compression garments enhance recovery from muscle damage in rugby players. *Journal of Strength and Conditioning Research*. doi: 10.1519/jsc.0000000000003408.

Brown, M. A., Stevenson, E. J. and Howatson, G. (2019) Montmorency tart cherry (Prunus cerasus L.) supplementation accelerates recovery from exercise-induced muscle damage in females. *European Journal of Sport Science*. doi: 10.1080/17461391.2018.1502360.

Brown, N. and Scurr, J. (2016) Do women with smaller breasts perform better in long distance running? *European Journal of Sports Science*, 16(8), pp. 965–971.

Brown, N., Smith, J., Brasher, A., Risius, D., Marczyk, A. and Wakefield-Scurr, J. (2018) Breast health education for schoolgirls: Why, what, when and how? *The Breast Journal*, 24(3), pp. 377–382.

Brown, N., White, J., Brasher, A. and Scurr, J. (2014a) The experience of breast pain (mastalgia) in female runners of the 2012 London Marathon and its effect on exercise behaviour. *British Journal of Sports Medicine*, 48(4), pp. 320–325.

Brown, N., White, J., Brasher, A. and Scurr, J. (2014b) An investigation into breast support and sports bra use in female runners of the 2012 London Marathon. *Journal of Sports Sciences*, 32(9), pp. 801–809.

Brueckner, J. C., Atchou, G., Capelli, C., Duvallet, A., Barrault, D., Jousselin, E., Rieu, M. and di Prampero, P. E. (1991) The energy cost of running increases with the distance covered. *European Journal of Applied Physiology*, 62(6), pp. 385–389.

Bruinvels, G., Burden, R., Brown, N., Richards, T. and Pedlar, C. (2016) The prevalence and impact of heavy menstrual bleeding (menorrhagia) in elite and non-elite athletes. *PLoS One*, 11(2), p. e0149881. doi: 10.1371/JOURNAL.PONE.0149881.

Bruton, A. M., Diss, C. E., Moore, I. S. and Mellalieu, S. D. (2017) Examining the effects of combined gait-retraining and video self-modelling on habitual runners experiencing knee pain. *Research in Imagery and Observation*. Roehampton, UK.

Bryant, A. L., Crossley, K. M., Bartold, S., Hohmann, E. and Clark, R. A. (2011) Estrogen-induced effects on the neuro-mechanics of hopping in humans. *European Journal of Applied Physiology*, 111(2), pp. 245–252.

Buchheit, M. and Laursen, P. B. (2013a) High-intensity interval training, solutions to the programming puzzle: Part I: Cardiopulmonary emphasis. *Sports Medicine*, 43(5), pp. 313–338.

Buchheit, M. and Laursen, P. B. (2013b) High-intensity interval training, solutions to the programming puzzle: Part II: Anaerobic energy, neuromuscular load and practical applications. *Sports Medicine*, 43(10), pp. 927–954.

Buchheit, M. and Mendez-Villanueva, A. (2014) Changes in repeated-sprint performance in relation to change in locomotor profile in highly-trained young soccer players. *Journal of Sports Sciences*, 32(13), pp. 1309–1317.

Buckalew, D. P., Barlow, D. A., Fischer, J. W. and Richards, J. G. (1985) Biomechanical profile of elite women marathoners. *International Journal of Sport Biomechanics*, 1(4), pp. 330–347.

Buckthorpe, M., Morris, J. and Folland, J. P. (2012) Validity of vertical jump measurement devices. *Journal of Sports Sciences*, 30(1), pp. 63–69.

Buczek, F. L. and Cavanagh, P. R. (1990) Stance phase knee and ankle kinematics and kinetics during level and downhill running. *Medicine and Science in Sports and Exercise*, 22(5), pp. 669–677.

Buick, F. J., Gledhill, N., Froese, A. B., Spriet, L. and Meyers, E. C. (1980) Effect of induced erythrocythemia on aerobic work capacity. *Journal of Applied Physiology: Respiratory, Environmental and Exercise Physiology*, 48(4), pp. 636–642.

Buist, I., Bredeweg, S. W., Van Mechelen, W., Lemmink, K. A., Pepping, G. J. and Diercks, R. L. (2008) No effect of a graded training program on the number of running-related injuries in novice runners: A randomized controlled trial. *American Journal of Sports Medicine*, 36, pp. 33–39.

Bula, J. E., Rhodes, E. C., Langill, R. H., Sheel, A. W. and Taunton, J. E. (2008) Effects of interindividual variation, state of training, and prolonged work on running economy. *Biology of Sport*, 25, pp. 197–210.

Bull, J. R., Rowland, S. P., Scherwitzl, E. B., Scherwitzl, R., Danielsson, K. G. and Harper, J. (2019) Real-world menstrual cycle characteristics of more than 600,000 menstrual cycles. *NPJ Digital Medicine*, 2(1), p. 83.

Bulun, S. E., Yilmaz, B. D., Sison, C., Miyazaki, K., Bernardi, L., Liu, S., Kohlmeier, A., Yin, P., Milad, M. and Wei, J. (2019) Endometriosis. *Endocrine Reviews*, 40(4), pp. 1048–1079.

Bundle, M. W., Hoyt, R. W. and Weyand, P. G. (2003) High-speed running performance: A new approach to assessment and prediction. *Journal of Applied Physiology*, 95(5), pp. 1955–1962.

Burd, N. A. et al. (2012) Greater stimulation of myofibrillar protein synthesis with ingestion of whey protein isolate v. micellar casein at rest and after resistance exercise in elderly men. *British Journal of Nutrition*. doi: 10.1017/S0007114511006271.

Burd, N. A. et al. (2019) Food-first approach to enhance the regulation of post-exercise skeletal muscle protein synthesis and remodeling. *Sports Medicine*. doi: 10.1007/s40279-018-1009-y.

Burke, L. M. (2008) Caffeine and sports performance. *Applied Physiology, Nutrition, and Metabolism*, 33, pp. 1319–1334.

Burke, L. M. (2015) Re-examining high-fat diets for sports performance: Did we call the 'nail in the coffin' too soon? *Sports Medicine*, 45(1), pp. 33–49. doi: 10.1007/S40279-015-0393-9.

Burke, L. M. (2020) Ketogenic low-CHO, high-fat diet: The future of elite endurance sport? *The Journal of Physiology*. doi: 10.1113/JP278928.

Burke, L. M., Collier, G. R. and Hargreaves, M. (1993) Muscle glycogen storage after prolonged exercise: Effect of the glycemic index of carbohydrate feedings. *Journal of Applied Physiology*, 75(2), pp. 1019–1023. doi: 10.1152/JAPPL.1993.75.2.1019.

Burke, L. M., Hawley, J. A., Schabort, E. J., St Clair Gibson, A., Mujika, I. and Noakes, T. D. (2000) Carbohydrate loading failed to improve 100-km cycling performance in a placebo-controlled trial. *Journal of Applied Physiology*, 88(4), pp. 1284–1290.

Burke, L. M., Hawley, J. A., Wong, S. H. and Jeukendrup, A. E. (2011) Carbohydrates for training and competition. *Journal of Sports Sciences*, 29(Suppl. 1), pp. S17–S27. doi: 10.1080/02640414.2011.585473.

Burke, L. M., Kiens, B. and Ivy, J. L. (2004) Carbohydrates and fat for training and recovery. *Journal of Sports Sciences*. doi: 10.1080/0264041031000140527.

Burke, L. M., van Loon, L. J. C. and Hawley, J. A. (2017a) Postexercise muscle glycogen resynthesis in humans. *Journal of Applied Physiology*, 122(5), pp. 1055–1067. doi: 10.1152/JAPPLPHYSIOL.00860.2016.

Burke, L. M. et al. (2017b) Low carbohydrate, high fat diet impairs exercise economy and negates the performance benefit from intensified training in elite race walkers. *The Journal of Physiology*, 595(9), pp. 2785–2807. doi: 10.1113/JP273230.

Burke, L. M. et al. (2018) Toward a common understanding of diet-exercise strategies to manipulate fuel availability for training and competition preparation in endurance sport. *International Journal of Sport Nutrition and Exercise Metabolism*, 28(5), pp. 451–463. doi: 10.1123/IJSNEM.2018-0289.

Burnett, E., White, J. and Scurr, J. (2015) The influence of the breast on physical activity participation in females. *Journal of Physical Activity and Health*, 12(4), pp. 588–594.

Burnley, M., Doust, J. H. and Vanhatalo, A. (2006) A 3-min all-out test to determine peak oxygen uptake and the maximal steady state. *Medicine & Science in Sports & Exercise*, 38(11), pp. 1995–2003.

Burnley, M. and Jones, A. M. (2007) Oxygen uptake kinetics as a determinant of sports performance. *European Journal of Sport Science*, 7(2), pp. 63–79.

Burnley, M. and Jones, A. M. (2018) Power-duration relationship: Physiology, fatigue, and the limits of human performance. *European Journal of Sport Science*, 18(1), pp. 1–12.

Burr, D. B., Martin, R. B., Schaffler, M. B. and Radin, E. L. (1985) Bone remodeling in response to in vivo fatigue microdamage. *Journal of Biomechanics*, 18, pp. 189–200.

Burton, D., Pickering, M. A., Weinberg, R. S., Yukelson, D. and Weigand, D. (2010) The competitive goal effectiveness paradox revisited: Examining the goal practices of prospective Olympic athletes. *Journal of Applied Sport Psychology*, 22, pp. 72–86.

Burton, D. and Weiss, C. (2008) The fundamental goal concept: The path to process and performance success. In Horn, T. S. (ed.) *Advances in sport psychology*. Champaign, IL: Human Kinetics, pp. 339–375.

Bushnell, T. and Hunter, I. (2007) Differences in technique between sprinters and distance runners at equal and maximal speeds. *Sports Biomechanics*, 6(3), pp. 261–268.

Bussmann, G. and Alfermann, D. (1994) Drop out in the female athlete: A study with track and field athletes. In Hackford, D. (ed.) *Psycho-social issues and interventions in elite sport*. Frankfurt: Lang, pp. 90–123.

Butler, R. J., Crowell III, H. P. and McClay Davis, I. (2003) Lower extremity stiffness: Implications for performance and injury. *Clinical Biomechanics*, 18(6), pp. 511–517.

Cade, J. R. et al. (1991) Dietary intervention and training in swimmers. *European Journal of Applied Physiology*, 63(3), pp. 210–215. doi: 10.1007/BF00233850.

Calabrese, E. J. (2018) Hormesis: Path and progression to significance. *International Journal of Molecular Sciences*, 19.

Calbet, J. A. L., Lundby, C., Koskolou, M. and Boushel, R. (2006) Importance of hemoglobin concentration to exercise: Acute manipulations. *Respiratory Physiology and Neurobiology*, 151(2–3), pp. 132–140.

Canova, R. (1998) Can cross-country running be considered an athletics event in its own right? *New Studies in Athletics*, 13(4), pp. 13–19.

Carr, A. J., Slater, G. J., Gore, C. J., Dawson, B. and Burke, L. M. (2011) Effect of sodium bicarbonate on [HCO$_3^-$], pH, and gastrointestinal symptoms. *International Journal of Sport Nutrition and Exercise Metabolism*, 21(3), pp. 189–194.

Carrick-Ranson, G., Hastings, J. L., Bhella, P. S., Shibata, S., Fujimoto, N., Palmer, D., Boyd, K. and Levine, B. D. (2012) The effect of age-related differences in body size and composition on cardiovascular determinants of VO2max. *The Journals of Gerontology: Series A*, 68(5), pp. 608–616.

Carter, H., Jones, A. M. and Doust, J. H. (1999) Effect of 6 weeks of endurance training on the lactate minimum speed. *Journal of Sports Sciences*, 17(12), pp. 957–967.

Carter, J. M., Jeukendrup, A. E. and Jones, D. A. (2004) The effect of carbohydrate mouth rinse on 1-h cycle time trial performance. *Medicine and Science in Sports and Exercise*, 36, pp. 2107–2112.

Casadio, J. R., Kilding, A. E., Cotter, J. D. and Laursen, P. B. (2017) From lab to real world: Heat acclimation considerations for elite athletes. *Sports Medicine*, 47(8), pp. 1467–1476. doi: 10.1007/s40279 016 0668 9.

Casado, A., Hanley, B. and Ruiz-Pérez, L. M. (2019a) Deliberate practice in training differentiates the best Kenyan and Spanish long-distance runners. *European Journal of Sport Science*, published ahead of print. doi: 10.1080/17461391.2019.1694077.

Casado, A., Hanley, B., Santos-Concejero, J. and Ruiz-Pérez, L. M. (2019b) World-class long-distance running performances are best predicted by volume of easy runs and deliberate practice of short-interval and tempo runs. *Journal of Strength and Conditioning Research*. https://doi.org/10.1519/jsc.0000000000003176.

Casado, A. and Renfree, A. (2018) Fortune favors the brave: Tactical behaviors in the middle-distance running events at the 2017 IAAF World Championships. *International Journal of Sports Physiology and Performance*, 13(10), pp. 1386–1391.

Casey, E., Hameed, F. and Dhaher, Y. Y. (2014) The muscle stretch reflex throughout the menstrual cycle. *Medicine & Science in Sports & Exercise*, 46(3), pp. 600–609.

Casoni, I. et al. (1990) Changes of magnesium concentrations in endurance athletes. *International Journal of Sports Medicine*, 11(3), pp. 234–237. doi: 10.1055/s-2007-1024798.

Cauci, S., Buligan, C., Marangone, M. and Francescato, M. P. (2016) Oxidative stress in female athletes using combined oral contraceptives. *Sports Medicine–Open*, 2(1), p. 40.

Cauci, S., Francescato, M. P. and Curcio, F. (2017) Combined oral contraceptives increase high-sensitivity C-reactive protein but not haptoglobin in female athletes. *Sports Medicine*, 47(1), pp. 175–185.

Cavagna, G. A., Dusman, B. and Margaria, R. (1968) Positive work done by a previously stretched muscle. *Journal of Applied Physiology*, 24, pp. 21–32. https://doi.org/10.1152/jappl.1968.24.1.21.

Cavagna, G. A. and Kaneko, M. (1977) Mechanical work and efficiency in level walking and running. *The Journal of Physiology*, 268(2), pp. 467–481.

Cavagna, G. A., Saibene, F. P. and Margaria, R. (1964) Mechanical work in running. *Journal of Applied Physiology*, 19(2), pp. 249–256.

Cavanagh, P. R. (ed.) (1990) *Biomechanics of distance running*. Champaign, IL: Human Kinetics.

Cavanagh, P. R. and Kram, R. (1989) Stride length in distance running: Velocity, body dimensions, and added mass effects. *Medicine and Science in Sports and Exercise*, 21, pp. 467–479.

Cavanagh, P. R. and Lafortune, M. A. (1980) Ground reaction forces in distance running. *Journal of Biomechanics*, 13(5), pp. 397–406.

Cavanagh, P. R., Pollock, M. L. and Landa, J. (1977) A biomechanical comparison of elite and good distance runners. *Annals of New York Academy Science*, 301, pp. 328–345.

Cavanagh, P. R. and Williams, K. R. (1982) The effect of stride length variation on oxygen uptake during distance running. *Medicine and Science in Sports and Exercise*, 14, pp. 30–35.

Ceyssens, L., Vanelderen, R., Barton, C., Malliaras, P. and Dingenen, B. (2019) Biomechanical risk factors associated with running-related injuries: A systematic review. *Sports Medicine*, 49(7), pp. 1095–1115. doi: 10.1007/S40279-019-01110-Z.

Chaabene, H. et al. (2019) Acute effects of static stretching on muscle strength and power: An attempt to clarify previous caveats. *Frontiers in Physiology*, 10.

Chalabaev, A., Radel, R., Ben Mahmoud, I., Massiera, B., Deroche, T. and d'Arripe-Longueville, F. (2017) Is motivation for marathon a protective factor or a risk factor of injury? *Scandinavian Journal of Medicine & Science in Sports*, 27(12), pp. 2040–2047.

Chambers, T. L., Burnett, T. R., Raue, U., Lee, G. A., Finch, W. H., Graham, B. M., Trappe, T. A. and Trappe, S. (2020) Skeletal muscle size, function, and adiposity with lifelong aerobic exercise. *Journal of Applied Physiology*, 128(2), pp. 368–378.

Chan, Z. Y. S., Zhang, J. H., Au, I. P. H., An, W. W., Shum, G. L. K., Ng, G. Y. F. and Cheung, R. T. H. (2018) Gait retraining for the reduction of injury occurrence in novice distance runners: 1-year follow-up of a randomized controlled trial. *American Journal of Sports Medicine*, 46, pp. 388–395.

Chang, Y.-H. and Kram, R. (1999) Metabolic cost of generating horizontal forces during human running. *Journal of Applied Physiology*, 86(5), pp. 1657–1662.

Chan-Roper, M., Hunter, I., Myrer, J. W., Eggett, D. L. and Seeley, M. K. (2012) Kinematic changes during a marathon for fast and slow runners. *Journal of Sport Science and Medicine*, 11(1), pp. 77–82.

Chapman, A. R., Vicenzino, B., Blanch, P. and Hodges, P. W. (2008) Is running less skilled in triathletes than runners matched for running training history? *Medicine & Science in Sports & Exercise*, 40(3), pp. 557–565.

Chase, J. D. et al. (2017) One night of sleep restriction following heavy exercise impairs 3-km cycling time-trial performance in the morning. *Applied Physiology, Nutrition and Metabolism*. doi: 10.1139/apnm-2016-0698.

Cheatham, S. W. et al. (2015) The effects of self-myofascial release using a foam roll or roller massager on joint range of motion, muscle recovery, and performance: A systematic review. *International Journal of Sports Physical Therapy*, 10(6), pp. 827–838.

Chen, T. C., Nosaka, K. and Tu, J.-H. (2007) Changes in running economy following downhill running. *Journal of Sports Sciences*, 25(1), pp. 55–63.

Chen, X., Gho, S. A., Wang, J. and Steele, J. R. (2016) Effect of sports bra type and gait speed on breast discomfort, bra discomfort and perceived breast movement in Chinese women. *Ergonomics*, 59, pp. 130–142.

Chen, X., Wang, J., Wang, Y., Gho, S. A. and Steele, J. R. (2019) Breast pain and sports bra usage reported by Chinese women: Why sports bra education programs are needed in China. *Fibres & Textiles in Eastern Europe*, 27(4), pp. 17–22.

Cheung, R. T. H. and Davis, I. S. (2011) Landing pattern modification to improve patellofemoral pain in runners: A case series. *Journal of Orthopaedic & Sports Physical Therapy*, 41, pp. 914–919.

Cheuvront, S. N., Carter, R. and Sawka, M. N. (2003) Fluid balance and endurance exercise performance. *Current Sports Medicine Reports*, 2(4), pp. 202–208. doi: 10.1249/00149619-200308000-00006.

Cheuvront, S. N., Montain, S. J. and Sawka, M. N. (2007) Fluid replacement and performance during the marathon. *Sports Medicine*, 37(4–5), pp. 353–357.

Chilibeck, P. D., Syrotuik, D. G. and Bell, G. J. (1999) The effect of strength training on estimates of mitochondrial density and distribution throughout muscle fibres. *European Journal of Applied Physiology*, 80(6), pp. 604–609.

Chistiakov, D. A., Sobenin, I. A., Revin, V. V., Orekhov, A. N. and Bobryshev, Y. V. (2014) Mitochondrial aging and age-related dysfunction of Mitochondria. *BioMed Research International*, 2014, p. 238463.

Chiu, J. K. W. et al. (2012) The effects of quadriceps strengthening on pain, function, and patellofemoral joint contact area in persons with patellofemoral pain. *American Journal of Physical Medicine & Rehabilitation*, 91(2), pp. 98–106. doi: 10.1097/PHM.0B013E318228C505.

Chow, J. W. and Darling, W. G. (1999) The maximum shortening velocity of muscle should be scaled with activation. *Journal of Applied Physiology*, 86(3), pp. 1025–1031.

Chow, J.-Y., Woo, M. and Koh, M. (2014) Effects of external and internal attention focus training on foot-strike patterns in running. *International Journal of Sports Science and Coaching*, 9, pp. 307–320.

Christopher, S. M., McCullough, J., Snodgrass, S. J. and Cook, C. (2019) Do alterations in muscle strength, flexibility, range of motion, and alignment predict lower extremity injury in runners: A systematic review. *Arch Physiother*, 9, p. 2.

Christou, D. D. and Seals, D. R. (2008) Decreased maximal heart rate with aging is related to reduced β-adrenergic responsiveness but is largely explained by a reduction in intrinsic heart rate. *Journal of Applied Physiology*, 105(1), pp. 24–29.

Chu, A. et al. (2018) Lower serum zinc concentration despite higher dietary zinc intake in athletes: A systematic review and meta-analysis. *Sports Medicine*, 48(2), pp. 327–336. doi: 10.1007/S40279-017-0818-8.

Chu, J. J. and Caldwell, G. E. (2004) Stiffness and damping response associated with shock attenuation in downhill running. *Journal of Applied Biomechanics*, 20(3), pp. 291–308.

Chumanov, E. S., Heiderscheit, B. C. and Thelen, D. G. (2011) Hamstring musculotendon dynamics during stance and swing phases of high-speed running. *Medicine and Science in Sports and Exercise*, 43(3), pp. 525–532.

Chumanov, E. S. et al. (2012) Changes in muscle activation patterns when running step rate is increased. *Gait & Posture*, 36(2), pp. 231–235.

Cichanowski, H. R. et al. (2007) Hip strength in collegiate female athletes with patellofemoral pain. *Medicine & Science in Sports & Exercise*, 39(8), pp. 1227–1232.

Clansey, A. C., Hanlon, M., Wallace, E. S., Nevill, A. and Lake, M. J. (2014) Influence of tibial shock feedback training on impact loading and running economy. *Medicine and Science in Sports and Exercise*, 46, pp. 973–981.

Clifford, T. et al. (2018) Cryotherapy reinvented: Application of phase change material for recovery in elite soccer. *International Journal of Sports Physiology and Performance*. doi: 10.1123/ijspp.2017-0334.

Clifford, T. et al. (2019) The effects of vitamin C and E on exercise-induced physiological adaptations: A systematic review and meta-analysis of randomized controlled trials. *Critical Reviews in Food Science and Nutrition*. doi: 10.1080/10408398.2019.1703642.

Close, G. L. and Morton, J. P. (2016) Nutrition for human performance. In Jeffreys, I. and Moody, J. (eds.) *Strength and conditioning for sports performance*. Oxon, UK: Routledge, pp. 143–177.

Close, G. L. et al. (2013) Assessment of vitamin D concentration in non-supplemented professional athletes and healthy adults during the winter months in the UK: Implications for skeletal muscle function. *Journal of Sports Sciences*, 31(4), pp. 344–353. doi: 10.1080/02640414.2012.733822.

Coakley, J. (1992) Burnout among adolescent athletes: A personal failure or social problem? *Sociology in Sport Journal*, 9, pp. 271–285.

Coates, A., Mountjoy, M. and Burr, J. (2017) Incidence of iron deficiency and iron deficient anemia in elite runners and triathletes. *Clinical Journal of Sport Medicine*, 27(5), pp. 493–498. doi: 10.1097/JSM.0000000000000390.

Coffey, V. G. and Hawley, J. A. (2017) Concurrent exercise training: Do opposites distract? *The Journal of Physiology*, 595(9), pp. 2883–2896. doi: 10.1113/JP272270.

Coggan, A. R., Abduljalil, A. M., Swanson, S. C., Earle, M. S., Farris, J. W., Mendenhall, L. A. and Robitaille, P. M. (1993) Muscle metabolism during exercise in young and older untrained and endurance-trained men. *Journal of Applied Physiology*, 75(5), pp. 2125–2133.

Coggan, A. R., Spina, R. J., Rogers, M. A., King, D. S., Brown, M., Nemeth, P. M. and Holloszy, J. O. (1990) Histochemical and enzymatic characteristics of skeletal muscle in master athletes. *Journal of Applied Physiology*, 68(5), pp. 1896–1901.

Cole, A. S., Woodruff, M. E., Horn, M. P. and Mahon, A. D. (2006) Strength, power, and aerobic exercise correlates of 5-km cross-country running performance in adolescent runners. *Pediatric Exercise Science*, 18(3), pp. 374–384.

Collins, D., MacNamara, A. and McCarthy, N. (2016) Super champions, champions, and almosts: Important differences and commonalities on the rocky road. *Frontiers in Psychology*, 6, pp. 1–11.

Coltman, C. E., McGhee, D. E. and Steele, J. R. (2015) Bra strap orientations and designs to minimise bra strap discomfort and pressure during sport and exercise in women with large breasts. *Sports Medicine Open*, 1(1), p. 21.

Coltman, C. E., Steele, J. R. and McGhee, D. E. (2017) Effect of aging on breast skin thickness and elasticity: Implications for breast support. *Skin Research Technology*, 23, pp. 303–311.

Comfort, P. and Kasim, P. (2007) Optimizing squat technique. *Strength & Conditioning Journal*, 29(6), pp. 10–13.

Conley, D. L. and Krahenbuhl, G. S. (1980) Running economy and distance running performance of highly trained athletes. *Medicine and Science in Sports and Exercise*, 12(5), pp. 357–360. https://doi.org/10.1249/00005768-198025000-00010.

Conley, D. L., Krahenbuhl, G. S., Burkett, L. N. and Millar, A. L. (1984) Following Steve Scott: Physiological changes accompanying training. *The Physician and Sportsmedicine*, 12(1), pp. 103–106.

Connolly, D. A., Sayers, S. P. and McHugh, M. P. (2003) Treatment and prevention of delayed onset muscle soreness. *Journal of Strength and Conditioning Research*, 17(1), pp. 197–208. doi: 10.1519/00124278-200302000-00030.

Conradsson, D., Friden, C., Nilsson-Wikmar, L. and Ang, B. O. (2010) Ankle-joint mobility and standing squat posture in elite junior cross-country skiers: A pilot study. *The Journal of Sports Medicine & Physical Fitness*, 50(2), pp. 132–138.

Cook, G., Burton, L., Hoogenboom, B. J. and Voight, M. (2014) Functional movement screening: The use of fundamental movements as an assessment of function-part 1. *International Journal of Sports Physical Therapy*, 9(3), pp. 396–409.

Cook, J. L. and Docking, S. (2015) 'Rehabilitation will increase the "capacity" of your . . . insert musculoskeletal tissue here . . .' Defining 'tissue capacity': A core concept for clinicians. *British Journal of Sports Medicine*, 49, pp. 1484–1485.

Cook, J. L. and Purdam, C. R. (2009) Is tendon pathology a continuum? A pathology model to explain the clinical presentation of load-induced tendinopathy. *British Journal of Sports Medicine*, 43, pp. 409–416.

Cook, J. L., Rio, E., Purdam, C. R. and Docking, S. I. (2016) Revisiting the continuum model of tendon pathology: What is its merit in clinical practice and research? *British Journal of Sports Medicine*, 50, pp. 1187–1191.

Coppack, R. J., Etherington, J. and Wills, A. K. (2011) The effects of exercise for the prevention of overuse anterior knee pain a randomized controlled trial. *American Journal of Sports Medicine*, 39(5), pp. 940–948.

Cormie, P., McGuigan, M. R. and Newton, R. U. (2010) Influence of strength on magnitude and mechanisms of adaptation to power training. *Medicine and Science in Sports and Exercise*, 42(8), pp. 1566–1581. doi: 10.1249/MSS.0b013e3181cf818d.

Costa, R. J. S., Hoffman, M. D. and Stellingwerff, T. (2019a) Considerations for ultra-endurance activities: Part 1-nutrition. *Research in Sports Medicine*, 27(2), pp. 166–118.

Costa, R. J. S., Knechtle, B., Tarnopolsky, M. and Hoffman, M. D. (2019b) Nutrition for ultramarathon running: Trail, track, and road. *International Journal of Sport Nutrition and Exercise Metabolism*, 29(2), pp. 130–140.

Costa, R. J. S., Snipe, R. M. J., Kitic, C. M. and Gibson, P. R. (2017) Systematic review: Exercise-induced gastrointestinal syndrome-implications for health and intestinal disease. *Alimentary Pharmacology and Therapeutics*, 46(3), pp. 246–265.

Costello, J. T. et al. (2012) Muscle, skin and core temperature after -110°c cold air and 8°c water treatment. *PLoS One*. doi: 10.1371/journal.pone.0048190.

Costill, D. L., Bowers, R., Branam, G. and Sparks, K. (1971) Muscle glycogen utilization during prolonged exercise on successive days. *Journal of Applied Physiology*, 31(6), pp. 834–838.

Costill, D. L., Dalsky, G. P. and Fink, W. J. (1978) Effects of caffeine ingestion on metabolism and exercise performance. *Medicine and Science in Sports*, 10, pp. 155–158.

Costill, D. L. and Miller, J. M. (1980) Nutrition for endurance sport: Carbohydrate and fluid balance. *International Journal of Sports Medicine*, 1, pp. 2–14.

Costill, D. L., Thomason, H. and Roberts, E. (1973) Fractional utilization of the aerobic capacity during distance running. *Medicine & Science in Sports & Exercise*, 5(4), pp. 248–252.

Côté, J. and Erickson, K. (2015) Diversification and deliberate play during the sampling years. In Baker, J. and Farrow, D. (eds.) *Routledge handbook of sport expertise: Deliberate practice in sport*. Florence: Routledge, pp. 305–316.

Côté, J., Lidor, R. and Hackfort, D. (2009) ISSP position stand: To sample or to specialize? Seven postulates about youth sport activities that lead to continued participation and elite performance. *International Journal of Sport and Exercise Psychology*, 7, pp. 7–17.

Cox, G. R., Clark, S. A., Cox, A. J., Halson, S. L., Hargreaves, M., Hawley, J. A. et al. (2010) Daily training with high carbohydrate availability increases exogenous carbohydrate oxidation during endurance cycling. *Journal of Applied Physiology*, 109(1), pp. 126–134.

Coyle, E. F. (1991) Timing and method of increased carbohydrate intake to cope with heavy training, competition and recovery. *Journal of Sports Sciences*, 9, pp. 29–52. doi: 10.1080/02640419108729865.

Coyle, E. F. (1995) Integration of the physiological factors determining endurance performance ability. *Exercise and Sport Sciences Reviews*, 23(1), pp. 25–63. https://doi.org/10.1249/00003677-199500230-00004.

Coyle, E. F. et al. (1983) Carbohydrate feeding during prolonged strenuous exercise can delay fatigue. *Journal of Applied Physiology*, 55(1), pp. 230–235. doi: 10.1152/JAPPL.1983.55.1.230.

Craib, M. W. et al. (1996) The association between flexibility and running economy in sub-elite male distance runners. *Medicine & Science in Sports & Exercise*, 28(6), pp. 737–743.

Craig, I. and Morgan, D. (1998) Relationship between 800-m running performance and accumulated oxygen deficit in middle-distance runners. *Medicine & Science in Sports & Exercise*, 30(11), pp. 1631–1636.

Craighead, D. H., Lehecka, N. and King, D. L. (2014) A novel running mechanic's class changes kinematics but not running economy. *Journal of Strength & Conditioning Research*, 28, pp. 3137–3145.

Creaby, M. W. and Franettovich Smith, M. M. (2016) Retraining running gait to reduce tibial loads with clinician or accelerometry guided feedback. *Journal of Science and Medicine in Sport*, 19, pp. 288–292.

Creagh, U. and Reilly, T. (1997) Physiological and biomechanical aspects of orienteering. *Sports Medicine*, 24(6), pp. 409–418.

Creinin, M. D., Meyn, L. A., Borgatta, L., Barnhart, K., Jensen, J., Burke, A. E., Westhoff, C., Gilliam, M., Dutton, C. and Ballagh, S. A. (2008) Multicenter comparison of the contraceptive ring and patch: A randomized controlled trial. *Obstetrics and Gynecology*, 111(2 Pt 1), pp. 267–277.

Crewe, H., Tucker, R. and Noakes, T. D. (2008) The rate of increase in rating of perceived exertion predicts the duration of exercise to fatigue at a fixed power output in different environmental conditions. *European Journal of Applied Physiology*, 103, pp. 569–577.

Crill, M. T., Kolba, C. P. and Chleboun, G. S. (2004) Using lunge measurements for baseline fitness testing. *Journal of Sport Rehabilitation*, 13(1), pp. 44–53.

Critchley, H. O. D., Maybin, J. A., Armstrong, G. M. and Williams, A. R. W. (2020) Physiology of the endometrium and regulation of menstruation. *Physiological Reviews*, 100(3), pp. 1149–1179.

Crossley, K. M., Stefanik, J. J., Selfe, J., Collins, N. J., Davis, I. S., Powers, C. M., McConnell, J., Vicenzino, B., Bazett-Jones, D. M., Esculier, J. F., Morrissey, D. and Callaghan, M. J. (2016) 2016 patellofemoral pain consensus statement from the 4th International Patellofemoral Pain Research Retreat, Manchester: Part 1: Terminology, definitions, clinical examination, natural history, patellofemoral osteoarthritis and patient-reported outcome measures. *British Journal of Sports Medicine*, 50, pp. 839–843.

Crossley, K. M., Zhang, W. J., Schache, A. G., Bryant, A. and Cowan, S. M. (2011) Performance on the single-leg squat task indicates hip abductor muscle function. *American Journal of Sports Medicine*, 39(4), pp. 866–873.

Crowell, H. P. and Davis, I. S. (2011) Gait retraining to reduce lower extremity loading in runners. *Clinical Biomechanics*, 26, pp. 78–83.

Crowell, H. P., Milner, C. E., Hamill, J. and Davis, I. S. (2010) Reducing impact loading during running with the use of real-time visual feedback. *Journal of Orthopaedic & Sports Physical Therapy*, 40, pp. 206–213.

Cunningham, L. N. (1990) Relationship of running economy, ventilatory threshold, and maximal oxygen consumption to running performance in high school females. *Research Quarterly for Exercise and Sport*, 61(4), pp. 369–374.

Cureton, K. J., Warren, G. L., Millard-Stafford, M. L., Wingo, J. E., Trilk, J. and Buyckx, M. (2007) Caffeinated sports drink: Ergogenic effects and possible mechanisms. *International Journal of Sport Nutrition and Exercise Metabolism*, 17, pp. 35–55.

Currell, K. and Jeukendrup, A. E. (2008) Superior endurance performance with ingestion of multiple transportable carbohydrates. *Medicine and Science in Sports and Exercise*, 40, pp. 275–281.

Cushion, E., Howe, L., Read, P. and Spence, A. (2017) A process for error correction for strength and conditioning coaches. *Strength & Conditioning Journal*, 39(6), pp. 84–92.

Dalleau, G., Belli, A., Bourdin, M. and Lacour, J.-R. (1998) The spring-mass model and the energy cost of treadmill running. *European Journal of Applied Physiology*, 77, pp. 257–263.

Damasceno, M. V. et al. (2015) Effects of resistance training on neuromuscular characteristics and pacing during 10-km running time trial. *European Journal of Applied Physiology*, 24/02/2015, 115(7), pp. 1513–1522. doi: 10.1007/s00421-015-3130-z.

Damsted, C., Glad, S., Nielsen, R. O., Sorensen, H. and Malisoux, L. (2018) Is there evidence for an association between changes in training load and running-related injuries? A systematic review. *International Journal of Sports Physical Therapy*, 13, pp. 931–942.

Damsted, C., Parner, E. T., Sørensen, H., Malisoux, L., Hulme, A. and Nielsen, R. (2019a) The association between changes in weekly running distance and running-related injury: Preparing for a half marathon. *Journal of Orthopaedic & Sports Physical Therapy*, 49, pp. 230–238.

Damsted, C., Parner, E. T., Sørensen, H., Malisoux, L. and Nielsen, R. O. (2019b) ProjectRun21: Do running experience and running pace influence the risk of running injury-A 14-week prospective cohort study. *Journal of Science and Medicine in Sport*, 22, pp. 281–287.

Daniels, J. T. (1985) A physiologist's view of running economy. *Medicine and Science in Sports and Exercise*, 17(3), pp. 332–338.

Daniels, J. T. and Daniels, N. (1992) Running economy of elite male and elite female runners. *Medicine and Science in Sports and Exercise*, 24(4), pp. 483–489.

Daniels, J. T., Yarbrough, R. and Foster, C. (1978) Changes in $\dot V$ O2 max and running performance with training. *European Journal of Applied Physiology and Occupational Physiology*, 39(4), pp. 249–254.

Dankel, S. J. et al. (2017) A critical review of the current evidence examining whether resistance training improves time trial performance. *Journal of Sports Science*, 36(13), pp. 1–7.

Dáttilo, M. et al. (2020) Effects of sleep deprivation on acute skeletal muscle recovery after exercise. *Medicine and Science in Sports and Exercise*. doi: 10.1249/mss.0000000000002137.

Davies, C. T. M. (1980) Effects of wind assistance and resistance on the forward motion of a runner. *Journal of Applied Physiology*, 48(4), pp. 702–709.

Davies, J. and Kadir, R. A. (2017) Heavy menstrual bleeding: An update on management. *Thrombosis Research*, 151, pp. S70–S77.

Davis, I. S., Bowser, B. J. and Mullineaux, D. R. (2016) Greater vertical impact loading in female runners with medically diagnosed injuries: A prospective investigation. *British Journal of Sports Medicine*, 50, pp. 887–892.

Davis, I. S. and Futrell, E. (2016) Gait retraining: Altering the fingerprint of gait. *Physical Medicine and Rehabilitation Clinics of North America*, 27, pp. 339–355.

Davis, J. M. (1995) Carbohydrates, branched-chain amino acids, and endurance: The central fatigue hypothesis. *International Journal of Sport Nutrition*, 5, pp. S29–S38.

Dawood, M. Y. (1987) Dysmenorrhea and prostaglandins. In Gold, J. J. and Josimovich, J. B. (eds.) *Gynecologic endocrinology*. Boston, MA: Springer.

De Blaiser, C., Roosen, P., Willems, T., Danneels, L., Bossche, L. V. and De Ridder, R. (2018) Is core stability a risk factor for lower extremity injuries in an athletic population? A systematic review. *Physical Therapy in Sport*, 30, pp. 48–56.

De Jonge, J., Balk, Y. A. and Taris, T. W. (2020) Mental recovery and running-related injuries in recreational runners: The moderating role of passion for running. *International Journal of Environmental Research and Public Health*, 17.

De Jonge, J., Van Iperen, L., Gevers, J. and Vos, S. (2018) 'Take a mental break!' Study: Role of mental aspects in running-related injuries using a randomised controlled trial. *BMJ Open Sport & Exercise Medicine*, 4, p. e000427.

De Marneffe, M., Jacobs, P., Haardt, R. and Englert, M. (1986) Variations of normal sinus node function in relation to age: Role of autonomic influence. *European Heart Journal*, 7(8), pp. 662–672.

de Oliveira, E. P., Burini, R. C. and Jeukendrup, A. (2014) Gastrointestinal complaints during exercise: Prevalence, etiology, and nutritional recommendations. *Sports Medicine*, 44(Suppl. 1), pp. S79–S85.

De Ruiter, C. J., Verdijk, P. W., Werker, W., Zuidema, M. J. and De Haan, A. (2013) Stride frequency in relation to oxygen consumption in experienced and novice runners. *European Journal of Sport Science*, 14, pp. 251–258.

De Souza, M. J., Nattiv, A., Joy, E., Misra, M., Williams, N. I., Mallinson, R. J., Gibbs, J. C., Olmsted, M., Goolsby, M. and Matheson, G. (2014) 2014 female athlete triad coalition consensus statement on treatment and return to play of the female athlete triad: 1st international conference held in San Francisco, California, May 2012 and 2nd international conference held in Indianapolis, Indiana, May 2013. *British Journal of Sports Medicine*, 48(4), p. 289.

De Souza, M. J., Nattiv, A., Joy, E. et al. (2014a) 2014 female athlete triad coalition consensus statement on treatment and return to play of the female athlete triad: 1st international conference held in San Francisco, California, May 2012, and 2nd international conference held in Indianapolis, Indiana, May 2013. *Clinical Journal of Sport Medicine*, 24(2), pp. 96–119.

De Souza, M. J., Williams, N. I., Koltun, K. J. and Strock, N. C. A. (2020) Female athlete triad coalition risk assessment tool is an evidenced-based tool that is reliable and well-described. *Journal of Sports Sciences*, 38(9), pp. 996–999.

De Souza, M. J., Williams, N. I., Nattiv, A. et al. (2014b) Misunderstanding the female athlete triad: Refuting the IOC consensus statement on relative energy deficiency in sport (RED-S). *British Journal of Sports Medicine*, 48(20), pp. 1461–1465.

de Villarreal, E. S., Requena, B. and Cronin, J. B. (2012) The effects of plyometric training on sprint performance: A meta-analysis. *The Journal of Strength & Conditioning Research*, 26(2), pp. 575–584.

De Witt, J. K., English, K. L., Crowell, J. B., Kalogera, K. L., Guilliams, M. E., Nieschwitz, B. E., Hanson, A. M. and Ploutz-Snyder, L. L. (2018) Isometric midthigh pull reliability and relationship to deadlift one repetition maximum. *The Journal of Strength & Conditioning Research*, 32(2), pp. 528–533.

Deaner, R. O., Addona, V. and Hanley, B. (2019) Risk taking runners slow more in the marathon. *Frontiers in Psychology*, 10, p. 333.

Deaner, R. O., Carter, R. E., Joyner, M. J. and Hunter, S. K. (2015) Men are more likely than women to slow in the marathon. *Medicine and Science in Sports and Exercise*, 47(3), pp. 607–616.

Debenham, J., Travers, M., Gibson, W., Campbell, A. and Allison, G. (2016) Eccentric fatigue modulates stretch-shortening cycle effectiveness: A possible role in lower limb overuse injuries. *International Journal of Sports Medicine*, 37(1), pp. 50–55.

Deci, E. L. and Ryan, R. M. (2000) The 'what' and 'why' of goal pursuits: Human needs and the self-determination of behavior. *Psychological Inquiry*, 11, pp. 227–268.

Decker, M. J., Torry, M. R., Noonan, T. J., Riviere, A. M. Y. and Sterett, W. I. (2002) Landing adaptations after ACL reconstruction. *Medicine & Science in Sports & Exercise*, 34(9), pp. 1408–1413.

Dedrick, G. S., Sizer, P. S., Merkle, J. N., Hounshell, T. R., Robert-McComb, J. J., Sawyer, S. F., Brismée, J.-M. and James, C. R. (2008) Effect of sex hormones on neuromuscular control patterns during landing. *Journal of Electromyography and Kinesiology*, 18(1), pp. 68–78.

Degens, H., Maden-Wilkinson, T. M., Ireland, A., Korhonen, M. T., Suominen, H., Heinonen, A., Radak, Z., McPhee, J. S. and Rittweger, J. (2013) Relationship between ventilatory function and age in master athletes and a sedentary reference population. *Age*, 35(3), pp. 1007–1015.

Deldicque, L. and Francaux, M. (2015) Recommendations for healthy nutrition in female endurance runners: An update. *Frontiers in Nutrition*, 2, p. 17. doi: 10.3389/FNUT.2015.00017.

Dempsey, J. A., Hanson, P. G. and Henderson, K. S. (1984) Exercise-induced arterial hypoxaemia in healthy human subjects at sea level. *The Journal of Physiology*, 355, pp. 161–175.

Denadai, B. S. et al. (2017) Explosive training and heavy weight training are effective for improving running economy in endurance athletes: A systematic review and meta-analysis. *Sports Medicine*, 47(3), pp. 545–554. doi: 10.1007/s40279-016-0604-z.

Denison, J. (2004) *The greatest: The Haile Gebrselassie story*. Halcottsville, NY: Breakaway Books.

Dennis, R. J., Finch, C. F., Elliott, B. C. and Farhart, P. J. (2008) The reliability of musculoskeletal screening tests used in cricket. *Physical Therapy in Sport*, 9(1), pp. 25–33.

Derrick, T. R., Caldwell, G. E. and Hamill, J. (2000) Modeling the stiffness characteristics of the human body while running with various stride lengths. *Journal of Applied Biomechanics*, 16, pp. 36–51.

Desbrow, B. and Leveritt, M. (2007) Well-trained endurance athletes' knowledge, insight, and experience of caffeine use. *International Journal of Sport Nutrition and Exercise Metabolism*, 17, pp. 328–339.

Díaz, J. J., Fernández-Ozcorta, E. J. and Santos-Concejero, J. (2018) The influence of pacing strategy on marathon world records. *European Journal of Sport Science*, 18(6), pp. 781–786.

Di Caprio, F., Buda, R., Mosca, M., Calabro, A. and Giannini, S. (2010) Foot and lower limb diseases in runners: Assessment of risk factors. *Journal of Sports Science and Medicine*, 9, pp. 587–596.

Díaz, J. J., Renfree, A., Fernández-Ozcorta, E. J., Torres, M. and Santos-Concejero, J. (2019) Pacing and performance in the 6 World Marathon Majors. *Frontiers in Sports and Active Living*, 1, p. 54.

Diebal, A. R., Gregory, R., Alitz, C. and Gerber, J. P. (2012) Forefoot running improves pain and disability associated with chronic exertional compartment syndrome. *American Journal of Physiology*, 40, pp. 1060–1067.

Dieën, J. H. Van, Ogita, F. and Haan, A. De (2003) Reduced neural drive in bilateral exertions: A performance-limiting factor? *Medicine & Science in Sports & Exercise*, 35(1), pp. 111–118. doi: 10.1097/00005768-200301000-00018.

Dierks, T. A., Manal, K. T., Hamill, J. and Davis, I. S. (2008) Proximal and distal influences on hip and knee kinematics in runners with patellofemoral pain during a prolonged run. *Journal of Orthopaedic & Sports Physical Therapy*, 38(8), pp. 448–456.

DiFiori, J. P., Benjamin, H. J., Brenner, J. S. et al. (2014) Overuse injuries and burnout in youth sports: A position statement from the American Medical Society for Sports Medicine. *British Journal of Sports Medicine*, 48(4), pp. 287–288.

Dill, K. E., Begalle, R. L., Frank, B. S., Zinder, S. M. and Padua, D. A. (2014) Altered knee and ankle kinematics during squatting in those with limited weight-bearing-lunge ankle-dorsiflexion range of motion. *Journal of Athletic Training*, 49(6), pp. 723–732.

DiLorenzo, F. M., Drager, C. J. and Rankin, J. W. (2014) Docosahexaenoic acid affects markers of inflammation and muscle damage after eccentric exercise. *Journal of Strength and Conditioning Research*. doi: 10.1519/JSC.0000000000000617.

DiMenna, F. J. and Jones, A. M. (2016) Developing endurance for sports performance. In *Strength and conditioning for sports performance*. New York, USA: Routledge, p. 377.

Di Michele, R. and Merni, F. (2014) The concurrent effects of strike pattern and ground-contact time on running economy. *Journal of Science and Medicine in Sport*, 17(4), pp. 414–418.

di Prampero, P. E. (1985) Metabolic and circulatory limitations to VO2 max at the whole animal level. *Journal of Experimental Biology*, 115(1), pp. 319–331.

Dis, D. M., Stellingwerff, T., Kitic, C. M., Fell, J. W. and Ahuja, K. D. K. (2018) Low FODMAP: A preliminary strategy to reduce gastrointestinal distress in athletes. *Medicine and Science in Sports and Exercise*, 50(1), pp. 116–123.

Diss, C. E., Doyle, S., Moore, I. S., Mellalieu, S. D. and Bruton, A. M. (2018) Examining the effects of combined gait retraining and video self-modeling on habitual runners experiencing knee pain: A pilot study. *Translational Sports Medicine*, 1, pp. 273–282.

Diss, C. E., Gittoes, M., Tong, R. and Kerwin, D. (2015) Stance limb kinetics of older male athletes endurance running performance. *Sports Biomechanics*, 14(3), pp. 300–309.

Dixon, J. B. (2009) Gastrocnemius vs. soleus strain: How to differentiate and deal with calf muscle injuries. *Current Reviews in Musculoskeletal Medicine*, 2(2), pp. 74–77.

Dixon, S. J., Collop, A. C. and Batt, M. E. (2000) Surface effects on ground reaction forces and lower extremity kinematics in running. *Medicine & Science in Sports & Exercise*, 32, pp. 1919–1926.

Doma, K., Deakin, G. B. and Bentley, D. J. (2017) Implications of impaired endurance performance following single bouts of resistance training: An alternate concurrent training perspective. *Sports Medicine*. doi: 10.1007/s40279-017-0758-3.

Donaldson, C. M., Perry, T. L. and Rose, M. C. (2010) Glycemic index and endurance performance. *International Journal of Sport Nutrition and Exercise Metabolism*, 20(2), pp. 154–165. doi: 10.1123/IJSNEM.20.2.154.

Donnelly, G., Brockwell, E. and Goom, T. (2020) Return to running postnatal-guideline for medical, health and fitness professionals managing this population. *Physiotherapy*, 107, pp. e188–e189.

Donohue, M. R., Ellis, S. M., Heinbaugh, E. M., Stephenson, M. L., Zhu, Q. and Dai, B. (2015) Differences and correlations in knee and hip mechanics during single-leg landing, single-leg squat, double-leg landing, and double-leg squat tasks. *Research in Sports Medicine*, 23(4), pp. 394–411.

Donovan, J. and Williams, K. J. (2003) Missing the mark: Effects of time and causal attributions on goal revision in response to goal-performance discrepancies. *Journal of Applied Psychology*, 88, pp. 379–390.

Dorn, T. W., Schache, A. G. and Pandy, M. G. (2012) Muscular strategy shift in human running: Dependence of running speed on hip and ankle muscle performance. *The Journal of Experimental Biology*, 215(11), pp. 1944–1956. doi: 10.1242/JEB.064527.

Dowrick, P. W. (1999) A review of self modeling and related interventions. *Applied and Preventive Psychology*, 8, pp. 23–39.

Drew, K. (2020) Investigating the junior-to-senior transition in sport: Interventions to support the transitional process (Doctoral Dissertation). Liverpool John Moores University, Liverpool, UK.

Drobnic, F. et al. (2014) Reduction of delayed onset muscle soreness by a novel curcumin delivery system (Meriva®): A randomised, placebo-controlled trial. *Journal of the International Society of Sports Nutrition*. doi: 10.1186/1550-2783-11-31.

Duan, Y. et al. (2016) The role of leucine and its metabolites in protein and energy metabolism. *Amino Acids*, 48(1), pp. 41–51. doi: 10.1007/S00726-015-2067-1.

Dubey, R. K. and Jackson, E. K. (2001) Estrogen-induced cardiorenal protection: Potential cellular, biochemical, and molecular mechanisms. *American Journal of Physiology-Renal Physiology*, 280(3), pp. F365–F388.

Duffield, R. and Dawson, B. (2003) Energy system contribution in track running. *New Studies in Athletics*, 18(4), pp. 47–56.

Duffield, R., Dawson, B. and Goodman, C. (2005) Energy system contribution to 400-metre and 800-metre track running. *Journal of Sports Sciences*, 23(3), pp. 299–307. doi: 10.1080/02640410410001730043.

Dumke, C. L., Pfaffenroth, C. M., McBride, J. M. and McCauley, G. O. (2010) Relationship between muscle strength, power and stiffness and running economy in trained male runners. *International Journal of Sports Physiology and Performance*, 5(2), pp. 249–261.

Dutto, D. J. and Smith, G. A. (2002) Changes in spring-mass characteristics during treadmill running to exhaustion. *Medicine and Science in Sports and Exercise*, 34(8), pp. 1324–1331.

Dye, S. F. (2005) The pathophysiology of patellofemoral pain: A tissue homeostasis perspective. *Clinical Orthopaedics and Related Research*, 436(436), pp. 100–110.

Eapen, C., Nayak, C. D. and Zulfeequer, C. P. (2011) Effect of eccentric isotonic quadriceps muscle exercises on patellofemoral pain syndrome: An exploratory pilot study. *Asian Journal of Sports Medicine*, 2(4), pp. 227–234. doi: 10.5812/ASJSM.34747.

Earl, J. E. and Hoch, A. Z. (2011) A proximal strengthening program improves pain, function, and biomechanics in women with patellofemoral pain syndrome. *American Journal of Sports Medicine*, 39(1), pp. 154–163. doi: 10.1177/0363546510379967.

Edouard, P., Navarro, L., Branco, P., Gremeaux, V., Timpka, T. and Junge, A. (2020) Injury frequency and characteristics (location, type, cause and severity) differed significantly among athletics ('track and field') disciplines during 14 international championships (2007–2018): Implications for medical service planning. *British Journal of Sports Medicine*, 54, pp. 159–167.

Eiling, E., Bryant, A. L., Petersen, W., Murphy, A. and Hohmann, E. (2007) Effects of menstrual-cycle hormone fluctuations on musculotendinous stiffness and knee joint laxity. *Knee Surgery, Sports Traumatology, Arthroscopy*, 15(2), pp. 126–132.

Eisenmann, J. C., Pivarnik, J. M. and Malina, R. M. (2001) Scaling peak Vo2 to body mass in young male and female distance runners. *Journal of Applied Physiology*, 90(6), pp. 2172–2180.

El-Hemaidi, I., Gharaibeh, A. and Shehata, H. (2007) Menorrhagia and bleeding disorders. *Current Opinion in Obstetrics and Gynecology*, 19(6), pp. 513–520.

Elliot, B. and Ackland, T. (1981) Biomechanical effects of fatigue on 10,000 meter running technique. *Research Quarterly for Exercise and Sport*, 52(2), pp. 160–166.

Elliott-Sale, K. J., McNulty, K. L., Ansdell, P., Goodall, S., Hicks, K. M., Thomas, K., Swinton, P. A. and Dolan, E. (2020) The effects of oral contraceptives on exercise performance in women: A systematic review and meta-analysis. *Sports Medicine*, pp. 1–28.

Elliott-Sale, K. J., Tenforde, A. S., Parziale, A. L., Holtzman, B. and Ackerman, K. E. (2018) Endocrine effects of relative energy deficiency in sport. *International Journal of Sport Nutrition and Exercise Metabolism*, 28(4), pp. 335–349.

Ely, M. R., Martin, D. E., Cheuvront, S. N. and Montain, S. J. (2008) Effect of ambient temperature on marathon pacing is dependent on runner ability. *Medicine and Science in Sports and Exercise*, 40(9), pp. 1675–1680.

Emery, C. A. (2003) Risk factors for injury in child and adolescent sport: A systematic review of the literature. *Clinical Journal of Sport Medicine*, 13, pp. 256–268.

Enoka, R. M. (2008) *Neuromechanics of human movement*. 4th edn. Champaign, IL: Human Kinetics.

Enoksen, E. (2011) Drop-out rate and drop-out reasons among promising Norwegian track and field athletes: A 25 year study. *Scandinavian Sports Studies Forum*, 2, pp. 19–43.

Enoksen, E., Tjelta, A. R. and Tjelta, L. I. (2011) Distribution of training volume and intensity of elite male and female track and marathon runners. *International Journal of Sports Science and Coaching*. https://doi.org/10.1260/1747-9541.6.2.273.

Enomoto, Y., Kadono, H., Suzuki, Y., Chiba, T. and Koyama, K. (2008) Biomechanical analysis of the medalists in the 10,000 metres at the 2007 World Championship in athletics. *New Studies in Athletics*, 23(3), pp. 61–66.

Ericsson, K. A., Krampe, R. T. and Tesch-Römer, C. (1993) The role of deliberate practice in the acquisition of expert performance. *Psychological Review*, 100(3), pp. 363–406.

Eriksson, M., Halvorsen, K. A. and Gullstrand, L. (2011) Immediate effect of visual and auditory feedback to control the running mechanics of well-trained athletes. *Journal of Sports Sciences*, 29, pp. 253–262.

Esculier, J. F., Bouyer, L. J., Dubois, B., Fremont, P., Moore, L., McFadyen, B. and Roy, J. S. (2017) Is combining gait retraining or an exercise programme with education better than education alone in treating runners with patellofemoral pain? A randomised clinical trial. *British Journal of Sports Medicine*, 52, pp. 659–666.

Esculier, J.-F. et al. (2018) Is combining gait retraining or an exercise programme with education better than education alone in treating runners with patellofemoral pain? A randomised clinical trial. *British Journal of Sports Medicine*, 52(10), pp. 659–666.

Esposito, F., Reese, V., Shabetai, R., Wagner, P. D. and Richardson, R. S. (2011) Isolated quadriceps training increases maximal exercise capacity in chronic heart failure: The role of skeletal muscle convective and diffusive oxygen transport. *Journal of the American College of Cardiology*, 58(13), pp. 1353–1362.

Essen-Gustavsson, B. and Borges, O. (1986) Histochemical and metabolic characteristics of human skeletal muscle in relation to age. *Acta Physiologica Scandinavica*, 126(1), pp. 107–114.

Esteve-Lanao, J., Foster, C., Seiler, S. and Lucia, A. (2007) Impact of training intensity distribution on performance in endurance athletes. *Journal of Strength and Conditioning Research*, 21(3), pp. 943–949. https://doi.org/10.1519/R-19725.1.

Esteve-Lanao, J., Larumbe-Zabala, E., Dabab, A., Alcocer-Gamboa, A. and Ahumada, F. (2014) Running world cross-country championships: A unique model for pacing. *International Journal of Sports Physiology and Performance*, 9(6), pp. 1000–1005.

Esteve-Lanao, J., San Juan, A. F., Earnest, C. P., Foster, C. and Lucia, A. (2005) How do endurance runners actually train? Relationship with competition performance. *Medicine and Science in Sports and Exercise*. https://doi.org/10.1249/01.MSS.0000155393.78744.86.

Eston, R. G., Lemmey, A. B., McHugh, P., Byrne, C. and Walsh, S. E. (2000) Effect of stride length on symptoms of exercise-induced muscle damage during a repeated bout of downhill running. *Scandinavian Journal of Medicine and Science in Sports*, 10(4), pp. 199–204.

Eston, R. G., Mickleborough, J. and Baltzopoulos, V. (1995) Eccentric activation and muscle damage: Biomechanical and physiological considerations during downhill running. *British Journal of Sports Medicine*, 29(2), pp. 89–94.

Evans, G. H. et al. (2017) Optimizing the restoration and maintenance of fluid balance after exercise-induced dehydration. *Journal of Applied Physiology*. doi: 10.1152/japplphysiol.00745.2016.

Evans, S. L., Davy, K. P., Stevenson, E. T. and Seals, D. R. (1995) Physiological determinants of 10-km performance in highly trained female runners of different ages. *Journal of Applied Physiology*, 78(5), pp. 1931–1941.

Evans, W. J. and Lexell, J. (1995) Human aging, muscle mass, and fiber type composition. *The Journals of Gerontology: Series A*, 50A(Special_Issue), pp. 11–16.

Everman, S., Farris, J. W., Bay, R. C. and Daniels, J. T. (2018) Elite distance runners. *Medicine & Science in Sports & Exercise*, 50(1), pp. 73–78.

Fagerberg, P. (2017) Negative consequences of low energy availability in natural male bodybuilding: A review. *International Journal of Sport Nutrition and Exercise Metabolism*, 28(4), pp. 385–402. doi: 10.1123/IJSNEM.2016-0332.

Faigenbaum, A. D., Lloyd, R. S., MacDonald, J. and Myer, G. D. (2016) Citius, Altius, Fortius: Beneficial effects of resistance training for young athletes: Narrative review. *British Journal of Sports Medicine*, 50(1), pp. 3–7.

Fair, R. C. (2007) Estimated age effects in athletic events and chess. *Experimental Aging Research*, 33(1), pp. 37–57.

Fairclough, J., Hayashi, K., Toumi, H., Lyons, K., Bydder, G., Phillips, N., Best, T. M. and Benjamin, M. (2007) Is iliotibial band syndrome really a friction syndrome? *Journal of Science and Medicine in Sport*, 10, pp. 74–76.

Farley, C. T., Glasheen, J. and MacMahon, T. A. (1993) Running springs: Speed and animal size. *Journal of Experimental Biology*, 185, pp. 71–86.

Farrell, P. A., Wilmore, J. H., Coyle, E. F., Billing, J. E. and Costill, D. L. (1979) Plasma lactate accumulation and distance running performance. *Medicine & Science in Sports & Exercise*, 11(4), pp. 338–344.

Faude, O., Kindermann, W. and Meyer, T. (2009) Lactate threshold concepts. *Sports Medicine*, 39(6), pp. 469–490.

Faulkner, J. A. (1968) New perspectives in training for maximum performance. *JAMA: The Journal of the American Medical Association*. https://doi.org/10.1001/jama.1968.03140370043009.

Faust, L., Bradley, D., Landau, E., Noddin, K., Farland, L. V., Baron, A. and Wolfberg, A. (2019) Findings from a mobile application-based cohort are consistent with established knowledge of the menstrual cycle, fertile window, and conception. *Fertility and Sterility*, 112(3), pp. 450–457.e3.

Faustmann, G., Meinitzer, A., Magnes, C., Tiran, B., Obermayer-Pietsch, B., Gruber, H.-J., Ribalta, J., Rock, E., Roob, J. M. and Winklhofer-Roob, B. M. (2018) Progesterone-associated arginine decline at luteal phase of menstrual cycle and associations with related amino acids and nuclear factor kB activation. *PLoS One*, 13(7), p. e0200489.

Fay, L., Londeree, B. R., Lafontaine, T. P. and Volek, M. R. (1989) Physiological parameters related to distance running performance in female athletes. *Medicine and Science in Sports and Exercise*, 21(3), pp. 319–324.

Fehring, R. J., Schneider, M. and Raviele, K. (2006) Variability in the phases of the menstrual cycle. *Journal of Obstetric, Gynecologic, & Neonatal Nursing*, 35(3), pp. 376–384.

Feltz, D. L., Short, S. E. and Sullivan, P. J. (2008) *Self-efficacy in sport.* Champaign, IL: Human Kinetics.

Ferber, R. et al. (2010) Competitive female runners with a history of iliotibial band syndrome demonstrate atypical hip and knee kinematics. *Journal of Orthopaedic & Sports Physical Therapy*, 40(2), pp. 52–58. doi: 10.2519/JOSPT.2010.3028.

Ferber, R., Kendall, K. D. and Farr, L. (2011) Changes in knee biomechanics after a hip-abductor strengthening protocol for runners with patellofemoral pain syndrome. *Journal of Athletic Training*, 46(2), pp. 142–149.

Ferguson, C., Rossiter, H. B., Whipp, B. J., Cathcart, A. J., Murgatroyd, S. R. and Ward, S. A. (2010) Effect of recovery duration from prior exhaustive exercise on the parameters of the power-duration relationship. *Journal of Applied Physiology*, 108(4), pp. 866–874.

Fernández-Lázaro, D. et al. (2020) Modulation of exercise-induced muscle damage, inflammation, and oxidative markers by curcumin supplementation in a physically active population: A systematic review. *Nutrients*. doi: 10.3390/nu12020501.

Fernhall, B., Kohrt, W., Burkett, L. N. and Walters, S. (1996) Relationship between the lactate threshold and cross-country run performance in high school male and female runners. *Pediatric Exercise Science*, 8(1), pp. 37–47.

Ferrauti, A., Bergermann, M. and Fernandez-Fernandez, J. (2010) Effects of a concurrent strength and endurance training on running performance and running economy in recreational marathon runners. *Journal of Strength and Conditioning Research*, 24(10), pp. 2770–2778. doi: 10.1519/JSC.0b013e3181d64e9c.

Ferreira, A., Dias, J., Fernandes, R., Sabino, G., Anjos, M. and Felício, D. (2012) Prevalence and associated risks of injury in amateur street runners from Belo Horizonte, MG. *Revista Brasileira de Medicina do Esporte*, 18, pp. 252–255.

Ferreira, R. and Rolim, R. (2006) The evolution of marathon training: A comparative analysis of elite runners' training programmes. *New Studies in Athletics*, 21(1), p. 29.

Ferreira-Junior, J. B. et al. (2015) One session of partial-body cryotherapy (-110°C) improves muscle damage recovery. *Scandinavian Journal of Medicine and Science in Sports*. doi: 10.1111/sms.12353.

Ferri, A., Adamo, S., La Torre, A., Marzorati, M., Bishop, D. J. and Miserocchi, G. (2012) Determinants of performance in 1,500-m runners. *European Journal of Applied Physiology*, 112(8), pp. 3033–3043.

Ferris, D. P., Liang, K. and Farley, C. T. (1999) Runners adjust leg stiffness for their first step on a new running surface. *Journal of Biomechanics*, 32, pp. 787–794.

Festa, L. et al. (2019) Effects of flywheel strength training on the running economy of recreational endurance runners. *Journal of Strength and Conditioning Research*, 33(3), pp. 684–690. doi: 10.1519/JSC.0000000000002973.

Filipas, L., Ballati, E. N., Bonato, M., La Torre, A. and Piacentini, M. F. (2018a) Elite male and female 800-m runners' display of different pacing strategies during season-best performances. *International Journal of Sports Physiology and Performance*, 13(10), pp. 1344–1348.

Filipas, L., La Torre, A. and Hanley, B. (2018b) Pacing profiles of Olympic and IAAF World Championship long-distance runners. *The Journal of Strength and Conditioning Research*. Published ahead of print. doi: 10.1519/jsc.0000000000002873.

Findlay, R. J., Macrae, E. H. R., Whyte, I. Y., Easton, C. and Whyte, L. J. F. (2020) How the menstrual cycle and menstruation affect sporting performance: Experiences and perceptions of elite female rugby players. *British Journal of Sports Medicine*, 54, pp. 1108–1113.

Finestone, A. and Milgrom, C. (2008) How stress fracture incidence was lowered in the Israeli army: A 25-yr struggle. *Medicine and Science in Sport and Exercise*, 40(11), pp. S623–S639.

Finnoff, J. T. et al. (2011) Hip strength and knee pain in high school runners: A prospective study. *Physical Medicine and Rehabilitation*, 3(9), pp. 792–801. doi: 10.1016/J.PMRJ.2011.04.007.

Flanagan, E. P., Ebben, W. P. and Jensen, R. L. (2008) Reliability of the reactive strength index and time to stabilization during depth jumps. *The Journal of Strength and Conditioning Research*, 22(5), pp. 1677–1682.

Fleischman, A., Makimura, H., Stanley, T. L. et al. (2010) Skeletal muscle phosphocreatine recovery after submaximal exercise in children and young and middle-aged adults. *Journal of Clinical Endocrinology and Metabolism*, 95, pp. e69–e74.

Fletcher, J. R., Esau, S. P. and Macintosh, B. R. (2009) Economy of running: Beyond the measurement of oxygen uptake. *Journal of Applied Physiology (1985)*, 107(6), pp. 1918–1922.

Fletcher, J. R., Esau, S. P. and MacIntosh, B. R. (2010) Changes in tendon stiffness and running economy in highly trained distance runners. *European Journal of Applied Physiology*, 110(5), pp. 1037–1046. doi: 10.1007/s00421-010-1582-8.

Fletcher, J. R. and MacIntosh, B. R. (2017) Running economy from a muscle energetics perspective. *Frontiers in Physiology*, 8, p. 433. doi: 10.3389/fphys.2017.00433.

Fletcher, J. R., Pfister, T. R. and Macintosh, B. R. (2013) Energy cost of running and Achilles tendon stiffness in man and woman trained runners. *Physiological Reports*, 1(7), p. e00178.

Folland, J. P., Allen, S. J., Black, M. I., Handsaker, J. C. and Forrester, S. E. (2017) Running technique is an important component of running economy and performance. *Medicine and Science in Sports and Exercise*, 49(7), pp. 1412–1423.

Folland, J. P. and Williams, A. G. (2007) The adaptations to strength training. *Sports Medicine*, 37(2), pp. 145–168. doi: 10.2165/00007256-200737020-00004.

Foss, J. L., Sinex, J. A. and Chapman, R. F. (2019) Career performance progressions of junior and senior elite track and field athletes. *Journal of Science in Sport and Exercise*, 1(2), pp. 168–175.

Foster, C., Daniels, J. T., de Koning, J. J. and Cotter, H. M. (2006) Field testing of athletes. In Maud, P. J. and Foster, C. (eds.) *Physiological assessment of human fitness*. Champaign, IL: Human Kinetics.

Foster, C., Florhaug, J. A., Franklin, J., Gottschall, L., Hrovatin, L. A., Parker, S., . . . Dodge, C. (2001) A new approach to monitoring exercise training. *Journal of Strength and Conditioning Research*. https://doi.org/10.1519/1533-4287(2001)015<0109:ANATME>2.0.CO;2.

Franch, J., Madsen, K., Djurhuus, M. S. and Pedersen, P. K. (1998) Improved running economy following intensified training correlates with reduced ventilatory demands. *Medicine & Science in Sports & Exercise*, 30(8), pp. 1250–1256.

Francis, P. et al. (2019) The proportion of lower limb running injuries by gender, anatomical location and specific pathology: A systematic review. *Journal of Sports Science and Medicine*, 18(1), pp. 21–31.

Franettovich, M. M. S. et al. (2014) Neuromotor control of gluteal muscles in runners with Achilles tendinopathy. *Medicine and Science in Sports and Exercise*, 46(3), pp. 594–599.

Franklyn, M. and Oakes, B. (2015) Aetiology and mechanisms of injury in medial tibial stress syndrome: Current and future developments. *World Journal of Orthopedics*, 6, pp. 577–589.

Franklyn-Miller, A. (2016) The athletic shin. In Joyce, D. and Lewindon, D. (eds.) *Sports injury prevention and rehabilitation*. Oxon, UK: Routledge.

Freckleton, G., Cook, J. and Pizzari, T. (2014) The predictive validity of a single leg bridge test for hamstring injuries in Australian rules football players. *British Journal of Sports Medicine*, 48(8), pp. 713–717.

Frederick, E. C. (1984) Physiological and ergonomics factors in running shoe design. *Applied Ergonomics*, 15, pp. 281–287.

Fredericson, M., Cookingham, C. L., Chaudhari, A. M., Dowdell, B. C., Oestreicher, N. and Sahrmann, S. A. (2000) Hip abductor weakness in distance runners with iliotibial band syndrome. *Clinical Journal of Sport Medicine*, 10(3), pp. 169–175.

Freemas, J. A., Baranauskas, M. N., Constantini, K., Constantini, N., Greenshields, J. T., Mickleborough, T. D., Raglin, J. S. and Schlader, Z. J. (2020) Exercise performance is impaired during the mid-luteal phase of the menstrual cycle. *Medicine & Science in Sports & Exercise*, Publish Ahead of Print.

Freitas, L. L. D. S. N. et al. (2020) Sleep debt induces skeletal muscle injuries in athletes: A promising hypothesis. *Medical Hypotheses*. doi: 10.1016/j.mehy.2020.109836.

Friedmann-Bette, B. (2008) Classical altitude training. *Scandinavian Journal of Medicine and Science in Sports*, 18, pp. 11–20. doi: 10.1111/j.1600-0838.2008.00828.x.

Frohm, A., Heijne, A., Kowalski, J., Svensson, P. and Myklebust, G. (2012) A nine test screening battery for athletes: A reliability study. *Scandinavian Journal of Medicine & Science in Sports*, 22(3), pp. 306–315.

Frost, D. M., Beach, T. A., Callaghan, J. P. and McGill, S. M. (2015) FMS scores change with performers' knowledge of the grading criteria: Are general whole-body movement screens capturing 'Dysfunction'? *The Journal of Strength & Conditioning Research*, 29(11), pp. 3037–3044.

Frost, G., Dowling, J., Dyson, K. et al. (1997) Cocontraction in three age groups of children during treadmill locomotion. *Journal of Electromyography and Kinesiology*, 7, pp. 179–186.

Fuchs, C. J. et al. (2016) Sucrose ingestion after exhaustive exercise accelerates liver, but not muscle glycogen repletion compared with glucose ingestion in trained athletes. *Journal of Applied Physiology*. doi: 10.1152/japplphysiol.01023.2015.

Fuglsang, E. I., Telling, A. S. and Sørensen, H. (2017) Effect of ankle mobility and segment ratios on trunk lean in the barbell back squat. *The Journal of Strength & Conditioning Research*, 31(11), pp. 3024–3033.

Fujimoto, N., Hastings, J. L., Bhella, P. S., Shibata, S., Gandhi, N. K., Carrick-Ranson, G., Palmer, D. and Levine, B. D. (2012) Effect of ageing on left ventricular compliance and distensibility in healthy sedentary humans. *The Journal of Physiology*, 590(8), pp. 1871–1880.

Fukuba, Y. and Whipp, B. J. (1999) A metabolic limit on the ability to make up for lost time in endurance events. *Journal of Applied Physiology*, 87(2), pp. 853–861.

Fukuchi, R. K., Stefanyshyn, D. J., Stirling, L., Duarte, M. and Ferber, R. (2014) Flexibility, muscle strength and running biomechanical adaptations in older runners. *Clinical Biomechanics*, 29, pp. 304–310.

Fullagar, H. H., Skorski, S., Duffield, R., Hammes, D., Coutts, A. J. and Meyer, T. (2015) Sleep and athletic performance: The effects of sleep loss on exercise performance, and physiological and cognitive responses to exercise. *Sports Medicine*, 45, pp. 161–186.

Fuller, J. T., Bellenger, C. R., Thewlis, D., Tsiros, M. D. and Buckley, J. D. (2014) The effect of footwear on running performance and running economy in distance runners. *Sports Medicine*, pp. 1–12.

Fuller, J. T., Bellenger, C. R., Thewlis, D., Tsiros, M. D. and Buckley, J. D. (2015) The effect of footwear on running performance and running economy in distance runners. *Sports Medicine*, 45(3), pp. 411–422.

Fuller, J. T., Thewlis, D., Buckley, J. D., Brown, N. A., Hamill, J. and Tsiros, M. D. (2017) Body mass and weekly training distance influence the pain and injuries experienced by runners using minimalist shoes: A randomized controlled trial. *American Journal of Sports Medicine*, 45, pp. 1162–1170.

Fullerton, C. L., Lane, A. M. and Devonport, T. J. (2017) The influence of a pacesetter on psychological responses and pacing behavior during a 1600 m run. *Journal of Sports Science & Medicine*, 16(4), p. 551.

Funnell, M. P. et al. (2019) Blinded and unblinded hypohydration similarly impair cycling time trial performance in the heat in trained cyclists. *Journal of Applied Physiology*. doi: 10.1152/japplphysiol.01026.2018.

Gabbett, T. J. (2016) The training-injury prevention paradox: Should athletes be training smarter and harder? *British Journal of Sports Medicine*, 50, pp. 273–280.

Gabbett, T. J. (2020) Debunking the myths about training load, injury and performance: Empirical evidence, hot topics and recommendations for practitioners. *British Journal of Sports Medicine*, 54, pp. 58–66.

Gaesser, G. A. and Wilson, L. A. (1988) Effects of continuous and interval training on the parameters of the power-endurance time relationship for high-intensity exercise. *International Journal of Sports Medicine*, 9(6), pp. 417–421.

Galbraith, A., Hopker, J. G., Cardinale, M., Cunniffe, B. and Passfield, L. (2014a) A 1-year study of endurance runners: Training, laboratory tests, and field tests. *International Journal of Sports Physiology and Performance*, 9(6), pp. 1019–1025.

Galbraith, A., Hopker, J. G., Jobson, S. A. and Passfield, L. (2011) A novel field test to determine critical speed. *Journal of Sports Medicine & Doping Studies*, 1(1), pp. 1–4.

Galbraith, A., Hopker, J. G., Lelliott, S., Diddams, L. and Passfield, L. (2014b) A single-visit field test of critical speed. *International Journal of Sports Physiology and Performance*, 9(6), pp. 931–935.

Galbraith, A., Hopker, J. G. and Passfield, L. (2015) Modeling intermittent running from a single-visit field test. *International Journal of Sports Medicine*, 36(5), pp. 365–370.

Gao, C., Kuklane, K. and Holmér, I. (2010) Cooling vests with phase change material packs: The effects of temperature gradient, mass and covering area. *Ergonomics*. doi: 10.1080/00140130903581649.

Gao, Y. et al. (2018) Muscle atrophy induced by mechanical unloading: Mechanisms and potential countermeasures. *Frontiers in Physiology*, 9, p. 235.

Garcia-Pinillos, F., Carton-Llorente, A., Jaen-Carrillo, D., Delgado-Floody, P., Carrasco-Alarcon, V., Martinez, C. and Roche-Seruendo, L. E. (2020) Does fatigue alter step characteristics and stiffness during running? *Gait Posture*, 76, pp. 259–263.

Gaskell, S. K. and Costa, R. J. S. (2019) Applying a low-FODMAP dietary intervention to a female ultraendurance runner with irritable bowel syndrome during a multistage ultramarathon. *International Journal of Sport Nutrition and Exercise Metabolism*, 29(1), pp. 61–67.

Gaskins, A. J., Wilchesky, M., Mumford, S. L., Whitcomb, B. W., Browne, R. W., Wactawski-Wende, J., Perkins, N. J. and Schisterman, E. F. (2012) Endogenous reproductive hormones and C-reactive protein across the menstrual cycle the biocycle study. *American Journal of Epidemiology*, 175(5), pp. 423–431.

Gastin, P. B. (2001) Energy system interaction and relative contribution during maximal exercise. *Sports Medicine*, 31(10), pp. 725–741.

Gates, P. E., Strain, W. D. and Shore, A. C. (2009) Human endothelial function and microvascular ageing. *Experimental Physiology*, 94(3), pp. 311–316.

Gazeau, F., Koralsztein, J. P. and Billat, V. (1997) Biomechanical events in the time to exhaustion at maximum aerobic speed. *Archives of Physiology and Biochemistry*, 105(6), pp. 583–590.

Gefen, A. and Dilmoney, B. (2007) Mechanics of the normal woman's breast. *Technology and Health Care*, 15(4), pp. 259–271.

Gehlsen, G. and Albohm, M. (1980) Evaluation of sports bras. *The Physician and Sports Medicine*, 8(10), pp. 88–97.

Geithner, C. A., Woynarowska, B. and Malina, R. M. (1998) The adolescent spurt and sexual maturation in girls active and not active in sport. *Annals of Human Biology*, 25, pp. 415–423.

Gent, D. N. and Norton, K. (2013) Aging has greater impact on anaerobic versus aerobic power in trained masters athletes. *Journal of Sports Sciences*, 31(1), pp. 97–103.

Gibbs, J. C., Williams, N. I. and Souza, M. J. De (2013) Prevalence of individual and combined components of the female athlete triad. *Medicine and Science in Sport and Exercise*, 45(5), pp. 985–996. doi: 10.1249/MSS.0B013E31827E1BDC.

Giffin, K. L. et al. (2017) Predisposing risk factors and stress fractures in Division I cross country runners. *Journal of Strength and Conditioning Research*. doi: 10.1519/JSC.0000000000002408.

Gifford, J. R., Garten, R. S., Nelson, A. D., Trinity, J. D., Layec, G., Witman, M. A. H., Weavil, J. C., Mangum, T., Hart, C., Etheredge, C., Jessop, J., Bledsoe, A., Morgan, D. E., Wray, D. W., Rossman, M. J. and Richardson, R. S. (2016) Symmorphosis and skeletal muscle: In vivo and in vitro measures reveal differing constraints in the exercise-trained and untrained human. *The Journal of Physiology*, 594(6), pp. 1741–1751.

Giovanelli, N. et al. (2017) Effects of strength, explosive and plyometric training on energy cost of running in ultra-endurance athletes. *European Journal of Sport Science*, 17(7), pp. 805–813. doi: 10.1080/17461391.2017.1305454.

Giovanelli, N., Scaini, S., Billat, V. and Lazzer, S. (2019) A new field test to estimate the aerobic and anaerobic thresholds and maximum parameters. *European Journal of Sport Science*. https://doi.org/10.1080/17461391.2019.1640289.

Girard, O., Millet, G. P., Slawinski, J., Racinais, S. and Micallef, J. P. (2013) Changes in running mechanics and spring-mass behaviour during a 5-km time trial. *International Journal of Sports Medicine*, 34(9), pp. 832–840.

Girman, A., Lee, R. and Kligler, B. (2002) An integrative medicine approach to premenstrual syndrome. *Clinical Journal of Women's Health*, 2(3), pp. 116–127.

Glace, B. W., Murphy, C. A. and McHugh, M. P. (2002) Food intake and electrolyte status of ultramarathoners competing in extreme heat. *Journal of the American College of Nutrition*, 21(6), pp. 553–559.

Gleeson, M., Nieman, D. C. and Pedersen, B. K. (2004) Exercise, nutrition and immune function. *Journal of Sports Sciences*, 22(1), pp. 115–125. doi: 10.1080/0264041031000140590.

Gleim, G. W., Stachenfeld, N. S. and Nicholas, J. A. (1990) The influence of flexibility on the economy of walking and jogging. *Journal of Orthopaedic Research*, 8(6), pp. 814–823.

Goldberg, R. J. and Katz, J. (2007) A meta-analysis of the analgesic effects of omega-3 polyunsaturated fatty acid supplementation for inflammatory joint pain. *Pain*. doi: 10.1016/j.pain.2007.01.020.

Golf, S. W., Bender, S. and Grüttner, J. (1998) On the significance of magnesium in extreme physical stress. *Cardiovascular Drugs and Therapy*, 12, pp. 197–202. doi: 10.1023/a:1007708918683.

Gollwitzer, P. M. and Oettingen, G. (2019) Goal attainment. In Ryan, R. M. (ed.) *The Oxford handbook of human motivation*. New York, NY: Oxford University Press, pp. 247–268.

Gomez-Cabrera, M.-C., Domenech, E. and Viña, J. (2008a) Moderate exercise is an antioxidant: Upregulation of antioxidant genes by training. *Free Radical Biology and Medicine*, 44(2), pp. 126–131. doi: 10.1016/J.FREERADBIOMED.2007.02.001.

Gomez-Cabrera, M.-C. et al. (2008b) Oral administration of vitamin C decreases muscle mitochondrial biogenesis and hampers training-induced adaptations in endurance performance. *The American Journal of Clinical Nutrition*, 87(1), pp. 142–149. doi: 10.1093/AJCN/87.1.142.

Gomez-Molina, J., Ogueta-Alday, A., Camara, J., Stickley, C. and Garcia-Lopez, J. (2018) Effect of 8 weeks of concurrent plyometric and running training on spatiotemporal and physiological variables of novice runners. *European Journal of Sport Science*, 18, pp. 162–169.

Gonzalez-Mohino, F., Santos-Concejero, J., Yustres, I. and Gonzalez-Rave, J. M. (2020) The effects of interval and continuous training on the oxygen cost of running in recreational runners: A systematic review and meta-analysis. *Sports Medicine*, 50(2), pp. 283–294.

Goodwin, J. E. and Cleather, D. J. (2016) The biomechanical principles underpinning strength and conditioning. In Jeffreys, I. and Moody, J. A. (eds.) *Strength and conditioning for sports performance*. London, UK: Routledge.

Goom, T. S., Malliaras, P., Reiman, M. P. and Purdam, C. R. (2016) Proximal hamstring tendinopathy: Clinical aspects of assessment and management. *Journal of Orthopaedic & Sports Physical Therapy*, 46, pp. 483–493.

Goose, M. and Winter, S. (2012) The coach's impact on long distance runners' training and competition motivation. *International Journal of Sport Science and Coaching*, 7, pp. 383–398.

Gordon, D., Wightman, S., Basevitch, I., Johnstone, J., Espejo-Sanchez, C., Beckford, C., Boal, M., Scruton, A., Ferrandino, M. and Merzbach, V. (2017) Physiological and training characteristics of recreational marathon runners. *Open Access Journal of Sports Medicine*, 8, p. 231.

Gordon, D., Wood, M., Porter, A., Vetrivel, V., Gernigon, M., Caddy, O., Merzbach, V., Keiller, D., Baker, J. and Barnes, R. (2014) Influence of blood donation on the incidence of plateau at VO2max. *European Journal of Applied Physiology*, 114(1), pp. 21–27.

Gorissen, S. H. M. and Witard, O. C. (2018) Characterising the muscle anabolic potential of dairy, meat and plant-based protein sources in older adults. *Proceedings of the Nutrition Society*. doi: 10.1017/S002966511700194X.

Gottschall, J. S. and Kram, R. (2005) Ground reaction forces during downhill and uphill running. *Journal of Biomechanics*, 38(3), pp. 445–452.

Gould, D., Carson, S., Fifer, A. et al. (2009) Social-emotional and life skill development issues characterizing today's high school sport experience. *Journal of Coaching Education*, 2, pp. 1–25.

Gould, Z. I., Oliver, J., Lloyd, R. S., Read, P. and Neil, R. (2017) Intra and inter-rater reliability of the Golf Movement Screen (GMS). *International Journal of Golf Science*, 6, pp. 118–129.

Grabiner, M. D. and Enoka, R. M. (1995) Changes in movement capabilities with aging. *Exercise and Sport Science Reviews*, 23, pp. 65–104.

Graham, T. E., Battram, D. S., Dela, F., El-Sohemy, A. and Thong, F. S. (2008) Does caffeine alter muscle carbohydrate and fat metabolism during exercise? *Applied Physiology, Nutrition, and Metabolism*, 33, pp. 1311–1318.

Granacher, U., Lesinski, M., Büsch, D. et al. (2016) Effects of resistance training in youth athletes on muscular fitness and athletic performance: A conceptual model for long-term athlete development. *Frontiers in Physiology*, 7, p. 164.

Granata, C., Jannick, N. A. and Bishop, D. J. (2018) Training-induced changes in mitochondrial content and respiratory function in human skeletal muscle. *Sports Medicine*, 48(8), pp. 1809–1828.

Green, B., Bourne, M. N., Van Dyk, N. and Pizzari, T. (2020) Recalibrating the risk of hamstring strain injury (HSI): A 2020 systematic review and meta-analysis of risk factors for index and recurrent hamstring strain injury in sport. *British Journal of Sports Medicine*, 54(18), pp. 1081–1088.

Green, B. and Pizzari, T. (2017) Calf muscle strain injuries in sport: A systematic review of risk factors for injury. *British Journal of Sports Medicine*, 51, pp. 1189–1194.

Green, L. J., O'Brien, P. M. S., Panay, N., Craig, M. on behalf of the Royal College of Obstetricians and Gynaecologists (2017) Management of premenstrual syndrome. *British Journal of Obstetrics and Gynaecology*, 124, pp. e73–e105.

Green, S. (1994) A definition and systems view of anaerobic capacity. *European Journal of Applied Physiology and Occupational Physiology*, 69(2), pp. 168–173.

Greenbaum, A. R., Heslop, T., Morris, J. and Dunn, K. W. (2003) An investigation of the suitability of bra fit in women referred for reduction mammaplasty. *British Journal of Plastic Surgery*, 56(3), pp. 230–236.

Gregson, W. et al. (2011) Influence of cold water immersion on limb and cutaneous blood flow at rest. *American Journal of Sports Medicine*. doi: 10.1177/0363546510395497.

Gries, K. J., Raue, U., Perkins, R. K., Lavin, K. M., Overstreet, B. S., D'Acquisto, L. J., Graham, B., Finch, W. H., Kaminsky, L. A., Trappe, T. A. and Trappe, S. (2018) Cardiovascular and skeletal muscle health with lifelong exercise. *Journal of Applied Physiology*, 125(5), pp. 1636–1645.

Grindler, N. M. and Santoro, N. F. (2015) Menopause and exercise. *Menopause*, 22(12), pp. 1351–1358.

Groen, B. B. L., Hamer, H. M., Snijders, T., van Kranenburg, J., Frijns, D., Vink, H. and van Loon, L. J. C. (2014) Skeletal muscle capillary density and microvascular function are compromised with aging and type 2 diabetes. *Journal of Applied Physiology*, 116(8), pp. 998–1005.

Gruber, A. H., Silvernall, J. F., Brüggeman, G.-P., Rohr, E. and Hamill, J. (2013a) Footfall patterns during barefoot running on harder and softer surfaces. *Footwear Science*, 5, pp. 39–44.

Gruber, A. H., Umberger, B. R., Braun, B. and Hamill, J. (2013b) Economy and rate of carbohydrate oxidation during running with rearfoot and forefoot running patterns. *Journal of Applied Physiology*, 115(2), pp. 194–201.

Gulick, D. T. et al. (1996) Various treatment techniques on signs and symptoms of delayed onset muscle soreness. *Journal of Athletic Training*, 31(2), pp. 145–152.

Güllich, A. (2018) Sport-specific and non-specific practice of strong and weak responders in junior and senior elite athletics: A matched-pairs analysis. *Journal of Sports Sciences*, 36(19), pp. 2256–2264.

Gumbs, V. L., Segal, D., Halligan, J. B. and Lower, G. (1982) Bilateral distal radius and ulnar fractures in adolescent weight lifters. *American Journal of Sports Medicine*, 10(6), pp. 375–379.

Gunning, J. L., Callaghan, J. P. and McGill, S. M. (2001) Spinal posture and prior loading history modulate compressive strength and type of failure in the spine: A biomechanical study using a porcine cervical spine model. *Clinical Biomechanics*, 16(6), pp. 471–480.

Gupta, L., Morgan, K. and Gilchrist, S. (2017) Does elite sport degrade sleep quality? A systematic review. *Sports Medicine*, 47, pp. 1317–1333. doi: 10.1007/s40279-016-0650-6.

Gustafsson, H., Kentta, G., Hassmen, P. and Lundqvist, C. (2007) Prevalence of burnout in competitive adolescent athletes. *The Sports Psychologist*, 21, pp. 21–37.

Gustafsson, J.-Å. (2003) What pharmacologists can learn from recent advances in estrogen signalling. *Trends in Pharmacological Sciences*, 24(9), pp. 479–485.

Gustavsson, A. et al. (2006) A test battery for evaluating hop performance in patients with an ACL injury and patients who have undergone ACL reconstruction. *Knee Surgery Sports Traumatology Arthroscopy*, 14(8), pp. 778–788.

Habets, B., Smits, H. W., Backx, F. J. G., Van Cingel, R. E. H. and Huisstede, B. M. A. (2017) Hip muscle strength is decreased in middle-aged recreational male athletes with midportion Achilles tendinopathy: A cross-sectional study. *Physical Therapy in Sport*, 25, pp. 55–61.

Habte, K. et al. (2015) Iron, folate and vitamin B12 status of Ethiopian professional runners. *Nutrition & Metabolism*, 12(1), p. 62. doi: 10.1186/S12986-015-0056-8.

Hackney, A. C. (2008) Effects of endurance exercise on the reproductive system of men: The 'exercise-hypogonadal male condition'. *Journal of Endocrinological Investigation*, 31(10), pp. 932–938. doi: 10.1007/BF03346444.

Hackney, A. C., Sinning, W. E. and Bruot, B. C. (1988) Reproductive hormonal profiles of endurance-trained and untrained males. *Medicine & Science in Sports & Exercise*, 20(1), pp. 60–65.

Hagberg, J. M., Allen, W. K., Seals, D. R., Hurley, B. F., Ehsani, A. A. and Holloszy, J. O. (1985) A hemodynamic comparison of young and older endurance athletes during exercise. *Journal of Applied Physiology*, 58(6), pp. 2041–2046.

Hagberg, J. M. and Coyle, E. F. (1983) Physiological determinants of endurance performance as studied in competitive racewalkers. *Medicine and Science in Sports and Exercise*, 15(4), pp. 287–289.

Hall, R., Barber Foss, K., Hewett, T. E. and Myer, G. D. (2015) Sport specialization's association with an increased risk of developing anterior knee pain in adolescent female athletes. *Journal of Sport Rehabilitation*, 24, pp. 31–35.

Halson, S. L. (2013) Sleep and the elite athlete. *Sports Science Exchange*, 26(113), pp. 1–4.

Halson, S. L. (2014) Sleep in elite athletes and nutritional interventions to enhance sleep. *Sports Medicine*. doi: 10.1007/s40279-014-0147-0.

Halson, S. L. (2019) Sleep monitoring in athletes: Motivation, methods, miscalculations and why it matters. *Sports Medicine*, 49, pp. 1487–1497. doi: 10.1007/s40279-019-01119-4.

Halson, S. L., Bridge, M. W., Meeusen, R., Busschaert, B., Gleeson, M., Jones, D. A. and Jeukendrup, A. E. (2002) Time course of performance changes and fatigue markers during intensified training in trained cyclists. *Journal of Applied Physiology*, 93(3), pp. 947–956. doi: 10.1152/japplphysiol.01164.2001.

Halson, S. L. and Jeukendrup, A. E. (2004) Does overtraining exist? *Sports Medicine*, 34(14), pp. 967–981. doi: 10.2165/00007256-200434140-00003.

Halson, S. L. and Martin, D. T. (2013) Lying to win–placebos and sport science. *International Journal of Sports Physiology and Performance*. doi: 10.1123/ijspp.8.6.597.

Hamner, S. R., and Delp, S. L. (2013) Muscle contributions to fore-aft and vertical body mass center accelerations over a range of running speeds. *Journal of Biomechanics*, 46, pp. 780–787.

Hamner, S. R., Seth, A. and Delp, S. L. (2010) Muscle contributions to propulsion and support during running. *Journal of Biomechanics*, 43(14), pp. 2709–2716.

Hanley, B. (2014) Senior men's pacing profiles at the IAAF World Cross Country Championships. *Journal of Sports Sciences*, 32(11), pp. 1060–1065.

Hanley, B. (2015) Pacing profiles and pack running at the IAAF World Half Marathon Championships *Journal of Sports Sciences*, 33(11), pp. 1189–1195.

Hanley, B. (2016) Pacing, packing and sex-based differences in Olympic and IAAF World Championship marathons. *Journal of Sports Sciences*, 34(17), pp. 1675–1681.

Hanley, B. (2018) Pacing profiles of senior men and women at the 2017 IAAF World Cross Country Championships. *Journal of Sports Sciences*, 36(12), pp. 1402–1406.

Hanley, B., Bissas, A. and Merlino, S. (2020) Better water jump clearances were differentiated by longer landing distances in the 2017 IAAF World Championship 3000 m steeplechase finals. *Journal of Sports Sciences*, 38(3), pp. 330–335.

Hanley, B., Bissas, A., Merlino, S. and Gruber, A. H. (2019) Most marathon runners at the 2017 IAAF World Championships were rearfoot strikers, and most did not change footstrike pattern. *Journal of Biomechanics*, 92, pp. 54–60.

Hanley, B., Smith, L. C. and Bissas, A. (2011) Kinematic variations due to changes in pace during men's and women's 5 km road running. *International Journal of Sports Science and Coaching*, 6(2), pp. 243–252.

Hanley, B. and Tucker, C. B. (2018) Gait variability and symmetry remain consistent during 10,000 m treadmill running. *Journal of Biomechanics*, 79, pp. 129–134.

Hanley, B. and Williams, E. L. (2020) Successful pacing profiles of Olympic men and women 3,000 m steeplechasers. *Frontiers in Sports and Active Living*, 2, p. 21.

Hanon, C., Thépaut-Mathieu, C. and Vandewalle, H. (2005) Determination of muscular fatigue in elite runners. *European Journal of Applied Physiology*, 94, pp. 118–125.

Hardy, J. (2006) Speaking clearly: A critical review of the self-talk literature. *Psychology of Sport and Exercise*, 7(1), pp. 81–97.

Hargreaves, M., Hawley, J. A. and Jeukendrup, A. (2004) Pre-exercise carbohydrate and fat ingestion: Effects on metabolism and performance. *Journal of Sports Sciences*, 22(1), pp. 31–38.

Hargreaves, M. and Spriet, L. L. (2018) Exercise metabolism: Fuels for the fire. *Cold Spring Harbor Perspectives in Medicine*, 8(8). doi: 10.1101/CSHPERSPECT.A029744.

Hargreaves, M. and Spriet, L. L. (2020) Skeletal muscle energy metabolism during exercise. *Nature Metabolism*. doi: 10.1038/s42255-020-0251-4.

Harridge, S., Magnusson, G. and Saltin, B. (1997) Life-long endurance-trained elderly men have high aerobic power, but have similar muscle strength to non-active elderly men. *Aging Clinical and Experimental Research*, 9(1–2), pp. 80–87.

Harries, S. K., Lubans, D. R. and Callister, R. (2012) Resistance training to improve power and sports performance in adolescent athletes: A systematic review and meta-analysis. *Journal of Science and Medicine in Sport*, 15(6), pp. 532–540.

Hasegawa, H., Yamauchi, T. and Kraemer, W. J. (2007) Foot strike patterns of runners at the 15-km point during an elite-level half marathon. *The Journal of Strength and Conditioning Research*, 21(3), pp. 888–893.

Hasselstrøm, H., Hansen, S. E., Froberg, K. and Andersen, L. B. (2002) Physical fitness and physical activity during adolescence as predictors of cardiovascular disease risk in young adulthood. Danish youth and sports study: An eight-year follow-up study. *International Journal of Sports Medicine*, 23(S1), pp. 27–31.

Hassiotou, F. and Geddes, D. (2013) Anatomy of the human mammary gland: Current status of knowledge. *Clinical Anatomy*, 26, pp. 29–48.

Hatzigeorgiadis, A., Bartura, K., Argiropoulos, C., Comoutos, N., Galanis, E. and Flouris, D. A. (2018) Beat the heat: Effects of a motivational self-talk intervention on endurance performance. *Journal of Applied Sport Psychology*, 30(4), pp. 388–401.

Hatzigeorgiadis, A., Zourbanos, N., Mpoumpaki, S. and Theodorakis, Y. (2009) Mechanisms underlying the self-talk: Performance relationship: The effects of motivational self-talk on self-confidence and anxiety. *Psychology of Sport and Exercise*, 10(1), pp. 186–192.

Haugen, T. A., Solberg, P. A., Foster, C. et al. (2018) Peak age and performance progression in world-class track-and-field athletes. *International Journal of Sports Physiology and Performance*, 13(9), pp. 1122–1129.

Haaswirth, C. et al. (2011) Effects of whole-body cryotherapy vs. far-infrared vs. passive modalities on recovery from exercise-induced muscle damage in highly-trained runners. *PLoS One*. doi: 10.1371/journal.pone.0027749.

Havemann, L. et al. (2006) Fat adaptation follwoed by carbohydrate-loading compromises high-intensity sprint performance. *Journal of Applied Physiology*, 100(1), pp. 194–202. doi: 10.1152/JAPPLPHYSIOL.00813.2005.

Hawkins, D. and Metheny, J. (2001) Overuse injuries in youth sports: Biomechanical considerations. *Medicine and Science in Sports and Exercise*, 33, pp. 1701–1707.

Hawkins, S. A., Marcell, T. J., Victoria Jaque, S. and Wiswell, R. A. (2001) A longitudinal assessment of change in $\dot{V}O2max$ and maximal heart rate in master athletes. *Medicine & Science in Sports & Exercise*, 33(10).

Hawkins, S. A. and Wiswell, R. A. (2003) Rate and mechanism of maximal oxygen consumption decline with aging. *Sports Medicine*, 33(12), pp. 877–888.

Hawley, J. A., Schabort, E. J., Noakes, T. D. and Dennis, S. C. (1997) Carbohydrate-loading and exercise performance: An update. *Sports Medicine*, 24(2), pp. 73–81.

Hayes, P. R., Bowen, S. J. and Davies, E. J. (2004) The relationships between local muscular endurance and kinematic changes during a run to exhaustion at $v\dot{V}O_2$ max. *The Journal of Strength and Conditioning Research*, 18(4), pp. 898–903.

Hayes, P. R. and Caplan, N. (2012) Foot strike patterns and ground contact times during high-calibre middle-distance races. *Journal of Sports Sciences*, 30(12), pp. 1275–1283.

Hayes, P. R. and Caplan, N. (2014) Leg stiffness decreases during a run to exhaustion at the speed at $\dot{V}O_2$ max. *European Journal of Sport Science*, 14(6), pp. 556–562.

Hayes, P. R., French, D. N. and Thomas, K. (2011) The effect of muscular endurance on running economy. *The Journal of Strength and Conditioning Research*, 25(9), pp. 2464–2469.

Haynes, T., Bishop, C., Antrobus, M. and Brazier, J. (2019) The validity and reliability of the My Jump 2 app for measuring the reactive strength index and drop jump performance. *The Journal of Sports Medicine and Physical Fitness*, 59(2), pp. 253–258.

Hébert-Losier, K., Schneiders, A. G., Newsham-West, R. J. and Sullivan, S. J. (2009) Scientific bases and clinical utilisation of the calf-raise test. *Physical Therapy in Sport*, 10(4), pp. 142–149.

Heiderscheit, B. C., Chumanov, E. S., Michalski, M. P., Wille, C. M. and Ryan, M. B. (2011) Effects of step rate manipulation on joint mechanics during running. *Medicine and Science in Sports and Exercise*, 43, pp. 296–302.

Heikura, I. A., Stellingwerff, T. and Burke, L. M. (2018a) Self-reported periodization of nutrition in elite female and male runners and race walkers. *Frontiers in Physiology*, 9. doi: 10.3389/FPHYS.2018.01732.

Heikura, I. A., Uusitalo, A. L. T., Stellingwerff, T., Bergland, D., Mero, A. A. and Burke, L. M. (2018b) Low energy availability is difficult to assess but outcomes have large impact on bone injury rates in elite distance athletes. *International Journal of Sport Nutrition and Exercise Metabolism*, 28, pp. 403–411.

Heikura, I. A. et al. (2017) Low energy availability is difficult to assess but outcomes have large impact on bone injury rates in elite distance athletes. *International Journal of Sport Nutrition and Exercise Metabolism*, 28(4), pp. 403–411. doi: 10.1123/IJSNEM.2017-0313.

Heinert, B. L., Kernozek, T. W., Greany, J. F. and Fater, D. C. (2008) Hip abductor weakness and lower extremity kinematics during running. *Journal of Sport Rehabilitation*, 17(3), pp. 243–256.

Heise, G. D., Smith, J. D. and Martin, P. E. (2011) Lower extremity mechanical work during stance phase of running partially explains interindividual variability of metabolic power. *European Journal of Applied Physiology*, 111, pp. 1777–1785.

Hellard, P., Avalos, M., Hausswirth, C., Pyne, D., Toussaint, J. F. and Mujika, I. (2013) Identifying optimal overload and taper in elite swimmers over time. *Journal of Sports Science and Medicine*, 12(4), pp. 668–678.

Hemmerich, A., Brown, H., Smith, S., Marthandam, S. S. K. and Wyss, U. P. (2006) Hip, knee, and ankle kinematics of high range of motion activities of daily living. *Journal of Orthopaedic Research*, 24(4), pp. 770–781.

Henschke, N. (2011) Stretching before or after exercise does not reduce delayed-onset muscle soreness. *British Journal of Sports Medicine*. doi: 10.1136/bjsports-2011-090599.

Heritage, A., Stumpf, W., Sar, M. and Grant, L. (1980) Brainstem catecholamine neurons are target sites for sex steroid hormones. *Science*, 207(4437), pp. 1377–1379.

Herzberg, S. D., Motu'apuaka, M. L., Lambert, W., Fu, R., Brady, J. and Guise, J.-M. (2017) The effect of menstrual cycle and contraceptives on ACL injuries and laxity: A systematic review and meta-analysis. *Orthopaedic Journal of Sports Medicine*, 5(7), 2325967117718781.

Hettinga, F. J., Edwards, A. M. and Hanley, B. (2019) The science behind competition and winning in athletics: Using world-level competition data to explore pacing and tactics. *Frontiers in Sports and Active Living*, 1, p. 11.

Hew-Butler, T., Rosner, M. H., Fowkes-Godek, S., Dugas, J. P., Hoffman, M. D., Lewis, D. P. et al. (2015) Statement of the third international exercise-associated hyponatremia consensus development conference, Carlsbad, California. *Clinical Journal of Sports Medicine*, 25(4), pp. 303–320.

Hickey, M. and Kaunitz, A. M. (2011) *Williams textbook of endocrinology*. 12th edn. Section V: Reproduction. London, UK: Elsevier, pp. 661–687.

Hill, A. V. and H. Lupton (1923) Muscular exercise, lactic acid, and the supply and utilization of oxygen. *QJM*, os-16(62), pp. 135–171.

Hill, D. W. (1999) Energy system contributions in middle-distance running events. *Journal of Sports Sciences*, 17(6), pp. 477–483.

Hill, J. A. et al. (2014) Compression garments and recovery from exercise-induced muscle damage: A meta-analysis. *British Journal of Sports Medicine*. doi: 10.1136/bjsports-2013-092456.

Hill, J. A. et al. (2015) The variation in pressures exerted by commercially available compression garments. *Sports Engineering*. doi: 10.1007/s12283-015-0170-x.

Hills, A. P., Mokhtar, N. and Byrne, N. M. (2014) Assessment of physical activity and energy expenditure: An overview of objective measures. *Frontiers in Nutrition*, 1, p. 5.

Hindle, W. (1991) The breast and exercise. In Hale, R. W. (ed.) *Caring for the exercising woman*. New York: Elsevier Science Publishing, pp. 83–92.

Hinrichs, R. N. (1987) Upper extremity function in running II: Angular momentum considerations. *International Journal of Sports Biomechanics*, 3(3), pp. 242–263.

Hirvonen, J., Rehunen, S., Rusko, H. and Harkonen, M. (1987) Breakdown of high-energy phosphate compounds and lactate accumulation during short supramaximal exercise. *European Journal of Applied Physiology and Occupational Physiology*, 56(3), pp. 253–259.

Hoch, A. Z., Pajewski, N. M., Moraski, L. et al. (2009) Prevalence of the female athlete triad in high school athletes and sedentary students. *Clinical Journal of Sports Medicine*, 19, pp. 421–428.

Hodge, K. and Petlichkoff, L. (2000) Goal profiles in sport motivation: A cluster analysis. *Journal of Sport and Exercise Psychology*, 22, pp. 256–272.

Hoffman, M. D., Hew-Butler, T. and Stuempfle, K. J. (2013) Exercise-associated hyponatremia and hydration status in 161-km ultramarathoners. *Medicine and Science in Sports and Exercise*, 45(4), pp. 784–791.

Hoffman, M. D. and Stuempfle, K. J. (2015) Sodium supplementation and exercise-associated hyponatremia during prolonged exercise. *Medicine and Science in Sports and Exercise*, 47(9), pp. 1781–1787.

Hofmeister, S. and Bodden, S. (2016) Premenstrual syndrome and premenstrual dysphoric disorder. *American Family Physician*, 94(3), pp. 236–240.

Hollings, S. C., Hopkins, W. G. and Hume, P. A. (2014) Age at peak performance of successful track & field athletes. *International Journal of Sports Science and Coaching*, 9(4), pp. 651–661.

Holloszy, J. O. and Coyle, E. F. (1984) Adaptations of skeletal muscle to endurance exercise and their metabolic consequences. *Journal of Applied Physiology*, 56(4), pp. 831–838.

Holmes, P. and Collins, D. (2001) The PETTLEP approach to motor imagery: A functional equivalence model for sport psychologists. *Journal of Applied Sport Psychology*, 13, pp. 60–83.

Hoogkamer, W. et al. (2016) Altered running economy directly translates to altered distance-running performance. *Medicine and Science in Sports and Exercise*, 48(11), pp. 2175–2180. doi: 10.1249/MSS.0000000000001012.

Hoon, M. W., Jones, A. M., Johnson, N. A., Blackwell, J. R., Broad, E. M., Lundy, B. et al. (2014) The effect of variable doses of inorganic nitrate-rich beetroot juice on simulated 2000-m rowing performance in trained athletes. *International Journal of Sports Physiology and Performance*, 9(4), pp. 615–620.

Hopkins, W. G. (2000) Measures of reliability in sports medicine and science. *Sports Medicine*, 30(1), pp. 1–15.

Horga, L. M., Henckel, J., Fotiadou, A., Hirschmann, A., Torlasco, C., Di Laura, A., Silva, A., Sharma, S., Moon, J. and Hart, A. (2019) Can marathon running improve knee damage of middle-aged adults? A prospective cohort study. *BMJ Open Sport and Exercise Medicine*, 5, p. e000586.

Horn, E., Gergen, N. and McGarry, K. A. (2014) The female athlete triad. *The Rhode Island Medical Journal*, 97, pp. 18–21.

Horowitz, J., Sidossis, L. and Coyle, E. (1994) High efficiency of type I muscle fibers improves performance. *International Journal of Sports Medicine*, 15(3), pp. 152–157.

Hotta, T., Nishiguchi, S., Fukutani, N., Tashiro, Y., Adachi, D., Morino, S., Shirooka, H., Nozaki, Y., Hirata, H., Yamaguchi, M. and Aoyama, T. (2015) Functional movement screen for predicting running injuries in 18-to 24-year-old competitive male runners. *The Journal of Strength & Conditioning Research*, 29(10), pp. 2808–2815.

Houmard, J. A. (1991) Impact of reduced training on performance in endurance athletes. *Sports Medicine*, 12(6), pp. 380–393. doi: 10.2165/00007256-199112060-00004.

Houmard, J. A., Costill, D. L., Mitchell, J. B., Park, S. H., Hickner, R. C. and Roemmich, J. N. (1990) Reduced training maintains performance in distance runners. *International Journal of Sports Medicine*, 11(1), pp. 46–52. doi: 10.1055/s-2007-1024761.

Houmard, J. A., Scott, B. K., Justice, C. L. and Chenier, T. C. (1994) The effects of taper on performance in distance runners. *Medicine and Science in Sports and Exercise*, 26(5), pp. 624–631. doi: 0795-9131/94/2605-0624.

Houmard, J. A. et al. (1991) The role of anaerobic ability in middle distance running performance. *European Journal of Applied Physiology and Occupational Physiology*, 62(1), pp. 40–43.

House, J. R. et al. (2013) The impact of a phase-change cooling vest on heat strain and the effect of different cooling pack melting temperatures. *European Journal of Applied Physiology*. doi: 10.1007/s00421-012-2534-2.

Housh, T. J., Cramer, J. T., Bull, A. J., Johnson, G. O. and Housh, D. J. (2001) The effect of mathematical modeling on critical velocity. *European Journal of Applied Physiology*, 84(5), pp. 469–475.

Housh, T. J., Thorland, W. G., Johnson, G. O. et al. (1984) Body composition variables as discriminators of sports participation of elite adolescent female athletes. *Research Quarterly in Exercise and Sport*, 55, pp. 302–305.

Howatson, G. and Van Someren, K. A. (2008) The prevention and treatment of exercise-induced muscle damage *Sports Medicine*. doi: 10.2165/00007256-200838060-00004.

Howatson, G. et al. (2010) Influence of tart cherry juice on indices of recovery following marathon running. *Scandinavian Journal of Medicine and Science in Sports*. doi: 10.1111/j.1600-0838.2009.01005.x.

Howden, E. J., Carrick-Ranson, G., Sarma, S., Hieda, M., Fujimoto, N. and Levine, B. D. (2018) Effects of sedentary aging and lifelong exercise on left ventricular systolic function. *Medicine & Science in Sports & Exercise*, 50(3), pp. 494–501.

Howe, L. P., Bampouras, T. M., North, J. S. and Waldron, M. (2020) Reliability of two-dimensional measures associated with bilateral drop-landing performance. to be published in *Movement & Sport Sciences-Science & Motricité* [Preprint]. doi: 10.1051/sm/2019037.

Howe, L. P. and Blagrove, R. C. (2015) Shoulder function during overhead lifting tasks: Implications for screening athletes *Strength & Conditioning Journal*, 37(5), pp. 84–96.

Howe, L. P. and Cushion, E. (2017) A problem-solving process to identify the origins of poor movement. *Professional Strength & Conditioning Journal*, 45, pp. 7–15.

Howe, L. P., Goodwin, J. and Blagrove, R. (2014) The integration of unilateral strength training for the lower extremity within an athletic performance programme. *Professional Strength and Conditioning*, 33, pp. 19–24.

Howe, L. P. and Read, P. (2015) Thoracic spine function: Assessment and self-management. *Professional Journal of Strength & Conditioning*, 39, pp. 21–31.

Howe, L. P. and Waldron, M. (2019) Measuring range of motion: An S&C coach's guide to assessing mobility. *Professional Strength & Conditioning*, 55, pp. 7–17.

Hreljac, A. (2000) Stride smoothness evaluation of runners and other athletes. *Gait & Posture*, 11, pp. 199–206.

Hreljac, A. (2005) Etiology, prevention, and early intervention of overuse injuries in runners: A biomechanical perspective. *Physical Medicine and Rehabilitation Clinics of North America*, 16(3), pp. 651–667. doi: 10.1016/J.PMR.2005.02.002.

Hreljac, A., Marshall, R. N. and Hume, P. A. (2000) Evaluation of lower extremity overuse injury potential in runners. *Medicine and Science in Sports and Exercise*, 32, pp. 1635–1641.

Hudgins, B. et al. (2013) Relationship between jumping ability and running performance in events of varying distance. *The Journal of Strength & Conditioning Research*, 27(3), pp. 563–567.

Hughson, R. L., Orok, C. J. and Staudt, L. E. (1984) A high velocity treadmill running test to assess endurance running potential. *International Journal of Sports Medicine*, 5(1), pp. 23–25.

Hulin, B. T., Gabbett, T. J., Lawson, D. W., Caputi, P. and Sampson, J. A. (2016) The acute: Chronic workload ratio predicts injury: High chronic workload may decrease injury risk in elite rugby league players. *British Journal of Sports Medicine*, 50, pp. 231–236.

Hulme, A., Nielsen, R. O., Timpka, T., Verhagen, E. and Finch, C. (2017) Risk and protective factors for middle- and long-distance running-related injury. *Sports Medicine*, 47, pp. 869–886.

Hulme, A., Thompson, J., Nielsen, R. O., Read, G. J. M. and Salmon, P. M. (2019) Towards a complex systems approach in sports injury research: Simulating running-related injury development with agent-based modelling. *British Journal of Sports Medicine*, 53, pp. 560–569.

Hulston, C. J. and Jeukendrup, A. E. (2008) Substrate metabolism and exercise performance with caffeine and carbohydrate intake. *Medicine and Science in Sports and Exercise*, 40, pp. 2096–2104.

Hulston, C. J. et al. (2010) Training with low muscle glycogen enhances fat metabolism in well-trained cyclists. *Medicine and Science in Sports and Exercise*, 42(11), pp. 2046–2055. doi: 10.1249/MSS.0B013E3181DD5070.

Hulteen, R. M., Smith, J. J., Morgan, P. J., Barnett, L. M., Hallal, P. C., Colyvas, K. and Lubans, D. R. (2017) Global participation in sport and leisure-time physical activities: A systematic review and meta-analysis. *Preventive Medicine*, 95, pp. 14–25.

Hunter, G. R. et al. (2011) Tendon length and joint flexibility are related to running economy. *Medicine and Science in Sports and Exercise*, 43(8), pp. 1492–1499.

Hunter, I. and Smith, G. A. (2007) Preferred and optimal stride frequency, stiffness and economy: Changes with fatigue during a 1-h high-intensity run. *European Journal of Applied Physiology*, 100(6), pp. 653–661.

Hunter, J. P., Marshall, R. N. and McNair, P. J. (2004) Interaction of step length and cadence during sprint running. *Medicine and Science in Sport and Exercise*, 36(2), pp. 261–271.

Hunter, L., Louw, Q. A. and Van Niekerk, S. M. (2014) Effect of running retraining on pain, function, and lower-extremity biomechanics in a female runner with iliotibial band syndrome. *Journal of Sport Rehabilitation*, 23, pp. 145–157.

Huxley, D. J., O'Connor, D. and Bennie, A. (2018) Olympic and World Championship track and field athletes' experiences during the specialising and investment stages of development: A qualitative study with Australian male and female representatives. *Qualitative Research in Sport, Exercise and Health*, 10(2), pp. 256–272.

Huxley, D. J., O'Connor, D. and Healey, P. A. (2014) An examination of the training profiles and injuries in elite youth track and field athletes. *European Journal of Sport Science*, 14(2), pp. 185–192.

Huxley, D. J., O'Connor, D. and Larkin, P. (2017) The pathway to the top: Key factors and influences in the development of Australian Olympic and World Championship Track and field athletes. *International Journal of Sports Science and Coaching*, 12(2), pp. 264–275.

Hyman, M. (1970) Diet and athletics. *British Medical Journal*, 4(5726), p. 52. doi: 10.1136/BMJ. 4.5726.52-B.

Iaia, F. M. and Bangsbo, J. (2010) Speed endurance training is a powerful stimulus for physiological adaptations and performance improvements of athletes. *Scandinavian Journal of Medicine & Science in Sports*, 20(2), pp. 11–23.

Ibegbuna, V. et al. (2003) Effect of elastic compression stockings on venous hemodynamics during walking. *Journal of Vascular Surgery*. doi: 10.1067/mva.2003.104.

Impey, S. G. et al. (2018) Fuel for the work required: A theoretical framework for carbohydrate periodization and the glycogen threshold hypothesis. *Sports Medicine*, 48(5), pp. 1031–1048. doi: 10.1007/S40279-018-0867-7.

Ingham, S. A. et al. (2008) Determinants of 800-m and 1500-m running performance using allometric models. *Medicine and Science in Sports and Exercise*, 40(2), pp. 345–350. doi: 10.1249/mss. 0b013e31815a83dc.

Ingham, S. A., Fudge, B. W. and Pringle, J. S. (2011) Training distribution, physiological profile and performance for a male. *International Journal of Sports Physiology and Performance*, 2, Human Kinetics, Inc.

Ingham, S. A., Fudge, B. W. and Pringle, J. S. (2012) Training distribution, physiological profile, and performance for a male international 1500-m runner. *International Journal of Sports Physiology and Performance*, 7(2), pp. 193–195. https://doi.org/10.1123/ijspp.7.2.193.

Ingle, S. (2018) Interview: Laura Muir: 'I would have a lot easier life if I didn't say stuff'. www. theguardian.com/sport/2018/jul/19/laura-muir-interview-scottish-runner-athletics Accessed on: 08/09/2020.

Inman, V. T., Ralston, H. J. and Todd, F. (1981) *Human walking*. Baltimore, MD: Williams & Wilkins.

Isacco, L. and Boisseau, N. (2017) Sex hormones and substrate metabolism during endurance exercise. In Hackney, A. C. (ed.) *Sex hormones, exercise and women, scientific and clinical aspects*. Cham, Switzerland: Springer International, pp. 35–58.

Issurin, V. B. (2010) New horizons for the methodology and physiology of training periodization. *Sports Medicine*. https://doi.org/10.2165/11319770-000000000-00000.

Ito, A., Komi, P. V., Sjodin, B., Bosco, C. and Karlsson, J. (1983) Mechanical efficiency of positive work in running at different speeds. *Medicine & Science in Sports & Exercise*, 15(4), pp. 299–308.

Ito, R., Nakano, M., Yamane, M., Amano, M. and Matsumoto, T. (2013) Effects of rain on energy metabolism while running in a cold environment. *International Journal of Sports Medicine*, 34(8), pp. 707–711.

Iversen, N., Krustrup, P., Rasmussen, H. N., Rasmussen, U. F., Saltin, B. and Pilegaard, H. (2011) Mitochondrial biogenesis and angiogenesis in skeletal muscle of the elderly. *Experimental Gerontology*, 46(8), pp. 670–678.

Ivy, J. L., Costill, D. L., Fink, W. J. and Lower, R. (1979) Influence of caffeine and carbohydrate feedings on endurance performance. *Medicine and Science in Sports*, 11, pp. 6–11.

Ivy, J. L. et al. (1988) Muscle glycogen synthesis after exercise: Effect of time of carbohydrate ingestion. *Journal of Applied Physiology*. doi: 10.1152/jappl.1988.64.4.1480.

Iwaoka, K., Fuchi, T., Higuchi, M. and Kobayashi, S. (1988) Blood lactate accumulation during exercise in older endurance runners. *International Journal of Sports Medicine*, 9(4), pp. 253–256.

Izquierdo, M., Ibanez, J., González-Badillo, J. J., Hakkinen, K., Ratamess, N. A., Kraemer, W. J., French, D. N., Eslava, J., Altadill, A., Asiain, X. and Gorostiaga, E. M. (2006) Differential effects of strength training leading to failure versus not to failure on hormonal responses, strength, and muscle power gains. *Journal of Applied Physiology*, 100(5), pp. 647–1656. doi: 10.1152/japplphysiol.01400.2005.

Jacobson, T. L., Febbraio, M. A., Arkinstall, M. J. and Hawley, J. A. (2001) Effect of caffeine co-ingested with carbohydrate or fat on metabolism and performance in endurance-trained men. *Experimental Physiology*, 86, pp. 137–144.

Jäger, R. et al. (2017) International society of sports nutrition position stand: Protein and exercise. *Journal of the International Society of Sports Nutrition*, 14, pp. 20–45. doi: 10.1186/s12970-017-0177-8.

Jakeman, J. R., Byrne, C. and Eston, R. G. (2010) Lower limb compression garment improves recovery from exercise-induced muscle damage in young, active females. *European Journal of Applied Physiology*. doi: 10.1007/s00421-010-1464-0.

James, D. V. and Doust, J. H. (1998) Oxygen uptake during moderate intensity running: Response following a single bout of interval training. *European Journal of Applied Physiology and Occupational Physiology*, 77(6), pp. 551–555.

James, L. J., Funnell, M. P. et al. (2019a) Does hypohydration really impair endurance performance? methodological considerations for interpreting hydration research. *Sports Medicine*. doi: 10.1007/s40279-019-01188-5.

James, L. J., Stevenson, E. J. et al. (2019b) Cow's milk as a post-exercise recovery drink: Implications for performance and health. *European Journal of Sport Science*. doi: 10.1080/17461391.2018.1534989.

James, L. P. et al. (2018) The impact of strength level on adaptations to combined weightlifting, plyometric and ballistic training. *Scandinavian Journal of Medicine and Science in Sports*, 28(5), pp. 1494–1505.

Jamnick, N. A., Botella, J., Pyne, D. B. and Bishop, D. J. (2018) Manipulating graded exercise test variables affects the validity of the lactate threshold and V O 2 peak. *PLoS One*, 13(7), p. e0199794.

Janssen, I., Heymsfield, S. B., Wang, Z. M. and Ross, R. (2000) Skeletal muscle mass and distribution in 468 men and women aged 18–88 yr. *Journal of Applied Physiology*, 89(1), pp. 81–88.

Jaspers, A., Kuyvenhoven, J. P., Staes, F., Frencken, W. G. P., Helsen, W. F. and Brink, M. S. (2018) Examination of the external and internal load indicators' association with overuse injuries in professional soccer players. *Journal of Science and Medicine in Sport*, 21, pp. 579–585.

Jayanthi, N. A., LaBella, C. R., Fischer, D. et al. (2015) Sports-specialized intensive training and the risk of injury in young athletes: A clinical case-control study. *American Journal of Sports Medicine*, 43, pp. 794–801.

Jelsing, E. J., Finnoff, J. T., Cheville, A. L., Levy, B. A. and Smith, J. (2013) Sonographic evaluation of the iliotibial band at the lateral femoral epicondyle: Does the iliotibial band move? *Journal of Ultrasound in Medicine*, 32, pp. 1199–1206.

Jenkins, D. G. and Quigley, B. M. (1992) Endurance training enhances critical power. *Medicine and Science in Sports and Exercise*, 24(11), pp. 1283–1289.

Jenkins, D. G. and Quigley, B. M. (1993) The influence of high-intensity exercise training on the Wlim-Tlim relationship. *Medicine and Science in Sports and Exercise*, 25(2), pp. 275–282.

Jentjens, R. L. and Jeukendrup, A. E. (2005) High rates of exogenous carbohydrate oxidation from a mixture of glucose and fructose ingested during prolonged cycling exercise. *British Journal of Nutrition*, 93, pp. 485–492.

Jentjens, R. L., Moseley, L., Waring, R. H., Harding, L. K. and Jeukendrup, A. E. (2004) Oxidation of combined ingestion of glucose and fructose during exercise. *Journal of Applied Physiology*, 96, pp. 1277–1284.

Jentjens, R. L., Underwood, K., Achten, J., Currell, K., Mann, C. H. and Jeukendrup, A. E. (2006) Exogenous carbohydrate oxidation rates are elevated after combined ingestion of glucose and fructose during exercise in the heat. *Journal of Applied Physiology*, 100, pp. 807–816.

Jeukendrup, A. E. (2004) Carbohydrate intake during exercise and performance. *Nutrition*, 20, pp. 669–677.

Jeukendrup, A. E. (2011) Nutrition for endurance sports: Marathon, triathlon, and road cycling. *Journal of Sports Sciences*, 29(Suppl. 1), pp. S91–S99.

Jeukendrup, A. E. (2013) Multiple transportable carbohydrates and their benefits. *GSSI Sports Science Exchange*, 26(108), pp. 1–5.

Jeukendrup, A. E. (2014) A step towards personalized sports nutrition: Carbohydrate intake during exercise. *Sports Medicine*, 44(Suppl. 1), pp. S25–S33.

Jeukendrup, A. E. (2017a) Personalized nutrition for athletes. *Sports Medicine*, 47(Suppl. 1), pp. S51–S63. doi: 10.1007/s40279-017-0694-2.

Jeukendrup, A. E. (2017b) Training the gut for athletes. *Sports Medicine*, 47(Suppl. 1), pp. S101–S110.

Jeukendrup, A. E., Jentjens, R. L. P. G. and Moseley, L. (2005) Nutritional considerations in triathlon. *Sports Medicine*, 35, pp. 163–181.

Jeukendrup, A. E. and Moseley, L. (2010) Multiple transportable carbohydrates enhance gastric emptying and fluid delivery. *Scandanavian Journal of Medicine and Science in Sports*, 20, pp. 112–121.

Jeukendrup, A. E., Vet-Joop, K., Sturk, A., Stegen, J. H., Senden, J., Saris, W. H. et al. (2000) Relationship between gastro-intestinal complaints and endotoxaemia, cytokine release and the acute-phase reaction during and after a long-distance triathlon in highly trained men. *Clinical Science (London)*, 98, pp. 47–55.

Johnston, R. E., Quinn, T. J., Kertzer, R. and Vroman, N. B. (1997) Strength training in female distance runners: Impact on running economy. *Journal of Strength and Conditioning Research*, 11(4), pp. 224–229.

Jones, A. M. (1998) A five year physiological case study of an Olympic runner. *British Journal of Sports Medicine*, 32(1), pp. 39–43.

Jones, A. M. (2002) Running economy is negatively related to sit-and-reach test performance in international-standard distance runners. *International Journal of Sports Medicine*, 23(1), pp. 40–43.

Jones, A. M. (2006a) Middle and long distance running. *Sport and Exercise Physiology Testing Guidelines*, 1, pp. 147–154.

Jones, A. M. (2006b) The physiology of the world record holder for the women's marathon. *International Journal of Sports Science and Coaching*, 1(2), pp. 101–116. doi: 10.1260/174795406777 641258.

Jones, A. M. (2014) Dietary nitrate supplementation and exercise performance. *Sports Medicine*, 44(1), pp. 35–45.

Jones, A. M., Burnley, M., Black, M. I., Poole, D. C. and Vanhatalo, A. (2019) The maximal metabolic steady state: Redefining the 'gold standard'. *Physiological Reports*, 7(10), p. e14098.

Jones, A. M. and Carter, H. (2000) The effect of endurance training on parameters of aerobic fitness. *Sports Medicine*, 29(6), pp. 373–386.

Jones, A. M., Carter, H. and Doust, J. H. (1999) Effect of six weeks of endurance training on parameters of aerobic fitness. *Medicine & Science in Sports & Exercise*, 31(5), p. S280.

Jones, A. M. and Doust, J. H. (1996) A 1% treadmill grade most accurately reflects the energetic cost of outdoor running. *Journal of Sports Sciences*, 14(4), pp. 321–327.

Jones, A. M. and Doust, J. H. (1998) The validity of the lactate minimum test for determination of the maximal lactate steady state. *Medicine and Science in Sports and Exercise*, 30(8), pp. 1304–1313.

Jones, A. M., Thompson, C., Wylie, L. J. and Vanhatalo, A. (2018) Dietary nitrate and physical performance. *Annual Review of Nutrition*, 38, pp. 303–328.

Jones, A. M., Vanhatalo, A., Burnley, M., Morton, R. H. and Poole, D. C. (2010) Critical power: Implications for determination of V O2max and exercise tolerance. *Medicine & Science in Sports & Exercise*, 42(10), pp. 1876–1890.

Jones, A. M. and Whipp, B. J. (2002) Bioenergetic constraints on tactical decision making in middle distance running. *British Journal of Sports Medicine*, 36(2), pp. 102–104.

Jones, A. M., Wilkerson, D. P., Vanhatalo, A. and Burnley, M. (2008) Influence of pacing strategy on O2 uptake and exercise tolerance. *Scandinavian Journal of Medicine and Science in Sports*, 18(5), pp. 615–626.

Jones, R. A., Mahoney, J. W. and Gucciardi, D. F. (2014) On the transition into elite rugby league: Perceptions of players and coaching staff. *Sport, Exercise, and Performance Psychology*, 3, pp. 28–45.

Jonge, X. A. K. J. D., Thompson, M. W., Chuter, V. H., Silk, L. N. and Thom, J. M. (2012) Exercise performance over the menstrual cycle in temperate and hot, humid conditions. *Medicine & Science in Sports & Exercise*, 44(11), pp. 2190–2198.

Joy, E., De Souza, M. J., Nattiv, A. et al. (2014) 2014 female athlete triad coalition consensus statement on treatment and return to play of the female athlete triad. *Current Sports Medicine Reports*, 13(4), pp. 219–232.

Joyner, M. J. (1991) Modeling: Optimal marathon performance on the basis of physiological factors. *Journal of Applied Physiology*, 70(2), pp. 683–687.

Joyner, M. J. (2016) Fatigue: Where did we come from and how did we get here? *Medicine & Science in Sports & Exercise*, 48(11), pp. 2224–2227.

Joyner, M. J., Hunter, S. K., Lucia, A. and Jones, A. M. (2020) Physiology and fast marathons. *Journal of Applied Physiology*, 128(4), pp. 1065–1068.

Julian, R., Hecksteden, A., Fullagar, H. H. K. and Meyer, T. (2017) The effects of menstrual cycle phase on physical performance in female soccer players. *PLoS One*, 12(3), p. e0173951.

Juliff, L. E. et al. (2018) Longer sleep durations are positively associated with finishing place during a national multiday netball competition. *Journal of Strength and Conditioning Research*. doi: 10.1519/jsc.0000000000001793.

Julio, U. F., Panissa, V. L. G., Paludo, A. C., Alves, E. D., Campos, F. A. D. and Franchini, E. (2020) Use of the anaerobic speed reserve to normalize the prescription of high-intensity interval exercise intensity. *European Journal of Sport Science*, 20(2), pp. 166–173.

Kaggestad, J. (1987) So trainiert Ingrid Kristiansen 1986. *Leichtatletik*, 38, pp. 831–834.

Kaiserauer, S. et al. (1989) Nutritional, physiological, and menstrual status of distance runners. *Medicine and Science in Sports and Exercise*, 21(2), pp. 120–125. doi: 10.1249/00005768-198904000-00002.

Kalkhoven, J. T., Watsford, M. L. and Impellizzeri, F. M. (2020) A conceptual model and detailed framework for stress-related, strain-related, and overuse athletic injury. *Journal of Science and Medicine in Sport*, 23, pp. 726–734.

Kang, J., Mangine, G. T., Ratamess, N. A., Faigenbaum, A. D. and Hoffman, J. R. (2014) Acute effect of intensity fluctuation on energy output and substrate utilization. *The Journal of Strength and Conditioning Research*, 28(8), pp. 2136–2144.

Karp, J. R. (2007) How they train. *Running Times*, 351, pp. 32–33.

Karsten, B. et al. (2016) The effects of a sport-specific maximal strength and conditioning training on critical velocity, anaerobic running distance, and 5-km race performance. *International Journal of Sports Physiology and Performance*, 11(1), pp. 80–85. doi: 10.1123/ijspp.2014-0559.

Kasch, F. W., Boyer, J. L., Van Camp, S. P., Verity, L. S. and Wallace, J. P. (1993) Effect of exercise on cardiovascular ageing. *Age and Ageing*, 22(1), pp. 5–10.

Kato, H. et al. (2016) Protein requirements are elevated in endurance athletes after exercise as determined by the indicator amino acid oxidation method. *PloS One*, 11(6), p. e0157406.

Katzel, L. I., Sorkin, J. D. and Fleg, J. L. (2001) A comparison of longitudinal changes in aerobic fitness in older endurance athletes and sedentary men. *Journal of the American Geriatrics Society*, 49(12), pp. 1657–1664.

Keane, K. M. et al. (2016) Phytochemical uptake following human consumption of Montmorency tart cherry (L. Prunus cerasus) and influence of phenolic acids on vascular smooth muscle cells in vitro. *European Journal of Nutrition*. doi: 10.1007/s00394-015-0988-9.

Kearney, P. E., Comyns, T. M. and Hayes, P. R. (2020) Coaches and parents hold contrasting perceptions of optimal youth development activities in track and field athletics. *International Journal of Sports Science and Coaching*, published ahead of print. doi: 10.1177/1747954119900052.

Kearney, P. E. and Hayes, P. R. (2018) Excelling at youth level in competitive track and field athletics is not a prerequisite for later success. *Journal of Sports Sciences*, 36(21), pp. 2502–2509.

Kearney, P. E., Hayes, P. R. and Nevill, A. (2018) Faster, higher, stronger, older: Relative age effects are most influential during the youngest age grade of track and field athletics in the United Kingdom. *Journal of Sports Sciences*, 36(20), pp. 2282–2288.

Keegan, R. (2019) Achievement goals in sport and physical activity. In Horn, T. S. and Smith, A. L. (eds.) *Advances in sport and exercise psychology*. Champaign, IL: Human Kinetics, pp. 265–288.

Kellis, E. and Liassou, C. (2009) The effect of selective muscle fatigue on sagittal lower limb kinematics and muscle activity during level running. *Journal of Orthopaedic and Sports Physical Therapy*, 39(3), pp. 210–220.

Kellmann, M., Bertollo, M., Bosquet, L., Brink, M., Coutts, A. J., Duffield, R., Erlacher, D., Halson, S. L., Hecksteden, A., Heidari, J. and Kallus, K. W. (2018) Recovery and performance in sport: Consensus statement. *International Journal of Sports Physiology and Performance*, 13(2), pp. 240–245. doi: 10.1123/ijspp.2017-0759.

Kellmann, M. and Kallus, K. W. (2001) *Recovery-stress questionnaire for athletes: User manual*. Champaign, IL: Human Kinetics.

Kemler, E., Blokland, D., Backx, F. and Huisstede, B. (2018) Differences in injury risk and characteristics of injuries between novice and experienced runners over a 4-year period. *The Physician and Sportsmedicine*, 46, pp. 485–491.

Kenefick, R. W. (2018) Drinking strategies: Planned drinking versus drinking to thirst. *Sports Medicine*, 48(Suppl. 1), pp. 31–37.

Kenneally, M., Casado, A. and Santos-Concejero, J. (2018) The effect of periodization and training intensity distribution on middle-and long-distance running performance: A systematic review. *International Journal of Sports Physiology and Performance*. https://doi.org/10.1123/ijspp.2017-0327.

Kenneally-Dabrowski, C. J. B., Brown, N. A. T., Lai, A. K. M., Perriman, D., Spratford, W. and Serpell, B. G. (2019) Late swing or early stance? A narrative review of hamstring injury mechanisms during high-speed running. *Scandinavian Journal of Medicine & Science in Sports*, 29, pp. 1083–1091.

Kerksick, C. M. et al. (2017) International society of sports nutrition position stand: Nutrient timing. *Journal of the International Society of Sports Nutrition*, 14, p. 33. doi: 10.1186/s12970-017-0189-4.

Kerksick, C. M. et al. (2018) ISSN exercise & sports nutrition review update: Research & recommendations. *Journal of the International Society of Sports Nutrition*, 15(1). doi: 10.1186/S12970-018-0242-Y.

Khan, D. and Ahmed, S. A. (2016) The immune system is a natural target for estrogen action: Opposing effects of estrogen in two prototypical autoimmune diseases. *Frontiers in Immunology*, 6, p. 635.

Kingston, K. M. and Wilson, K. M. (2009) The application of goal setting in sport. In Mellalieu, S. D. and Hanton, S. (eds.) *Advances in applied sport psychology: A review*. London, UK: Routledge, pp. 75–123.

Kjær, M. et al. (2009) From mechanical loading to collagen synthesis, structural changes and function in human tendon. *Scandinavian Journal of Medicine & Science in Sport*, 19(4), pp. 500–510.

Kleynen, M., Jie, L. J., Theunissen, K., Rasquin, S. M., Masters, R. S., Meijer, K., Beurskens, A. J. and Braun, S. M. (2019) The immediate influence of implicit motor learning strategies on spatiotemporal gait parameters in stroke patients: A randomized within-subjects design. *Clinical Rehabilitation*, 33, pp. 619–630.

Klitgaard, H., Mantoni, M., Schiaffino, S., Ausoni, S., Gorza, L., Laurent-Winter, C., Schnohr, P. and Saltin, B. (1990) Function, morphology and protein expression of ageing skeletal muscle: A cross-sectional study of elderly men with different training backgrounds. *Acta Physiologica Scandinavica*, 140(1), pp. 41–54.

Kluitenberg, B., Van Middelkoop, M., Diercks, R. and Van Der Worp, H. (2015) What are the differences in injury proportions between different populations of runners? A systematic review and meta-analysis. *Sports Medicine*, 45, pp. 1143–1161.

Knapik, J. J., Trone, D. W., Tchandja, J. and Jones, B. H. (2014) Injury-reduction effectiveness of prescribing running shoes on the basis of foot arch height: Summary of military investigations. *Journal of Orthopaedic & Sports Physical Therapy*, 44, pp. 805–812.

Knapik, J. J. et al. (1991) Preseason strength and flexibility imbalances associated with athletic injuries in female collegiate athletes. *Clinical Journal of Sport Medicine*, 1(3). doi: 10.1097/00042752-199107000-00023.

Knechtle, B., Rüst, B., Knechtle, P. and Rosemann, T. (2012) Does muscle mass affect running times in male long-distance master runners? *Asian Journal of Sports Medicine*, 3(4), pp. 247–256.

Knudson, R. J., Lebowitz, M. D., Holberg, C. J. and Burrows, B. (1983) Changes in the normal maximal expiratory flow-volume curve with growth and aging. *American Review of Respiratory Disease*, 127(6), pp. 725–734.

Koehler, K. et al. (2016) Low energy availability in exercising men is associated with reduced leptin and insulin but not with changes in other metabolic hormones. *Journal of Sports Sciences*, 34(20), pp. 1921–1929. doi: 10.1080/02640414.2016.1142109.

Kölling, S., Duffield, R., Erlacher, D., Venter, R. and Halson, S. L. (2019) Sleep-related issues for recovery and performance in athletes. *International Journal of Sports Physiology and Performance*, 14(2), pp. 144–148. doi: 10.1123/ijspp.2017-0746.

Komi, P. V. (2000) Stretch-shortening cycle: A powerful model to study normal and fatigued muscle. *Journal of Biomechanics*, 33(10), pp. 1197–1206.

Kondepudi, D. (2008) *Introduction to modern thermodynamics*. West Sussex, UK: Wiley.

Kong, P. W. and de Heer, H. (2008) Anthropometric, gait and strength characteristics of Kenyan distance runners. *Journal of Sports Science and Medicine*, 7(4), pp. 499–504.

Konttinen, N., Toskala, A., Laakso, L. and Konttinen, R. (2013) Predicting sustained participation in competitive sports: A longitudinal study young track and field athletes. *IAAF New Studies in Athletics*, 28(1/2), pp. 23–32.

Kordi, M., Menzies, C. and Galbraith, A. (2019) Comparison of critical speed and D' derived from 2 or 3 maximal tests. *International Journal of Sports Physiology and Performance*, 14(5), pp. 685–688.

Korhonen, M. T., Cristea, A., Alén, M., Häkkinen, K., Sipilä, S., Mero, A., Viitasalo, J. T., Larsson, L. and Suominen, H. (2006) Aging, muscle fiber type, and contractile function in sprint-trained athletes. *Journal of Applied Physiology*, 101(3), pp. 906–917.

Korhonen, M. T., Mero, A. and Suominen, H. (2003) Age-related differences in 100-m sprint performance in male and female master runners. *Medicine & Science in Sports & Exercise*, 35(8), pp. 1419–1428.

Koziel, S. and Malina, R. M. (2018) Modified maturity offset prediction equations: Validation in independent longitudinal samples of boys and girls. *Sports Medicine*, 48(1), pp. 221–236.

Kraemer, W. J. et al. (2010) Effects of awhole body compression garment on markers of recovery after a heavy resistance workout in men and women. *Journal of Strength and Conditioning Research*. doi: 10.1519/JSC.0b013e3181d33025.

Kram, R. and Taylor, C. R. (1990) Energetics of running: A new perspective. *Nature*, 346, pp. 265–267.

Kraus, E., Tenforde, A. S., Nattiv, A., Sainani, K. L., Kussman, A., Deakins-Roche, M., Singh, S., Kim, B. Y., Barrack, M. T. and Fredericson, M. (2019) Bone stress injuries in male distance runners: Higher modified female athlete triad cumulative risk assessment scores predict increased rates of injury. *British Journal of Sports Medicine*, 53(4), pp. 237–242.

Kubo, K., Kanehisa, H., Ito, M. and Fukunaga, T. (2001a) Effects of isometric training on the elasticity of human tendon structures in vivo. *Journal of Applied Physiology*, (1985), 91(1), pp. 26–32.

Kubo, K., Kanehisa, H. and Fukunaga, T. (2001b) Effects of different duration isometric contractions on tendon elasticity in human quadriceps muscles. *The Journal of Physiology*, 536, pp. 649–655.

Kubo, K., Kanehisa, H., Kawakami, Y. and Fukunaga, T. (2001c) Influences of repetitive muscle contractions with different modes on tendon elasticity in vivo. *Journal of Applied Physiology*, (1985), 91(1), pp. 277–282.

Kubo, K., Kanehisa, H. and Fukunaga, T. (2002) Effects of resistance and stretching training programmes on the viscoelastic properties of human tendon structures in vivo. *The Journal of Physiology*, 538(1), pp. 219–226.

Kubo, K., Miyazaki, D., Tanaka, S., Shimoju, S. and Tsunoda, N. (2015) Relationship between Achilles tendon properties and foot strike patterns in long-distance runners. *Journal of Sport Science*, 33(7), pp. 665–669.

Kubukeli, Z. N., Noakes, T. D. and Dennis, S. C. (2002) Training techniques to improve endurance exercise performances. *Sports Medicine*, 32(8), pp. 489–509. doi: 10.2165/00007256-200232080-00002.

Kujala, U. M., Sarna, S. and Kaprio, J. (2005) Cumulative incidence of Achilles tendon rupture and tendinopathy in male former elite athletes. *Clinical Journal of Sport Medicine*, 15, pp. 133–135.

Kulmala, J.-P., Avela, J., Pasanen, K. and Parkkari, J. (2013) Forefoot strikers exhibit lower running-induced knee loading than rearfoot strikers. *Medicine and Science in Sports and Exercise*, 45(12), pp. 2306–2313.

Kwiecien, S. Y., McHugh, M. P. and Howatson, G. (2018) The efficacy of cooling with phase change material for the treatment of exercise-induced muscle damage: Pilot study. *Journal of Sports Sciences*. doi: 10.1080/02640414.2017.1312492.

Kwiecien, S. Y. et al. (2019) Exploring the efficacy of a safe cryotherapy alternative: Physiological temperature changes from cold-water immersion versus prolonged cooling of phase-change material. *International Journal of Sports Physiology and Performance*. doi: 10.1123/ijspp.2018-0763.

Kyle, C. R. (1979) Reduction of wind resistance and power output of racing cyclists and runners travelling in groups. *Ergonomics*, 22(4), pp. 387–397.

Kyrolainen, H., Avela, J. and Komi, P. V. (2005) Changes in muscle activity with increasing running speed. *Journal of Sports Sciences*, 23(10), pp. 1101–1109.

Lack, S., Neal, B., De Oliveira Silva, D. and Barton, C. (2018) How to manage patellofemoral pain: Understanding the multifactorial nature and treatment options. *Physical Therapy in Sport*, 32, pp. 155–166.

Laffite, L. P., Mille-Hamard, L., Koralsztein, J. P. and Billat, V. L. (2003) The effects of interval training on oxygen pulse and performance in supra-threshold runs. *Archives of Physiology and Biochemistry*, 111(3), pp. 202–210.

Lai, A. et al. (2015) In vivo behavior of the human soleus muscle with increasing walking and running speeds. *Journal of Applied Physiology*, 118(10), pp. 1266–1275. doi: 10.1152/JAPPLPHYSIOL.00128.2015.

Lambert, C. et al. (2020) Regional changes in indices of bone strength of upper and lower limbs in response to high-intensity impact loading or high-intensity resistance training. *Bone*, 132. doi: 10.1016/J.BONE.2019.115192.

Lambert, G. P., Lang, J., Bull, A., Pfeifer, P. C., Eckerson, J., Moore, G. et al. (2008) Fluid restriction during running increases GI permeability. *International Journal of Sports Medicine*, 29(3), pp. 194–198.

Lancha, Jr., A. H., De Salles Painelli, V., Saunders, B. and Artioli, G. G. (2015) Nutritional strategies to modulate intracellular and extracellular buffering capacity during high-intensity exercise. *Sports Medicine*, 45(1), pp. 71–81.

Lane, A. M. and Terry, P. C. (2016) *Online mood profiling and self-regulation of affective responses*. New York: Routledge/Taylor & Francis Group.

Lane, A. M., Totterdell, P., MacDonald, I., Devonport, T. J., Friesen, A. P., Beedie, C. J., Stanley, D. and Nevill, A. (2016) Brief online training enhances competitive performance: Findings of the BBC Lab UK psychological skills intervention study. *Frontiers in Psychology*, 7, p. 413.

Lane, A. R., Hackney, A. C., Smith-Ryan, A., Kucera, K., Registar-Mihalik, J. and Ondrak, K. (2019) Prevalence of low energy availability in competitively trained male endurance athletes. *Medicina (Kaunas)*, 55(10).

Lanza, I. R. and Sreekumaran Nair, K. (2010) Regulation of skeletal muscle mitochondrial function: Genes to proteins. *Acta Physiologica*, 199(4), pp. 529–547.

LaRoche, D. P. and Connolly, D. A. J. (2006) Effects of stretching on passive muscle tension and response to eccentric exercise. *American Journal of Sports Medicine*. doi: 10.1177/0363546505284238.

Larsen, H. B. (2003) Kenyan dominance in distance running. *Comparative Biochemistry and Physiology - Part A: Molecular & Integrative Physiology*, 136(1), pp. 161–170.

Larsen, H. B., Christensen, D. L., Nolan, T. and Sondergaard, H. (2004) Body dimensions, exercise capacity and physical activity level of adolescent Nandi boys in western Kenya. *Annals of Human Biology*, 31(2), pp. 159–173.

Larson, P., Higgins, E., Kaminski, J., Decker, T., Preble, J., Lyons, D., McIntyre, K. and Normile, A. (2011) Foot strike patterns of recreational and sub-elite runners in a long-distance road race. *Journal of Sports Sciences*, 29(15), pp. 1665–1673.

Latorre Román, P. Á., Pinillos, F. G. and Robles, J. L. (2018) Early sport dropout: High performance in early years in young athletes is not related with later success. *Nuevas Tendencias en Educación Física, Deporte y Recreación*, 33, pp. 210–212.

Lauersen, J. B., Andersen, T. E. and Andersen, L. B. (2018) Strength training as superior, dose-dependent and safe prevention of acute and overuse sports injuries: A systematic review, qualitative analysis and meta-analysis. *British Journal of Sports Medicine*, 52(24), pp. 1557–1563. doi: 10.1136/BJSPORTS-2018-099078.

Lauersen, J. B., Bertelsen, D. M. and Andersen, L. B. (2014) The effectiveness of exercise interventions to prevent sports injuries: A systematic review and meta-analysis of randomised controlled trials. *British Journal of Sports Medicine*, 48(11), pp. 871–877. doi: 10.1136/bjsports-2013-092538.

Laurence, G., Wallman, K. and Guelfi, K. (2012) Effects of caffeine on time trial performance in sedentary men. *Journal of Sports Sciences*, 30, pp. 1235–1240.

Laursen, P. B. and Jenkins, D. G. (2002) The scientific basis for high-intensity interval training: Optimising training programmes and maximising performance in highly trained endurance athletes. *Sports Medicine*, 32(1), pp. 53–73.

Lawson, L. and Lorentzen, D. (1990) Selected sports bras: Comparisons of comfort and support. *Clothing & Textiles Research Journal*, 8, pp. 55–60.

Lazarus, R. S. (1999) *Stress and emotion: A new synthesis*. New York: Springer Publishing Company.

Lazarus, R. S. (2000) How emotions influence performance in competitive sports. *The Sport Psychologist*, 14(3), pp. 229–252.

Le Bars, H., Gernigon, C. and Ninot, G. (2009) Personal and contextual determinants of elite young athletes' persistence or dropping out over time. *Scandinavian Journal of Medicine and Science in Sports*, 19, pp. 274–285.

Lebrun, C. M., Joyce, S. M. and Constantini, N. W. (2013) Effects of female reproductive hormones on sports performance. In Constantini, N. and Hackney, A. C. (eds.) *Endocrinology of physical activity and sport*. 2nd edn. New York, NY: Springer Science, pp. 281–322.

Lee, M. J. C., Hammond, K. M., Vasdev, A., Poole, K. L., Impey, S. G., Close, G. L. et al. (2014) Self-selecting fluid intake while maintaining high carbohydrate availability does not impair half-marathon performance. *International Journal of Sports Medicine*, 35(14), pp. 1216–1222.

Lee, Y. H., Bae, S. C. and Song, G. G. (2012) Omega-3 polyunsaturated fatty acids and the treatment of rheumatoid arthritis: A meta-analysis. *Archives of Medical Research*. doi: 10.1016/j.arcmed.2012.06.011.

Leeder, J. D., Glaister, M., Pizzoferro, K., Dawson, J. and Pedlar, C. (2012a) Sleep duration and quality in elite athletes measured using wristwatch actigraphy. *Journal of Sports Sciences*, 30, pp. 541–545.

Leeder, J. D. et al. (2012b) Cold water immersion and recovery from strenuous exercise: A meta-analysis. *British Journal of Sports Medicine*. doi: 10.1136/bjsports-2011-090061.

Leeder, J. D. et al. (2015) Effects of seated and standing cold water immersion on recovery from repeated sprinting. *Journal of Sports Sciences*. doi: 10.1080/02640414.2014.996914.

Leetun, D. T., Ireland, M. L., Willson, J. D., Ballantyne, B. T. and Davis, I. M. (2004) Core stability measures as risk factors for lower extremity injury in athletes. *Medicine & Science in Sports & Exercise*, 36(6), pp. 926–934.

Legaz Arrese, A., Serrano Ostariz, E., Jcasajus Mallen, J. A. and Munguia Izquierdo, D. (2005) The changes in running performance and maximal oxygen uptake after long-term training in elite athletes. *The Journal of Sports Medicine and Physical Fitness*, 45(4), pp. 435–440.

Léger, L. and Mercier, D. (1984) Gross energy cost of horizontal treadmill and track running. *Sports Medicine*, 1, pp. 270–277.

Legwold, G. and Kummant, I. (1982) Does lifting weights harm a prepubescent athlete? *The Physician and Sports Medicine*, 10(7), pp. 141–144.

Leite, G. S. F., Resende, A. S., West, N. P. and Lancha, A. H. (2019) Probiotics and sports: A new magic bullet? *Nutrition*, 60, pp. 152–160.

Leknes, T. (2013) The training process in 800 m from adolescent to intenational level (in Norwegian: Treningsprosessen på 800 m fra ungdomsår til internasjonalt nivå). In Tjelta, L. I., Enoksen, E. and Tønnesen, E. (eds.) *Endurance training: Research and best practice (in Norwegian: Utholdenhetstrening. Forskning og beste praksis)*. Oslo: Cappelen Damm Akademisk.

Le Meur, Y., Hausswirth, C. and Mujika, I. (2012) Tapering for competition: A review. *Science and Sports*, 27(2), pp. 77–87. doi: 10.1016/j.scispo.2011.06.013.

Lenhart, R. L., Thelen, D. G., Wille, C. M., Chumanov, E. S. and Heiderscheit, B. C. (2014) Increasing running step rate reduces patellofemoral joint forces. *Medicine and Science in Sports and Exercise*, 46(3), pp. 557–564.

Lesinski, M., Prieske, O. and Granacher, U. (2016) Effects and dose–response relationships of resistance training on physical performance in youth athletes: A systematic review and meta-analysis. *British Journal of Sports Medicine*, 50(13), pp. 781–795.

Leskinen, A., Häkkinen, K., Virmavirta, M., Isolehto, J. and Kyröläinen, H. (2009) Comparison of running kinematics between elite and national-standard 1500-m runners. *Sports Biomechanics*, 8(1), pp. 1–9.

Levine, B. D. (2008) V̇O2max: What do we know, and what do we still need to know? *Journal of Physiology*, 586(1), pp. 25–34.

Levine, D., Richards, J. and Whittle, M. W. (2012) *Whittle's gait analysis*. 5th edn. Edinburgh: Churchill Livingstone.

Lewis, N. A., Daniels, D., Calder, P. C., Castell, L. M. and Pedlar, C. R. (2020) Are there benefits from the use of fish oil supplements in athletes? A systematic review. *Advances in Nutrition*, 11(5), pp. 1300–1314.

Li, F. et al. (2019) Correlation of eccentric strength, reactive strength, and leg stiffness with running economy in well-trained distance runners. *Journal of Strength and Conditioning Research*. United States. doi: 10.1519/JSC.0000000000003446.

Liao, T. C., Yin, L. and Powers, C. M. (2018) The influence of isolated femur and tibia rotations on patella cartilage stress: A sensitivity analysis. *Clin Biomech (Bristol, Avon)*, 54, pp. 125–131.

Lieber, R. I. and Fridén, J. (1993) Muscle damage is not a function of muscle force but active muscle strain. *Journal of Applied Physiology*, 74(2), pp. 520–526. https://doi.org/10.1152/jappl.1993.74.2.520.

Lieberman, D. E., Venkadesan, M., Werbel, W. A., Daoud, A. I., D'Andrea, S., Davis, I. S., Mang'eni, R. O. and Pitsiladis, Y. (2010) Foot strike patterns and collision forces in habitually barefoot versus shod runners. *Nature*, 463(7280), pp. 531–535.

Lieberman, D. E., Warrener, A. G., Wang, J. and Castillo, E. R. (2015) Effects of stride frequency and foot position at landing on braking force, hip torque, impact peak force and the metabolic cost of running in humans. *Journal of Experimental Biology*, 218, pp. 3406–3414.

Lillegard, W. A., Brown, E. W., Wilson, D. J. et al. (1997) Efficacy of strength training in prepubescent to early postpubescent males and females: Effects of gender and maturity. *Pediatric Rehabilitation*, 1(3), pp. 147–157.

Lindholm, C., Hirschberg, A. L., Carlstrom, K. and von Schoultz, B. (1995) Altered adrenal steroid metabolism underlying hypercortisolism in female endurance athletes. *Fertility and Sterility*, 63, pp. 1190–1194.

Linton, L. and Valentin, S. (2018) Running with injury: A study of UK novice and recreational runners and factors associated with running related injury. *Journal of Science and Medicine in Sport*, 21, pp. 1221–1225.

List, R., Gülay, T., Stoop, M. and Lorenzetti, S. (2013) Kinematics of the trunk and the lower extremities during restricted and unrestricted squats. *The Journal of Strength & Conditioning Research*, 27(6), pp. 1529–1538.

Lloyd, R. S., Cronin, J. B., Faigenbaum, A. D. et al. (2016) National Strength and Conditioning Association position statement on long-term athletic development. *Journal of Strength and Conditioning Research*, 30(6), pp. 1491–1509.

Lloyd, R. S., Faigenbaum, A. D., Stone, M. H. et al. (2014) Position statement on youth resistance training: The 2014 International Consensus. *British Journal of Sports Medicine*, 48(7), pp. 498–505.

Lloyd, R. S. and Oliver, J. L. (2012) The youth physical development model: A new approach to long-term athletic development. *Strength and Conditioning Journal*, 34(3), pp. 61–72.

Lobby Havey, M. (2020) Positive self talk: Inside the heads of America's top runners. www.active.com/running/articles/positive-self-talk-inside-the-heads-of-america-s-top-runners Accessed on: 08/09/2020.

Lobo, R. A. (2017) Hormone-replacement therapy: Current thinking. *Nature Reviews Endocrinology*, 13(4), pp. 220–231.

Logan, S., Hunter, I., Hopkins, J. T., Feland, J. B. and Parcell, A. C. (2010) Ground reaction force differences between running shoes, racing flats, and distance spikes in runners. *Journal of Sports Science and Medicine*, 9, pp. 147–153.

Lohse, K. R., Sherwood, D. E. and Healy, A. F. (2010) How changing the focus of attention affects performance, kinematics, and electromyography in dart throwing. *Human Movement Science*, 29, pp. 542–555.

Lolli, L., Batterham, A. M., Weston, K. L. and Atkinson, G. (2017) Size exponents for scaling maximal oxygen uptake in over 6500 humans: A systematic review and meta-analysis. *Sports Medicine*, 47(7), pp. 1405–1419.

Londeree, B. R. (1986) The use of laboratory test results with long distance runners. *Sports Medicine*, 3(3), pp. 201–213.

Lopes, A. D., Hespanhol, Jr., L. C., Yeung, S. S. and Costa, L. O. (2012) What are the main running-related musculoskeletal injuries? A systematic review. *Sports Medicine*, 42, pp. 891–905.

Lopez, L. M., Chen, M., Long, S. M., Curtis, K. M. and Helmerhorst, F. M. (2015) Steroidal contraceptives and bone fractures in women: Evidence from observational studies. *Cochrane Database of Systematic Reviews*, 7(7), p. CD009849.

Lorentzen, D. and Lawson, L. (1987) Selected sports bras: A biomechanical analysis of breast motion while jogging. *The Physician and Sports Medicine*, 15, pp. 128–139.

Loucks, A. B. (2004) Energy balance and body composition in sports and exercise. *Journal of Sports Sciences*, 22(1), pp. 1–14.

Loucks, A. B., Kiens, B. and Wright, H. H. (2011) Energy availability in athletes. *Journal of Sports Sciences*, 29(Suppl. 1), pp. 15–24. doi: 10.1080/02640414.2011.588958.

Loucks, A. B., Laughlin, G. A., Mortola, J. F., Girton, L., Nelson, J. C. and Yen, S. S. (1992) Hypothalamic-pituitary-thyroidal function in eumenorrheic and amenorrheic athletes. *The Journal of Clinical Endocrinology and Metabolism*, 75(2), pp. 514–518.

Loucks, A. B., Mortola, J. F., Girton, L. and Yen, S. S. (1989) Alterations in the hypothalamic-pituitary-ovarian and the hypothalamic-pituitary-adrenal axes in athletic women. *Journal of Clinical Endocrinology and Metabolism*, 68, pp. 402–411.

Loucks, A. B. and Thuma, J. R. (2003) Luteinizing hormone pulsatility is disrupted at a threshold of energy availability in regularly menstruating women. *The Journal of Clinical Endocrinology & Metabolism*, 88(1), pp. 297–311.

Low, J. L. et al. (2019) Prior band-resisted squat jumps improves running and neuromuscular performance in middle-distance runners. *Journal of Sports Science and Medicine*, 18(2), pp. 301–315.

Lowery, E. M., Brubaker, A. L., Kuhlmann, E. and Kovacs, E. J. (2013) The aging lung. *Clinical Interventions in Aging*, 8, pp. 1489–1496.

Lubahn, A. J. et al. (2011) Hip muscle activation and knee frontal plane motion during weight bearing therapeutic exercises. *The International Journal of Sports Physical Therapy*, 6(2), pp. 92–103.

Lubans, D. R., Morgan, P. J., Cliff, D. P., Barnett, L. M. and Okely, A. D. (2010) Fundamental movement skills in children and adolescents. *Sports Medicine*, 40(12), pp. 1019–1035.

Lucia, A., Esteve-Lanao, J., Olivan, J., Gomez-Gallego, F., San Juan, A. F., Santiago, C., Perez, M., Chamorro-Vina, C. and Foster, C. (2006) Physiological characteristics of the best Eritrean runners-exceptional running economy. *Applied Physiology, Nutrition, and Metabolism*, 31(5), pp. 530–540.

Luedke, L. E., Heiderscheit, B. C., Williams, D. S. and Rauh, M. J. (2015) Association of isometric strength of hip and knee muscles with injury risk in high school cross country runners. *The International Journal of Sports Physical Therapy*, 10(6), pp. 868–876.

Lukaski, H. C. (2004) Vitamin and mineral status: Effects on physical performance. *Nutrition*, 20(7), pp. 632–644. doi: 10.1016/J.NUT.2004.04.001.

Lund, H. et al. (2007) The effect of passive stretching on delayed onset muscle soreness, and other detrimental effects following eccentric exercise. *Scandinavian Journal of Medicine & Science in Sports*. doi: 10.1111/j.1600-0838.1998.tb00195.x.

Lundberg, J. O. and Weitzberg, E. (2009) NO generation from inorganic nitrate and nitrite: Role in physiology, nutrition and therapeutics. *Archives of Pharmacal Research*, 32(8), pp. 1119–1126.

Lundberg, T. R. and Howatson, G. (2018) Analgesic and anti-inflammatory drugs in sports: Implications for exercise performance and training adaptations. *Scandinavian Journal of Medicine and Science in Sports*. doi: 10.1111/sms.13275.

Lundby, C., Montero, D. and Joyner, M. (2017) Biology of VO2 max: Looking under the physiology lamp. *Acta Physiologica (Oxf)*, 220(2), pp. 218–228.

Lundgren, L. E., Tran, T. T., Nimphius, S., Raymond, E., Secomb, J. L., Farley, O. R., Newton, R. U. and Sheppard, J. M. (2016) Comparison of impact forces, accelerations and ankle range of motion in surfing-related landing tasks. *Journal of Sports Sciences*, 34(11), pp. 1051–1057.

Lussiana, T., Patoz, A., Gindre, C., Mourot, L. and Hébert-Losier, K. (2019) The implications of time on the ground on running economy: Less is not always better. *Journal of Experimental Biology*. doi: 10.1242/jeb.192047.

Lutz, G. J. and Rome, L. C. (1994) Built for jumping: The design of the frog muscular system. *Science*, 263(5145), pp. 370–372.

Lye, M. and Donnellan, C. (2000) General cardiology: Heart disease in the elderly. *Heart*, 84(5), pp. 560–566.

Macera, C. A., Pate, R. R., Powell, K. E., Jackson, K. L., Kendrick, J. S. and Craven, T. E. (1989) Predicting lower-extremity injuries among habitual runners. *Archives of Internal Medicine*, 149, pp. 2565–2568.

Machin, D. R. et al. (2014) Effects of differing dosages of pomegranate juice supplementation after eccentric exercise. *Physiology Journal*. doi: 10.1155/2014/271959.

MacInnis, M. J., Skelly, L. E. and Gibala, M. J. (2019) Rebuttal from Martin MacInnis, Lauren Skelly and Martin Gibala. *The Journal of Physiology*, 597(16), pp. 4119–4120.

Mackay, K., González, C., Zbinden-Foncea, H. and Peñailillo, L. (2019) Effects of oral contraceptive use on female sexual salivary hormones and indirect markers of muscle damage following eccentric cycling in women. *European Journal of Applied Physiology*, 119(11–12), pp. 2733–2744.

Macnaughton, L. S. et al. (2016) The response of muscle protein synthesis following whole-body resistance exercise is greater following 40 g than 20 g of ingested whey protein. *Physiological Reports*. doi: 10.14814/phy2.12893.

MacPhail, A. and Kirk, D. (2006) Young people's socialisation into sport: Experiencing the specialising phase. *Leisure Studies*, 25(1), pp. 57–74.

MacRae, B. A., Cotter, J. D. and Laing, R. M. (2011) Compression garments and exercise: Garment considerations, physiology and performance. *Sports Medicine*. doi: 10.2165/11591420-000000000-00000.

Maffulli, N., Baxter-Jones, A. D. and Grieve, A. (2005) Long term sport involvement and sport injury rate in elite young athletes. *Archives of Disease in Childhood*, 90, pp. 525–527.

Magnusson, S. P., Langberg, H. and Kjaer, M. (2010) The pathogenesis of tendinopathy: Balancing the response to loading. *Nature Reviews Rheumatology*, 6, pp. 262–268.

Mahieu, N. N. et al. (2006) Intrinsic risk Factors for the development of Achilles tendon overuse injury a prospective study. *American Journal of Sports Medicine*, 34(2), pp. 226–235. doi: 10.1177/0363546505279918.

Mahon, A., Del Corral, P., Howe, C. et al. (1996) Physiological correlates of 3-kilometer running performance in male children. *International Journal of Sports Medicine*, 17(8), pp. 580–584.

Malina, R. M. (1994) Physical growth and biological maturation of young athletes. *Exercise and Sport Science Reviews*, 22, pp. 389–434.

Malisoux, L., Chambon, N., Delattre, N., Gueguen, N., Urhausen, A. and Theisen, D. (2016) Injury risk in runners using standard or motion control shoes: A randomised controlled trial with participant and assessor blinding. *British Journal of Sports Medicine*, 50, pp. 481–487.

Malisoux, L., Ramesh, J., Mann, R., Seil, R., Urhausen, A. and Theisen, D. (2015) Can parallel use of different running shoes decrease running-related injury risk? *Scandinavian Journal of Medicine and Science in Sports*, 25, pp. 110–115.

Malliaras, P. et al. (2013) Achilles and patellar tendinopathy loading programmes : A systematic review comparing clinical outcomes and identifying potential mechanisms for effectiveness. *Sports Medicine*, 43(4), pp. 267–286. doi: 10.1007/S40279-013-0019-Z.

Malliaropoulos, N., Mendiguchia, J., Pehlivanidis, H., Papadopoulou, S., Valle, X., Malliaras, P. and Maffulli, N. (2012) Hamstring exercises for track and field athletes: Injury and exercise biomechanics, and possible implications for exercise selection and primary prevention. *British Journal of Sports Medicine*, 46(12), pp. 846–851.

Mandhane, P. J., Hanna, S. E., Inman, M. D., Duncan, J. M., Greene, J. M., Wang, H.-Y. and Sears, M. R. (2009) Changes in exhaled nitric oxide related to estrogen and progesterone during the menstrual cycle. *Chest*, 136(5), pp. 1301–1307.

Manore, M. M., Kam, L. C., Loucks, A. B. and International Association of Athletics, F. (2007) The female athlete triad: Components, nutrition issues, and health consequences. *Journal of Sports Sciences*, 25(Suppl 1), pp. S61–S71.

Manzi, V., Iellamo, F., Impellizzeri, F., D'ottavio, S. and Castagna, C. (2009) Relation between individualized training impulses and performance in distance runners. *Medicine & Science in Sports & Exercise*, 41, pp. 2090–2096.

Marc, A., Sedeaud, A., Guillaume, M., Rizk, M., Schipman, J., Antero-Jacquemin, J., Haida, A., Berthelot, G. and Toussaint, J. F. (2014) Marathon progress: Demography, morphology and environment. *Journal of Sports Sciences*, 32, pp. 524–532.

Marcell, T. J., Hawkins, S. A., Tarpenning, K. M., Hyslop, D. A. N. M. and Wiswell, R. A. (2003) Longitudinal analysis of lactate threshold in male and female master athletes. *Medicine & Science in Sports & Exercise*, 35(5).

March, D. S., Vanderburgh, P. M., Titlebaum, P. J. and Hoops, M. L. (2011) Age, sex, and finish time as determinants of pacing in the marathon. *The Journal of Strength and Conditioning Research*, 25(2), pp. 386–391.

Margaria, R., Oliva, R. D., Di Prampero, P. E. and Cerretelli, P. (1969) Energy utilization in intermittent exercise of supramaximal intensity. *Journal of Applied Physiology*, 26(6), pp. 752–756.

Marika, M. et al. (2019) Effect of cocoa products and its polyphenolic constituents on exercise performance and exercise-induced muscle damage and inflammation: A review of clinical trials. *Nutrients*. doi: 10.3390/nu11071471.

Marret, H., Fauconnier, A., Chabbert-Buffet, N., Cravello, L., Golfier, F., Gondry, J., Agostini, A., Bazot, M., Brailly-Tabard, S., Brun, J.-L., Raucourt, E. D., Gervaise, A., Gompel, A., Graesslin, O., Huchon, C., Lucot, J.-P., Plu-Bureau, G., Roman, H., Fernandez, H. and CNGOF, O. (2010) Clinical practice guidelines on menorrhagia: Management of abnormal uterine bleeding before menopause. *European Journal of Obstetrics & Gynecology and Reproductive Biology*, 152(2), pp. 133–137.

Marshall, J. (1963) Thermal changes in the normal menstrual cycle. *British Medical Journal*, 1(5323), p. 102.

Marti, B. and Howald, H. (1990) Long-term effects of physical training on aerobic capacity: Controlled study of former elite athletes. *Journal of Applied Physiology*, 69(4), pp. 1451–1459.

Martin, D. E. and Coe, P. N. (1991) *Training distance runners*. Champaign, IL: Leisure Press.

Martin, D. E. and Coe, P. N. (1997) *Better training for distance runners*. 2nd edn. Champaign, IL: Human Kinetics.

Martin, D. E., Sale, C., Cooper, S. B. and Elliott-Sale, K. J. (2018) Period prevalence and perceived side effects of hormonal contraceptive use and the menstrual cycle in elite athletes. *International Journal of Sports Physiology and Performance*, 13(7), pp. 926–932.

Martin, D. E., Vroon, D. H., May, D. F. and Pilbeam, S. P. (1986) Physiological changes in elite male distance runners training for Olympic competition. *The Physician and Sportsmedicine*, 14(1), pp. 152–206.

Martin, K. A., Moritz, S. E. and Hall, C. R. (1999) Imagery use in sport: A literature review and applied model. *The Sport Psychologist*, 13, pp. 245–268.

Martin, P. E. (1985) Mechanical and physiological responses to lower extremity loading during running. *Medicine and Science in Sports and Exercise*, 17(4), pp. 427–433.

Martinez, S., Aguilo, A., Rodas, L., Lozano, L., Moreno, C. and Tauler, P. (2018) Energy, macronutrient and water intake during a mountain ultramarathon event: The influence of distance. *Journal of Sports Sciences*, 36(3), pp. 333–339.

Mascher, H. et al. (2007) Changes in signalling pathways regulating protein synthesis in human muscle in the recovery period after endurance exercise. *Acta Physiologica*. doi: 10.1111/j.1748-1716.2007.01712.x.

Mason, B. R., Page, K. A. and Fallon, K. (1999) An analysis of movement and discomfort of the female breast during exercise and the effects of breast support in three cases. *Journal of Science and Medicine in Sport*, 2(2), pp. 134–144.

Matos, N., Winsley, R. J. and Williams, C. A. (2011) Prevalence of non-functional overreaching/overtraining in young English athletes. *Medicine and Science in Sport and Exercise*, 43, pp. 1287–1294.

Mattern, C. O., Gutilla, M. J., Bright, D. L., Kirby, T. E., Hinchcliff, K. W. and Devor, S. T. (2003) Maximal lactate steady state declines during the aging process. *Journal of Applied Physiology*, 95(6), pp. 2576–2582.

Maud, P. J. and Foster, C. (2006) *Physiological assessment of human fitness*. Champagne, IL: Human Kinetics.

Maughan, R. J. (2013) Quality assurance issues in the use of dietary supplements, with special reference to protein supplements. *Journal of Nutrition*, 143(11), pp. 1843S–1847S. doi: 10.3945/JN.113.176651.

Maughan, R. J., Burke, L. M., Dvorak, J., Larson-Meyer, D. E., Peeling, P., Phillips, S. M. et al. (2018) IOC consensus statement: Dietary supplements and the high-performance athlete. *International Journal of Sport Nutrition and Exercise Metabolism*, 28(2), pp. 104–125.

Maughan, R. J., Leiper, J. B. and Shirreffs, S. M. (1996) Restoration of fluid balance after exercise-induced dehydration: Effects of food and fluid intake. *European Journal of Applied Physiology*, 73(3), pp. 317–325. doi: 10.1007/BF02425493.

Mawhinney, C. et al. (2013) Influence of cold-water immersion on limb and cutaneous blood flow after exercise. *Medicine and Science in Sports and Exercise*. doi: 10.1249/MSS.0b013e31829d8e2e.

Maybin, J. A. and Critchley, H. O. D. (2015) Menstrual physiology: Implications for endometrial pathology and beyond. *Human Reproduction Update*, 21(6), pp. 748–761.

Maybin, J. A., Critchley, H. O. D. and Jabbour, H. N. (2011) Inflammatory pathways in endometrial disorders. *Molecular and Cellular Endocrinology*, 335(1), pp. 42–51.

Mayers, N. and Gutin, B. (1979) Physiological characteristics of elite prepubertal cross-country runners. *Medicine and Science in Sports*, 11(2), pp. 172–176.

Mayhew, J. L., Piper, F. C. and Etheridge, G. L. (1979) Oxygen cost and energy requirement of running in trained and untrained males and females. *Journal of Sports Medicine and Physical Fitness*, 19(1), p. 39.

McCambridge, T. and Stricker, P. (2008) Strength training by children and adolescents. *Pediatrics*, 121(4), pp. 835–840.

McClaran, S. R., Babcock, M. A., Pegelow, D. F., Reddan, W. G. and Dempsey, J. A. (1995) Longitudinal effects of aging on lung function at rest and exercise in healthy active fit elderly adults. *Journal of Applied Physiology*, 78(5), pp. 1957–1968.

McColl, E. M., Wheeler, G. D., Gomes, P., Bhambhani, Y. and Cumming, D. C. (1989) The effects of acute exercise on pulsatile LH release in high-mileage male runners. *Clinical Endocrinology (Oxf)*, 31(5), pp. 617–621.

McConell, G. K., Costill, D. L., Widrick, J. J., Hickey, M. S., Tanaka, H. and Gastin, P. B. (1993) Reduced training volume and intensity maintain aerobic capacity but not performance in distance runners. *International Journal of Sports Medicine*, 14(1), pp. 33–37. doi: 10.1055/s-2007-1021142.

McCormick, A. and Hatzigeorgiadis, A. (2019) Self-talk and endurance performance. In Meijen, C. (ed.) *Endurance performance in sport: Psychological theory and interventions*. Oxon, UK: Routledge, pp. 153–167.

McCormick, A., Meijen, C. and Marcora, S. (2015) Psychological determinants of whole-body endurance performance. *Sports Medicine*, 45(7), pp. 997–1015.

McCormick, A., Meijen, C. and Marcora, S. (2018) Effects of a motivational self-talk intervention for endurance athletes completing an ultramarathon. *The Sport Psychologist*, 32(1), pp. 42–50.

McCurdy, K. et al. (2010) Comparison of lower extremity EMG between the 2-leg squat and modified single-leg squat in female athletes. *Journal of Sport Rehabilitation*, 19(1), pp. 57–70. doi: 10.1123/JSR.19.1.57.

McGhee, D. E. and Steele, J. R. (2010a) Breast elevation and compression decrease exercise-induced breast discomfort. *Medicine and Science in Sports and Exercise*, 42, pp. 1333–1338.

McGhee, D. E. and Steele, J. R. (2010b) Optimising breast support in female patients through correct bra fit: A cross-sectional study. *Journal of Science and Medicine in Sport*, 13(6), pp. 568–572.

McGhee, D. E. and Steele, J. R. (2020a) Breast biomechanics: What do we really know? *Physiology*, 35(2), pp. 144–156.

McGhee, D. E. and Steele, J. R. (2020b) Biomechanics of breast support for active women. *Exercise and Sport Sciences Reviews*, 48(3), pp. 99–109.

McGhee, D. E., Steele, J. R. and Munro, B. J. (2010) Education improves bra knowledge and fit, and level of breast support in adolescent female athletes: A cluster-randomised trial. *Journal of Physiotherapy*, 56(1), pp. 19–24.

McGhee, D. E., Steele, J. R., Zealey, W. J. and Takacs, G. J. (2013) Bra-breast forces generated in women with large breasts while standing and during treadmill running: Implications for sports bra design. *Applied Ergonomics*, 44, pp. 112–118.

McHugh, M. P. et al. (2019) Countermovement jump recovery in professional soccer players using an inertial sensor. *International Journal of Sports Physiology and Performance*. doi: 10.1123/ijspp.2018-0131.

McKean, K. A., Manson, N. A. and Stanish, W. D. (2006) Musculoskeletal injury in the masters runners. *Clinical Journal of Sport Medicine*, 16(2), pp. 149–154.

McKeon, P. O., Hertel, J., Bramble, D. and Davis, I. (2015) The foot core system: A new paradigm for understanding intrinsic foot muscle function. *British Journal of Sports Medicine*, 49, p. 290.

McLaughlin, J. E., Howley, E. T., Bassett, Jr. D. R., Thompson, D. L. and Fitzhugh, E. C. (2010) Test of the classic model for predicting endurance running performance. *Medicine and Science in Sports and Exercise*, 42(5), pp. 991–997. https://doi.org/10.1249/MSS.0b013e3181c0669d.

McLay, R. T., Thomson, C. D., Williams, S. M. and Rehrer, N. J. (2007) Carbohydrate loading and female endurance athletes: Effect of menstrual-cycle phase. *International Journal of Sport Nutrition and Exercise Metabolism*, 17(2), pp. 189–205.

McLeay, Y. et al. (2012) Effect of New Zealand blueberry consumption on recovery from eccentric exercise-induced muscle damage. *Journal of the International Society of Sports Nutrition*. doi: 10.1186/1550-2783-9-19.

McLellan, C. P., Lovell, D. I. and Gass, G. C. (2011) The role of rate of force development on vertical jump performance. *The Journal of Strength & Conditioning Research*, 25(2), pp. 379–385.

McMahon, T. and Cheng, G. (1990) The mechanics of running: How does stiffness couple with speed? *Journal of Biomechanics*, 23, pp. 65–78.

McMillian, D. J., Rynders, Z. G. and Trudeau, T. R. (2016) Modifying the functional movement screen deep squat test: The effect of foot and arm positional variations. *The Journal of Strength & Conditioning Research*, 30(4), pp. 973–979.

McNair, D., Lorr, M. and Droppleman, L. (1971) *Manual for the profile of mood states (POMS)*. San Diego: Educational and Industrial Testing Service.

McNarry, M., Barker, A., Lloyd, R. S. et al. (2014) The BASES expert statement on trainability during childhood and adolescence. *The Sport and Exercise Scientist*, 41, pp. 22–23.

McNarry, M. and Jones, A. (2014) The influence of training status on the aerobic and anaerobic responses to exercise in children: A review. *European Journal of Sport Science*, 14(S1), pp. S57–S68.

Mcnaughton, L. R. (1992) Bicarbonate ingestion: Effects of dosage on 60 s cycle ergometry. *Journal of Sports Sciences*, 10(5), pp. 415–423.

Mcnaughton, L. R., Gough, L., Deb, S., Bentley, D. and Sparks, S. A. (2016) Recent developments in the use of sodium bicarbonate as an ergogenic aid. *Current Sports Medicine Reports*, 15(4), pp. 233–244.

McNulty, K. L., Elliott-Sale, K. J., Dolan, E., Swinton, P. A., Ansdell, P., Goodall, S., Thomas, K. and Hicks, K. M. (2020) The effects of menstrual cycle phase on exercise performance in eumenorrheic women: A systematic review and meta-analysis. *Sports Medicine*, 50, pp. 1813–1827.

Meardon, S. A. and Derrick, T. R. (2014) Effect of step width manipulation on tibial stress during running. *Journal of Biomechanics*, 47, pp. 2738–2344.

Medbø, J. I. and Burgers, S. (1990) Effect of training on the anaerobic capacity. *Medicine & Science in Sports & Exercise*, 22(4), pp. 501–507.

Medbø, J. I., Mohn, A. C., Tabata, I., Bahr, R., Vaage, O. and Sejersted, O. M. (1988) Anaerobic capacity determined by maximal accumulated O2 deficit. *Journal of Applied Physiology*, (1985), 64(1), pp. 50–60.

Meeusen, R., Duclos, M., Foster, C., Fry, A., Gleeson, M., Nieman, D., Raglin, J., Rietjens, G., Steinacker, J. and Urhausen, A. (2013a) Prevention, diagnosis, and treatment of the overtraining syndrome: Joint consensus statement of the European College of Sport Science and the American College of Sports Medicine. *Medicine and Science in Sports and Exercise*, 45(1), pp. 186–205. doi: 10.1249/MSS.0b013e318279a10a.

Meeusen, R., Duclos, M., Foster, C. et al. (2013b) Prevention, diagnosis and treatment of the overtraining syndrome: Joint consensus statement of the European College of Sport Science (ECSS) and the American College of Sports Medicine (ACSM). *European Journal of Sport Science*, 13, pp. 1–24.

Meijen, C. (2019) *Endurance performance in sport: Psychological theory and interventions*. Oxon, UK: Routledge.

Melin, A. K., Heikura, I. A., Tenforde, A. and Mountjoy, M. (2019) Energy availability in athletics: Health, performance, and physique. *International Journal of Sport Nutrition and Exercise Metabolism*, 29(2), pp. 152–164.

Melin, A. K., Tornberg, A. B., Skouby, S., Faber, J., Ritz, C., Sjödin, A. and Sundgot-Borgen, J. (2014) The LEAF questionnaire: A screening tool for the identification of female athletes at risk for the female athlete triad. *British Journal of Sports Medicine*, 48(7), pp. 540–545.

Mendiguchia, J., Conceição, F., Edouard, P., Fonseca, M., Pereira, R., Lopes, H., Morin, J. B. and Jiménez-Reyes, P. (2020) Sprint versus isolated eccentric training: Comparative effects on hamstring architecture and performance in soccer players. *PLoS One*, 15, p. e0228283.

Mercer, J. A., Vance, J., Hreljac, A. and Hamill, J. (2002) Relationship between shock attenuation and stride length during running at different velocities. *European Journal of Applied Physiology*, 87, p. 403–408.

Mercier, J., Vago, P., Ramonatxo, M. et al. (1987) Effect of aerobic training quantity on the VO2 max of circumpubertal swimmers. *International Journal of Sports Medicine*, 8, pp. 26–30.

Merrick, M. A. (2002) Secondary injury after musculoskeletal trauma: A review and update. *Journal of Athletic Training*, 37(2), pp. 209–217.

Messier, S. P., Martin, D. F., Mihalko, S. L., IP, E., Devita, P., Cannon, D. W., Love, M., Beringer, D., Saldana, S., Fellin, R. E. and Seay, J. F. (2018) A 2-year prospective cohort study of overuse running injuries: The Runners and Injury Longitudinal Study (TRAILS). *American Journal of Sports Medicine*, 46, pp. 2211–2221.

Mian, O., Baltzopoulos, V., Minetti, A. and Narici, M. (2007) The impact of physical training on loco-motion function in older people. *Sports Medicine*, 37(8), pp. 683–701.

Midgley, A. W., McNaughton, L. R. and Jones, A. M. (2007) Training to enhance the physiological determinants of long-distance running performance: Can valid recommendations be given to runners and coaches based on current scientific knowledge? *Sports Medicine*, 37(10), pp. 857–880. https://doi.org/10.2165/00007256-200737100-00003.

Midgley, A. W., McNaughton, L. R. and Wilkinson, M. (2006a) Is there an optimal training intensity for enhancing the maximal oxygen uptake of distance runners? Empirical research findings, current opinions, physiological rationale and practical recommendations. *Sports Medicine*, 36(2), pp. 117–132.

Midgley, A. W., McNaughton, L. R. and Wilkinson, M. (2006b) The relationship between the lactate turnpoint and the time at VO2max during a constant velocity run to exhaustion. *International Journal of Sports Medicine*, 27(4), pp. 278–282.

Midgely, A. W., McNaughton, L. R. and Wilkinson, M. (2006c) Criteria and other methodological considerations in the evaluation of time at VO2 max. *Journal of Sports Medicine and Physical Fitness*, 26, pp. 183–188.

Mikkola, J., Rusko, H., Nummela, A. et al. (2007) Concurrent endurance and explosive type strength training improves neuromuscular and anaerobic characteristics in young distance runners. *International Journal of Sports Medicine*, 28(7), pp. 602–611.

Milanović, Z., Sporiš, G. and Weston, M. (2015) Effectiveness of high-intensity interval training (HIT) and continuous endurance training for VO 2max improvements: A systematic review and meta-analysis of controlled trials. *Sports Medicine*, 45(10), pp. 1469–1481.

Milewski, M. D., Skaggs, D. L., Bishop, G. A., Pace, J. L., Ibrahim, D. A., Wren, T. A. and Barzdukas, A. (2014) Chronic lack of sleep is associated with increased sports injuries in adolescent athletes. *Journal of Pediatric Orthopaedics*, 34(2), pp. 129–133.

Milgrom, C., Radeva-Petrova, D. R., Finestone, A., Nyska, M., Mendelson, S., Benjuya, N., Simkin, A. and Burr, D. (2007) The effect of muscle fatigue on in vivo tibial strains. *Journal of Applied Biomechanics*, 40, pp. 845–850.

Miller, D. (1981) *Running free*. London, UK: Hodder & Stoughton Ltd.

Millet, G. P. et al. (2002) Effects of concurrent endurance and strength training on running economy and .VO(2) kinetics. *Medicine and Science in Sports and Exercise*, 34(8), pp. 1351–1359. www.ncbi.nlm.nih.gov/pubmed/12165692.

Milligan, A. (2013) The effect of breast support on running biomechanics (Unpublished Thesis). University of Portsmouth, Portsmouth, UK.

Milligan, A., Mills, C., Corbett, J. and Scurr, J. (2015) The influence of breast support on torso, pelvis and arm kinematics during a five kilometre treadmill run. *Human Movement Science*, 42, pp. 246–260.

Milligan, A., Mills, C. and Scurr, J. (2014) Within-participant variance in multiplanar breast kinematics during 5 km treadmill running. *Journal of Applied Niomechanics*, 30(2), pp. 244–249.

Mills, A., Butt, J., Maynard, I. and Harwood, C. (2012) Identifying factors perceived to influence the development of elite English football academy players. *Journal of Sports Sciences*, 30, pp. 1593–1604.

Milner, C. E., Ferber, R., Pollard, C. D., Hamill, J. and Davis, I. S. (2006) Biomechanical factors associated with tibial stress fracture in female runners. *Medicine and Science in Sports and Exercise*, 38, pp. 323–328.

Milner, C. E., Hamill, J. and Davis, I. S. (2010) Distinct hip and rearfoot kinematics in female runners with a history of tibial stress fracture. *Journal of Orthopaedic & Sports Physical Therapy*, 40(2), pp. 59–66. doi: 10.2519/JOSPT.2010.3024.

Milone, M. T., Bernstein, J., Freedman, K. B. and Tjoumakaris, F. (2013) There is no need to avoid resistance training (weight lifting) until physeal closure. *The Physician and Sports Medicine*, 41(4), pp. 101–105.

Minahan, C., Melnikoff, M., Quinn, K. and Larsen, B. (2017) Response of women using oral contraception to exercise in the heat. *European Journal of Applied Physiology*, 117(7), pp. 1383–1391.

Minetti, A. E., Ardigò, L. P. and Saibene, F. (1994) Mechanical determinants of the minimum energy cost of gradient running in humans. *The Journal of Experimental Biology*, 195(1), pp. 211–225.

Mirwald, R. L., Baxter-Jones, A. D., Bailey, D. A. and Beunen, G. P. (2002) An assessment of maturity from anthropometric measurements. *Medicine and Science in Sports and Exercise*, 34(4), pp. 689–694.

Mizrahi, J., Verbitsky, O. and Isakov, E. (2000) Fatigue-related loading imbalance on the shank in running: A possible factor in the stress fractures. *Annals of Biomedical Engineering*, 28, pp. 463–469.

Möck, S., Hartmann, R., Wirth, K., Rosenkranz, G. and Mickel, C. (2018) Correlation of dynamic strength in the standing calf raise with sprinting performance in consecutive sections up to 30 meters. *Research in Sports Medicine*, 26(4), pp. 474–481.

Modin, A., Björne, H., Herulf, M., Alving, K., Weitzberg, E. and Lundberg, J. O. N. (2001) Nitrite-derived nitric oxide: A possible mediator of 'acidic–metabolic' vasodilation. *Acta Physiologica Scandinavica*, 171(1), pp. 9–16.

Moen, M. H., Bongers, T., Bakker, E. W., Zimmermann, W. O., Weir, A., Tol, J. L. and Backx, F. J. G. (2012) Risk factors and prognostic indicators for medial tibial stress syndrome. *Scandinavian Journal of Medicine & Science in Sports,* 22, pp. 34–39.

Moesch, K., Elbe, A. M., Hauge, M. L. and Wikman, J. M. (2011) Late specialization: The key to success in centimeters, grams, or seconds (cgs) sports. *Scandinavian Journal of Sports Medicine*, 21, pp. e282–e290.

Molinari, C. A., Palacin, F., Poinsard, L. and Billat, V. L. (2020) Determination of submaximal and maximal training zones from a 3-stage, variable-duration, perceptually regulated track test. *International Journal of Sports Physiology and Performance*. https://doi.org/10.1123/ijspp.2019-0423

Montain, S. J., Sawka, M. N. and Wenger, C. B. (2001) Hyponatremia associated with exercise: Risk factors and pathogenesis. *Exercise and Sport Science Reviews*, 29(3), pp. 113–117.

Monteiro Rodrigues, L. A. et al. (2020) Lower limb massage in human increases local perfusion and impacts systemic hemodynamics. *Journal of Applied Physiology*. doi: 10.1152/japplphysiol.00437.2019.

Montero, D. and Díaz-Cañestro, C. (2015) Maximal cardiac output in athletes: Influence of age. *European Journal of Preventive Cardiology*, 22(12), pp. 1588–1600.

Montero, D., Diaz-Canestro, C. and Lundby, C. (2015) Endurance training and VO2max: Role of maximal cardiac output and oxygen extraction. *Medicine & Science in Sports & Exercise*, 47(10), pp. 2024–2033.

Montgomery, M. M., Shultz, S. J., Schmitz, R. J., Wideman, L. and Henson, R. A. (2012) Influence of lean body mass and strength on landing energetics. *Medicine & Science in Sports & Exercise*, 44(12), pp. 2376–2383.

Moore, D. R. (2015) Nutrition to support recovery from endurance exercise: Optimal carbohydrate and protein replacement. *Current Sports Medicine Reports*, 14(4), pp. 294–300. doi: 10.1249/JSR.0000000000000180.

Moore, D. R. et al. (2012a) Daytime pattern of post-exercise protein intake affects whole-body protein turnover in resistance-trained males. *Nutrition and Metabolism*. doi: 10.1186/1743-7075-9-91.

Moore, I. S., Jones, A. M. and Dixon, S. J. (2012b) Mechanisms for improved running economy in beginner runners. *Medicine and Science in Sports and Exercise*, 44, pp. 1756–1763.

Moore, D. R. et al. (2014a) Beyond muscle hypertrophy: Why dietary protein is important for endurance athletes. *Applied Physiology, Nutrition and Metabolism*. doi: 10.1139/apnm-2013-0591.

Moore, I. S., Jones, A. M. and Dixon, S. J. (2014b) The pursuit of improved running performance: Can changes in cushioning and somatosensory feedback influence running economy and injury risk? *Footwear Science*, 6, pp. 1–11.

Moore, I. S. (2016) Is there an economical running technique? A review of modifiable biomechanical factors affecting running economy. *Sports Medicine*, 46(6), pp. 793–807. doi: 10.1007/s40279-016-0474-4.

Moore, I. S. (2019) *Software to Determine the Modeled Optimal Gait Characteristic (Runtime Needed)*. doi: 10.25401/cardiffmet.8323283.v1.

Moore, I. S. (2020) *Predicting Optimal Gait Characteristics Spreadsheet*. doi: 10.25401/cardiffmet.12383897.v1.

Moore, I. S., Ashford, K. J., Cross, C., Hope, J., Jones, H. S. R. and McCarthy-Ryan, M. (2019a) Humans optimize ground contact time and leg stiffness to minimize the metabolic cost of running. *Frontiers in Sports and Active Living*, 1.

Moore, I. S., Phillips, D. J., Ashford, K. A., Mullen, R., Goom, T. and Gittoes, M. R. J. (2019b) An interdisciplinary examination of attentional focus strategies used during running gait retraining. *Scandinavian Journal of Medicine and Science in Sports*, 29, pp. 1572–1582.

Moore, I. S. and Dixon, S. J. (2014) Changes in sagittal plane kinematics with treadmill familiarization to barefoot running. *Journal of Applied Biomechanics*, 30, pp. 626–631.

Moore, I. S., Jones, A. M. and Dixon, S. J. (2016) Reduced oxygen cost of running is related to alignment of the resultant GRF and leg axis vector: A pilot study. *Scandinavian Journal of Medicine and Science in Sports*, 26, pp. 809–815.

Moore, I. S. and Willy, R. W. (2019) Use of wearables: Tracking and retraining in endurance runners. *Current Sports Medicine Reports*, 18, pp. 437–444.

Moore, S. A., McKay, H. A., Macdonald, H. et al. (2015) Enhancing a somatic maturity prediction model. *Medicine and Science in Sports and Exercise*, 47(8), pp. 1755–1764.

Mooses, M., Mooses, K., Haile, D. W., Durussel, J., Kaasik, P. and Pitsiladis, Y. P. (2015) Dissociation between running economy and running performance in elite Kenyan distance runners. *Journal of Sport Science*, 33(2), pp. 136–144.

MoradiFili, B., Ghiasvand, R., Pourmasoumi, M., Feizi, A., Shahdadian, F. and Shahshahan, Z. (2020) Dietary patterns are associated with premenstrual syndrome: Evidence from a case-control study. *Public Health Nutrition*, 23(5), pp. 833–842.

Morgan, D. W., Baldini, F. D., Martin, P. E. and Kohrt, W. M. (1989a) Ten kilometer performance and predicted velocity at VO2max among well-trained male runners. *Medicine and Science in Sports and Exercise*, 21(1), pp. 78–83.

Morgan, D. W., Martin, P. E. and Krahenbuhl, G. S. (1989b) Factors affecting running economy. *Sports Medicine*, 7(5), pp. 310–330.

Morgan, D. W., Bransford, D. R., Costill, D. L., Daniels, J. T., Howley, E. T. and Krahenbuhl, G. S. (1995) Variation in the aerobic demand of running among trained and untrained subjects. *Medicine and Science in Sports and Exercise*, 27(3), pp. 404–409.

Morgan, D. W. and Daniels, J. T. (1994) Relationship between VO2max and the aerobic demand of running in elite distance runners. *International Journal of Sports Medicine*, 15(7), pp. 426–429.

Morgan, D. W., Martin, P. E., Craib, M., Caruso, C., Clifton, R. and Hopewell, R. (1994) Effect of step length optimization on the aerobic demand of running. *Journal of Applied Physiology*, 77, pp. 245–251.

Morgan, W. P. and Pollock, M. L. (1977) Psychologic characterization of the elite distance runner. *Annals of the New York Academy of Sciences*, 301(1), pp. 382–403.

Moritani, T., Oddsson, L., Thorstensson, A. et al. (1989) Neural and biomechanical differences between men and young boys during a variety of motor tasks. *Acta Physiologica Scandinavia*, 137, pp. 347–355.

Moritz, S. E., Feltz, D. L., Fahrbach, K. R. and Mack, D. E. (2000) The relation of self-efficacy measures to sport performance: A meta-analytic review. *Research Quarterly for Exercise and Sport*, 7, pp. 280–294.

Morrison, D. et al. (2015) Vitamin C and E supplementation prevents some of the cellular adaptations to endurance-training in humans. *Free Radical Biology and Medicine*, 89, pp. 852–862. doi: 10.1016/J.FREERADBIOMED.2015.10.412.

Mortensen, S. P., Nyberg, M., Winding, K. and Saltin, B. (2012) Lifelong physical activity preserves functional sympatholysis and purinergic signalling in the ageing human leg. *The Journal of Physiology*, 590(23), pp. 6227–6236.

Morton, R. H. and Billat, L. V. (2004) The critical power model for intermittent exercise. *European Journal of Applied Physiology*, 91(2–3), pp. 303–307.

Mostafavifar, A. M., Best, T. M. and Myer, G. D. (2013) Early sport specialisation, does it lead to long-term problems? *British Journal of Sport Medicine*, 47, pp. 1060–1061.

Mountjoy, M., Sundgot-Borgen, J. K., Burke, L. M., Ackerman, K. E., Blauwet, C., Constantini, N., Lebrun, C., Lundy, B., Melin, A. K., Meyer, N. L., Sherman, R. T., Tenforde, A. S., Klungland Torstveit, M. and Budgett, R. (2018a) IOC consensus statement on relative energy deficiency in sport (RED-S): 2018 update. *British Journal of Sports Medicine*, 52(11), pp. 687–697.

Mountjoy, M. et al. (2018b) International Olympic Committee (IOC) consensus statement on relative energy deficiency in sport (RED-S): 2018 update. *International Journal of Sport Nutrition and Exercise Metabolism*, 28(4), pp. 316–331. doi: 10.1123/IJSNEM.2018-0136.

Mountjoy, M., Sundgot-Borgen, J., Burke, L. M., Carter, S., Constantini, N., Lebrun, C., Meyer, N., Sherman, R., Steffen, K., Budgett, R. and Ljungqvist, A. (2014) The IOC consensus statement: Beyond the female athlete triad: Relative energy deficiency in sport (RED-S). *British Journal of Sports Medicine*, 48(7), pp. 491–497.

Mountjoy, M., Sundgot-Borgen, J., Burke, L. et al. (2015a) RED-S CAT: Relative energy deficiency in sport (RED-S) Clinical Assessment Tool (CAT). *British Journal of Sports Medicine*, 49(7), pp. 421–423.

Mountjoy, M., Sundgot-Borgen, J., Burke, L. et al. (2015b) The IOC relative energy deficiency in sport clinical assessment tool (RED-S CAT). *British Journal of Sports Medicine*, 49(21), p. 1354.

Mousavi, S. H., Hijmans, J. M., Rajabi, R., Diercks, R., Zwerver, J. and Van Der Worp, H. (2019) Kinematic risk factors for lower limb tendinopathy in distance runners: A systematic review and meta-analysis. *Gait Posture*, 69, pp. 13–24.

Mozaffarian, D. et al. (2006) Trans fatty acids and cardiovascular disease. *Obstetrical & Gynecological Survey*, 61(8), pp. 525–526. doi: 10.1097/01.OGX.0000228706.09374.E7.

Mucha, M. D., Caldwell, W., Schlueter, E. L., Walters, C. and Hassen, A. (2017) Hip abductor strength and lower extremity running related injury in distance runners: A systematic review. *Journal of Science & Medicine in Sport*, 20(4), pp. 349–355.

Mujika, I. (1998) The influence of training characteristics and tapering on the adaptation in highly trained individuals: A review. *International Journal of Sports Medicine*, 19(7), pp. 439–446.

Mujika, I. (2010) Intense training: The key to optimal performance before and during the taper. *Scandinavian Journal of Medicine & Science in Sports*, 20, pp. 24–31. doi: 10.1111/j.1600-0838.2010.01189.x.

Mujika, I., Goya, A., Padilla, S., Grijalba, A., Gorostiaga, E. and Ibanez, J. (2000) Physiological responses to a 6-d taper in middle-distance runners: Influence of training intensity and volume. *Medicine and Science in Sports and Exercise*, 32(2), pp. 511–517.

Mujika, I. and Padilla, S. (2001a) Cardiorespiratory and metabolic characteristics of detraining in humans. *Medicine and Science in Sports and Exercise*, 33(3), pp. 413–421.

Mujika, I. and Padilla, S. (2001b) Muscular characteristics of detraining in humans. *Medicine and Science in Sports and Exercise*, 33(8), pp. 1297–1303.

Mujika, I. and Padilla, S. (2003) Scientific bases for precompetition tapering strategies. *Medicine and Science in Sports and Exercise*, 35(7), pp. 1182–1187. doi: 10.1249/01.MSS.0000074448.73931.11.

Mujika, I., Padilla, S. and Pyne, D. (2002) Swimming performance changes during the final 3 weeks of training leading to the Sydney 2000 Olympic games. *International Journal of Sports Medicine*, 23(8), pp. 582–587. doi: 10.1055/s-2002-35526.

Mujika, I., Padilla, S., Pyne, D. and Busso, T. (2004) Physiological changes associated with the pre-event taper in athletes. *Sports Medicine*, 34(13), pp. 891–927. doi: 10.2165/00007256-200434130-00003.

Mulvad, B., Nielsen, R. O., Lind, M. and Ramskov, D. (2018) Diagnoses and time to recovery among injured recreational runners in the RUN CLEVER trial. *PLoS One*, 13, p. e0204742.

Munoz, I., Seiler, S., Alcocer, A., Carr, N. and Esteve-Lanao, J. (2015) Specific intensity for peaking: Is race pace the best option? *Asian Journal of Sports Medicine*, 6(3) [online]. doi: 10.5812/asjsm.24900. Accessed on: 16/04/2020.

Muñoz, I., Seiler, S., Bautista, J., España, J., Larumbe, E. and Esteve-Lanao, J. (2014) Does polarized training improve performance in recreational runners? *International Journal of Sports Physiology and Performance*, 9(2), pp. 265–272. https://doi.org/10.1123/IJSPP.2012-0350.

Munro, C. F., Miller, D. I. and Fuglevand, A. J. (1987) Ground reaction forces in running: A reexamination. *Journal of Biomechanics*, 20(2), pp. 147–155.

Murray, N. B., Gabbett, T. J., Townshend, A. D. and Blanch, P. (2017a) Calculating acute: Chronic workload ratios using exponentially weighted moving averages provides a more sensitive indicator of injury likelihood than rolling averages. *British Journal of Sports Medicine,* 51, pp. 749–754.

Murray, N. B., Gabbett, T. J., Townshend, A. D., Hulin, B. T. and McLellan, C. P. (2017b) Individual and combined effects of acute and chronic running loads on injury risk in elite Australian footballers. *Scandinavian Journal of Medicine & Science in Sports,* 27, pp. 990–998.

Myburgh, K. H. (2014) Polyphenol supplementation: Benefits for exercise performance or oxidative stress? *Sports Medicine.* doi: 10.1007/s40279-014-0151-4.

Myer, G. D., Faigenbaum, A. D., Chu, D. A. et al. (2011) Integrative training for children and adolescents: Techniques and practices for reducing sports-related injuries and enhancing athletic performance. *The Physician and Sports Medicine*, 39(1), pp. 74–84.

Myer, G. D., Jayanthi, N., DiFiori, J. P. et al. (2015) Sports specialization, part I: Does early sports specialization increase negative outcomes and reduce the opportunity for success in young athletes? *Sports Health*, 7, pp. 437–442.

Myer, G. D., Jayanthi, N., DiFiori, J. P. et al. (2016) Sports specialization, part II: Alternative solutions to early sport specialization in youth athletes. *Sports Health*, 8(1), pp. 65–73.

Myer, G. D., Kushner, A. M., Brent, J. L., Schoenfeld, B. J., Hugentobler, J., Lloyd, R. S., Vermeil, A., Chu, D. A., Harbin, J. and McGill, S. M. (2014) The back squat: A proposed assessment of functional deficits and technical factors that limit performance. *Strength & Conditioning Journal*, 36(6), pp. 4–27.

Myers, A. M., Beam, N. W. and Fakhoury, J. D. (2017) Resistance training for children and adolescents. *Translational Pediatrics*, 6(3), pp. 137–143.

Myers, M. J. and Steudel, K. (1985) Effect of limb mass and its distribution on the energetic cost of running. *Journal of Experimental Biology*, 116, pp. 363–373.

Mytton, G. J., Archer, D. T., Turner, L., Skorski, S., Renfree, A., Thompson, K. G. and St Clair Gibson, A. (2015) Increased variability of lap speeds: Differentiating medalists and nonmedalists in middle-distance running and swimming events. *International Journal of Sports Physiology and Performance*, 10(3), pp. 369–373.

Napier, C., Maclean, C. L., Maurer, J., Taunton, J. E. and Hunt, M. A. (2018) Kinetic risk factors of running-related injuries in female recreational runners. *Scandinavian Journal of Medicine and Science in Sports*, 28, pp. 2164–2172.

Napier, C., Maclean, C. L., Maurer, J., Taunton, J. E. and Hunt, M. A. (2019) Real-time biofeedback of performance to reduce braking forces associated with running-related injury: An exploratory study. *Journal of Orthopaedic & Sports Physical Therapy*, 49, pp. 136–144.

Nattiv, A., Agostini, R., Drinkwater, B. and Yeager, K. K. (1994) The female athlete triad: The inter-relatedness of disordered eating, amenorrhea, and osteoporosis. *Clinics in Sports Medicine*, 13(2), pp. 405–418.

Nattiv, A., Loucks, A. B., Manore, M. M. et al. (2007) American College of Sports Medicine position stand: The female athlete triad. *Medicine & Science in Sports & Exercise*, 39(10), pp. 1867–1882.

Nazem, T. G. and Ackerman, K. E. (2012) The female athlete triad. *Sports Health: A Multidisciplinary Approach*, 4(4), pp. 302–311.

Neal, B. S., Barton, C. J., Gallie, R., O'Halloran, P. and Morrissey, D. (2016) Runners with patellofemoral pain have altered biomechanics which targeted interventions can modify: A systematic review and meta analysis. *Gait Posture*, 45, pp. 69–82.

Neal, B. S., Griffiths, I. B., Dowling, G. J., Murley, G. S., Munteanu, S. E., Franettovich Smith, M. M., Collins, N. J. and Barton, C. J. (2014) Foot posture as a risk factor for lower limb overuse injury: A systematic review and meta-analysis. *Journal of Foot and Ankle Research*, 7, p. 55.

Neamatallah, Z., Herrington, L. and Jones, R. (2020) An investigation into the role of gluteal muscle strength and EMG activity in controlling hip and knee motion during landing tasks. *Physical Therapy in Sport*, 43, pp. 230–235.

Neary, J., Martin, T., Reid, D., Burnham, R. and Quinney, H. (1992) The effects of a reduced exercise duration taper programme on performance and muscle enzymes of endurance cyclists. *European Journal of Applied Physiology and Occupational Physiology*, 65(1), pp. 30–36. doi: 10.1007/BF01466271.

Nebl, J. et al. (2019) Micronutrient status of recreational runners with vegetarian or non-vegetarian dietary patterns. *Nutrients*, 11(5). doi: 10.3390/NU11051146.

Nelson, R. C., Brooks, C. M. and Pike, N. L. (1977) Biomechanical comparison of male and female distance runners. *Annals of New York Academy Science*, 301, pp. 793–807.

Neto, W. K. et al. (2020) Gluteus maximus activation during common strength and hypertrophy exercises: A systematic review. *Journal of Sports Science and Medicine*, 19(1), pp. 195–203.

Newell, J., Korir, P., Moore, B. and Pedlar, C. (2015) App for the calculation of blood lactate markers. *Journal of Sports Sciences*, 33, pp. 568–569.

Newman, P., Witchalls, J., Waddington, G. and Adams, R. (2013) Risk factors associated with medial tibial stress syndrome in runners: A systematic review and meta-analysis. *Open Access Journal of Sports Medicine*, 4, pp. 229–241.

Newsholme, E. A., Blomstrand, E. and Ekblom, B. (1992) Physical and mental fatigue: Metabolic mechanisms and importance of plasma amino acids. *British Medical Bulletin*, 48, pp. 477–495.

Nicholls, J. G. (1984) Achievement motivation: Conceptions of ability, subjective experience, task choice, and performance. *Psychological Review*, 91(3), pp. 328–346.

Nichols, J. F., Rauh, M. J., Lawson, M. J. et al. (2006) Prevalence of the female athlete triad syndrome among high school athletes. *Archives of Paediatric and Adolescent Medicine*, 160, pp. 137–142.

Nicholson, A. N., Pascoe, P. A. and Stone, B. M. (1986) Modulation of catecholamine transmission and sleep in man. *Neuropharmacology*, 25, pp. 271–274.

Nicholson, R. M. and Sleivert, G. G. (2001) Indices of lactate threshold and their relationship with 10-km running velocity. *Medicine & Science in Sports & Exercise*, 33(2), pp. 339–342.

Nicol, C., Komi, P. V. and Marconnet, P. (1991a) Effects of marathon fatigue on running kinematics and economy. *Scandinavian Journal of Medicine and Science in Sports*, 1(4), pp. 195–204. doi: 10.1111/j.1600-0838.1991.tb00296.x.hal-01644944.

Nicol, C., Komi, P. V. and Marconnet, P. (1991b) Fatigue effects of marathon running on neuromuscular performance. *Scandinavian Journal of Medicine and Science in Sports*, 1(1), pp. 10–17.

Nicol, L. M. et al. (2015) Curcumin supplementation likely attenuates delayed onset muscle soreness (DOMS). *European Journal of Applied Physiology*. doi: 10.1007/s00421-015-3152-6.

Nicolas, M., Martinent, G., Millet, G., Bagneux, V. and Gaudino, M. (2019) Time courses of emotions experienced after a mountain ultra-marathon: Does emotional intelligence matter? *Journal of Sports Sciences*, 37(16), pp. 1831–1839.

Nielsen, F. H. and Lukaski, H. C. (2006) Update on the relationship between magnesium and exercise. *Magnesium Research*, 19(3), pp. 180–189. doi: 10.1684/MRH.2006.0060.

Nielsen, R. O., Buist, I., Sorensen, H., Lind, M. and Rasmussen, S. (2012) Training errors and running related injuries: A systematic review. *International Journal of Sports Physical Therapy*, 7, pp. 58–75.

Nielsen, R. O., Parner, E. T., Nohr, E. A., Sorensen, H., Lind, M. and Rasmussen, S. (2014a) Excessive progression in weekly running distance and risk of running-related injuries: An association which varies according to type of injury. *Journal of Orthopaedic & Sports Physical Therapy*, 44, pp. 739–747.

Nielsen, R. O., Rønnow, L., Rasmussen, S. and Lind, M. (2014b) A prospective study on time to recovery in 254 injured novice runners. *PLoS One*, 9, p. e99877.

Nieman, D. C. et al. (1989) Nutrient intake of marathon runners. *Journal of the American Dietetic Association*, 89(9), pp. 1273–1278.

Niemuth, P. E. et al. (2005) Hip muscle weakness and overuse injuries in recreational runners. *Clinical Journal of Sport Medicine*, 15(1), pp. 14–21.

Nieves, J. W. et al. (2010) Nutritional factors that influence change in bone density and stress fracture risk among young female cross-country runners. *Physical Medicine and Rehabilitation*, 2(8), pp. 740–750. doi: 10.1016/J.PMRJ.2010.04.020.

Nigg, B. M. (1997) Impact forces in running. *Current Opinion in Orthopedics*, 8(6), pp. 43–47.

Noakes, T. (2002) Hyponatremia in distance runners: Fluid and sodium balance during exercise. *Current Sports Medicine Reports*, 1(4), pp. 197–207.

Noakes, T. (2003) Fluid replacement during marathon running. *Clinical Journal of Sport Medicine*, 13(5), pp. 309–318.

Noakes, T. D., Lambert, M. I. and Hauman, R. (2009) Which lap is the slowest? An analysis of 32 world mile record performances. *British Journal of Sports Medicine*, 43(10), pp. 760–764.

Noehren, B., Davis, I. and Hamill, J. (2007) ASB clinical biomechanics award winner 2006 prospective study of the biomechanical factors associated with iliotibial band syndrome. *Clinical Biomechanics*, 22, pp. 951–956.

Noehren, B., Scholz, J. and Davis, I. (2011) The effect of real-time gait retraining on hip kinematics, pain and function in subjects with patellofemoral pain syndrome. *British Journal of Sports Medicine*, 45, pp. 691–696.

Noehren, B. et al. (2012) Proximal and distal kinematics in female runners with patellofemoral pain. *Clinical Biomechanics*, 27(4), pp. 366–371. doi: 10.1016/J.CLINBIOMECH.2011.10.005.

Novacheck, T. F. (1998) The biomechanics of running. *Gait & Posture*, 7(1), pp. 77–95.

Nowak, J., Borkowska, B. and Pawlowski, B. (2016) Leukocyte changes across menstruation, ovulation, and mid-luteal phase and association with sex hormone variation. *American Journal of Human Biology*, 28(5), pp. 721–728.

Nummela, A., Heath, K. A., Paavolainen, L. M., Lambert, M. I., St Clair Gibson, A., Rusko, H. K. and Noakes, T. D. (2008) Fatigue during a 5-km running time trial. *International Journal of Sports Medicine*, 29(9), pp. 738–745.

Nummela, A., Keränen, T. and Mikkelsson, L. O. (2007) Factors related to top running speed and economy. *International Journal of Sports Medicine*, 28(8), pp. 655–661.

Nummela, A. T. et al. (2006) Neuromuscular factors determining 5 km running performance and running economy in well-trained athletes. *European Journal of Applied Physiology*, 97(1), pp. 1–8. doi: 10.1007/s00421-006-0147-3.

Nunns, M., House, C., Fallowfield, J., Allsopp, A. and Dixon, S. (2013) Biomechanical characteristics of barefoot footstrike modalities. *Journal of Biomechanics*, 46, pp. 2603–2610.

Nunns, M., House, C., Rice, H., Mostazir, M., Davey, T., Stiles, V., Fallowfield, J., Allsopp, A. and Dixon, S. (2016) Four biomechanical and anthropometric measures predict tibial stress fracture: A prospective study of 1065 Royal Marines. *British Journal of Sports Medicine*, 50(19), pp. 1206–1210.

Nuzzo, J. L., McBride, J. M., Cormie, P. and McCaulley, G. O. (2008) Relationship between counter-movement jump performance and multijoint isometric and dynamic tests of strength. *The Journal of Strength & Conditioning Research*, 22(3), pp. 699–707.

O'Brien, M. J., Viguie, C. A., Mazzeo, R. S. and Brooks, G. A. (1993) Carbohydrate dependence during marathon running. *Medicine and Science in Sports and Exercise*, 25(9), pp. 1009–1017.

Onate, J. A., Dewey, T., Kollock, R. O., Thomas, K. S., Van Lunen, B. L., DeMaio, M. and Ringleb, S. I. (2012) Real-time intersession and interrater reliability of the functional movement screen. *The Journal of Strength & Conditioning Research*, 26(2), pp. 408–415.

O'Neill, S., Barry, S. and Watson, P. (2019) Plantarflexor strength and endurance deficits associated with mid-portion Achilles tendinopathy: The role of soleus. *Physical Therapy in Sport*, 37, pp. 69–76. doi: 10.1016/J.PTSP.2019.03.002.

O'Neill, S., Watson, P. J. and Barry, S. (2016) A Delphi study of risk factors for Achilles tendinopathy-opinions of world tendon experts. *The International Journal of Sports Physical Therapy*, 11(5), pp. 684–697.

Oosthuyse, T. and Bosch, A. N. (2010) The effect of the menstrual cycle on exercise metabolism. *Sports Medicine*, 40(3), pp. 207–227.

Osu, R., Franklin, D. W., Kato, H., Gomi, H., Domen, K., Yoshioka, T. and Kawato, M. (2002) Short- and long-term changes in joint co-contraction associated with motor learning as revealed from surface EMG. *Journal of Neurophysiology*, 88(2), pp. 991–1004.

Otis, C. L., Drinkwater, B., Johnson, M., Loucks, A. and Wilmore, J. (1997) American College of Sports Medicine position stand: The female athlete triad. *Medicine & Science in Sports & Exercise*, 29(5), pp. i–ix.

Paavolainen, L. M., Hakkinen, K., Hamalainen, I., Nummela, A. and Rusko, H. (1999a) Explosive-strength training improves 5-km running time by improving running economy and muscle power. *Journal of Applied Physiology*, 86(5), pp. 1527–1533.

Paavolainen, L. M., Nummela, A. T. and Rusko, H. K. (1999b) Neuromuscular characteristics and muscle power as determinants of 5-km running performance. *Medicine and Science in Sports and Exercise*, 31(1), pp. 124–130.

Page, K. A. and Steele, J. R. (1999) Breast motion and sports brassiere design. *Sports Medicine*, 27(4), pp. 205–211.

Papoti, M., Martins, L. E., Cunha, S. A., Zagatto, A. M. and Gobatto, C. A. (2007) Effects of taper on swimming force and swimmer performance after an experimental ten-week training program. *The Journal of Strength and Conditioning Research*, 21(2), pp. 538–542. doi: 10.1519/00124278-200705000-00043.

Paradisis, G. P. and Cooke, C. B. (2001) Kinematic and postural characteristics of sprint running on sloping surfaces. *Journal of Sports Sciences*, 19(2), pp. 149–159.

Parkin, J. A. M. et al. (1997) Muscle glycogen storage following prolonged exercise: Effect of timing of ingestion of high glycemic index food. *Medicine and Science in Sports and Exercise*. doi: 10.1097/00005768-199702000-00009.

Parmar, C., West, M., Pathak, S., Nelson, J. and Martin, L. (2011) Weight versus volume in breast surgery: An observational study. *JRSM Short Reports*, 2(11), pp. 1–5.

Pasadyn, S. R., Soudan, M., Gillinov, M., Houghtaling, P., Phelan, D., Gillinov, N., Bittel, B. and Desai, M. Y. (2019) Accuracy of commercially available heart rate monitors in athletes: A prospective study. *Cardiovascular Diagnosis and Therapy*, 9, pp. 379–385.

Pasricha, S.-R. S. et al. (2010) Diagnosis and management of iron deficiency anaemia: A clinical update. *The Medical Journal of Australia*, 193(9), pp. 525–532. doi: 10.5694/J.1326-5377.2010.TB04038.X.

Pate, R. R., Macera, C. A., Bailey, S. P., Bartoli, W. P. and Powell, K. E. (1992) Physiological, anthropometric, and training correlates of running economy. *Medicine and Science in Sports and Exercise*, 24(10), pp. 1128–1133.

Patterson, E. et al. (2012) Health implications of high dietary omega-6 polyunsaturated fatty acids. *Journal of Nutrition and Metabolism*, 2012, p. 539426. doi: 10.1155/2012/539426.

Paulsen, G. et al. (2014a) Vitamin C and E supplementation alters protein signalling after a strength training session, but not muscle growth during 10 weeks of training. *Journal of Physiology*. doi: 10.1113/jphysiol.2014.279950.

Paulsen, G. et al. (2014b) Vitamin C and E supplementation hampers cellular adaptation to endurance training in humans: A double-blind, randomised, controlled trial. *The Journal of Physiology*, 592(8), pp. 1887–1901. doi: 10.1113/JPHYSIOL.2013.267419.

Payne, V. G. and Morrow, J. R. (1993) Exercise and VO2 max in children: A meta-analysis. *Research Quarterly for Exercise and Sport*, 64, pp. 305–313.

Payton, C. J. (2007) Motion analysis using video. In Payton, C. J. and Bartlett, R. M. (eds.) *Biomechanical evaluation of movement in sport and exercise*. New York: Routledge, pp. 8–32.

Peake, J. M., Kerr, G. and Sullivan, J. P. (2018) A critical review of consumer wearables, mobile applications, and equipment for providing biofeedback, monitoring stress, and sleep in physically active populations. *Frontiers in Physiology*, 9.

Peake, J. M., Markworth, J. F., Nosaka, K., Raastad, T., Wadley, G. D. and Coffey, V. G. (2015) Modulating exercise-induced hormesis: Does less equal more? *Journal of Applied Physiology (1985)*, 119, pp. 172–189. doi: 10.1152/japplphysiol.01055.2014.

Pearcey, G. E. P. et al. (2015) Foam rolling for delayed-onset muscle soreness and recovery of dynamic performance measures. *Journal of Athletic Training*. doi: 10.4085/1062-6050-50.1.01.

Pechter, E. A. (1998) A new method for determining bra size and predicting postaugmentation breast size. *Plastic and Reconstructive Surgery*, 102(4), pp. 1259–1265.

Pedlar, C. R., Newell, J. and Lewis, N. A. (2019) Blood biomarker profiling and monitoring for high-performance physiology and nutrition: Current perspectives, limitations and recommendations. *Sports Medicine*, 49, pp. 185–198.

Pedlar, C. R. et al. (2018) Iron balance and iron supplementation for the female athlete: A practical approach. *European Journal of Sport Science*, 18(2), pp. 295–305. doi: 10.1080/17461391.2017.1416178.

Pedley, J. S., Lloyd, R. S., Read, P., Moore, I. S. and Oliver, J. L. (2017) Drop jump: A technical model for scientific application. *Strength & Conditioning Journal*, 39.

Pedret, C., Rodas, G., Balius, R., Capdevila, L., Bossy, M., Vernooij, R. W. and Alomar, X. (2015) Return to play after soleus muscle injuries. *Orthopaedic Journal of Sports Medicine*, 3, p. 2325967115595802.

Peeling, P., Binnie, M. J., Goods, P. S., Sim, M. and Burke, L. M. (2018) Evidence-based supplements for the enhancement of athletic performance. *International Journal of Sport Nutrition and Exercise Metabolism*, 28(2), pp. 178–187.

Peeling, P., Dawson, B., Goodman, C., Landers, G. and Trinder, D. (2008) Athletic induced iron deficiency: New insights into the role of inflammation, cytokines and hormones. *European Journal of Applied Physiology*, 103(4), p. 381.

Peeling, P. et al. (2009) Effects of exercise on hepcidin response and iron metabolism during recovery. *International Journal of Sport Nutrition and Exercise Metabolism*, 19(6), pp. 583–597. doi: 10.1123/ IJSNEM.19.6.583.

Pellegrino, J., Ruby, B. C. and Dumke, C. L. (2016) Effect of plyometrics on the energy cost of running and MHC and titin isoforms. *Medicine and Science in Sports and Exercise*, 48(1), pp. 49–56. doi: 10.1249/MSS.0000000000000747.

Pereira, E. R., de Andrade, M. T., Mendes, T. T., Ramos, G. P., Maia-Lima, A., Melo, E. S. et al. (2017) Evaluation of hydration status by urine, body mass variation and plasma parameters during an official half-marathon. *Journal of Sports Medicine and Physical Fitness*, 57(11), pp. 1499–503.

Peronnet, F. and Massicotte, D. (1991) Table of nonprotein respiratory quotient: An update. *Canadian Journal of Sport Sciences*, 16(1), pp. 23–29.

Petkus, D. L., Murray-Kolb, L. E. and De Souza, M. J. (2017) The unexplored crossroads of the female athlete triad and iron deficiency: A narrative review. *Sports Medicine*, 47(9), pp. 1721–1737.

Pettitt, R. W., Jamnick, N. A. and Clark, I. E. (2012) 3-min all-out exercise test for running. *International Journal of Sports Medicine*, 33(6), pp. 426–431.

Pettitt, R. W., Jamnick, N. A., Kramer, M. and Dicks, N. D. (2019) A different perspective of the 3-minute all-out exercise test. *The Journal of Strength and Conditioning Research*, 33(8), pp. e223–e224.

Phillips, D., Ashford, K. J., Gittoes, M. J. R. and Moore, I. S. (2017) The effectiveness of different motor learning strategies to retrain running gait: Innovative interventions for tibial stress fractures. *British Association of Sport and Exercise Medicine*. Bath, UK.

Phillips, J. (2018) Learning from the greats: Eliud Kipchoge. https://jhprunning.com/2018/05/18/ learning-from-the-greats-eliud-kipchoge/. Accessed on 08/09/2020.

Phillips, J. et al. (2018) Effect of varying self-myofascial release duration on subsequent athletic performance. *Journal of Strength and Conditioning Research*. doi: 10.1519/jsc.0000000000002751.

Phillips, S. M., Chevalier, S. and Leidy, H. J. (2016) Protein 'requirements' beyond the RDA: Implications for optimizing health. *Applied Physiology, Nutrition, and Metabolism = Physiologie appliquee, nutrition et metabolisme*. doi: 10.1139/apnm-2015-0550.

Phillips, S. M., Tang, J. E. and Moore, D. R. (2009) The role of milk- and soy-based protein in support of muscle protein synthesis and muscle protein accretion in young and elderly persons. *Journal of the American College of Nutrition*, 28(4), pp. 343–354. doi: 10.1080/07315724.2009.10718096.

Philpott, J. D., Witard, O. C. and Galloway, S. D. R. (2019) Applications of omega-3 polyunsaturated fatty acid supplementation for sport performance. *Research in Sports Medicine*. doi: 10.1080/ 15438627.2018.1550401.

Philpott, J. D. et al. (2018) Adding fish oil to whey protein, leucine, and carbohydrate over a six-week supplementation period attenuates muscle soreness following eccentric exercise in competitive soccer players. *International Journal of Sport Nutrition and Exercise Metabolism*. doi: 10.1123/ijsnem.2017-0161.

Phinney, S. D. et al. (1983) The human metabolic response to chronic ketosis without caloric restriction: Preservation of submaximal exercise capability with reduced carbohydrate oxidation☆. *Metabolism Clinical and Experimental*, 32(8), pp. 769–776. doi: 10.1016/0026-0495(83)90106-3.

Piacentini, M. F. et al. (2013) Concurrent strength and endurance training effects on running economy in master endurance runners. *Journal of Strength and Conditioning Research*, 27(8), pp. 2295–2303. doi: 10.1519/JSC.0b013e3182794485.

Pingitore, A., Lima, G. P., Mastorci, F., Quinones, A., Iervasi, G. and Vassalle, C. (2015) Exercise and oxidative stress: Potential effects of antioxidant dietary strategies in sports. *Nutrition*, 31, pp. 916–922.

Pinnington, H. C. and Dawson, B. (2001) The energy cost of running on grass compared to soft dry beach sand. *Journal of Science and Medicine in Sport*, 4(4), pp. 416–430.

Pinshaw, R., Atlas, V. and Noakes, T. D. (1984) The nature and response to therapy of 196 consecutive injuries seen at a runners' clinic. *South African Medical Journal*, 65, pp. 291–298.

Pobiruchin, M., Suleder, J., Zowalla, R. and Wiesner, M. (2017) Accuracy and adoption of wearable technology used by active citizens: A marathon event field study. *JMIR Mhealth Uhealth*, 5, p. e24.

Pohl, M. B., Hamill, J. and Davis, I. S. (2009) Biomechanical and anatomic factors associated with a history of plantar fasciitis in female runners. *Clinical Journal of Sports Medicine*, 19, pp. 372–376.

Pohl, M. B., Mullineaux, D. R., Milner, C. E., Hamill, J. and Davis, I. S. (2008) Biomechanical predictors of retrospective tibial stress fractures in runners. *Journal of Biomechanics*, 41, pp. 1160–1165.

Pontzer, H., Holloway III, J. H. H., Raichlen, D. A. and Lieberman, D. E. (2009) Control and function of arm swing in human walking and running. *The Journal of Experimental Biology*, 212(4), pp. 523–534.

Poole, D. C., Ward, S. A. and Whipp, B. J. (1990) The effects of training on the metabolic and respiratory profile of high-intensity cycle ergometer exercise. *European Journal of Applied Physiology and Occupational Physiology*, 59(6), pp. 421–429.

Poppendieck, W. et al. (2013) Cooling and performance recovery of trained athletes: A meta-analytical review. *International Journal of Sports Physiology and Performance*. doi: 10.1123/ijspp.8.3.227.

Post, E. G., Trigsted, S. M., Schaefer, D. A. et al. (2018) Knowledge, attitudes, and beliefs of youth sports coaches regarding sport volume recommendations and sport specialization. *Journal of Strength and Conditioning Research*, published ahead of print. doi: 10.1519/JSC.0000000000002529.

Potvin, J. R., Norman, R. W. and McGill, S. M. (1991) Reduction in anterior shear forces on the L4/L5 disc by the lumbar musculature. *Clinical Biomechanics*, 6(2), pp. 88–96.

Prasad, A., Popovic, Z. B., Arbab-Zadeh, A., Fu, Q., Palmer, D., Dijk, E., Greenberg, N. L., Garcia, M. J., Thomas, J. D. and Levine, B. D. (2007) The effects of aging and physical activity on doppler measures of diastolic function. *American Journal of Cardiology*, 99(12), pp. 1629–1636.

Proctor, D. N. and Parker, B. A. (2006) Vasodilation and vascular control in contracting muscle of the aging human. *Microcirculation*, 13(4), pp. 315–327.

Pugh, J. N., Sparks, A. S., Doran, D. A., Fleming, S. C., Langan-Evans, C., Kirk, B. et al. (2019) Four weeks of probiotic supplementation reduces GI symptoms during a marathon race. *European Journal of Applied Physiology*, 119(7), pp. 1491–1501.

Pugh, L. G. C. E. (1971) The influence of wind resistance in running and walking and the mechanical efficiency of work against horizontal or vertical forces. *The Journal of Physiology*, 213(2), pp. 255–276.

Pummell, B., Harwood, C. and Lavallee, D. (2008) Jumping to the next level: A qualitative examination of within career transition in adolescent event riders. *Psychology of Sport and Exercise*, 9, pp. 427–447.

Pummell, E. K. L. and Lavallee, D. (2019) Preparing UK tennis academy players for the junior-to-senior transition: Development, implementation, and evaluation of an intervention program. *Psychology of Sport and Exercise*, 40, pp. 156–164.

Quatman-Yates, C. C., Quatman, C. E., Meszaros, A. J. et al. (2012) A systematic review of sensorimotor function during adolescence: A developmental stage of increased motor awkwardness? *British Journal of Sports Medicine*, 46(9), pp. 649–655.

Quesnele, J. J., Laframboise, M. A., Wong, J. J., Kim, P. and Wells, G. D. (2014) The effects of beta-alanine supplementation on performance: A systematic review of the literature. *International Journal of Sport Nutrition and Exercise Metabolism*, 24(1), pp. 14–27.

Quinn, T. J., Dempsey, S. L., Laroche, D. P., Mackenzie, A. M. and COOK, S. B. (2019) Step frequency training improves running economy in well-trained female runners. *Journal of Strength & Conditioning Research*. doi: 10.1519/JSC.0000000000003206.

Quinn, T. J., Manley, M. J., Aziz, J., Padham, J. L. and MacKenzie, A. M. (2011) Aging and factors related to running economy. *The Journal of Strength & Conditioning Research*, 25(11), pp. 2971–2979.

Quotetab.com (2020) Haile Gebrselassie quotes. www.quotetab.com/quote/by-haile-gebrselassie/i-love-running-and-i-will-always-run. Accessed on 08/09/2020.

Rabadán, M., Díaz, V., Calderón, F. J., Benito, P. J., Peinado, A. B. and Maffulli, N. (2011) Physiological determinants of speciality of elite middle-and long-distance runners. *Journal of Sports Sciences*, 29(9), pp. 975–982.

Racinais, S., Alonso, J. M., Coutts, A. J., Flouris, A. D., Girard, O., González-Alonso, J., Hausswirth, C., Jay, O., Lee, J. K., Mitchell, N. and Nassis, G. P. (2015) Consensus recommendations on training and competing in the heat. *Scandinavian Journal of Medicine and Science in Sports*, 25, pp. 6–19. doi: 10.1111/sms.12467.

Radowicka, M., Pietrzak, B. and Wielgos, M. (2013) Assessment of the occurrence of menstrual disorders in female flight attendants: Preliminary report and literature review. *Neuro Endocrinology Letters*, 34(8), pp. 809–813.

Rae, D. E. et al. (2017) One night of partial sleep deprivation impairs recovery from a single exercise training session. *European Journal of Applied Physiology*. doi: 10.1007/s00421-017-3565-5.

Raglin, J., Sawamura, S., Alexiou, S. et al. (2000) Training practices and staleness in 13–18-year-old swimmers: A cross-cultural study. *Paediatric Exercise Science*, 12, pp. 61–70.

Ramírez-Campillo, R., Álvarez, C., Henríquez-Olguín, C., Baez, E. B., Martínez, C., Andrade, D. C. and Izquierdo, M. (2014) Effects of plyometric training on endurance and explosive strength performance in competitive middle-and long-distance runners. *The Journal of Strength & Conditioning Research*, 28(1), pp. 97–104. doi: 10.1519/JSC.0b013e3182a1f44c.

Ramsay, J. A., Blimkie, C., Smith, K. et al. (1990) Strength training effects in prepubescent boys. *Medicine and Science in Sports and Exercise*, 22(5), pp. 605–614.

Ramsbottom, R., Nevill, A., Nevill, M., Newport, S. and Williams, C. (1994) Accumulated oxygen deficit and short-distance running performance. *Journal of Sports Sciences*, 12(5), pp. 447–453.

Ramskov, D., Barton, C., Nielsen, R. O. and Rasmussen, S. (2015) High eccentric hip abduction strength reduces the risk of developing patellofemoral pain among novice runners initiating a self-structured running program: A 1-year observational study. *Journal of Orthopaedic & Sports Physical Therapy*, 45(3), pp. 153–161.

Ratel, S. and Blazevich, A. J. (2017) Are prepubertal children metabolically comparable to well-trained adult endurance athletes? *Sports Medicine*, 47(8), pp. 1477–1485.

Rauh, M. J., Margherita, A. J., Rice, S. G., Koepsell, T. D. and Rivara, F. P. (2000) High school cross country running injuries: A longitudinal study. *Clinical Journal of Sport Medicine*, 10, pp. 110–116.

Rauh, M. J., Nichols, J. F. and Barrack, M. T. (2010) Relationships among injury and disordered eating, menstrual dysfunction, and low bone mineral density in high school athletes: A prospective study. *Journal of Athletic Training*, 45, pp. 243–252.

Ray, M. L. et al. (1998) Effect of sodium in a rehydration beverage when consumed as a fluid or meal. *Journal of Applied Physiology*, 85(4), pp. 1329–1336. doi: 10.1152/JAPPL.1998.85.4.1329.

Raysmith, B. P. and Drew, M. K. (2016) Performance success or failure is influenced by weeks lost to injury and illness in elite Australian track and field athletes: A 5-year prospective study. *Journal of Science and Medicine in Sport*, 19, pp. 778–783.

Reaburn, P. and Dascombe, B. (2008) Endurance performance in masters athletes. *European Review of Aging and Physical Activity*, 5(1), pp. 31–42.

Reaburn, P. and Dascombe, B. (2009) Anaerobic performance in masters athletes. *European Review of Aging and Physical Activity*, 6(1), pp. 39–53.

Read, P. J., Oliver, J. L., Croix, M. B. D. S., Myer, G. D. and Lloyd, R. S. (2016) Assessment of injury risk factors in male youth soccer players. *Strength & Conditioning Journal*, 38(1), pp. 12–21.

Reardon, J. (2013) Optimal pacing for running 400-and 800-m track races. *American Journal of Physics*, 81(6), pp. 428–435.

Reed, C. A., Ford, K. R., Myer, G. D. and Hewett, T. E. (2012) The effects of isolated and integrated 'core stability' training on athletic performance measures: A systematic review. *Sports Medicine*, 42, pp. 697–706.

Reid, M. B. (2016) Redox interventions to increase exercise performance. *Journal of Physiology*. doi: 10.1113/JP270653.

Reilly, T. (2000) The menstrual cycle and human performance: An overview. *Biological Rhythm Research*, 31, pp. 29–40.

Reiman, M. P., Bolgla, L. A. and Loudon, J. K. (2012) A literature review of studies evaluating gluteus maximus and gluteus medius activation during rehabilitation exercises. *Physiotherapy Theory and Practice*, 28(4), pp. 257–268.

Reisman, S., Walsh, L. D. and Proske, U. (2005) Warm-up stretches reduce sensations of stiffness and soreness after eccentric exercise. *Medicine and Science in Sports and Exercise*. doi: 10.1249/01. mss.0000170471.98084.70.

Reiss, M., Ernest, O. and Gohlitz, D. (1993) Analysis of the 1989–1992 Olympic cycle with conclusions for coaching distance running and walking events. *New Studies in Athletics*, 8(4), pp. 7–18.

Renfree, A., Crivoi do Carmo, E., Martin, L. and Peters, D. M. (2015) The influence of collective behavior on pacing in endurance competitions. *Frontiers in Physiology*, 6, p. 373.

Renfree, A., Mytton, G. J., Skorski, S. and St Clair Gibson, A. (2014a) Tactical considerations in the middle-distance running events at the 2012 Olympic Games: A case study. *International Journal of Sports Physiology and Performance*, 9(2), pp. 362–364.

Renfree, A., Martin, L., Micklewright, D. and St Clair Gibson, A. (2014b) Application of decision-making theory to the regulation of muscular work rate during self-paced competitive endurance activity. *Sports Medicine*, 44(2), pp. 147–158.

Renfree, A. and St Clair Gibson, A. (2013) Influence of different performance levels on pacing strategy during the women's World Championship marathon race. *International Journal of Sports Physiology and Performance*, 8(3), pp. 279–285.

Res, P. T. et al. (2012) Protein ingestion before sleep improves postexercise overnight recovery. *Medicine and Science in Sports and Exercise*, 44(8), pp. 1560–1569. doi: 10.1249/MSS.0B013E31824CC363.

Reynolds, J. M., Gordon, T. J. and Robergs, R. A. (2006) Prediction of one repetition maximum strength from multiple repetition maximum testing and anthropometry. *The Journal of Strength & Conditioning Research*, 20(3), pp. 584–592.

Riazati, S., Caplan, N., Matabuena, M. and Hayes, P. R. (2020) Fatigue induced changes in muscle strength and gait following two different intensity, energy expenditure matches runs. *Frontiers in Bioengineering and Biotechnology*, 8, p. 360.

Richardson, R. S., Grassi, B., Gavin, T. P., Haseler, L. J., Tagore, K., Roca, J. and Wagner, P. D. (1999) Evidence of O2 supply-dependent VO2 max in the exercise-trained human quadriceps. *Journal of Applied Physiology (1985)*, 86(3), pp. 1048–1053.

Risius, D., Milligan, A., Berns, J., Brown, N. and Scurr, J. (2016) Understanding key performance indicators for breast support: An analysis of breast support effects on biomechanical, physiological and subjective measures during running. *Journal of Sports Sciences*, 35(9), pp. 842–851.

Risius, D., Milligan, A., Mills, C. and Scurr, J. (2015) Multiplanar breast kinematics during different exercise modalities. *European Journal of Sport Science*, 15, pp. 111–117.

Rivera, A. M., Pels, A. E., Sady, S. P., Sady, M. A., Cullinane, E. M. and Thompson, P. D. (1989) Physiological factors associated with the lower maximal oxygen consumption of master runners. *Journal of Applied Physiology*, 66(2), pp. 949–954.

Robazza, C., Pellizzari, M., Bertollo, M. and Hanin, Y. L. (2008) Functional impact of emotions on athletic performance: Comparing the IZOF model and the directional perception approach. *Journal of Sports Sciences*, 26(10), pp. 1033–1047.

Roberts, G. C. and Ommundsen, Y. (1996) Effect of goal orientations on achievement beliefs, cognitions, and strategies in team sport. *Scandinavian Journal of Medicine and Science in Sport*, 6, pp. 46–56.

Roberts, J. D., Suckling, C. A., Peedle, G. Y., Murphy, J. A., Dawkins, T. G. and Roberts, M. G. (2016) An exploratory investigation of endotoxin levels in novice long distance triathletes, and the effects of a multi-strain probiotic/prebiotic, antioxidant intervention. *Nutrients*, 8(11), pp. 733, 1–18.

Roberts, J. D., Tarpey, M. D., Kass, L. S., Tarpey, R. J. and Roberts, M. G. (2014) Assessing a commercially available sports drink on exogenous carbohydrate oxidation, fluid delivery and sustained exercise performance. *Journal of the International Society of Sports Nutrition*, 11(8), pp. 1–14.

Robinson, D. M., Robinson, S. M., Hume, P. A. and Hopkins, W. G. (1991) Training intensity of elite male distance runners. *Medicine and Science in Sports and Exercise*. https://doi.org/10.1249/00005768-199109000-00013.

Rodriguez, N. R. et al. (2009) Position of the American Dietetic Association, Dietitians of Canada, and the American College of Sports Medicine: Nutrition and athletic performance. *Journal of the American Dietetic Association*, 109(3), pp. 509–527. doi: 10.1016/J.JADA.2009.01.005.

Rogers, S. A., Whatman, C. S., Pearson, S. N. and Kilding, A. E. (2017) Assessments of mechanical stiffness and relationships to performance determinants in middle-distance runners. *International Journal of Sports Physiology and Performance*, 12(10), pp. 1329–1334.

Rollo, I., Williams, C., Gant, N. and Nute, M. (2008) The influence of carbohydrate mouth rinse on self-selected speeds during a 30-min treadmill run. *International Journal of Sport Nutrition and Exercise*, 18, pp. 585–600.

Rollo, I., Williams, C. and Nevill, M. (2011) Influence of ingesting versus mouth rinsing a carbohydrate solution during a 1-h run. *Medicine and Science in Sports and Exercise*, 43(3), pp. 468–475.

Romero-Parra, N., Alfaro-Magallanes, V. M., Rael, B., Cupeiro, R., Rojo-Tirado, M. A., Benito, P. J., Peinado, A. B. and Group, I. S. (2020) Indirect markers of muscle damage throughout the menstrual cycle. *International Journal of Sports Physiology and Performance*, online ahead of print. doi: 10.1123/ijspp.2019-0727.

Rooney, B. D. and Derrick, T. R. (2013) Joint contact loading in forefoot and rearfoot strike patterns during running. *Journal of Biomechanics*, 46(13), pp. 2201–2206.

Roos, L., Taube, W., Tuch, C., Frei, K. M. and Wyss, T. (2018) Factors that influence the rating of perceived exertion after endurance training. *International Journal of Sports Physiology and Performance*, 13, pp. 1042–1049.

Roper, J. L., Harding, E. M., Doerfler, D., Dexter, J. G., Kravitz, L., Dufek, J. S. and Mermier, C. M. (2016) The effects of gait retraining in runners with patellofemoral pain: A randomized trial. *Clinical Biomechanics*, 35, pp. 14–22.

Rowland, T. W. (1985) Aerobic responses to endurance training in prepubescent children: A critical analysis. *Medicine Sport and Exercise Science*, 17, pp. 493–497.

Rowlands, D. S., Swift, M., Ros, M. and Green, J. G. (2012) Composite versus single transportable carbohydrate solution enhances race and laboratory cycling performance. *Applied Physiology Nutrition and Metabolism*, 37, pp. 425–436.

Rowlands, D. S. et al. (2014) Protein-leucine fed dose effects on muscle protein synthesis after endurance exercise. *Medicine and Science in Sports and Exercise*. doi: 10.1249/MSS.0000000000000447.

Rubaltelli, E., Agnoli, S. and Leo, I. (2018) Emotional intelligence impact on half marathon finish times. *Personality and Individual Differences*, 128, pp. 107–112.

Rubeor, A. et al. (2018) Does iron supplementation improve performance in iron-deficient nonanemic athletes? *Sports Health a Multidisciplinary Approach*, 10(5), pp. 400–405. doi: 10.1177/1941738118777488.

Ryan, M. B., Elashi, M., Newsham-West, R. and Taunton, J. (2014) Examining injury risk and pain perception in runners using minimalist footwear. *British Journal of Sports Medicine*, 48, pp. 1257–1262.

Ryan, M. B., Valiant, G. A., McDonald, K. and Taunton, J. E. (2011) The effect of three different levels of footwear stability on pain outcomes in women runners: A randomised control trial. *British Journal of Sports Medicine*, 45, pp. 715–721.

Ryan, R. M. and Deci, E. L. (2000) Self-determination theory and the facilitation of intrinsic motivation, social development, and well-being. *American Psychologist*, 55, pp. 68–78.

Sabatier, J. P., Guaydier-Souquières, G., Laroche, D. et al. (1996) Bone mineral acquisition during adolescence and early adulthood: A study in 574 healthy females 10–24 years of age. *Osteoporosis International*, 6, pp. 141–148.

Sabetta, J. R. et al. (2010) Serum 25-hydroxyvitamin d and the incidence of acute viral respiratory tract infections in healthy adults. *PLoS One*, 5(6). doi: 10.1371/JOURNAL.PONE.0011088.

Sahin, K. et al. (2016) Curcumin prevents muscle damage by regulating NF-κB and Nrf2 pathways and improves performance: An in vivo model. *Journal of Inflammation Research*. doi: 10.2147/JIR.S110873.

Sahlin, K., Tonkonogi, M. and Söderlund, K. (1998) Energy supply and muscle fatigue in humans. *Acta Physiol Scand*, 162(3), pp. 261–266.

Salive, M. E., Cornoni-Huntley, J., Guralnik, J. M., Phillips, C. L., Wallace, R. B., Ostfeld, A. M. and Cohen, H. J. (1992) Anemia and hemoglobin levels in older persons: Relationship with age, gender, and health status. *Journal of the American Geriatrics Society*, 40(5), pp. 489–496.

Saltin, B., Larsen, H., Terrados, N., Bangsbo, J., Bak, T., Kim, C. K., Svedenhag, J. and Rolf, C. J. (1995) Aerobic exercise capacity at sea level and at altitude in Kenyan boys, junior and senior runners compared with Scandinavian runners. *Scandinavian Journal of Medicine & Science in Sports*, 5(4), pp. 209–221.

Samson, A. (2014) Sources of self-efficacy during marathon training: A qualitative, longitudinal investigation. *The Sport Psychologist*, 28(2), pp. 164–175.

Samson, A., Simpson, D., Kamphoff, C. and Langlier, A. (2017) Think aloud: An examination of distance runners' thought processes. *International Journal of Sport and Exercise Psychology*, 15(2), pp. 176–189.

Sandford, G. N., Allen, S. V., Kilding, A. E., Ross, A. and Laursen, P. B. (2019a) Anaerobic speed reserve: A key component of elite male 800-m running. *International Journal of Sports Physiology and Performance*, 14(4), pp. 501–508. doi: 10.1123/IJSPP.2018-0163.

Sandford, G. N., Day, B. T. and Rogers, S. A. (2019b) Racing fast and slow: Defining the tactical behavior that differentiates medalists in elite men's 1,500 m championship racing. *Front Sports Act Living*, 1(43).

Sandford, G. N., Kilding, A. E., Ross, A. and Laursen, P. B. (2019c) Maximal sprint speed and the anaerobic speed reserve domain: The untapped tools that differentiate the world's best male 800 m runners. *Sports Medicine*, 49(6), pp. 843–852.

Sandford, G. N., Pearson, S., Allen, S. V., Malcata, R. M., Kilding, A. E., Ross, A. and Laursen, P. B. (2018) Tactical behaviors in men's 800-m Olympic and World-Championship medalists: A changing of the guard. *International Journal of Sports Physiology and Performance*, 13(2), pp. 246–249.

Sandford, G. N., Rogers, S. A., Sharma, A. P., Kilding, A. E., Ross, A. and Laursen, P. B. (2019d). Implementing anaerobic speed reserve testing in the field: Validation of v-VO2max prediction from 1500-m race performance in elite middle-distance runners. *International Journal of Sports Physiology and Performance*, 14(8), pp. 1147–1150.

Sandford, G. N. and Stellingwerff, T. (2019) 'Question your categories': The misunderstood complexity of middle-distance running profiles with implications for research methods and application. *Frontiers in Sports and Active Living*, 1, p 28. https://doi.org/10.3389/fspor.2019.00028.

Santos, I. S., Minten, G. C., Valle, N. C., Tuerlinckx, G. C., Silva, A. B., Pereira, G. A. and Carriconde, J. F. (2011) Menstrual bleeding patterns: A community-based cross-sectional study among women aged 18–45 years in Southern Brazil. *BMC Women's Health*, 11(1), p. 26.

Santos-Concejero, J., Olivan, J., Mate-Munoz, J. L., Muniesa, C., Montil, M., Tucker, R. and Lucia, A. (2015) Gait-cycle characteristics and running economy in elite Eritrean and European runners. *International Journal of Sports Physiology and Performance*, 10(3), pp. 381–387.

Santos-Lozano, A., Collado, P. S., Foster, C., Lucia, A. and Garatachea, N. (2014) Influence of sex and level on marathon pacing strategy: Insights from the New York City race. *International Journal of Sports Medicine*, 35(11), pp. 1–6.

Saragiotto, B. T. et al. (2014) What are the main risk factors for running-related injuries? *Sports Medicine*, 44(8), pp. 1153–1163. doi: 10.1007/S40279-014-0194-6.

Saunders, J. B., Ellott-Sale, K., Artiolo, G. G., Swinton, P. A., Dolan, E., Roschel, H., Sale, C. and Gualano, B. (2017) β-alanine supplementation to improve exercise capacity and performance: A systematic review and meta-analysis. *British Journal of Sports Medicine*, 51(8), pp. 658–669.

Saunders, J. B., Inman, V. T. and Eberhart, H. D. (1953) The major determinants in normal and pathological gait. *The Journal of Bone and Joint Surgery*, 35(3), pp. 543–558.

Saunders, P. U., Pyne, D. B., Telford, R. D. and Hawley, J. A. (2004) Factors effecting running economy in trained distance runners. *Sports Medicine*, 34(7), pp. 465–485.

Saunders, P. U. et al. (2006) Short-term plyometric training improves running economy in highly trained middle and long distance runners. *Journal of Strength and Conditioning Research*, 08/12/2006, 20(4), pp. 947–954. doi: 10.1519/r-18235.1.

Saunders, P. U. et al. (2010) Physiological measures tracking seasonal changes in peak running speed. *International Journal of Sports Physiology and Performance*, 5(2), pp. 230–238.

Saw, A. E., Main, L. C. and Gastin, P. B. (2016) Monitoring the athlete training response: Subjective self-reported measures trump commonly used objective measures: A systematic review. *British Journal of Sports Medicine*, 50, pp. 281–291.

Sawka, M. N., Burke, L. M., Eichner, E. R., Maughan, R. J., Montain, S. J. and Stachenfeld, N. S. (2007) American College of Sports Medicine position stand: Exercise and fluid replacement. *Medicine and Science in Sports and Exercise.* United States, 39(2), pp. 377–390. doi: 10.1249/mss.0b013e31802ca597.

Schache, A., Blanch, P., Rath, D., Wrigley, T. I. M. and Bennell, K. I. M. (2003) Differences between the sexes in the three-dimensional angular rotations of the lumbo-pelvic-hip complex during treadmill running. *Journal of Sports Sciences*, 21, pp. 105–118.

Schieber, M. and Chandel, N. S. (2014) ROS function in redox signaling and oxidative stress. *Current Biology*, 24(10). doi: 10.1016/J.CUB.2014.03.034.

Schmidt, W. and Prommer, N. (2010) Impact of alterations in total hemoglobin mass on VO2max. *Exercise and Sport Sciences Reviews*, 38(2), pp. 68–75.

Schmitz, A., Russo, K., Edwards, L. and Noehren, B. (2014) Do novice runners have weak hips and bad running form? *Gait & Posture*, 40, pp. 82–86.

Schoeller, D. A., Taylor, P. B. and Shay, K. (1995) Analytic requirements for the doubly labeled water method. *Obesity research*, 3(Suppl. 1), pp. 15–20.

Schoene, R. B. (2001) Limits of human lung function at high altitude. *The Journal of Experimental Biology*, 204(18), pp. 3121–3127.

Scholz, M. N., Bobbert, M. F., van Soest, A. J., Clark, J. R. and van Heerden, J. (2008) Running biomechanics: Shorter heels, better economy. *The Journal of Experimental Biology*, 211(20), pp. 3266–3271.

Schücker, L., Knopf, C., Strauss, B. and Hagemann, N. (2014) An internal focus of attention is not always as bad as its reputation: How specific aspects of internally focused attention do not hinder running efficiency. *Journal of Sport and Exercise Psychology*, 36(3), pp. 233–243.

Schuermans, J., Danneels, L., Van Tiggelen, D., Palmans, T. and Witvrouw, E. (2017a) Proximal neuromuscular control protects against hamstring injuries in male soccer players: A prospective study with electromyography time-series analysis during maximal sprinting. *American Journal of Sports Medicine*, 45, pp. 1315–1325.

Schuermans, J., Van Tiggelen, D., Palmans, T., Danneels, L. and Witvrouw, E. (2017b) Deviating running kinematics and hamstring injury susceptibility in male soccer players: Cause or consequence? *Gait Posture*, 57, pp. 270–277.

Schwanbeck, S., Chilibeck, P. D. and Binsted, G. (2009) A comparison of free weight squat to Smith machine squat using electromyography. *Journal of Strength and Conditioning Research*, 23(9), pp. 2588–2591. doi: 10.1519/JSC.0b013e3181b1b181.

Schweickle, M., Groves, S., Vella, S. and Swann, C. (2017) The effects of open vs. specific goals on flow and clutch states in a cognitive task. *Psychology of Sport and Exercise*, 33, pp. 45–54.

Scurr, J. C., Brown, N., Smith, J., Brasher, A., Risius, D. and Marczyk, A. (2016) The influence of the breast on sport and exercise participation in school girls in the United Kingdom. *Journal of Adolescent Health*, 58(2), pp. 167–173.

Scurr, J. C., White, J. L. and Hedger, W. (2009) Breast displacement in three dimensions during the walking and running gait cycles. *Journal of Applied Biomechanics*, 25(4), pp. 322–329.

Scurr, J. C., White, J. L. and Hedger, W. (2010) The effect of breast support on the kinematics of the breast during the running gait cycle. *Journal of Sports Sciences*, 28, pp. 1103–1109.

Scurr, J. C., White, J. L. and Hedger, W. (2011) Supported and unsupported breast displacement in three dimensions across treadmill activity levels. *Journal of Sports Sciences*, 29(1), pp. 55–61.

Seiler, S. (2010) What is best practice for training intensity and duration distribution in endurance athletes? *International Journal of Sports Physiology and Performance.* https://doi.org/10.1123/ijspp.5.3.276.

Seiler, S. and Tønnessen, E. (2009) Intervals, thresholds, and long slow distance: The role of intensity and duration in endurance training. *Sportscience*, 13.

Seitz, L. B. et al. (2014) Increases in lower-body strength transfer positively to sprint performance: A systematic review with meta-analysis. *Sports Medicine*, 44(12), pp. 1693–1702.

Seki, H. et al. (2010) The anti-inflammatory and proresolving mediator resolvin e1 protects mice from bacterial pneumonia and acute lung injury. *The Journal of Immunology.* doi: 10.4049/jimmunol.0901809.

Serafini, M. and Peluso, I. (2017) Functional foods for health: The interrelated antioxidant and anti-inflammatory role of fruits, vegetables, herbs, spices and cocoa in humans. *Current Pharmaceutical Design*, 22(44), pp. 6701–6715.

Serhan, C. N. and Petasis, N. A. (2011) Resolvins and protectins in inflammation resolution. *Chemical Reviews*. doi: 10.1021/cr100396c.

Serpell, B. G., Ball, N. B., Scarvell, J. M. and Smith, P. N. (2012) A review of models of vertical, leg, and knee stiffness in adults for running, jumping or hopping tasks. *Journal of Sports Sciences*, 30(13), pp. 1347–1363.

Sharma, A. P., Saunders, P. U., Garvican-Lewis, L. A., Périard, J. D., Clark, B., Gore, C. J., Raysmith, B. P., Stanley, J., Robertson, E. Y. and Thompson, K. G. (2018) Training quantification and periodization during live high train high at 2100 M in elite runners: An observational cohort case study. *Journal of Sports Science and Medicine*, 17(4), pp. 607–616.

Shaw, A. J., Ingham, S. A. and Folland, J. P. (2014) The valid measurement of running economy in runners. *Medicine & Science in Sports & Exercise*, 46(10), pp. 1968–1973.

Shaw, D. M. et al. (2019) Effect of a ketogenic diet on submaximal exercise capacity and efficiency in runners. *Medicine and Science in Sports and Exercise*, 51(10), pp. 2135–2146. doi: 10.1249/MSS.0000000000002008.

Sheerin, K. R., Reid, D., Taylor, D. and Besier, T. F. (2020) The effectiveness of real-time haptic feedback gait retraining for reducing resultant tibial acceleration with runners. *Physical Therapy in Sport*, 43, pp. 173–180.

Shepley, B., MacDougall, J. D., Cipriano, N., Sutton, J. R., Tarnopolsky, M. A. and Coates, G. (1992) Physiological effects of tapering in highly trained athletes. *Journal of Applied Physiology*, 72(2), pp. 706–711. doi: 10.1152/jappl.1992.72.2.706.

Sherman, W. M., Costill, D. L., Fink, W. J. and Miller, J. M. (1981) Effect of exercise-diet manipulation on muscle glycogen and its subsequent utilization during performance. *International Journal of Sports Medicine*, 2(2), pp. 114–118.

Shibli, S. and Barrett, D. (2011) *Bridging the gap: Research to provide insight into the development and retention of young athletes*. London: Sport Industry Research Centre for England Athletics.

Shih, Y., Lin, K.-L. and Shiang, T.-Y. (2013) Is the foot striking pattern more important than barefoot or shod conditions in running? *Gait and Posture*, 38(3), pp. 490–494.

Shimizu, K., Suzuki, N., Nakamura, M. et al. (2012) Mucosal immune function comparison between amenorrheic and eumenorrheic distance runners. *The Journal of Strength and Conditioning Research*, 26(5), pp. 1402–1406.

Shing, C. M., Peake, J. M., Lim, C. L., Briskey, D., Walsh, N. P., Fortes, M. B. et al. (2014) Effects of probiotics supplementation on gastrointestinal permeability, inflammation and exercise performance in the heat. *European Journal of Applied Physiology*, 114(1), pp. 93–103.

Shirreffs, S. M. and Maughan, R. J. (1998) Volume repletion after exercise-induced volume depletion in humans: Replacement of water and sodium losses. *American Journal of Physiology Renal Physiology*, 274(5). doi: 10.1152/AJPRENAL.1998.274.5.F868.

Shirreffs, S. M., Taylor, A. J., Leiper, J. B. and Maughan, R. J. (1996) Post-exercise rehydration in man: Effects of volume consumed and drink sodium content. *Medicine and Science in Sports and Exercise*, 28(10), pp. 1260–1271.

Shivitz, N. L. (2001) Adaptation of vertical ground reaction force due to changes in breast support in running (Master of Science Thesis). Oregon State University, Corvallis, OR, USA.

Shrier, I. (2004) Does stretching improve performance?: A systematic and critical review of the literature. *Clinical Journal of Sport Medicine*, 14(5), pp. 267–273.

Siegel, A. J., Hennekens, C. H., Solomon, H. S. and Boeckel, B. V. (1979) Exercise-related hematuria: Findings in a group of marathon runners. *Journal of the American Medical Association*, 241(4), pp. 391–392.

Siewe, J., Rudat, J., Röllinghoff, M., Schlegel, U. J., Eysel, P. and Michael, J. P. (2011) Injuries and overuse syndromes in powerlifting. *International Journal of Sports Medicine*, 32(9), pp. 703–711.

Silva, T. d. A. e., de Souza, M. E. D. C. A., de Amorim, J. F., Stathis, C. G., Leandro, C. G. and Lima-Silva, A. E. (2013) Can carbohydrate mouth rinse improve performance during exercise? A systematic review. *Nutrients*, 6, pp. 1–10.

Sim, M. et al. (2019) Iron considerations for the athlete: A narrative review. *European Journal of Applied Physiology*, 119(7), pp. 1463–1478. doi: 10.1007/S00421-019-04157-Y.

Sinnett, A. M., Berg, K., Latin, R. W. and Noble, J. M. (2001) The relationship between field tests of anaerobic power and 10-km run performance. *The Journal of Strength & Conditioning Research*, 15(4), pp. 405–412.

Sjödin, B., Jacobs, I. and Svedenhag, J. (1982) Changes in onset of blood lactate accumulation (OBLA) and muscle enzymes after training at OBLA. *European Journal of Applied Physiology and Occupational Physiology*, 49(1), pp. 45–57.

Skinner, J. S. and McLellan, T. H. (1980) The transition from aerobic to anaerobic metabolism. *Research Quarterly for Exercise and Sport.* https://doi.org/10.1080/02701367.1980.10609285.

Skovgaard, C. et al. (2014) Concurrent speed endurance and resistance training improves performance, running economy, and muscle NHE1 in moderately trained runners. *Journal of Applied Physiology*, 117(10), pp. 1097–1109. doi: 10.1152/japplphysiol.01226.2013.

Smith, B. E., Selfe, J., Thacker, D., Hendrick, P., Bateman, M., Moffatt, F., Rathleff, M. S., Smith, T. O. and Logan, P. (2018) Incidence and prevalence of patellofemoral pain: A systematic review and meta-analysis. *PLoS One*, 13, p. e0190892.

Smith, C. G. and Jones, A. M. (2001) The relationship between critical velocity, maximal lactate steady-state velocity and lactate turnpoint velocity in runners. *European Journal of Applied Physiology*, 85(1–2), pp. 19–26.

Smith, D., Telford, R., Peltola, E. and Tumilty, D. (2000) Protocols for the physiological assessment of high performance runners. In Gore, C. J. (ed.) *Physiological test for elite athletes*. Champagne, IL: Human Kinetics, pp. 334–344.

Smith, D. J. (2003) A framework for understanding the training process leading to elite performance. *Sports Medicine*, 33(15), pp. 1103–1126. doi: 10.2165/00007256-200333150-00003.

Smith, E. P., Boyd, J., Frank, G. R., Takahashi, H., Cohen, R. M., Specker, B., Williams, T. C., Lubahn, D. B. and Korach, K. S. (1995) Estrogen resistance caused by a mutation in the estrogen-receptor gene in a man. *Obstetrical & Gynecological Survey*, 50(3), pp. 201–204.

Smith, J. J., Eather, N., Morgan, P. J. et al. (2014) The health benefits of muscular fitness for children and adolescents: A systematic review and meta-analysis. *Sports Medicine*, 44(9), pp. 1209–1223.

Smith, L. L. et al. (1994) The effects of athletic massage on delayed onset muscle soreness, creatine kinase, and neutrophil count: A preliminary report. *Journal of Orthopaedic and Sports Physical Therapy.* doi: 10.2519/jospt.1994.19.2.93.

Smith, L. C. and Hanley, B. (2013) Comparisons between swing phase characteristics of race walkers and distance runners. *International Journal of Exercise Science*, 6(4), pp. 269–277.

Smith, S., Chester, N. and Close, G. (2015) Supplement use in sport: A worrying game of Russian roulette for athletes today. *Professional Strength and Conditioning*, 38, pp. 9–15.

Snyder, K. L., Kram, R. and Gottschall, J. S. (2012) The role of elastic energy storage and recovery in downhill and uphill running. *The Journal of Experimental Biology*, 215(13), pp. 2283–2287.

Soligard, T., Schwellnus, M., Alonso, J. M., Bahr, R., Clarsen, B., Dijkstra, H. P., Gabbett, T., Gleeson, M., Hägglund, M., Hutchinson, M. R., Janse Van Rensburg, C., Khan, K. M., Meeusen, R., Orchard, J. W., Pluim, B. M., Raftery, M., Budgett, R. and Engebretsen, L. (2016) How much is too much? (Part 1) International Olympic Committee consensus statement on load in sport and risk of injury. *British Journal of Sports Medicine*, 50, pp. 1030–1041.

Solinas, M., Ferré, S., You, Z. B., Karcz-Kubicha, M., Popoli, P. and Goldberg, S. R. (2002) Caffeine induces dopamine and glutamate release in the shell of the nucleus accumbens. *Journal of Neuroscience*, 22, pp. 6321–6324.

Sorbini, C. A., Grassi, V., Solinas, E. and Muiesan, G. (1968) Arterial oxygen tension in relation to age in healthy subjects. *Respiration*, 25(1), pp. 3–13.

Souza, A., Fillenbaum, G. and Blay, S. (2015) Prevalence and correlates of physical inactivity among older adults in Rio Grande do Sul, Brazil. *PLoS One*, 10(2), p. e0117060. https://doi.org/10.1371/journal.pone.0117060.

Souza, R. B. and Powers, C. M. (2009) Differences in hip kinematics, muscle strength, and muscle activation between subjects with and without patellofemoral pain. *Journal of Orthopaedic & Sports Physical Therapy*, 39, pp. 12–19.

Spencer, M. R. and Gastin, P. B. (2001) Energy system contribution during 200- to 1500-m running in highly trained athletes. *Medicine and Science in Sports and Exercise*, 33(1), pp. 157–162. https://doi.org/10.1097/00005768-200101000-00024.

Spilsbury, K. L., Fudge, B. W., Ingham, S. A., Faulkner, S. H. and Nimmo, M. A. (2015) Tapering strategies in elite British endurance runners. *European Journal of Sport Science*, 15(5), pp. 367–373. doi: 10.1080/17461391.2014.955128.

Spilsbury, K. L., Nimmo, M. A., Fudge, B. W., Pringle, J. S., Orme, M. W. and Faulkner, S. H. (2019) Effects of an increase in intensity during tapering on 1500-m running performance. *Applied Physiology, Nutrition, and Metabolism*, 44(7), pp. 783–790. doi: 10.1139/apnm-2018-0551.

Spriet, L. L. (2014) New insights into the interaction of carbohydrate and fat metabolism during exercise. *Sports Medicine*, 44(1), pp. 87–96. doi: 10.1007/S40279-014-0154-1.

Spurrs, R. W., Murphy, A. J. and Watsford, M. L. (2003) The effect of plyometric training on distance running performance. *European Journal of Applied Physiology*, 89(1), pp. 1–7.

Stanley, D. M., Lane, A. M., Devonport, T. J. and Beedie, C. J. (2012) I run to feel better, so why am I thinking so negatively. *International Journal of Psychology and Behavioral Sciences*, 2(6), pp. 208–213.

Starr, C., Branson, D., Shehab, R., Farr, C., Ownbey, S. and Swinney, J. (2005) Biomechanical analysis of a prototype sports bra. *Journal of Textile and Apparel, Technology and Management*, 4(3), pp. 1–14.

Statista (2018) Share of children aged 11 to 15 participating in sports in the last 4 weeks in England in 2017/18, by activity. www.statista.com/statistics/421571/children-11-15-sport-activity-involvment-england-uk/. Accessed on 08/01/2020.

St Clair Gibson, A., Lambert, E. V., Rauch, L. H., Tucker, R., Baden, D. A., Foster, C. and Noakes, T. D. (2006) The role of information processing between the brain and peripheral physiological systems in pacing and perception of effort. *Sports Medicine*, 36(8), pp. 705–722.

Stearne, S. M., Alderson, J. A., Green, B. A., Donnelly, C. J. and Rubenson, J. (2014) Joint kinetics in rearfoot versus forefoot running: Implications of switching technique. *Medicine and Science in Sports and Exercise*, 46(8), pp. 1578–1587.

Stegeman, B. H., Bastos, M. de, Rosendaal, F. R., Vlieg, A. van H., Helmerhorst, F. M., Stijnen, T. and Dekkers, O. M. (2013) Different combined oral contraceptives and the risk of venous thrombosis: Systematic review and network meta-analysis. *British Medical Journal*, 347, p. f5298.

Steib, S. et al. (2017) Dose-response relationship of neuromuscular training for injury prevention in youth athletes: A meta-analysis. *Frontiers in Physiology*, 8, p. 920.

Stellingwerff, T. (2012) Case study: Nutrition and training periodization in three elite marathon runners. *International Journal of Sport Nutrition and Exercise Metabolism*, 22(5), pp. 392–400. doi: 10.1123/IJSNEM.22.5.392.

Stellingwerff, T. (2018) Case study: Body composition periodization in an Olympic-level female middle-distance runner over a 9-year career. *International Journal of Sport Nutrition and Exercise Metabolism*, 28(4), pp. 428–433. doi: 10.1123/ijsnem.2017-0312.

Stellingwerff, T. et al. (2006) Decreased PDH activation and glycogenolysis during exercise following fat adaptation with carbohydrate restoration. *American Journal of Physiology Endocrinology and Metabolism*, 290(2). doi: 10.1152/AJPENDO.00268.2005.

Stellingwerff, T., Morton, J. P. and Burke, L. M. (2019) A framework for periodized nutrition for athletics. *International Journal of Sport Nutrition and Exercise Metabolism*, 29(2), pp. 141–151. doi: 10.1123/IJSNEM.2018-0305.

Ste-Marie, D., Vertes, K., Rymal, A. and Martini, R. (2011) Feedforward self-modeling enhances skill acquisition in children learning trampoline skills. *Frontiers in Psychology*, 2.

Stepto, N. K., Patten, R. K., Tassone, E. C., Misso, M. L., Brennan, L., Boyle, J., Boyle, R. A., Harrison, C. L., Hirschberg, A. L., Marsh, K., Moreno-Asso, A., Redman, L., Thondan, M., Wijeyaratne, C., Teede, H. J. and Moran, L. J. (2019) Exercise recommendations for women with polycystic ovary syndrome: Is the evidence enough? *Sports Medicine*, 49(8), pp. 1143–1157.

Stickler, L., Finley, M. and Gulgin, H. (2015) Relationship between hip and core strength and frontal plane alignment during a single leg squat. *Physical Therapy in Sport*, 16(1), pp. 66–71.

Stiles, V. H., Pearce, M., Moore, I. S., Langford, J. and Rowlands, A. V. (2018) Wrist-worn accelerometry for runners: Objective quantification of training load. *Medicine and Science in Sports and Exercise*, 50, pp. 2277–2284.

Stodden, D. F., True, L. K., Langendorfer, S. J. and Gao, Z. (2013) Associations among selected motor skills and health-related fitness: Indirect evidence for Seefeldt's proficiency barrier in young adults? *Research Quarterly for Exercise and Sport*, 84(3), pp. 397–403.

Stöggl, T. L. and Sperlich, B. (2014) Polarized training has greater impact on key endurance variables than threshold, high intensity, or high volume training. *Frontiers in Physiology*. https://doi.org/10.3389/fphys.2014.00033.

Stöggl, T. L. and Sperlich, B. (2015) The training intensity distribution among well-trained and elite endurance athletes. *Frontiers in Physiology*. https://doi.org/10.3389/fphys.2015.00295.

Stone, A. A., Bachrach, C. A., Jobe, J. B., Kurtzman, H. S. and Cain, V. S. (1999) *The science of self-report: Implications for research and practice*. London, UK: Psychology Press.

Storen, O. et al. (2008) Maximal strength training improves running economy in distance runners. *Medicine and Science in Sports and Exercise*, 40(6), pp. 1087–1092. doi: 10.1249/MSS.0b013e318168da2f.

Stratton, G. and Oliver, J. L. (2014) The impact of growth and maturation on physical performance. In Lloyd, R. S. and Oliver, J. L. (eds.) *Strength and conditioning for young athletes*. London, UK: Routledge, p. 4.

Stuart, S. D. F., Wang, L., Woodard, W. R., Ng, G. A., Habecker, B. A. and Ripplinger, C. M. (2018) Age-related changes in cardiac electrophysiology and calcium handling in response to sympathetic nerve stimulation. *The Journal of Physiology*, 596(17), pp. 3977–3991.

Sung, E., Han, A., Hinrichs, T., Vorgerd, M., Manchado, C. and Platen, P. (2014) Effects of follicular versus luteal phase-based strength training in young women. *SpringerPlus*, 3(1), p. 668.

Svedenhag, J. and Sjödin, B. (1984) Maximal and submaximal oxygen uptakes and blood lactate levels in elite male middle-and long-distance runners. *International Journal of Sports Medicine*, 5(5), pp. 255–261.

Svedenhag, J. and Sjodin, B. (1985) Physiological characteristics of elite male runners in and off-season. *Canadian Journal of Applied Sport Sciences*, 10(3), pp. 127–133.

Swinton, P. A., Lloyd, R., Keogh, J. W., Agouris, I. and Stewart, A. D. (2012) A biomechanical comparison of the traditional squat, powerlifting squat, and box squat. *The Journal of Strength & Conditioning Research*, 26(7), pp. 1805–1816.

Tachtsis, B., Camera, D. and Lacham-Kaplan, O. (2018) Potential roles of n-3 PUFAs during skeletal muscle growth and regeneration. *Nutrients*. doi: 10.3390/nu10030309.

Talanian, J. L. and Spriet, L. L. (2016) Low and moderate doses of caffeine late in exercise improve performance in trained cyclists. *Applied Physiology, Nutrition, and Metabolism*, 41(8), pp. 850–855.

Tanabe, Y. et al. (2015) Attenuation of indirect markers of eccentric exercise-induced muscle damage by curcumin. *European Journal of Applied Physiology*. doi: 10.1007/s00421-015-3170-4.

Tanaka, H. and Seals, D. R. (2003) Invited review: Dynamic exercise performance in masters athletes: Insight into the effects of primary human aging on physiological functional capacity. *Journal of Applied Physiology*, 95(5), pp. 2152–2162.

Tanaka, H. and Seals, D. R. (2008) Endurance exercise performance in masters athletes: Age-associated changes and underlying physiological mechanisms. *Journal of Physiology*, 586(1), pp. 55–63.

Tanaka, K., Matsuura, Y., Matsuzaka, A., Hirakoba, K., Kumagai, S., Sun, S. O. and Asano, K. (1984) A longitudinal assessment of anaerobic threshold and distance-running performance. *Medicine and Science in Sports and Exercise*, 16(3), pp. 278–282.

Tanaka, K., Takeshima, N., Kato, T., Niihata, S. and Ueda, K. (1990) Critical determinants of endurance performance in middle-aged and elderly endurance runners with heterogeneous training habits. *European Journal of Applied Physiology and Occupational Physiology*, 59(6), pp. 443–449.

Tang, J. E. et al. (2009) Ingestion of whey hydrolysate, casein, or soy protein isolate: Effects on mixed muscle protein synthesis at rest and following resistance exercise in young men. *Journal of Applied Physiology*. doi: 10.1152/japplphysiol.00076.2009.

Tanner, J. (1949) Fallacy of per-weight and per-surface area standards, and their relation to spurious correlation. *Journal of Applied Physiology*, 2(1), pp. 1–15.

Tarnopolsky, M. A. (2004) Protein requirements for endurance athletes. *European Journal of Sport Science*, 4(1), pp. 1–15.

Tarnopolsky, M. A. (2008) Effect of caffeine on the neuromuscular system-potential as an ergogenic aid. *Applied Physiology, Nutrition, and Metabolism*, 33, pp. 1284–1289.

Tarnopolsky, M. A. (2010) Caffeine and creatine use in sport. *Annals of Nutrition and Metabolism*, 57, pp. 1–8.

Telford, R. D., Sly, G. J., Hahn, A. G., Cunningham, R. B., Bryant, C. and Smith, J. A. (2003) Foot-strike is the major cause of hemolysis during running. *Journal of Applied Physiology*, 94(1), pp. 38–42.

Telhan, G., Franz, J. R., Dicharry, J., Wilder, R. P., Riley, P. O. and Kerrigan, D. C. (2010) Lower limb joint kinetics during moderately sloped running. *Journal of Athletic Training*, 45(1), pp. 16–21.

Tenenbaum, G., Spence, R. and Christensen, S. (1999) The effect of goal difficulty and goal orientation on running performance in young female athletes. *Australian Journal of Psychology*, 51, pp. 6–11.

Tenforde, A. S., Barrack, M. T., Nattiv, A. and Fredericson, M. (2016) Parallels with the female athlete triad in male athletes. *Sports Medicine*, 46(2), pp. 171–182. doi: 10.1007/S40279-015-0411-Y.

Tenforde, A. S., Sayres, L. C., McCurdy, M. L., Sainani, K. L. and Fredericson, M. (2013) Identifying sex-specific risk factors for stress fractures in adolescent runners. *Medicine & Science in Sports & Exercise*, 45, pp. 1843–1851.

Tenforde, A. S. et al. (2018) Sport and triad risk factors influence bone mineral density in collegiate athletes. *Medicine and Science in Sport and Exercise*, 50(12), pp. 2536–2543. doi: 10.1249/MSS.0000000000001711.

Terblanche, S. et al. (1992) Failure of magnesium supplementation to influence marathon running performance or recovery in magnesium-replete subjects. *International Journal of Sport Nutrition*, 2, pp. 154–164. doi: 10.1123/ijsn.2.2.154.

Thaloor, D. et al. (1999) Systemic administration of the NF-κB inhibitor curcumin stimulates muscle regeneration after traumatic injury. *American Journal of Physiology-Cell Physiology*. doi: 10.1152/ajpcell.1999.277.2.c320.

Thein-Nissenbaum, J. (2013) Long term consequences of the female athlete triad. *Maturitas*, 75, pp. 107–112.

Thiel, C., Foster, C., Banzer, W. and de Koning, J. (2012) Pacing in Olympic track races: Competitive tactics versus best performance strategy. *Journal of Sports Sciences*, 30(11), pp. 1107–1115.

Thijs, Y., Pattyn, E., Van Tiggelen, D., Rombaut, L. and Witvrouw, E. (2011) Is hip muscle weakness a predisposing factor for patellofemoral pain in female novice runners? A prospective study. *American Journal of Sports Medicine*, 39, pp. 1877–1882.

Thomas, D. Q., Fernhall, B. and Granat, H. (1999) Changes in running economy during a 5-km run in trained men and women runners. *Journal of Strength and Conditioning Research*, 13(2), pp. 162–167.

Thomas, D. T., Erdman, K. A. and Burke, L. M. (2016a) American College of Sports Medicine joint position statement: Nutrition and athletic performance. *Medicie and Science in Sports and Exercise*. doi: 10.1249/MSS.0000000000000852.

Thomas, D. T., Erdman, K. A. and Burke, L. M. (2016b) Position of the academy of nutrition and dietetics, dietitians of Canada, and the American College of Sports Medicine: Nutrition and athletic performance. *Journal of the Academy of Nutrition and Dietetics*, 116, pp. 501–528.

Thomas, L., Mujika, I. and Busso, T. (2008) A model study of optimal training reduction during pre-event taper in elite swimmers. *Journal of Sports Sciences*, 26(6), pp. 643–652. doi: 10.1080/02640410701716782.

Thomas, L., Mujika, I. and Busso, T. (2009) Computer simulations assessing the potential performance benefit of a final increase in training during pre-event taper. *The Journal of Strength and Conditioning Research*, 23(6), pp. 1729–1736. doi: 10.1519/JSC.0b013e3181b3dfa1.

Thompson, M. A. (2017) Physiological and biomechanical mechanisms of distance specific human running performance. *Integrative and Comparative Biology*, 57(2), pp. 293–300.

Thompson, P. J. L. (2007) Perspectives on coaching pace skill in distance running: A commentary. *International Journal of Sports Science and Coaching*, 2(3), pp. 219–221.

Thurlbeck, W. M. and Angus, G. E. (1975) Growth and aging of the normal human lung. *Chest*, 67(Suppl. 2), pp. 3S–6S.

Tiller, N. B., Roberts, J. D., Beasley, L., Chapman, S., Pinto, J. M., Smith, L. (2019) International society of sports nutrition position stand: Nutritional considerations for single-stage ultra-marathon training and racing. *Journal of the International Society of Sports Nutrition*, 16(1 & 50), pp. 1–23. doi: 10.1186/S12970-019-0312-9.

Tillin, N. A. and Folland, J. P. (2014) Maximal and explosive strength training elicit distinct neuromuscular adaptations, specific to the training stimulus. *European Journal of Applied Physiology*, 114(2), pp. 365–374.

Timeoutdoors.com (2020) How to achieve your running goal. www.timeoutdoors.com/expert-advice/running/training/how-to-achieve-your-running-goal. Accessed on 08/09/2020.

Tipton, K. D., Hamilton, D. L. and Gallagher, I. J. (2018) Assessing the role of muscle protein breakdown in response to nutrition and exercise in humans. *Sports Medicine*. doi: 10.1007/s40279-017-0845-5.

Tipton, K. D. and Wolfe, R. R. (2001) Exercise, protein metabolism, and muscle growth. *International Journal of Sport Nutrition*. doi: 10.1123/ijsnem.11.1.109.

Tjelta, L. I. (2013) A longitudinal case study of the training of the 2012 European 1500 m track champion. *International Journal of Applied Sports Sciences*, 25(1), pp. 11–18.

Tjelta, L. I. (2016) The training of international level distance runners. *International Journal of Sports Science & Coaching*, 11(1), pp. 122–134. https://doi.org/10.1177/1747954115624813.

Tjelta, L. I. (2019) Three Norwegian brothers all European 1500 m champions: What is the secret? *International Journal of Sports Science & Coaching*, 14(5), pp. 694–700. https://doi.org/10.1177/1747954119872321.

Tjelta, L. I. and Enoksen, E. (2001) Training volume and intensity. In Bangsbo, J. and Larsen, H. B. (eds.) *Running and science: In an interdisciplinary perspective*. Copenhagen: Institute of Exercise and Sport Sciences, University of Copenhagen, Munksgaard, pp. 149–177.

Tjelta, L. I. and Kristiansen, I. (2015) Analysis of Ingrid Kristiansens training diary from the season 1985. Unpublished material.

Tjelta, L. I., Tønnessen, E. and Enoksen, E. (2014) A case study of the training of nine times New York marathon winner Grete Waitz. *International Journal of Sports Science and Coaching*. https://doi.org/10.1260/1747-9541.9.1.139.

Toner, J. and Moran, A. (2015) Enhancing performance proficiency at the expert level: Considering the role of 'somaesthetic awareness'. *Psychology of Sport and Exercise*, 16, pp. 110–117.

Tong, J. W. and Kong, P. W. (2013) Association between foot type and lower extremity injuries: Systematic literature review with meta-analysis. *Journal of Orthopaedic & Sports Physical Therapy*, 43, pp. 700–714.

Toresdahl, B. G. et al. (2020) A randomized study of a strength training program to prevent injuries in runners of the New York City marathon. *Sports Health: A Multidisciplinary Approach*, 12(1). doi: 10.1177/1941738119877180.

Torres, R., Appell, H. J. and Duarte, J. A. (2007) Acute effects of stretching on muscle stiffness after a bout of exhaustive eccentric exercise. *International Journal of Sports Medicine*, 28(7), pp. 590–594.

Townsend, R. et al. (2017) The effect of postexercise carbohydrate and protein ingestion on bone metabolism. *Medicine and Science in Sports and Exercise*. doi: 10.1249/MSS.0000000000001211.

Trappe, S. W. (2007) Marathon runners: How do they age? *Sports Medicine*, 37(4–5), pp. 302–305.

Trappe, S. W., Costill, D. L., Fink, W. J. and Pearson, D. R. (1995) Skeletal muscle characteristics among distance runners: A 20-yr follow-up study. *Journal of Applied Physiology*, 78(3), pp. 823–829.

Trappe, S. W., Costill, D. L., Vukovich, M. D., Jones, J. and Melham, T. (1996) Aging among elite distance runners: A 22-yr longitudinal study. *Journal of Applied Physiology*, 80(1), pp. 285–290.

Trappe, T. (2009) Influence of aging and long-term unloading on the structure and function of human skeletal muscle. *Applied Physiology of Nutrition and Metabolism*, 34(3), pp. 459–464.

Trehearn, T. L. and Buresh, R. J. (2009) Sit-and-reach flexibility and running economy of men and women collegiate distance runners. *The Journal of Strength & Conditioning Research*, 23(1), pp. 158–162.

Trenchard, H., Renfree, A. and Peters, D. M. (2016) A computer model of drafting effects on collective behavior in elite 10,000 m runners. *International Journal of Sports Physiology and Performance*, 12(3), pp. 345–350.

Trenell, M. I. et al. (2006) Compression garments and recovery from eccentric exercise: A31P-MRS study. *Journal of Sports Science and Medicine*, 5(1), pp. 106–114.

Trengrove, A. (2018) *The Golden Mile: Herb Elliotts biography as told by Alan Tengrove*. 2nd edn. South Fremantle, Western Australia: Runners Tribe Books.

Trexler, E. T., Smith-Ryan, A. E., Stout, J. R., Hoffman, J. R., Wilborn, C. D., Sale, C. et al. (2015) International society of sports nutrition position stand: Beta-Alanine. *Journal of the International Society of Sports Nutrition*, 12(30), pp. 1–14.

Triska, C., Karsten, B., Nimmerichter, A. and Tschan, H. (2017) Iso-duration determination of D' and CS under laboratory and field conditions. *International Journal of Sports Medicine*, 38(7), pp. 527–533.

Trombold, J. R. et al. (2010) Ellagitannin consumption improves strength recovery 2–3 d after eccentric exercise. *Medicine and Science in Sports and Exercise*. doi: 10.1249/MSS.0b013e3181b64edd.

Trombold, J. R. et al. (2011) The effect of pomegranate juice supplementation on strength and soreness after eccentric exercise. *Journal of Strength and Conditioning Research*. doi: 10.1519/JSC. 0b013e318220d992.

Trowell, D. et al. (2020) Effect of strength training on biomechanical and neuromuscular variables in distance runners: A systematic review and meta-analysis. *Sports Medicine*, 50(1), pp. 133–150. doi: 10.1007/S40279-019-01184-9.

Tschakovsky, M. E., Sujirattanawimol, K., Ruble, S. B., Valic, Z. and Joyner, M. J. (2002) Is sympathetic neural vasoconstriction blunted in the vascular bed of exercising human muscle? *Journal of Physiology*, 541(2), pp. 623–635.

Tseh, W., Caputo, J. L. and Morgan, D. W. (2008) Influence of gait manipulation on running economy in female distance runners. *Journal of Sports Science and Medicine*, 7, pp. 91–95.

Tucker, R., Lambert, M. I. and Noakes, T. D. (2006) An analysis of pacing strategies during men's world-record performances in track athletics. *International Journal of Sports Physiology and Performance*, 1(3), pp. 233–245.

Tucker, R. and Noakes, T. D. (2009) The physiological regulation of pacing strategy during exercise: A critical review. *British Journal of Sports Medicine*, 43(6) [online]. doi: 10.1136/bjsm.2009.057562. Accessed on: 16/04/2020.

Turner, A. M., Owings, M. and Schwane, J. A. (2003) Improvement in running economy after 6 weeks of plyometric training. *Journal of Strength and Conditioning Research*, 13/02/2003, 17(1), pp. 60–67.

Turner, C. H. (1998) Three rules for bone adaptation to mechanical stimuli. *Bone*, 23(5), pp. 399–407. doi: 10.1016/S8756-3282(98)00118-5.

Ulger, H. V., Erdogan, N., Kumanlioglu, S. and Unur, E. (2003) Effect of age, breast size, menopausal and hormonal status on mammographic skin thickness. *Skin Research Technology*, 9, pp. 284–289.

Ulmer, H. V. (1996) Concept of an extracellular regulation of muscular metabolic rate during heavy exercise in humans by psychophysiological feedback. *Experientia*, 52(5), pp. 416–420.

Umemura, Y. et al. (1997) Five jumps per day increase bone mass and breaking force in rats. *Journal of Bone and Mineral Research*, 12(9), pp. 1480–1485.

Unnithan, V., Timmons, J., Paton, J. and Rowland, T. (1995) Physiologic correlates to running performance in pre-pubertal distance runners. *International Journal of Sports Medicine*, 16(8), pp. 528–533.

Urrutia, R. P., Coeytaux, R. R., McBroom, A. J., Gierisch, J. M., Havrilesky, L. J., Moorman, P. G., Lowery, W. J., Dinan, M., Hasselblad, V., Sanders, G. D. and Myers, E. R. (2013) Risk of acute thromboembolic events with oral contraceptive use: A systematic review and meta-analysis. *Obstetrics and Gynecology*, 122(2 Pt 1), pp. 380–389.

Vaghela, N., Mishra, D., Sheth, M. and Dani, V. B. (2019) To compare the effects of aerobic exercise and yoga on premenstrual syndrome. *Journal of Education and Health Promotion*, 8, p. 199.

Vaitkevicius, P. V., Fleg, J. L., Engel, J. H., O'Connor, F. C., Wright, J. G., Lakatta, L. E., Yin, F. C. and Lakatta, E. G. (1993) Effects of age and aerobic capacity on arterial stiffness in healthy adults. *Circulation*, 88(4), pp. 1456–1462.

Valenzuela, P. L., Maffiuletti, N. A., Joyner, M. J., Lucia, A. and Lepers, R. (2020) Lifelong endurance exercise as a countermeasure against age-related V̇O2max decline: Physiological overview and insights from masters athletes. *Sports Medicine*, 50(4), pp. 703–716.

Van Der Worp, M. P., Ten Haaf, D. S., Van Cingel, R., De Wijer, A., Nijhuis-Van Der Sanden, M. W. and Staal, J. B. (2015) Injuries in runners: A systematic review on risk factors and sex differences. *PLoS One*, 10, p. e0114937.

Van Der Worp, M. P., Van Der Horst, N., De Wijer, A., Backx, F. J. G. and Nijhuis-Van Der Sanden, M. W. G. (2012) Iliotibial band syndrome in runners: A systematic review. *Sports Medicine*, 42, pp. 969–992.

Van der Zwaard, S., De Ruiter, C. J., Noordhof, D. A., Sterrenburg, R., Bloemers, F. W., De Koning, J. J., Jaspers, R. T. and Van der Laarse, W. J. (2016) Maximal oxygen uptake is proportional to muscle fiber oxidative capacity, from chronic heart failure patients to professional cyclists. *Journal of Applied Physiology*, 121(3), pp. 636–645.

Van Gent, R. N., Siem, D., Van Middelkoop, M., Van Os, A. G., Bierma-Zeinstra, S. M. A., Koes, B. W. and Taunton, J. E. (2007) Incidence and determinants of lower extremity running injuries in long distance runners: A systematic review. *British Journal of Sports Medicine*, 41, pp. 469–480.

Vanhatalo, A., Bailey, S. J., Blackwell, J. R., Dimenna, F. J., Pavey, T. G., Wilkerson, D. P. et al. (2010) Acute and chronic effects of dietary nitrate supplementation on blood pressure and the physiological responses to moderate-intensity and incremental exercise. *American Journal of Physiology-Regulatory, Integrative and Comparative Physiology*, 299(4), pp. R1121–R1131.

Vanhatalo, A., Doust, J. H. and Burnley, M. (2008) A 3-min all-out cycling test is sensitive to a change in critical power. *Medicine & Science in Sports & Exercise*, 40(9), pp. 1693–1699.

Van Leeuwen, K. D., Rogers, J., Winzenberg, T. and Van Middelkoop, M. (2016) Higher body mass index is associated with plantar fasciopathy/'plantar fasciitis': Systematic review and meta-analysis of various clinical and imaging risk factors. *British Journal of Sports Medicine*, 50, pp. 972–981.

Van Loon, L. J. C. et al. (2000) Maximizing postexercise muscle glycogen synthesis: Carbohydrate supplementation and the application of amino acid or protein hydrolysate mixtures. *American Journal of Clinical Nutrition*. doi: 10.1093/ajcn/72.1.106.

van Loon, L. J. C. et al. (2001) The effects of increasing exercise intensity on muscle fuel utilisation in humans. *The Journal of Physiology*, 536(1), pp. 295–304. doi: 10.1111/J.1469-7793.2001.00295.X.

Van Mechelen, W. (1992) Running injuries: A review of the epidemiological literature. *Sports Medicine*, 14, pp. 320–335.

Vannatta, C. N., Heinert, B. L. and Kernozek, T. W. (2020) Biomechanical risk factors for running-related injury differ by sample population: A systematic review and meta-analysis. *Clinical Biomechanics*, 75. doi: 10.1016/J.CLINBIOMECH.2020.104991.

Van Raalte, J. L., Morrey, R. B., Cornelius, A. E. and Brewer, B. W. (2015) Self-talk of marathon runners. *The Sport Psychologist*, 29(3), pp. 258–260.

Van Someren, K. A., Howatson, G., Nunan, D., Thatcher, R. and Shave, R. (2005) Comparison of the Lactate Pro and Analox GM7 blood lactate analysers. *International Journal of Sports Medicine*, 26, pp. 657–661.

van Vliet, S., Burd, N. A. and van Loon, L. J. (2015) The skeletal muscle anabolic response to plant- versus animal-based protein consumption. *The Journal of Nutrition*. doi: 10.3945/jn.114.204305.

Vardaxis, V. and Hoshizaki, T. B. (1989) Power patterns of the leg during the recovery phase of the sprinting stride for advanced and intermediate sprinters. *International Journal of Sports Biomechanics*, 5(3), pp. 332–349.

Vealey, R. S. and Greenleaf, C. A. (2006) Seeing is believing: Understanding and using imagery in sports. In Williams, J. M. (ed.) *Applied sport psychology: Personal growth to peak performance*. Boston, MA: McGraw-Hill, pp. 306–348.

Verdijk, L. B., Van Loon, L., Meijer, K. and Savelberg, H. H. (2009) One-repetition maximum strength test represents a valid means to assess leg strength in vivo in humans. *Journal of Sports Sciences*, 27(1), pp. 59–68.

Verrelst, R., Willems, T. M., De Clercq, D., Roosen, P., Goossens, L. and Witvrouw, E. (2014) The role of hip abductor and external rotator muscle strength in the development of exertional medial tibial pain: A prospective study. *British Journal of Sports Medicine*, 48, pp. 1564–1569.

Versey, N. G., Halson, S. L. and Dawson, B. T. (2011) Effect of contrast water therapy duration on recovery of cycling performance: A dose-response study. *European Journal of Applied Physiology*. doi: 10.1007/s00421-010-1614-4.

Versey, N. G., Halson, S. L. and Dawson, B. T. (2013) Water immersion recovery for athletes: Effect on exercise performance and practical recommendations. *Sports Medicine*. doi: 10.1007/s40279-013-0063-8.

Vesterinen, V., Häkkinen, K., Hynynen, E., Mikkola, J., Hokka, L. and Nummela, A. (2013) Heart rate variability in prediction of individual adaptation to endurance training in recreational endurance runners. *Scandinavian Journal of Medicine & Science in Sports*, 23, pp. 171–180.

Vieira, A. et al. (2016) The effect of water temperature during cold-water immersion on recovery from exercise-induced muscle damage. *International Journal of Sports Medicine*. doi: 10.1055/s-0042-111438.

Vikmoen, O. et al. (2016) Effects of heavy strength training on running performance and determinants of running performance in female endurance athletes. *PLoS One*, 10/03/2016, 11(3), p. e0150799. doi: 10.1371/journal.pone.0150799.

Vikmoen, O. et al. (2020) Adaptations to strength training differ between endurance-trained and untrained women. *European Journal of Applied Physiology*, pp. 1–9. doi: 10.1007/S00421-020-04381-X.

Vinet, A., Nottin, S., Lecoq, A. M. et al. (2002) Cardiovascular responses to progressive cycle exercise in healthy children and adults. *International Journal of Sports Medicine*, 23, pp. 242–246.

Vitale, K. and Getzin, A. (2019) Nutrition and supplement update for the endurance athlete: Review and recommendations. *Nutrients*, 11(6 & 1289), pp. 1–20. doi: 10.3390/NU11061289.

Volek, J. S., Noakes, T. and Phinney, S. D. (2015) Rethinking fat as a fuel for endurance exercise. *European Journal of Sport Science*, 15(1), pp. 13–20.

Voloshina, A. S. and Ferris, D. P. (2015) Biomechanics and energetics of running on uneven terrain. *The Journal of Experimental Biology*, 218(5), pp. 711–719.

Wade, G. N. and Jones, J. E. (2004) Neuroendocrinology of nutritional infertility. *American Journal of Physiology-Regulatory, Integrative and Comparative Physiology*, 287(6), pp. R1277–R1296.

Wakefield, C. and Smith, D. (2012) Perfecting practice: Applying the PETTLEP model of motor imagery. *Journal of Sport Psychology in Action*, 3, pp. 1–11.

Waldhelm, A. and Li, L. (2012) Endurance tests are the most reliable core stability related measurements. *Journal of Sport & Health Science*, 1(2), pp. 121–128.

Waldron, S., DeFreese, J. D., Pietrosimone, B., Register-Mihalik, J. and Barczak, N. (2019) Exploring early sport specialization: Associations with psychosocial outcomes. *Journal of Clinical Sport Psychology*, 14(2), pp. 182–202.

Walker, J. L., Heigenhauser, G. J., Hultman, E. and Spriet, L. L. (2000) Dietary carbohydrate, muscle glycogen content, and endurance performance in well-trained women. *Journal of Applied Physiology*, 88(6), pp. 2151–2158. doi: 10.1152/jappl.2000.88.6.2151.

Wallace, M., Hashim, Y. Z. H.-Y., Wingfield, M., Culliton, M., McAuliffe, F., Gibney, M. J. and Brennan, L. (2010) Effects of menstrual cycle phase on metabolomic profiles in premenopausal women. *Human Reproduction*, 25(4), pp. 949–956.

Walter, S. D., Hart, L. E., McIntosh, J. M. and Sutton, J. R. (1989) The Ontario cohort study of running-related injuries. *Archives of Internal Medicine*, 149, pp. 2561–2564.

Wang, L. et al. (2011) Resistance exercise enhances the molecular signaling of mitochondrial biogenesis induced by endurance exercise in human skeletal muscle. *Journal of Applied Physiology*, 111(5), pp. 1335–1344. doi: 10.1152/japplphysiol.00086.2011.

Wang, Q., Würtz, P., Auro, K., Morin-Papunen, L., Kangas, A. J., Soininen, P., Tiainen, M., Tynkkynen, T., Joensuu, A., Havulinna, A. S., Aalto, K., Salmi, M., Blankenberg, S., Zeller, T., Viikari, J., Kähönen, M., Lehtimäki, T., Salomaa, V., Jalkanen, S., Järvelin, M.-R., Perola, M., Raitakari, O. T., Lawlor, D. A., Kettunen, J. and Ala-Korpela, M. (2016) Effects of hormonal contraception on systemic metabolism: Cross-sectional and longitudinal evidence. *International Journal of Epidemiology*, 45(5), pp. 1445–1457.

Wang, R. et al. (2017) The effect of magnesium supplementation on muscle fitness: A meta-analysis and systematic review. *Magnesium Research*, 30(4), pp. 120–132. doi: 10.1684/MRH.2018.0430.

Warden, S. J., Davis, I. S. and Fredericson, M. (2014) Management and prevention of bone stress injuries in long-distance runners. *Journal of Orthopaedic and Sports Physical Therapy*, 44(10), pp. 749–765.

Ware, J. H., Dockery, D. W., Louis, T. A., Xu, X., Ferris, B. G. and Speizer, F. E. (1990) Longitudinal and cross-sectional estimates of pulmonary function decline in never-smoking adults. *American Journal of Epidemiology*, 132(4), pp. 685–700.

Watkins, J. (2010) *Structure and function of the musculoskeletal system*. 2nd edn. Champaign, IL: Human Kinetics.

Watson, A. M. (2017) Sleep and athletic performance. *Current Sports Medicine Reports*. doi: 10.1249/JSR.0000000000000418.

Watson, S. L. et al. (2018) High-intensity resistance and impact training improves bone mineral density and physical function in postmenopausal women with osteopenia and osteoporosis: The LIFTMOR randomized controlled trial. *Journal of Bone and Mineral Research*, 33(2), pp. 211–220. doi: 10.1002/JBMR.3284.

Weerapong, P., Hume, P. A. and Kolt, G. S. (2005) The mechanisms of massage and effects on performance, muscle recovery and injury prevention. *Sports Medicine*. doi: 10.2165/00007256-200535030-00004.

Wei, C. et al. (2020) A Plyometric warm-up protocol improves running economy in recreational endurance athletes. *Frontiers in Physiology*, 11. doi: 10.3389/FPHYS.2020.00197.

Weinberg, R. S. (2010) Making goals an effective primer for coaches. *Journal of Sport Psychology in Action*, 1, pp. 57–65.

Weinberg, R. S., Morrison, D., Loftin, M., Horn, T., Goodwin, E., Wright, E. and Block, C. (2019) Writing down goals: Does it actually improve performance? *The Sport Psychologist*, 33, pp. 35–41.

Weippert, M., Petelczyc, M., Thürkow, C. et al (2020) Individual performance progression of German elite female and male middle-distance runners. *European Journal of Sport Science*, published ahead of print. doi: 10.1080/17461391.2020.1736182.

Weiss Kelly, A. K., Hecht, S. and Council on Sports Medicine and Fitness (2016) The female athlete triad. *Pediatrics*, 138, pp. e1–e10.

Wen, D., Utesch, T., Wu, T., Robertson, S., Liu, J., Hu, G. and Chen, H. (2019) Effects of different protocols of high intensity interval training for VO2max improvements in adults: A meta-analysis of randomised controlled trials. *Journal of Science and Medicine in Sport*, 22(8), pp. 941–947.

Weston, M., Taylor, K. L., Batterham, A. M. and Hopkins, W. G. (2014) Effects of low-volume high-intensity interval training (HIT) on fitness in adults: A meta-analysis of controlled and non-controlled trials. *Sports Medicine*, 44(7), pp. 1005–1017.

Weyand, P. G. and Davis, J. A. (2005) Running performance has a structural basis. *Journal of Experimental Biology*, 208(14), pp. 2625–2631.

Weyand, P. G. et al. (2000) Faster top running speeds are achieved with greater ground forces not more rapid leg movements. *Journal of Applied Physiology*, 89(5), pp. 1991–1999.

Whatman, C., Hing, W. and Hume, P. (2011) Kinematics during lower extremity functional screening tests: Are they reliable and related to jogging? *Physical Therapy in Sport*, 12(1), pp. 22–29.

Wheeler, G. D., Wall, S. R., Belcastro, A. N., Conger, P. and Cumming, D. C. (1986) Are anorexic tendencies prevalent in the habitual runner? *British Journal of Sports Medicine*, 20(2), pp. 77–81.

White, G. E., Rhind, S. G. and Wells, G. D. (2014) The effect of various cold-water immersion protocols on exercise-induced inflammatory response and functional recovery from high-intensity sprint exercise. *European Journal of Applied Physiology*. doi: 10.1007/s00421-014-2954-2.

White, J. L., Lunt, H. and Scurr, J. (2011a) The effect of breast support on ventilation and breast comfort perception at the onset of exercise. *Proceedings of the BASES annual conference*. Essex: BASES, p. S74.

White, J. L., Mills, C., Ball, N. and Scurr, J. (2015) The effect of breast support and breast pain on upper-extremity kinematics during running: Implications for females with large breasts. *Journal of Sports Sciences*, 33, pp. 2043–2050.

White, J. L. and Scurr, J. C. (2012) Evaluation of professional bra fitting criteria for bra selection and fitting in the UK. *Ergonomics*, 55(6), pp. 704–711.

White, J. L., Scurr, J. and Hedger, W. (2011b) A comparison of three-dimensional breast displacement and breast comfort during overground and treadmill running. *Journal of Applied Biomechanics*, 27, pp. 47–53.

White, J. L., Scurr, J. C. and Smith, N. A. (2009) The effect of breast support on kinetics during overground running performance. *Ergonomics*, 52, pp. 492–498.

White, S. C. and Winter, D. (1985) Mechanical power analysis of the lower limb musculature in race walking. *International Journal of Sport Biomechanics*, 1(1), pp. 15–24.

Whiteside, D., Deneweth, J. M., Pohorence, M. A., Sandoval, B., Russell, J. R., McLean, S. G., Zernicke, R. F. and Goulet, G. C. (2016) Grading the functional movement screen: A comparison of manual (real-time) and objective methods. *The Journal of Strength & Conditioning Research*, 30(4), pp. 924–933.

Whittle, M. W. (1999) Generation and attenuation of transient impulsive forces beneath the foot: A review. *Gait and Posture*, 10(3), pp. 264–275.

Wiese-Bjornstal, D. M. (2010) Psychology and socioculture affect injury risk, response, and recovery in high-intensity athletes: A consensus statement. *Scandinavian Journal of Medicine & Science in Sports*, 20(Suppl. 2), pp. 103–111.

Wiewelhove, T. et al. (2019) A meta-analysis of the effects of foam rolling on performance and recovery. *Frontiers in Physiology*. doi: 10.3389/fphys.2019.00376.

Wiffin, M., Smith, L., Antonio, J., Johnstone, J., Beasley, L. and Roberts, J. (2019) Effect of a short-term low fermentable oligiosaccharide, disaccharide, monosaccharide and polyol (FODMAP) diet on exercise-related gastrointestinal symptoms. *Journal of the International Society of Sports Nutrition*, 16(1), pp. 1–9.

Wihlbäck, A.-C., Poromaa, I. S., Bixo, M., Allard, P., Mjörndal, T. and Spigset, O. (2004) Influence of menstrual cycle on platelet serotonin uptake site and serotonin2A receptor binding. *Psychoneuroendocrinology*, 29(6), pp. 757–766.

Wilcock, I. M., Cronin, J. B. and Hing, W. A. (2006) Physiological response to water immersion: A method for sport recovery? *Sports Medicine*. doi: 10.2165/00007256-200636090-00003.

Wilkinson, S. B. et al. (2007) Consumption of fluid skim milk promotes greater muscle protein accretion after resistance exercise than does consumption of an isonitrogenous and isoenergetic soy-protein beverage. *American Journal of Clinical Nutrition*. doi: 10.1093/ajcn/85.4.1031.

Williams, C. and Lamb, D. (2008) Do high-carbohydrate diets improve exercise performance? *GSSI Sports Science Exchange*, 21(1), pp. 1–6.

Williams, J. M. and Andersen, M. B. (1998) Psychosocial antecedents of sport injury: Review and critique of the stress and injury model. *Journal of Applied Sport Psychology*, 10, pp. 5–25.

Williams, K. R. and Cavanagh, P. R. (1987) Relationship between distance running mechanics, running economy, and performance. *Journal of Applied Physiology*, 63, pp. 1236–1245.

Williams, K. R., Cavanagh, P. R. and Ziff, J. L. (1987) Biomechanical studies of elite female distance runners. *International Journal of Sports Medicine*, 8(Suppl. 2), pp. 107–118.

Williams, S. E., Cooley, S. J., Newell, E., Weibull, F. and Cumming, J. (2013) Seeing the difference: Advice for developing effective imagery scripts for athletes. *Journal of Sport Psychology in Action*, 4, pp. 109–121.

Williams, T. D. et al. (2017) Comparison of periodized and non-periodized resistance training on maximal strength: A meta-analysis. *Sports Medicine*, 47(10), pp. 2083–2100. doi: 10.1007/S40279-017-0734-Y.

Willson, J., Bjorhus, J., Williams, B., Butler, R., Porcari, J. and Kernozek, T. (2014) Short-term changes in running mechanics and foot strike patterns after introduction to minimalistic footwear. *American Academy of Physical Medicine and Rehabilitation*, 6(1), pp. 34–43.

Willwacher, S., Sanno, M. and Brüggemann, G. P. (2020) Fatigue matters: An intense 10 km run alters frontal and transverse plane joint kinematics in competitive and recreational adult runners. *Gait Posture*, 76, pp. 277–283.

Willy, R. W. (2018) Innovations and pitfalls in the use of wearable devices in the prevention and rehabilitation of running related injuries. *Physical Therapy in Sport*, 29, pp. 26–33.

Willy, R. W., Buchenic, L., Rogacki, K., Ackerman, J., Schmidt, A. and Willson, J. D. (2016) In-field gait retraining and mobile monitoring to address running biomechanics associated with tibial stress fracture. *Scandinavian Journal of Medicine and Science in Sports*, 26, pp. 197–205.

Willy, R. W. and Davis, I. S. (2011) The effect of a hip-strengthening program on mechanics during running and during a single-leg squat. *Journal of Orthopaedic and Sports Physical Therapy*, 41(9), pp. 625–632.

Willy, R. W. and Davis, I. S. (2013) Varied response to mirror gait retraining of gluteus medius control, hip kinematics, pain, and function in 2 female runners with patellofemoral pain. *Journal of Orthopaedic & Sports Physical Therapy*, 43(12), pp. 864–874.

Willy, R. W., Manal, K. T., Witvrouw, E. E. and Davis, I. S. (2012a) Are mechanics different between male and female runners with patellofemoral pain? *Medicine and Science in Sports and Exercise*, 44, pp. 2165–2171.

Willy, R. W., Scholz, J. P. and Davis, I. S. (2012b) Mirror gait retraining for the treatment of patellofemoral pain in female runners. *Clinical Biomechanics*, 27, pp. 1045–1051.

Willy, R. W. and Paquette, M. R. (2019) The physiology and biomechanics of the master runner. *Sports Medicine and Arthroscopy Review*, 27(1), pp. 15–21.

Wilson, J. M. et al. (2012) Concurrent training: A meta-analysis examining interference of aerobic and resistance exercises. *Journal of Strength and Conditioning Research*, 26(8), pp. 2293–2307. doi: 10.1519/JSC.0b013e31823a3e2d.

Wilson, L. J. et al. (2018) Recovery following a marathon: A comparison of cold water immersion, whole body cryotherapy and a placebo control. *European Journal of Applied Physiology*. doi: 10.1007/s00421-017-3757-z.

Wilson, L. J. et al. (2019) Whole body cryotherapy, cold water immersion, or a placebo following resistance exercise: A case of mind over matter? *European Journal of Applied Physiology*. doi: 10.1007/s00421-018-4008-7.

Winter, D. A. (1980) Overall principle of lower limb support during stance phase of gait. *Journal of Biomechanics*, 13(11), pp. 923–927.

Winter, D. A. (1990) *Biomechanics and motor control of human movement*. New York: Wiley.

Winter, D. A. and Bishop, P. J. (1992) Lower extremity injury: Biomechanical factors associated with chronic injury to the lower extremity. *Sports Medicine*, 14, pp. 149–156.

Winter, E. M., Abt, G., Brookes, F. B. C., Challis, J. H., Fowler, N. E., Knudson, D. V., Knuttgen, H. G., Kraemer, W. J., Lane, A. M., van Mechelen, W., Morton, R. H., Newton, R. U., Williams, C. and Yeadon, M. R. (2016) Misuse of 'power' and other mechanical terms in sport and exercise science research. *The Journal of Strength and Conditioning Research*, 30(1), pp. 292–300.

Winter, E. M. and Fowler, N. (2009) Exercise defined and quantified according to the Systeme International d'Unites. *Journal of Sports Sciences*, 27(5), pp. 447–460.

Winter, S. C., Gordon, S., Brice, S. M., Lindsay, D. and Barrs, S. (2020) A multifactorial approach to overuse running injuries: A 1-year prospective study. *Sports Health*, 12, pp. 296–303.

Winter, S. C., Gordon, S. and Watt, K. (2017) Effects of fatigue on kinematics and kinetics during overground running: A systematic review. *Journal of Sports Medicine and Physical Fitness*, 57, pp. 887–899.

Winter, S. C., MacPherson, A. and Collins, D. (2014) To think, or not to think, that is the question. *Sport, Exercise, and Performance Psychology*, 32, pp. 102–115.

Winters, M., Bakker, E. W. P., Moen, M. H., Barten, C. C., Teeuwen, R. and Weir, A. (2017) Medial tibial stress syndrome can be diagnosed reliably using history and physical examination. *British Journal of Sports Medicine*, 52(19), pp. 1267–1272.

Winters, M., Burr, D. B., Van Der Hoeven, H., Condon, K. W., Bellemans, J. and Moen, M. H. (2019) Microcrack-associated bone remodeling is rarely observed in biopsies from athletes with medial tibial stress syndrome. *Journal of Bone and Mineral Metabolism*, 37, pp. 496–502.

Wiswell, R. A., Hawkins, S. A., Jaque, S. V., Hyslop, D., Constantino, N., Tarpenning, K., Marcell, T. and Schroeder, E. T. (2001) Relationship between physiological loss, performance decrement, and age in master athletes. *The Journals of Gerontology: Series A*, 56(10), pp. M618–M626.

Wiswell, R. A., Jaque, S. V., Marcell, T. J., Hawkins, S. A., Tarpenning, K. M., Constantino, N. and Hyslop, D. (2000) Maximal aerobic power, lactate threshold, and running performance in master athletes. *Medicine & Science in Sports & Exercise*, 32(6).

Wittig, A. F., Houmard, J. A. and Costill, D. L. (1989) Psychological effects during reduced training in distance runners. *International Journal of Sports Medicine*, 10(2), pp. 97–100. doi: 10.1055/s-2007-1021305.

Wood, C., Lane, L. C. and Cheetham, T. (2019) Normal physiology (brief overview). *Best Practice & Research Clinical Endocrinology & Metabolism*, 33(3), p. 101265.

Wood, K., Cameron, M. and Fitzgerald, K. (2008) Breast size, bra fit and thoracic pain in young women: A correlational study. *Chiropractic & Osteopathy*, 16(1), p. 1.

Wood, L. E., White, J., Milligan, A., Ayres, B., Hedger, W. and Scurr, J. (2012) Predictors of three-dimensional breast kinematics during bare-breasted running. *Medicine & Science in Sports & Exercise*, 44, pp. 1351–1357.

Woolf, K. and Manore, M. M. (2006) B-vitamins and exercise: Does exercise alter requirements? *International Journal of Sport Nutrition and Exercise Metabolism*, 16(5), pp. 453–484. doi: 10.1123/IJSNEM.16.5.453.

Wu, W. F., Porter, J. M. and Brown, L. E. (2012) Effect of attentional focus strategies on peak force and performance in the standing long jump. *Journal of Strength & Conditioning Research*, 26, pp. 1226–1231.

Wulf, G. and Dufek, J. S. (2009) Increased jump height with an external focus due to enhanced lower extremity joint kinetics. *Journal of Motor Behavior*, 41, pp. 401–409.

Wulf, G. and Lewthwaite, R. (2016) Optimizing performance through intrinsic motivation and attention for learning: The OPTIMAL theory of motor learning. *Psychonomic Bulletin & Review*, 23, pp. 1382–1414.

Wylie, L. J., Kelly, J., Bailey, S. J., Blackwell, J. R., Skiba, P. F., Winyard, P. G. et al. (2013) Beetroot juice and exercise: Pharmacodynamic and dose-response relationships. *Journal of Applied Physiology*, 115(3), pp. 325–336.

Yamada, K. and Takeda, T. (2018) Low proportion of dietary plant protein among athletes with pre-menstrual syndrome-related performance impairment. *The Tohoku Journal of Experimental Medicine*, 244(2), pp. 119–122.

Yamato, T. P., Saragiotto, B. T. and Lopes, A. D. (2015) A consensus definition of running-related injury in recreational runners: A modified delphi approach. *Journal of Orthopaedic & Sports Physical Therapy*, 45, pp. 375–380.

Yeh, M. P., Gardner, R. M., Adams, T. D., Yanowitz, F. G. and Crapo, R. O. (1983) Anaerobic thresh-old: Problems of determination and validation. *Journal of Applied Physiology*, 55(4), pp. 1178–1186.

Yeo, S. E., Jentjens, R. L., Wallis, G. A. and Jeukendrup, A. E. (2005) Caffeine increases exogenous carbohydrate oxidation during exercise. *Journal of Applied Physiology*, 99(3), pp. 844–850.

Yeung, E. H., Zhang, C., Mumford, S. L., Ye, A., Trevisan, M., Chen, L., Browne, R. W., Wactawski-Wende, J. and Schisterman, E. F. (2010) Longitudinal study of insulin resistance and sex hormones over the menstrual cycle: The biocycle study. *The Journal of Clinical Endocrinology & Metabolism*, 95(12), pp. 5435–5442.

Yeung, S. S., Yeung, E. W. and Gillespie, L. D. (2011) Interventions for preventing lower limb soft-tissue running injuries. *Cochrane Database of Systematic Reviews*, 6(7), p. CD001256. doi: 10.1002/14651858. CD001256.pub2.

Yfanti, C. et al. (2011) Effect of antioxidant supplementation on insulin sensitivity in response to endur-ance exercise training. *American Journal of Physiology: Endocrinology and Metabolism*. doi: 10.1152/ajpendo.00207.2010.

Yoshida, T., Udo, M., Chida, M., Ichioka, M., Makiguchi, K. and Yamaguchi, T. (1990) Specificity of physiological adaptation to endurance training in distance runners and competitive walkers. *European Journal of Applied Physiology and Occupational Physiology*, 61(3–4), pp. 197–201.

Young, B. W. and Salmela, J. H. (2010) Examination of practice activities related to the acquisition of elite performance in Canadian middle distance running. *International Journal of Sport Psychology*, 41(1), pp. 73–90.

Young, B. W. and Starkes, J. L. (2005) Career-span analyses of track performance: Longitudinal data present a more optimistic view of age-related performance decline. *Experimental Aging Research*, 31(1), pp. 69–90.

Yu, W. and Zhou, J. (2016) Sports bras and breast kinetics. In Yu Wing Man (ed.) *Advances in women's intimate apparel technology*. London, UK: Elsevier, pp. 135–146.

Zello, G. A. (2006) Dietary reference intakes for the macronutrients and energy: Considerations for physical activity. *Applied Physiology Nutrition and Metabolism*, 31(1), pp. 74–79. doi: 10.1139/H05-022.

Zhang, J. H., Chan, Z. Y., Au, I. P., An, W. W., Shull, P. B. and Cheung, R. T. (2019) Transfer learning effects of biofeedback running retraining in untrained conditions. *Medicine and Science in Sports and Exercise*, 51, pp. 1904–1908.

Zhang, S., Osumi, H., Uchizawa, A., Hamada, H., Park, I., Suzuki, Y., Tanaka, Y., Ishihara, A., Yajima, K., Seol, J., Satoh, M., Omi, N. and Tokuyama, K. (2020) Changes in sleeping energy metabolism and thermoregulation during menstrual cycle. *Physiological Reports*, 8(2).

Zhang, Y. et al. (2017) Can magnesium enhance exercise performance? *Nutrients*, 9(9), p. 946. https://doi.org/10.3390/nu9090946.

Zhao, R., Zhang, M. and Zhang, Q. (2017) The effectiveness of combined exercise interventions for preventing postmenopausal bone loss: A systematic review and meta-analysis. *Journal of Orthopaedic & Sports Physical Therapy*, 47(4), pp. 241–251.

Zhou, J., Yu, W. and Ng, S. (2013) Identifying effective design features of commercial sports bras. *Textiles Research Journal*, 83(14), pp. 1500–1513.

Ziemann, E. et al. (2012) Five-day whole-body cryostimulation, blood inflammatory markers, and performance in high-ranking professional tennis players. *Journal of Athletic Training*. doi: 10.4085/1062-6050-47.6.13.

Zuhl, M., Schneider, S., Lanphere, K., Conn, C., Dokladny, K. and Moseley, P. (2014) Exercise regula-tion of intestinal tight junction proteins. *British Journal of Sports Medicine*, 48(12), pp. 980–986.

INDEX

Page numbers in *italics* indicate figures; page numbers in **bold** indicate tables.

Made in the USA
Las Vegas, NV
26 September 2024

95836075R00247